DRUG INTERACTIONS

DRUG INTERACTIONS

a source book of adverse interactions, their
mechanisms, clinical importance and management

IVAN H. STOCKLEY

BPharm, PhD, MPS
Lecturer in Clinical Pharmacy and Pharmacology
University of Nottingham, England

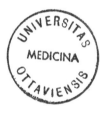

Blackwell Scientific Publications

OXFORD LONDON EDINBURGH

BOSTON MELBOURNE

© 1981 Ivan H. Stockley

Blackwell Scientific Publications
Osney Mead, Oxford, OX2 OEL
8 John Street, London, WCIN 2ES
9 Forrest Road, Edinburgh, EHI 2QH
52 Beacon Street, Boston,
    Massachusetts 02108, USA
214 Berkeley Street, Carlton,
    Victoria 3053, Australia

First published 1981

Printed in Great Britain at
the Alden Press, Oxford
and bound at
Kemp Hall Bindery

DISTRIBUTORS

USA
  Blackwell Mosby Book Distributors
  11830 Westline Industrial Drive,
  St Louis, Missouri 53141

Canada
  Blackwell Mosby Book Distributors
  120 Melford Drive, Scarborough,
  Ontario, MIB 2X4

Australia
  Blackwell Scientific Book Distributors
  214 Berkeley Street, Carlton,
  Victoria 3053

British Library
Cataloguing in Publication Data

Stockley, Ivan H.
  Drug interactions.
  1. Drug interactions
  I. Title
  615'704   RM302
  ISBN 0-632-008431

CONTENTS

PREFACE

Plans for this book were drawn up as long ago as 1971, but they were shelved in favour of writing a series of articles on interactions for *The Pharmaceutical Journal* at the invitation of the editor. Later in 1974 these articles were reprinted in facsimile form, with an index, and published under the title of *Drug Interactions and their Mechanisms*, so that there seemed little point at that time in writing another book on the same subject. A supplement on the oral contraceptives was added to the 1978 reprint, but eventually it became clear that a complete rewrite was necessary, incorporating the old material as well as the mass of new data published since the articles were first written. This book is therefore the up-dated successor to the familiar yellow-backed reprinted series of articles.

My aim, as before, has been to present to the practising doctor, pharmacist, surgeon, nurse, or anyone else who has neither the time nor the facilities to carry out detailed literature searches of their own, what is known about the hundreds of drug interactions now on record. I have attempted not only to answer the question of what is likely to happen if two drugs are given concurrently, but also the important associated questions such as these: Is it a genuine, reported, interaction or is it still only theoretical? Has it been described many times or only once? Is the interaction, when it occurs, serious or not? Are all patients affected or only a few? Is it best to avoid the concurrent use of the drugs altogether, or can the interaction be accommodated in some way? And what alternative drugs can be used which do not interact?

So that these questions can be answered succinctly, the material has been organized into a series of individual drug–drug or drug-food synopses—600 or so in all—and categorized into 20 chapters. A very brief outline of the most common mechanisms of interaction has been included at the beginning of the book and a few chapters also include a very short pharmacological introduction for the benefit of those whose pharmacology is not as fresh as it might be. The synopses have a common format with a summary for rapid reading, but very extensive bibliographies are included for those who wish to study the original literature in depth. The synopses are assembled into chapters according to the drugs whose activity is changed, although where the same drug is the affecting or interacting agent, it is usually categorized elsewhere. For this reason the index *must* be used to ensure that the whole range of interactions can be identified.

Through the generosity of the Leverhulme Trust in particular, and a number of Pharmaceutical Companies—Boots, Geistlich, Glaxo, Janssen, Lepetit, Leo, Ortho, Pfizer, Roche, Upjohn and Warner-Lambert—I was able to accumulate sufficient funds for my University to pay a temporary replacement member of staff to undertake my teaching duties for a year, thus enabling me to take sabbatical leave to write this book. I am grateful to all of those, within and without the university, who in one way or another gave me the support I needed.

I also owe a debt of gratitude to many other people: the library staff of the Science and Medical Libraries in the University of Nottingham; the staff of the drug information and medical departments of many of the pharmaceutical companies in the UK; numerous individuals who have drawn my attention to obscure papers and articles which I might otherwise have missed; Dr J. S. B. Stuart for some of the documentation of chapter 12; Boehringer Ingelheim for allowing me to reproduce the *Drug Interaction Alert* chart on the jacket of this book; Mr Per Saugman and his staff at Blackwell Scientific Publications in particular John Robson and Dominic Vaughan; and my wife Bridget, and children Alex, Rosalind, Ben and Beth who with such good grace put up with my acquisition of an intended playroom for a study, and a house strewn, seemingly for ever, with papers.

University of Nottingham   Ivan H Stockley

BEFORE USING THIS BOOK . . .

. . . it is important to have an appreciation of the extent and limitations of knowledge about interactions, so that the date summarized in these pages can be applied correctly.

What is known about interactions between drugs is derived from a number of sources of widely varying quality and reliability. The best information comes from clinical studies with large numbers of patients where the conditions are scrupulously controlled and the results statistically analysed. From data of this kind a very good idea of the extent and incidence of the interaction can be deduced.

However, what is known about some interactions comes from much less reliable sources: from observations on only one or two patients, possibly in uncontrolled situations and when it would be undesirable or unethical to rechallenge the patients with both drugs to confirm the interaction. It may be confined to the results of animal experiments or even based on only purely theoretical considerations. Not that such poorly established information is to be despised. Quite the contrary. Many of the now very well-confirmed interactions were detected initially in only one patient, without experimental controls, by an observant physician, or even in a laboratory on experimental animals, but observations like these require formal and careful confirmation before their clinical importance can be adequately categorized, and a clear distinction must be drawn between these possible interactions and those which are now well-established.

In addition to the variable quality of data on interactions, it must also be remembered that patients are not like selected batches of laboratory animals, of the same age, weight, sex and strain which can be expected to respond with a degree of uniformity. Any ward or surgery contains a heterogeneous group of individuals who are most unlikely to respond uniformly to one or more drugs because their genetic make up, renal and hepatic functions, disease states, ages and other conditions are all different. By the same token, the drug dosages, their form, route, duration and order of administration can have a vital bearing on the way a patient responds, and on whether an interaction develops or not.

The sum of all these variables is that while it is possible to describe what has already been seen to occur when drugs are administered together, the outcome of giving the same drugs to other patients is never totally predictable. Despite this, some idea of the probable outcome of using the drugs in other patients can be based on the clinical and experimental information available (the more extensive the data, the firmer the conclusions) and the 'importance and management' subsections of each synopsis are intended as assessments of the interactions which readers may set alongside their own evaluation of the data presented.

As the body of knowledge about interactions grows, so it becomes possible to make increasingly positive and less tentative statements about them, and informative and constructive comments, or reports of hitherto unpublished data on interactions, which would increase the practical day-to-day usefulness of future editions of this book are invited.

CHAPTER 1. AN OUTLINE SURVEY OF SOME BASIC DRUG INTERACTION MECHANISMS

Some drugs interact together in totally unique ways but, as the many examples in this book amply illustrate, there are certain mechanisms of interaction which are encountered time and time again. It is these common mechanisms which are discussed in detail in this chapter so that only the briefest reference need be made to them in the drug–drug interaction synopses throughout the book. Mechanisms which are more unusual or are peculiar to particular pairs of drugs are dealt with in the individual synopses. It is becoming increasingly clear that the interactions which occur when drugs are given concurrently are often the result, not of a single mechanism, but of two or more mechanisms acting in concert, although in this chapter most of the mechanisms of interaction are dealt with as though they occur in isolation.

1. Drugs with similar effects

The most obvious type of interaction occurs when drugs which have similar activity are used together, the result being the sum of their effects. For example, alcohol depresses the central nervous system and, if taken in moderate amounts with normal therapeutic doses of any of a large number of drugs such as the barbiturates, tranquillizers, neuroleptics, antiemetics, sedatives, antidepressants, antihistamines, and many others, can result in excessive drowsiness.

Many of the interactions of this type are predictable on the basis of their known pharmacology, but it is important not to lose sight of the fact that few if any drugs have a single pharmacological action. Additive interactions can occur with the incidental and undesirable side-effects of drugs as well as with the main effects. Thus an additive anticholinergic interaction can take place between the anticholinergic antiparkinson drugs (main effect) with the tricyclic antidepressants (side-effect), phenothiazines (side-effect) or butyrophenonones (side-effect) which can result in serious anticholinergic toxicity. Examples of this type of interaction are listed in Table 1.1.

It is common to use the terms 'additive', 'summation', 'synergy' or 'potentiation' to describe this type of interaction. These words have fairly precise pharmacological definitions, but they are often used rather loosely as synonyms because in practice (in man) it is often very difficult to determine precisely the extent of the increased activity (that is to say, whether the effects are greater or smaller than the sum of the individual effects).

2. Drugs with dissimilar or opposing effects

In contrast to the additive interactions, there are some pairs of drugs with activities

1

Table 1.1. Interactions between drugs with similar effects

Drug 1	Drug 2	Result of interaction
Anticholinergics + Anticholinergics (antiparkinsonian agents, tricyclic antidepressants, phenothiazines, butyrophenones)		Enhanced anticholinergic effects; heat stroke in hot and humid conditions; toxic psychosis; adynamic ileus
CNS depressants + CNS depressants (alcohol, antiemetics, antihistamines, antidepressants, hypnotics, sedatives, tranquilizers, etc)		Enhanced CNS depression; drowsiness
Nephrotoxic drugs + Nephrotoxic drugs (gentamicin or tobramycin with cephalothin)		Enhanced nephrotoxicity
Neuromuscular blockers + Neuromuscular blockers (conventional neuromuscular blockers and aminoglycoside antibiotics)		Enhanced neuromuscular blockade; prolonged apnoea
Ototoxic drugs + Ototoxic drugs (aminoglycoside antibiotics and ethacrynic acid)		Enhanced ototoxicity

which are opposed to one another. For example, the oral anticoagulants are able to prolong the blood clotting time by competitively inhibiting the effects of dietary vitamin K (see p. 113). If the intake of vitamin K is increased (this has occurred accidentally in patients who took chilblain preparations or health-foods which contained significant amounts of vitamin K), the effects of the oral anticoagulant are antagonized and the clotting time can return to normal, thus negating the therapeutic benefits of the anticoagulant therapy. Other examples of this type of interaction are listed in Table 1.2.

There is a certain obviousness and predictability about the two types of interaction mechanism discussed so far, but the interactions which occur in the pharmacokinetic phase of drug activity (sometimes referred to as the absorption/distribution/metabolism/excretion—ADME—interactions) were, when they were first encountered, very ill-understood. Much research has now gone into their elucidation, and for the most part the basic principles are now clear.

Table 1.2. Interactions between drugs with dissimilar or opposing effects

Drug 1	Drug 2	Result of interaction
Sulphonamides	PABA or local anaesthetics hydrolyzed to PABA	Antimicrobial effects of the sulphonamide antagonized
Beta-adrenoreceptor stimulating bronchodilator	Non-selective beta-2-adrenoreceptor blocker	Bronchodilator effects antagonized
Hypnotics	Caffeine	Hypnosis antagonized

3. Absorption interactions

The majority of drugs are given by mouth, most of them being intended for absorption into the circulation by the gut. En route, their bioavailability can be drastically reduced. For example, the tetracycline antibiotics form less-easily absorbed chelates with a number of ions such as aluminium, calcium, magnesium, bismuth, iron and zinc which are present in antacids, milk products and anti-anaemic preparations (see Fig. 1.1). Cholestyramine is an ion-exchange compound used to take up excess bile acids, but it can also take up anticoagulants, digitalis, sulphasalazine and other drugs. Kaolin, charcoal and attapulgite similarly reduce bioavailability by adsorbing other

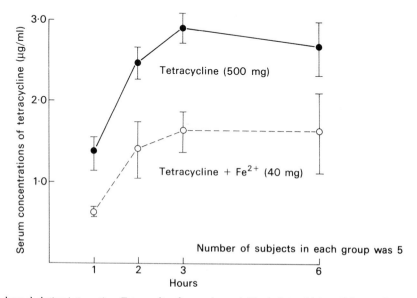

Fig. 1.1. A drug chelation interaction. Tetracycline forms a less-soluble chelate with iron if the two drugs are allowed to mix within the gut, which reduces the absorption and depresses the serum levels (after Neuvonen P J. *Brit Med J* (1970) **4**, 532, with permission).

drugs onto their surfaces. Most of these interactions can be accommodated by making sure that the administration of the interacting compounds is separated as much as possible to prevent their admixture in the gut.

If the general peristaltic rate, and the time occupied by the drug within the stomach is altered, the rate and extent of absorption of drugs can be changed by changes in mixing and dissolution. It is in this way that propantheline and metoclopramide, as well as other anticholinergic drugs which alter the motility of the gut, affect absorption. These and some other absorption interactions are listed in Table 1.3.

4. Drug displacement interactions

Following absorption, drugs are rapidly distributed around the body by the circulation. Some drugs become totally dissolved in the plasma water, but many others are transported with some proportion of its molecules in solution and the rest bound to the plasma proteins, particularly the albumins. The extent of this binding

Table 1.3. Absorption interactions

Drug 1	Drug 2	Result of interaction
Tetracycline antibiotics	Al^{3+}, Ca^{2+}, Mg^{2+} Fe^{2+}, Bi^{2+}, Zn^{2+}	Reduced absorption of the antibiotic due to the formation of poorly soluble chelates
Large number of drugs	Kaolin, attapulgite, charcoal	Reduced absorption of the drugs due to their adsorption onto the surface of these compounds
Anticoagulants Digitalis Thyroid	Cholestyramine	Reduced absorption due to the complexation of these drugs with cholestyramine
Digitalis	Propantheline and other anticholinergics	Reduced absorption due to reduced gut motility

varies enormously, but some drugs are extremely highly bound. For example, dicoumarol has only 4 out of every 1000 molecules remaining unbound at serum concentrations of 0·5 mg%. Other highly bound drugs include phenylbutazone, methotrexate, sulphinpyrazone, naldixic acid, diazoxide, phenytoin, ethacrynic acid, and sulphonamides. The binding is reversible, an equilibrium being established between those molecules which are bound, and those which are not. Only the unbound molecules remain free and pharmacologically active, while those which are bound form a pharmacologically inactive reservoir which is not immediately exposed to metabolism. As the free molecules become metabolized, so some of the bound molecules become unbound and pass into solution to exert their normal pharmacological actions, before they, in their turn, are metabolized and excreted.

The plasma albumins are not the only sites in the body where drugs become bound. There are static sites in the liver where pamaquine and mepacrine become bound, and highly lipid-soluble drugs rapidly become sequestered in fatty tissue throughout the body.

Depending on the concentrations and their relative affinities for the binding sites, one drug may successfully compete with another and displace it from the sites it is already occupying. The displaced (and now active) drug molecules pour into the plasma water where their concentration rapidly rises (see Fig. 1.2). So, for example, a drug which reduced the binding of another drug from (say) 99 to 96% would thereby increase the unbound concentration of free and active drug from 1 to 4% (a four-fold increase). This would seem to account for the increase in the effects of warfarin which can occur if patients are given chloral hydrate. The major metabolite of chloral, trichloroacetic acid, is a highly bound compound which can successfully displace warfarin thereby enhancing its anticoagulant effects. The effect is however very transient because the now free and active warfarin molecules become vulnerable to attack by the microsomal enzymes. Other processes can probably buffer any marked changes in drug concentrations, so that a new equilibrium rapidly becomes established.

The often quoted and 'classic' example of a drug displacement interaction is that

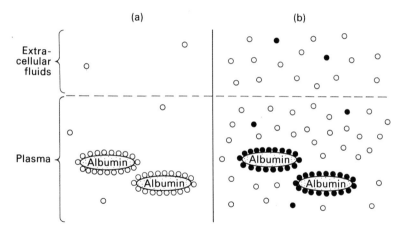

Fig. 1.2. A simple diagram to illustrate the displacement of one highly bound drug by another. (a) Drug (o) exists partly in solution in plasma water but mainly bound to the plasma albumins. (b) When drug (●) which has a greater affinity for the binding sites is introduced, drug (o) is displaced, resulting in a rise in the number of free and active molecules in solution. It should be emphasized that this is a deliberately exaggerated cartoon.

which occurs if phenylbutazone is given to patients stabilized on warfarin (see Fig. 1.3). However, in this case other mechanisms of interaction are almost certainly additionally involved. Warfarin is a mixture of two isomers, S and R. Phenylbutazone inhibits the metabolism of the S isomer but stimulates the metabolism of the R. Since the former is five times more potent than the latter, the result is that the inhibitory effects of the S isomer predominate and an enhancement of the warfarin-induced hypoprothrombinaemia occurs. It is doubtful if a displacement interaction mechanism, on its own, accounts for many (or even any) clinically important interactions, but in association with other mechanisms it appears to have some part to play.

5. Drug metabolism interactions

Although some drug molecules are excreted in the urine unchanged, a very large number are chemically altered within the body to less lipid-soluble metabolites which are more easily excreted by the kidneys. If this were not so, many drugs would remain in the body for extended periods of time, and might continue to exert their effects almost indefinitely. This chemical change is called metabolism, biotransformation, or sometimes detoxification. Some drug metabolism goes on in the serum, the kidneys, the skin or the intestines, but by far the greatest proportion is carried out by the enzymes which are found in the membranes of the endoplasmic reticulum of the liver cells. If the liver is homogenized and then centrifuged, the reticulum breaks up into small sacs called microsomes which carry the enzymes, and it is for this reason that the metabolizing enzymes in the liver are usually referred to as the 'liver microsomal enzymes'.

Enzyme induction

A phenomenon familiar to prescribers is the tolerance which develops to some drugs.

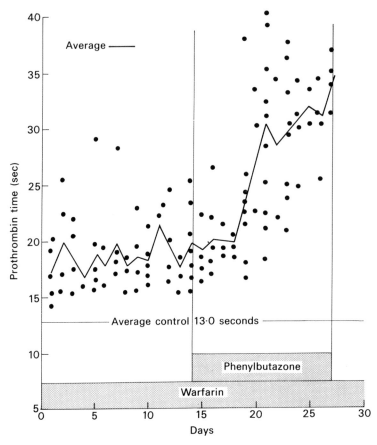

Fig. 1.3. A drug displacement interaction. The effect of phenylbutazone on the response of ten patients to warfarin therapy. Drug displacement has some part to play in this interaction, but changes in the metabolism of the warfarin are also involved (after Udall J. *Clin Med* (1970) **77**, 20).

For example, patients who are given barbiturate hypnotics require increasing doses if they receive them over a period of time because, as time goes by, the pace of the barbiturate metabolism and excretion increases. This is because the presence of the drug increases the activity of the microsomal enzymes. Enzyme stimulation, or induction, of this kind not only accounts for the phenomenon of tolerance, but if another drug is present as well which is metabolized by the same range of enzymes (a coumarin anticoagulant for example) its enzymic degradation is similarly increased and larger doses are needed to maintain the same therapeutic effect. Figure 1.4 illustrates the reduced response to dicoumarol demonstrated by a man on each of two occasions while concurrently being treated with phenobarbitone.

Figure 1.5 shows the effect of another enzyme-inducing agent, dichloralphenazone, on the metabolism of warfarin.

It is possible to maintain satisfactory anticoagulant control by using a higher dose of the anticoagulant, but the effects would require constant monitoring, and there are obvious dangers if the hypnotic is withdrawn. Just as the activity of the enzymes increases gradually over a period of days or weeks, so it gradually returns to its former levels when the inducing agent is removed. Unless the dosage of the anticoagulant is

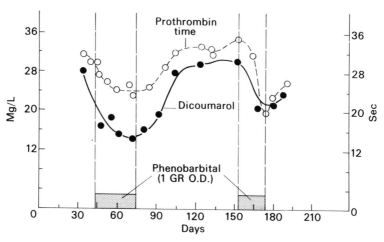

Fig. 1.4. An enzyme induction drug interaction. The effect of phenobarbitone on the plasma levels and prothrombin times of a man on long-term anticoagulant treatment with 75 mg dicoumarol daily (after Burns J J *et al*, in *Animal and Clinical Pharmacological Techniques in Drug Evaluation*. Edited by Siegler and Moyer, Vol 2 (1970) with permission).

then suitably reduced, the patient will be at risk of overdosage and, in this instance, of anticoagulant-induced haemorrhage. This is the kind of situation which can easily arise accidentally if a patient is stabilized on an anticoagulant in hospital while concurrently taking a hypnotic, and is then discharged without it.

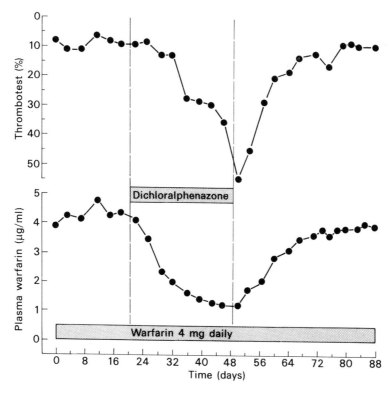

Fig. 1.5. An enzyme induction drug interaction. The effect of dichloralphenazone (*Welldorm*) 1300 mg nightly on the plasma levels and thrombotest percentages of a woman on long-term treatment with 4 mg warfarin daily (after Breckenridge A *et al. Clin Sci* (1971) **40**, 351, with permission).

Table 1.4. Enzyme induction interactions

Drug 1	Drug 2	Result of interaction
Anticoagulants (oral)	Barbiturates	Anticoagulant effects reduced
Contraceptives (oral)	Barbiturates Phenytoin Rifampicin	Contraceptive reliability reduced; pregnancies
Corticosteroids	Phenytoin	Corticosteroid effect reduced
Quinidine	Barbiturates Phenytoin	Quinidine effects reduced

An extremely large number of drugs interact together by this mechanism and numerous examples are to be found throughout this book (see Table 1.4 for some examples). Enzyme induction is not confined to drugs, but is also shown by a number of environmental chemical agents such as hydrocarbons, dyestuffs and halogenated insecticides.

Enzyme inhibition

Just as some drugs can stimulate the activity of the microsomal enzymes, so there are other drugs which have the opposite effect and act as inhibitors, and as a result the normal pace of drug metabolism is slackened. The metabolism of other drugs given concurrently can be reduced so that they are excreted more slowly and begin to accumulate within the body, the effect being essentially the same as when the dosage is increased. Figure 1.6 illustrates what happened when an epileptic patient on

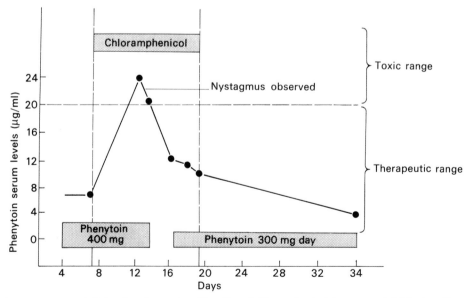

Fig. 1.6. An enzyme inhibition drug interaction. The effect of chloramphenicol (an enzyme inhibitor) on the serum phenytoin levels of a man (after Ballek R E *et al. Lancet* (1973) **i**, 150).

phenytoin was concurrently treated with chloramphenicol (an enzyme inhibitor). The accumulating phenytoin was not detected until it reached levels at which the patient began to manifest intoxication.

Some drugs manifest biphasic activity, that is to say they may initially cause enzyme inhibition, but later with continued use they cause enzyme induction. Table 1.5 lists some of the interactions due to the inhibition of microsomal and other enzymes. Numerous other examples are to be found throughout this book.

Table 1.5. Enzyme inhibition interactions

Drug 1	Drug 2	Result of interaction
Phenytoin	Chloramphenicol Disulfiram	Increased serum phenytoin levels; possible development of intoxication
Warfarin	Disulfiram	Increased serum warfarin levels; enhanced anticoagulant effects; bleeding
6-Mercaptopurine Azathioprine	Allopurinol	Enhanced cyotoxic effects; severe toxicity may develop
Suxamethonium	Ecothiophate iodide	Enhanced neuromuscular blockade; prolonged apnoea

6. Altered excretion interactions

With the exception of the inhalation anaesthetics, most drugs are excreted through the kidneys. Blood entering the kidneys along the renal arteries is, first of all, delivered to the glomeruli of the tubules where molecules small enough to pass through the pores of the glomerular membrane (e.g. water, salts, some drugs) are filtered through into the lumen of the kidney tubule. Larger molecules, such as the plasma proteins with drugs bound to them, and blood cells, are retained. The blood then passes to the remaining parts of the kidney tubules where active energy-using transport systems of the tubule cells are able to remove drugs and their metabolites from the blood, and secrete them into the tubular filtrate. The tubule cells additionally possess active and passive transport systems for the reabsorption of drugs, and it is here that drugs can interfere to alter the excretion or reabsorption of other drugs.

Changes in urinary pH

Although a very large number of drugs are either weak acids or bases, almost all of them are largely metabolized by the liver microsomal enzymes to inactive compounds and very few are excreted unchanged by the kidneys in significant amounts. In practice, therefore, normally only a handful of drugs are affected by changes in urinary pH, although in cases of overdosage, deliberate urinary pH changes have been used to hasten the loss of drugs such as phenobarbitone and salicylates.

Weak acids and bases exist in the urinary filtrate in both ionized and un-ionized forms, only the latter being lipid-soluble and able to diffuse back through the lipid-membranes of the tubule cells into the plasma. Since the pH of the urine determines how much of the drug exists in each form, it also determines whether the drug will be retained or lost in the urine. Thus, pH changes which increase the amount in the un-ionized form (acid urine for acidic drugs, alkaline for bases) increase the retention of the drug, whereas moving the pH in the opposite directions will hasten their loss. Figure 1.7 illustrates the situation with a weakly acidic drug, and Table 1.6 lists some of the drugs known to be affected by pH changes.

Changes in urinary pH do not affect the excretion of erythromycin or hexamine, but can affect the antibacterial activity of these two compounds.

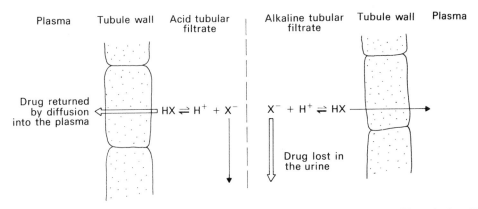

Fig. 1.7. An excretion interaction. Changes in urinary pH affect the retention or loss of a weakly acidic drug (HX). When the tubular filtrate is acidified, most of the drug exists in un-ionized lipid-soluble form (HX) which is able to diffuse through the lipid membranes of the tubule cells and is therefore retained. In alkaline urine most of the acidic drug exists in the ionized non-lipid soluble form (X^-) which is unable to diffuse freely through the cells back into the plasma and is therefore lost in the urine.

Table 1.6. The effect of changes in urinary pH on the excretion of acidic and basic drugs

Drug	Excretion	
	In acid urine	In alkaline urine
Acids		
Phenobarbitone	Decreased	Incresed
Salicylates		
Bases		
Amphetamines		
Mecamylamine	Increased	Decreased
Quinidine		

Competition for active tubular secretion

Drugs which use the same active transport systems in the kidney tubules can compete with one another for secretion. When penicillin was expensive, the successful competition by probenecid was used to reduce the secretion of penicillin and thereby

10

increase its retention in the body. The secreted probenecid molecules are passively reabsorbed further along the tubule (see Fig. 1.8). Competition of this kind occurs between probenecid and a number of acidic drugs which use the same secretory system, some of which are listed in Table 1.7.

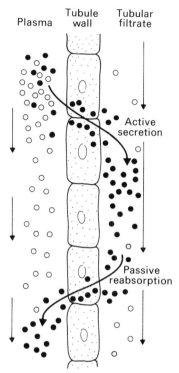

Fig. 1.8. Competition between drugs for active tubular secretion. Probenecid (●) is able to compete successfully with some other drugs (○) for an active secretory mechanism in the kidney tubule. This prevents them being secreted into the tubular filtrate and lost in the urine. The probenecid is later passively reabsorbed so that it too is retained.

Table 1.7. Drugs which can compete for active urinary tubule secretion

Drug 1	Drug 2	Results of interaction
Cephalosporins Dapsone Indomethacin Naldixic acid PAS Penicillins	Probenecid	Serum levels of drug 1 raised.
Acetohexamide	Phenylbutazone	Serum levels of the active metabolite of acetohexamide raised. Hypoglycaemia.

7. Interactions at adrenergic neurones

A very large number of drugs affect adrenergic neurones. The monoamine oxidase inhibitors, tricyclic antidepressants, beta-adrenergic receptor blockers, guanethidine-

11

like antihypertensives, methyldopa, clonidine, sympathomimetic amines and many others mediate their pharmacological and therapeutic effects at central and peripheral adrenergic neurones.

These neurones are found in the central nervous system (CNS) and are concerned with the transmission of nerve impulses across the brain. They are also the last link in the chain of nerves—the sympathetic nervous system—which commences in the brain and, after passing out along the spinal cord, spreads out and innervates most organs and tissues in the body.

Noradrenaline (norepinephrine) is synthesized within the neurone by a series of biochemical steps from tyrosine and is stored within vesicles in the area of the nerve ending. Using artist's licence these vesicles have been combined into one large vesicle in the diagrams in this book. Noradrenaline levels are kept constant by a balanced synthesis/destruction system: synthesis from tyrosine and destruction by monoamine oxidase (MAO).

When a nerve impulse arrives, small amounts of noradrenaline are released from the nerve ending and diffuse across the gap which separates the nerve from the receptor area. The noradrenaline attaches itself to the receptors, thereby stimulating them, and the organ or tissue with which they are associated, into appropriate activity. In the case of blood vessels this will be the contractions of their circular muscle by which blood pressure is maintained and increased. Bronchial muscle on the other hand is relaxed, whereas within the CNS the nerve impulse may be passed along yet another nerve chain.

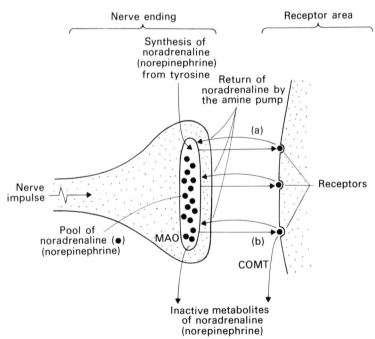

Fig. 1.9. A highly simplified diagram of an adrenergic neurone. Noradrenaline (norepinephrine) is synthesized from tyrosine and stored in vesicles or in a 'pool' at the nerve ending. The levels of noradrenaline are limited by the actions of MAO, an intracellular enzyme, which inactivates and deaminates the transmitter. The receptors are stimulated by the noradrenaline released from the pool by the arrival of a nerve impulse. The receptors are cleared by (a) the return of the noradrenaline into the nerve ending by means of the amine pump, and (b) inactivation by the extracellular enzyme catechol-O-methyltransferase (COMT).

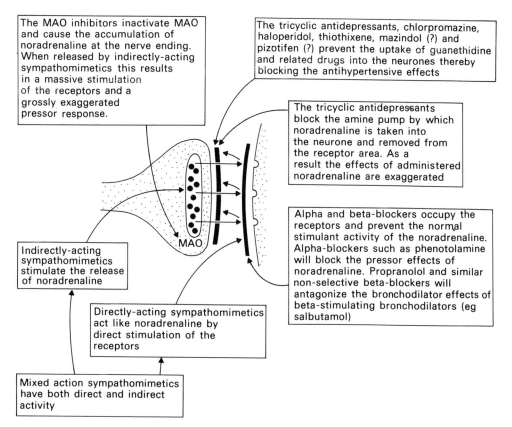

Fig. 1.10. Interactions at adrenergic neurones. A highly simplified diagram of an adrenergic neurone to indicate the different sites where various drugs interact. Further details of these interactions are to be found in the individual synopses.

The receptors are cleared in readiness for further stimulation by the return of the noradrenaline into the nerve endings by means of the amine pump, although a small proportion (about 10%) is destroyed by catechol-O-methyl transferase (COMT). The amine pump is also used by various drugs to enter the neurone (e.g. the guanethidine-like antihypertensives) and it can be inactivated or blocked by others (e.g. tricyclic antidepressants, chlorpromazine, etc.).

Figure 1.9 is an extremely simple diagram of an adrenergic neurone, and Fig. 1.10 illustrates some of the different sites on adrenergic neurones where various drugs interfere and interact. The details of these interactions are discussed in the individual synopses.

CHAPTER 2. ALCOHOL INTERACTIONS

For social and historical reasons alcohol is treated as a beverage and not as a drug, but pharmacologically speaking it has much in common with the other central nervous system depressants. The lay public tend to regard alcohol in small or moderate doses as a stimulant, because it can be used to liven up a party or some other social occasion, but objective tests show that alcohol is unquestionably a depressant which causes a progressive deterioration in the performance of a number of skills as blood-alcohol levels rise, reflecting a gradual and progressive disorganization of the central nervous system. The eminent pharmacologist Professor J. H. Gaddum put the matter amusingly and succinctly when, in describing the early effects of moderate amounts of alcohol, he said that '. . . logical thought is difficult but after-dinner speeches easy . . .'.

The mistaken belief in its stimulant effects has come about because alcohol relaxes the inhibitions imposed by upbringing and environment, so that otherwise well-controlled individuals lose their self-restraint and behave in a manner which, when sober again, they may have cause to regret. The expansiveness and loquaciousness which are socially acceptable lead on, with increasing amounts of alcohol, through drunkenness, eventually to unconsciousness, and finally to death from respiratory depression. Table 2.1 gives an indication of the reactions to different concentrations of alcohol.

Since alcohol impairs the skills needed to drive a car safely, national and state authorities have imposed maximum legal blood-alcohol limits. In the UK this is currently 80 mg% (80 mg per 100 ml) but impairment is detectable at 50 mg% (the

Table 2.1. Indication of reactions to different concentrations of alcohol

Blood-alcohol concentrations (mg%)	Effects	
50 (approximately 2 fl oz [60 ml] whisky in 2 h)	Some impairment of driving skills detectable	
80 (approximately 3 fl oz whisky in 2 h)	Definite impairment of driving skills	
100 (approximately)	'Dizzy and delightful'	
200 (approximately)	'Drunk and disorderly'	Gaddum's stages of alcoholic intoxication
300 (approximately)	'Dead drunk'	
400 (approximately)	'Danger of death'	
500 (approximately)	Dead	

legal limit in some other countries) and a measurable deterioration occurs in some individuals at even lower levels.

Interactions

Almost certainly the most common drug interaction of all occurs if alcohol is taken with other CNS depressants such as sedatives, hypnotics, antihistamines, analgesics, tranquillizers, neuroleptics, antidepressants, antinauseants and other drugs with which its depressant effects are additive. Even though the blood-alcohol levels remain well within the legal driving limits, the combined effects of moderate or even small amounts of alcohol with other drugs can be the same as the effects of blood-alcohol levels above the legal limit. Quite apart from the obvious consequences of this on the ability to drive safely, it may also make the performance of all kinds of other day-to-day tasks much more difficult and hazardous. A particular cause for concern is that the patient himself may be partially or totally unaware of the deterioration in his skills.

A less serious, but not uncommon, interaction between alcohol and some other drugs and chemical agents is the flushing reaction which is exploited in the case of disulfiram and calcium carbimide to treat alcoholism.

In addition to the interactions with alcohol which are described in this chapter, there are other interactions categorized elsewhere. For a full list reference should be made to the index.

Alcohol + antibiotics

Summary

Disulfiram-like reactions have been described after drinking alcohol in two patients on moxalactam, two patients on cefamandole, and volunteers on cefoperazone.

Interaction

A young man with cystic fibrosis was given 2 g moxalactam intravenously every 8 h for pneumonia. After 3 days' treatment he drank, as was his wont, a can of beer for dinner, and immediately he became flushed with a florid, macular eruption over his face and chest. This faded over the next 30 min but the patient complained of severe nausea and headache. A woman patient also on moxalactam became flushed, diaphoretic, and nauseated after drinking a cocktail of vodka and tomato juice.[1]

A similar flush reaction with shock has been described in a patient under treatment with cefamandole on each of two occasions when he drank wine,[2] in a woman on cefamandole when she drank chablis[5], in a volunteer on cefoperazone on three occasions when he drank beer[3], and in three other subjects on cefoperazone when alcohol was taken[4].

Mechanism

Not understood. The reactions described are superficially similar to the reaction described with disulfiram and alcohol (see page 25) but whether the mechanism is the same is not known.

Importance and management

Information appears to be limited to these reports. The incidence is not known but it is probably low. The report concerning moxalactam[1] states that 30 other patients on this antibiotic did not show this reaction. There seems to be no way of predicting which patients are likely to be affected, although the reaction would appear to be more unpleasant than dangerous in most patients.

References

1 Neu H C and Prince A S. Interaction between moxalactam and alcohol. *Lancet* (1980) 1, 1422.
2 Portier H, Chalopin J M, Freysz M and Tanter Y. Interaction between cephalosphorins and alcohol. *Lancet* (1980) 2, 263.
3 Foster T S, Raehl C L and Wilson H D. Disulfiram-like reaction associated with a parenteral cephalosporin. *Amer J Hosp Pharm* (1980) 37, 858.
4 Reeves D S and Davies A J. Alcohol-cephalosporin interaction. *Lancet* (1980) ii, 540.
5 Drummer S, Hauser W E and Remington J S. Antabuse-like effect of β-lactam antibiotics. *New Eng J Med* (1980) 303, 1417.

Alcohol + anticholinergics

Summary

A marked impairment of attention occurs if alcohol is taken in the presence of atropine or glycopyrrhonium which may make driving more hazardous.

Interaction, mechanism, importance and management

A study on healthy volunteers of the effects of 0·5 mg atropine or 1·0 mg glycopyrrhonium, in combination with alcohol (0·5 g/kg) or a placebo, on certain psychomotor skills (a choice reaction test, coordination tests and an attention test) showed that while reaction times and coordination were unaffected or even improved, there was marked impairment of attention which was large enough to make driving more hazardous.[1]

Reference

1 Linnoila M. Drug effects on psychomotor skills related to driving: interaction of atropine, glycopyrrhonium and alcohol. *Europ J clin Pharmacol* (1973) 6, 107.

Alcohol + antihistamines

Summary

The central depressant effects of alcohol and its detrimental effects on the skills related to driving are increased by the concurrent use of the more sedative antihistamines (e.g. promethazine, chlorpheniramine, diphenhydramine etc.), but in normal doses and with small amounts of alcohol some of the other antihistamines (clemizole, clemastine, pheniramine, tripelennamine, terfenadine, cyproheptadine) are reported not to interact.

Interaction

Alcohol + diphenhydramine, clemizole, tripelennamine, or clemastine

An investigation on 16 normal subjects examined the effects of alcohol (blood levels of about 50 mg%) and antihistamines alone or together on the performance of tests designed to assess mental and motor performances. Clemizole (40 mg), tripelennamine (50 mg) and diphenhydramine (50 mg) did not significantly affect the performance under the stress of delayed auditory feedback, but diphenhydramine enhanced the effects of alcohol on a pursuit meter test. The combined sedative effects of diphenhydramine and alcohol were apparent to all the subjects in this study, and confirmed in another.[9]

Diphenhydramine in doses of 25 or 50 mg was shown to increase the detrimental effects of alcohol on the performance of choice reaction and coordination tests by subjects who had taken 0·5 g/kg alcohol. Clemastine in 3 mg doses also affected coordination whereas 1·5 mg did not.[2]

The interaction of alcohol and diphenhydramine (100 mg) has been confirmed in other reports.[4,9]

Clemastine in doses of 1 mg has been shown not to interact.[5,6]

Alcohol + pheniramine or cyproheptadine

No interaction was detected in one study of the combined effects of pheniramine (4 mg) or cyproheptadine (4 mg) with alcohol (0·7 g/kg).[6]

Alcohol + chlorpheniramine

A double-blind study on the effects on 13 volunteers of alcohol (0·75 g/kg) and dexchlorpheniramine (4 mg/70 kg) showed that together they significantly impaired the performance of a number of tests (standing steadiness, reaction time, manual dexterity, perception etc).[7]

Alcohol + terfenadine

A double-blind study showed that terfenadine alone (60–240 mg) did not affect psychomotor skills, nor did it affect the adverse effects of alcohol.[9]

Mechanism

It seems reasonable to postulate that where an interaction is seen it arises from the combined central nervous depressant effects of both alcohol and the antihistamine.

Importance and management

Because many antihistamines, particularly the older ones, are central depressants and cause drowsiness it has become customary to issue a 'blanket' warning that alcohol will make certain activities such as driving, or handling machinery, more difficult and dangerous. This may not be appropriate for every antihistamine. For this reason some of them appear to be more suitable for general use as antihistamines than others. Thus with moderate amounts of alcohol and in the doses used clemizole (40 mg), tripelennamine (50 mg), clemastine (1 mg), pheniramine (4 mg), cyproheptadine (4 mg) and terfenadine (60–240 mg) failed to show an interaction in the tests cited. It is important, however, to appreciate that with larger doses and different amounts of alcohol it is possible that these antihistamines may also interact adversely.

However, some of the more sedative antihistamines such as diphenhydramine,[1,2,4] and chlorpheniramine[7] certainly interact adversely. A marked interaction with alcohol has also been described with promethazine[8] and I am aware of a double motor fatality attributed to the overwhelming sedative effects of this antihistamine with alcohol in a man who was also taking chlordiazepoxide. There appears to be no direct evidence of interactions between alcohol and the other antihistamines, but they may be expected to conform to the general pattern. In the absence of good evidence to the contrary, it would be prudent to assume that an adverse interaction is likely.

It is important not to lose sight of the fact that a number of antihistamines often appear 'in disguise' as antiemetics, sedatives, and as components of cough and cold remedies. Many of these can be bought 'over the counter' without prescription and the pharmacist who sells them should not overlook the potential seriousness of their interaction with alcohol.

References

1 Hughes F W and Forney R B. Comparative effect of three antihistamines and ethanol on mental and motor performance. *Clin Pharmacol Ther* (1961) **5**, 414.

2 Linnoila M. Effects of drugs on psychomotor skills related to driving: antihistamines, chlormezanone and alcohol. *Europ J Clin Pharmacol* (1973) **5**, 247.

3 Smith R B, Rossi G V and Orzechowski R F. Interactions of chlorpheniramine–ethanol combinations: acute toxicity and antihistamine activity. *Toxicol Appl Pharmacol* (1974) **28**, 240.

4 Tang P C and Rosenstein R. Influence of alcohol and dramamine alone and in combination on psychomotor performance. *Aerospace Med* (1967) **38**, 818.

5 Franks H M, Hensley V R, Hensley W J, Starmer G A & Teo R K C. The interaction between ethanol and antihistamines. 2. Clemastine. *Med J Aust* (1979) **1**, 185.

6 Landauer A A and Milner G. Antihistamines alone and together with alcohol in relation to driving safety. *J Forens Med* (1971) **18**, 127.

7 Franks H M, Hensley V R, Hensley W J, Starmer G A and Teo R K C. The interaction between ethanol and antihistamines 1: Dexchlorpheniramine. *Med J Aust* (1978) **1**, 449.

8 Hedges A, Hills M and Maclay W P. Some drug and peripheral effects of meclastine, a new antihistamine drug in man. *J Clin Pharmacol* (1971) **11**, 112.

9 Moser L, Hüther K J, Koch-Weser J and Lundt P V. Effects of terfenadine and diphenhydramine alone or in combination with diazepam or alcohol on psychomotor performance and subjective feelings. *Europ J Clin Pharmacol* (1978) **14**, 417

Alcohol + barbiturates

Summary

Alcohol and the barbiturates if taken together can have potentially serious central nervous system depressant effects. Patients should be warned about the hazards of driving, handling machinery, or undertaking other activities where alertness and good coordination are important.

Interactions

There are three different responses: (a) the CNS depressant effects of the barbiturates and alcohol are enhanced by concurrent use; (b) blood-alcohol levels are somewhat reduced by the barbiturates; (c) barbiturate metabolism is enhanced by chronic alcohol ingestion but inhibited if taken acutely.

(a) Combined central nervous depression

A study in man of the effects of alcohol (0·5 g/kg) taken on the morning following the use of 100 mg amylobarbitone as a hypnotic the night before showed that the performance of co-ordination skills was much more impaired than with either drug alone.[1]

Enhanced CNS depression has been described in a number of other clinical studies[2,3,4] and has featured very many times in coroners' reports of fatal accidents and suicides. There are far too many reports to quote here.

(b) Blood alcohol levels reduced by barbiturates
A study in human volunteers who were given 50 ml doses of vodka showed that the concurrent ingestion of 30 mg phenobarbitone caused a significant reduction in the blood alcohol levels measured 30 and 90 min later.[5]

Similar results are reported elsewhere.[3,9]

(c) Changes in barbiturate metabolism caused by alcohol
In-vitro and in-vivo studies in man and rats demonstrated that the chronic use of alcohol doubled the activity of the enzymes concerned with the metabolism of pentobarbitone, but that during acute ingestion the enzymic activity was inhibited.[4]
This has been described in other studies.[10]

Mechanisms
Both alcohol and the barbiturates have mutual CNS depressant effects which if sufficiently large can lead eventually to respiratory depression and death. It is not clear why blood-alcohol levels are depressed by the barbiturates but it would seem that alcohol can have enzyme-inducing effects which accelerate the metabolism of the barbiturates.[4,10]

Importance and management
The enhanced CNS depression is a very well-documented interaction of serious and practical importance. The most obvious hazards of drowsiness and impaired coordination are associated with handling machinery or driving, but it has also been rightly pointed out that '. . . many old people may have a whisky nightcap with their barbiturate sleeping pill. They then have to get out of bed

in the middle of the night to empty their bladder; they are unsteady, they fall, they are found in the morning with a fractured femur or in a hypothermic state. No figures are available to give us any reliable idea of the scale of this problem . . .'[7] There are many other day-to-day situations which can be made much more hazardous by CNS depression of this kind.

It should also be appreciated that the hangover effects of hypnotics such as amylobarbitone are still present next morning and can continue to interact significantly with alcohol. Patients should be warned of the dangers.

In addition it has been pointed out[8] that in man, blood-alcohol levels of 100 mg% combined with only 0·5 mg% barbiturate have proved fatal. This compares with lethal levels of alcohol alone of 500 mg% or more, and of phenobarbitone of 10–30 mg%.

References
1 Saario I and Linnoila M. Effect of subacute treatment with hypnotics, alone or in combination with alcohol, on psychomotor skills related to driving. *Acta pharmacol et toxicol* (1976) **38**, 382.
2 Kielholz P, Goldberg L, Obersteg J I, Pöldinger W, Ramseyer A and Schmid P. Fahrversuche zur Frage der Beeintrachtigung der Verkehrstüchtigkeit durch Alkohol, Tranquilizer und Hypnotika. *Deut Med Wochenschr* (1969) **94**, 301.
3 Morrelli P L, Veneroni E, Zaccala M and Bizzi A. Further observations on the interaction between ethanol and psychotropic drugs. *Arzneim-Forsch* (Drug Res) (1971) **21**, 20.
4 Wegener H and Kötter L. Analgetica und Verkehrstüchtigkeit Wirkung einer Kombination von 5-Allyl-5-isobutylsäure, Dimethylaminophenazon und Coffein nach einmaliger und wiederholter Applikation. *Arzneim-Forsch (Drug Res)* (1971) **21**, 47.
5 Mould G P, Curry S H and Binns T B. Interaction of glutethimide and phenobarbitone with ethanol in man. *J Pharm Pharmac* (1972) **24**, 894.
6 Rubin E and Lieber C S. Hepatic microsomal enzymes in man and rat: induction and inhibition of ethanol. *Science* (1968) **162**, 690.
7 Wilkes E. Are you still prescribing those outdated drugs? *MIMS Magazine* (1976) **27**, 84.
8 Seixas F A Alcohol and its drug interactions. *Ann Int Med* (1975) **83**, 86.
9 Mezey E and Robles E A. Effects of phenobarbital administration on rates of ethanol clearance and on ethanol-oxidizing enzymes in man. *Gastroenterology* (1974) **66**, 248.
10 Rubin E and Lieber C S. Inhibition of drug metabolism by acute ethanol intoxication. A hepatic microsomal mechanism. *Am J med* (1970) **49**, 801.

Alcohol + benzodiazepines

Summary
The central nervous depressant effects of alcohol and its detrimental effects on the skills related to driving are increased by the concurrent use of benzodiazepine

tranquillizers and hypnotics. Diazepam appears to interact in this way more consistently and to a greater extent than chlordiazepoxide. There is limited direct evidence about the other benzodiazepines.

Interaction
Direct comparability between the results of the extensive studies on this interaction is very difficult because of the differences between the tests, their duration, the doses of drug and alcohol used, whether administered chronically or acutely, and other variables, but the overall picture is that the performance of psychomotor skills related to driving is impaired by the concurrent use of alcohol and a benzodiazepine. A very large amount of data is documented, but only a summary is presented here.

Alcohol + chlordiazepoxide
Chlordiazepoxide has been variously reported as having no effect,[1,2,5] an additive effect[3,4,7] and even an antagonistic effect[6] on the detrimental activity of alcohol on the performance of psychomotor skill tests and others carried out in the laboratory, and on driving tests in cars on special test tracks.

Alcohol + diazepam
Unlike chlordiazepoxide, the majority of the reports on diazepam describe an additive effect on the detrimental activity of alcohol on the performance of psychomotor skills and other tests carried out.[6,8-13,16] The interaction with diazepam appears to be more potent than with chlordiazepoxide.

Alcohol + bromazepam, clobazam, medazepam or oxazepam
Far fewer studies have been carried out on these benzodiazepines. Bromazepam with alcohol is reported to have impaired coordination and divided attention in one series of tests[14] and clobazam interacts similarly.[15] Oxazepam is reported to interact to a lesser degree than diazepam[16] while single-dose experiments with medazepam indicate that it may not interact with alcohol significantly.[17]

Alcohol + flurazepam or nitrazepam
Next morning studies of the effects of alcohol on the performance of psychomotor skills of subjects who had had flurazepam[18] or nitrazepam[10,19] as a hypnotic the night before showed that a significant and detrimental 'hangover' interaction takes place.

Mechanism
Although the mechanism of this interaction is not known for certain, it seems not unreasonable to postulate that it results from the additive effects of two central nervous depressants.[21] There is also some evidence that alcohol increases the absorption and raises the serum levels of some of the benzodiazepines.[15,20]

Importance and management
The general picture which emerges from all these reports is that the benzodiazepines increase the central depressant activity of alcohol and increase its detrimental effects on the performance of certain psychomotor skills. Chlordiazepoxide appears to have a smaller and less consistent effect than diazapam, and this may also be true of oxazepam and medazepam, but the potency of bromazepam and clobazam are uncertain. There seems to be no direct evidence about the other benzodiazepines but they may be expected to conform to the general pattern.

It must be emphasized that the extent to which this adverse interaction develops will depend on the dosage, the amount of alcohol drunk and a number of other variables. With small amounts of alcohol the extent and importance of the interaction may be relatively small. However, patients should be warned that their usual response to a given amount of alcohol may be greater than expected, and their ability to drive a motor car safely may be impaired. This warning applies to the hypnotic as well as the tranquillizing benzodiazepines because, even though the drug is taken the night before, the body may still contain significant amounts of the drug, particularly during the early part of the next day. A 'hangover' effect like this is least evident in the young.[10]

References
1 Reggiani G, Hurlimann A and Theiss E. Some aspects of the experimental and clinical toxicology of chlordiazepoxide. *Acta pharmacol et toxicol* (1979) **45**, 257.
2 Hughes F W, Forney R B and Richards A B. Comparative effect in human subjects of chlordiazepoxide, diazepam, and placebo on mental and physical performance. *Clin Pharmacol Ther* (1965) **6**, 139.
3 Linnoila M. Effects of diazepam, chlordiazepoxide, thioridazine, haloperidol, flupenthixole and alcohol on psychomotor skills related to driving. *Ann Med Exp Biol Fenn* (1973) **51**, 125.
4 Linnoila M, Saario I, Olkoniemi J, Liljequist R, Himberg J J and Maki M. Effect of two weeks' treatment with chlordiazepoxide or flupenthixole, alone or in combination with

alcohol, on psychomotor skills related to driving. *Arzneim-Forsch (Drug Res)* (1975) **25**, 1088.

5 Hoffer A. Lack of potentiation by chlordiazepoxide (Librium) of depression or excitation due to alcohol. *Canad Med Ass J* (1962) **87**, 920.

6 Dundee J W and Isaac M. Interaction of alcohol with sedatives and tranquillisers (a study of blood levels at loss of consciousness following rapid infusion). *Med Sci Law* (1970) **10**, 220.

7 Kielholz P, Goldberg L, Obersteg J I, Pöldinger W, Ramseyer A and Schmid P. Fahrversuche zur frage der Beeintrachtigung der Verkehrstüchtigkeit durch Alkohol Tranquilizer und Hypnotika. *Deut Med Wochenschr* (1969) **94**, 301.

8 Morselli P L, Veneroni E, Zaccala M and Bizzi A. Further observations on the interaction between ethanol and psychotropic drugs. *Arzneim-Forsch* (Drug Res) (1971) **21**, 20.

9 Linnoila M and Hakkinen S. Effects of diazepam and codeine, alone and in combination with alcohol, on simulated driving. *Clin Pharmacol Ther* (1974) **15**, 368.

10 Linnoila M. Drug interaction on psychomotor skills related to driving: hypnotics and alcohol. *Ann Med Exp Biol Fenn* (1973) **51**, 118.

11 Missen A W, Cleary W, Eng L and McMillan S. Diazepam, alcohol and drivers. *New Zealand Med J* (1978) **87**, 275.

12 Laisi U, Linnoila M, Seppala T, Himberg J J and Matilla M J. Pharmacokinetic and Pharmacodynamic interactions of diazepam with different alcoholic beverages. *Europ J clin Pharmacol* (1979) **16**, 263.

13 Palva E S, Linnoila M, Saario I and Matilla M J. Acute and subacute effects of diazepam on psychomotor skills: interaction with alcohol. *Acta pharmacol et toxicol* (1979) **45**, 257.

14 Seppälä T, Saario I and Matilla M J. Two weeks' treatment with chlorpromazine, thioridazine, sulpiride or bromazepam: actions and interactions with alcohol on psychomotor skills related to driving. *Mod Probl Pharmacopsych* (1976) **11**, 85.

15 Taeuber K, Badian M, Brettell H F, Royen Th, Rupp K, Sittig W and Uihlein M. Kinetic and dynamic interaction of clobazam and alcohol. *Brit J Clin Pharmacol* (1979) **7**, 91S.

16 Molander L and Durhök C. Acute effects of oxazepam, diazepam and methylperone, alone and in combination with alcohol on sedation, coordination and mood. *Acta pharmacol et toxicol* (1976) **38**, 145.

17 Landauer A A, Pocock D A and Prott F W. The effect of medazepam and alcohol on cognitive and motor skills used in car driving. *Psychopharmacologia* (1974) **37**, 159.

18 Saario I and Matilla M. Effect of subacute treatment with hypnotics, alone or in combination with alcohol on psychomotor skills related to driving. *Acta pharmacol et toxicol* (1976) **38**, 382.

19 Saario I, Linnoila M and Maki M. Interaction of drugs with alcohol on human psychomotor skills related to driving: effect of sleep deprivation or two weeks' treatment with hypnotics. *J Clin Pharmacol* (1975) **15**, 52.

20 MacLeod S M, Giles H G, Patzalek G, Thiessen J J and Sellers E M. Diazepam actions and plasma concentrations following ethanol ingestion. *Europ J clin Pharmacol* (1977) **11**, 345.

21 Curry S H and Smith C M. Diazepam–ethanol interaction in humans: addition or potentiation? *Comm Psychopharmacol* (1979) **3**, 101.

Alcohol + Beta-blockers

Summary
Preliminary evidence suggests that propranolol may enhance the effects of alcohol.

Interaction, mechanism, importance and management

A double-blind random crossover study[1] on 12 moderate drinkers given 1·33 ml/kg alcohol and either a placebo or propranolol, 40 mg, showed that the propranolol enhanced the effects of alcohol on (a) mood (b) memory (c) neurological function, (d) global objective and subjective ratings, of inebriation, and (e) divided attention, but only the effects on the last two—(d) and (e)—were statistically significant. This suggests that driving may be made more hazardous but this has yet to be confirmed. Whether this also occurs with other beta-blockers is not known.

References
1 Noble E P, Parker E, Alkana R, Cohen H and Birch H. Propranolol–ethanol interaction in man. *Fed Proc* (1973) **32**, 724.

Alcohol + bromvaletone or ethinamate

Summary
The detrimental effects of alcohol on the performance of psychomotor skills related to driving are enhanced by bromvaletone. The interaction with ethinamate is mild. 'Hangover' effects also occur.

Interaction

A study on a very large number of subjects treated with 1 g ethinamate or 0·6 g bromvaletone, either alone or with 0·5 g/kg alcohol, showed that the performance of a number of psychomotor skills related to driving was slightly impaired by ethinamate. Its interaction with alcohol was mild, whereas the interaction of bromvaletone with alcohol was strong. There was sufficient 'hangover' for both drugs to interact with alcohol next morning after being used as a hypnotic the night before.[1]

Mechanism

Uncertain. Additive CNS depression?

Importance and management

The documentation is limited but these interactions appear to be well established. Patients should be warned of the potential hazards of combined use, and of the 'hangover' effects.

References

1 Linnoila M. Drug interaction on psychomotor skills related to driving: hypnotics and alcohol. *Ann Med Exp Biol Fenn* (1973) 51, 118.

Alcohol + caffeine

Summary

Despite popular belief, objective tests show that caffeine does not reverse the effects of alcohol.

Interaction

A study on a large number of subjects who were given caffeine, 300 mg, either alone or with alcohol, 0·75 mg/kg, showed that the caffeine did not antagonize the deleterious effects of alcohol on the performance of psychomotor skill tests. Only reaction times were reversed.[1]

Mechanism

None.

Importance and management

Information is very limited, but these results suggest that despite the time-hallowed use of black coffee to sober up those who have drunk too much, it is still not safe for them to drive or handle dangerous machinery.

Reference

1 Franks H M. Hagedorn H and Hensley V R. The effect of caffeine on human performance, alone and in combination with alcohol. *Psychopharmacology* (1975) 45, 177.

Alcohol + chloral hydrate

Summary

Both alcohol and chloral are CNS depressants and their effects may be additive, possibly even more than additive, if taken concurrently. Some patients may experience a disulfiram-like flushing reaction with alcohol after taking chloral for several days.

Interaction

Studies undertaken in 5 volunteers given chloral, 15 mg/kg, and alcohol, 0·5 mg/kg, showed that both drugs impaired their ability to carry out complex motor tasks. When taken together, the effects appeared to be additive, and possibly even more than additive. When chloral had been taken for 7 days, one individual showed a marked vasodilatory reaction after drinking alcohol (bright red-purple flushing of the face, tachycardia, hypotension, anxiety and persistent headache) which is similar to the alcohol/disulfiram reaction.[1,2]

The disulfiram-like reaction has been described in other reports.[3,4] One of these was published more than a century ago in 1872 and describes two

21

patients on chloral who experienced this reaction after drinking half a bottle of beer.[3]

Mechanisms
Alcohol, chloral and trichlorethanol (to which chloral is metabolized) are all CNS depressants. During concurrent use the metabolic pathways involved in their elimination are mutually inhibited. Blood-alcohol levels rise because the trichloroethanol competitively depresses the oxidation of alcohol to acetaldehyde, while the trichloroethanol levels are elevated because not only is its production from chloral enhanced, but its further conversion to the glucuronide is inhibited. As a result the blood levels of both alcohol and trichloroethanol rise higher than they would normally, and their effects are accordingly greater[1,2,5,6] (see Fig. 2.1).

The vasodilatory reaction, despite its superficial resemblance to the disulfiram reaction, may possibly have a different basis. Blood levels of acetaldehyde have been found to be elevated by only 50% during the use of chloral.[2]

Importance and management
A well-documented and well-established interaction. A comprehensive bibliography can be found in the references.[1,2] Patients given chloral should be warned about the extensive CNS depression which can follow the ingestion of alcohol, and of the disulfiram-like reaction which may occur after taking chloral for a period of time. The incidence of this reaction is uncertain. There seems to be little clinical evidence to support the idea of the legendary 'Mickey Finn', concocted of chloral and alcohol, which is reputed to be so potent that a deep sleep can be induced in the unsuspecting victim within minutes of ingestion—at least in normal therapeutic doses of 0·3–2·0 g. Larger doses may cause serious and potentially life-threatening CNS depression.

It seems probable that chloral betaine, triclofos and other compounds closely related to chloral hydrate will interact with alcohol in a similar way, but as yet there appear to be no confirmatory reports in the literature.

References
1 Sellers E M, Carr G, Bernstein J G, Sellers S and Koch-Weser J. Interaction of chloral hydrate and ethanol in man II. Haemodynamic and performance. *Clin Pharmacol Ther* (1972) **13**, 50.
2 Sellers E M, Lang M, Koch-Weser J, LeBlanc E and Kalant H. Interaction of chloral hydrate and ethanol in man I. Metabolism. *Clin Pharmacol Ther* (1972) **13**, 37.
3 Björström F. On the effect of alcoholic beverages and simultaneous use of chloral. *Uppsala Lakareforenings Forhandlingar* (1872) **8**, 114.
4 Bardoděj Z. Intolerance alkoholu po chloralhydratu. *Ceskolov farm* (1965) **14**, 478.
5 Owens A H, Marshall E K and Brown G O. A comparative evaluation of the hypnotic potency of chloral hydrate and trichloroethanol. *Bull Johns Hopkins Hosp* (1955) **96**, 71.
6 Wong L K and Biemann K. A study of drug interaction by gas chromatography–mass spectrometry. Synergism of chloral hydrate and ethanol. *Biochem Pharmacol* (1978) **27**, 1019.

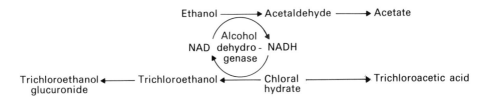

Fig. 2.1. The metabolism of alcohol (ethanol) and chloral hydrate

Alcohol + 'chlorodyne'

Summary
A case has been reported of severe hepatotoxicity in a heavy drinker who was taking large quantities of 'chlorodyne' (chloroform and morphine tincture BPC).

Interaction, mechanism, importance and management
Severe hepatotoxicity developed in a man who habitually took large quantities of chlorodyne to control chronic diarrhoea.[1] It was estimated that he was taking at least 100 ml a week, equivalent

to 32 mg morphine and 1·4 ml chloroform a day. He also had a history of fairly heavy rum intake. It is suggested that the alcohol induced the liver microsomal enzymes, thereby increasing the metabolism of the chloroform and resulting in the formation of hepatotoxic chloroform metabolites.[1] This would be consistent with the findings of animal experiments with alcohol and carbon tetrachloride, the latter compound being closely related chemically to chloroform and undergoing metabolism by a similar metabolic pathway.[2]

References
1 Stathers G M. The synergistic effect of ethanol and chlorodyne in producing hepatotoxicity. *Med J Aust* (1970) **2**, 1134.
2 Hasumura Y, Teschke R and Lieber C S. Increased carbon tetrachloride hepatotoxicity, and its mechanism, after chronic ethanol consumption. *Gastroenterol* (1974) **66**, 415.

Alcohol + codeine

Summary
Codeine both alone and with alcohol impairs the ability to drive safely.

Interaction
Double-blind studies on a very large number of professional army drivers showed that codeine, 50 mg, and alcohol, 0·5 g/kg, both alone and together impaired their ability to drive safely on a static driving simulator. The number of 'collisions', neglected instructions and the times they 'drove off the road' were increased.[1,2]

Mechanism
Uncertain.

Importance and management
A thoroughly examined and established interaction. The increased hazard due to this interaction is difficult to quantify precisely, but in the doses used codeine certainly added to the deleterious effects of alcohol on driving skills.

References
1 Linnoila M and Häkkinen S. Effects of diazepam and codeine, alone and in combination with alcohol, on simulated driving. *Clin Pharmacol Ther* (1974) **15**, 368.
2 Linnoila M and Mattila M J. Interaction of alcohol and drugs on psychomotor skills as demonstrated by a driving simulator. *Br J Pharmac* (1973) **47**, 671. P.

Alcohol + cycloserine

Summary
The effects of alcohol may be enhanced in the presence of cycloserine. The manufacturers state that concurrent use is contraindicated.

Interaction, mechanism, importance and management
A brief report describes an enhancement of the actions of alcohol in two patients on cycloserine.[1] One of the manufacturers of cycloserine, Lilley, states that cycloserine is contraindicated in patients who drink heavily, whereas Roche say that patients should be instructed to avoid alcohol since the individual response cannot be foreseen.

Martindale's Extra Pharmacopoeia, 27th ed, also states that great care is necessary in alcoholics. Most of these are secondary references so that it is not clear how strong the evidence is on which these statements are based.

References
1 Glass F, Mallach H J and Simsch A. Beobachtungen und Untersuchungen über die gemeinsame wirkung von Alkohol und D-Cycloserin. *Arzneim-Forsch* (*Drug Res*) (1965) **15**, 684.

Alcohol + dextropropoxyphene

Summary

The central nervous depressant effects of alcohol are enhanced to some extent by dextropropoxyphene in normal therapeutic doses.

Interaction

A study in 8 volunteers of the effects of alcohol and dextropropoxyphene on motor coordination, mental performance and stability of stance (using four pursuit meter patterns, nine verbal tests and four standing stability tests) showed that alcohol alone (blood levels of 50 mg%) impaired the performance of the tests to a greater degree than 65 mg dextropropoxyphene alone. When given together there was some evidence that the effects were greater than with either alone, but in some instances the impairment was no greater than with just alcohol. The effect of the alcohol clearly predominated.[1]

Mechanism

Both drugs are CNS depressants, and the effects appear to be additive.

Importance and management

There are numerous reports about the severe and sometimes fatal respiratory depression which can follow alcohol/dextropropoxyphene overdosage, but information about the combined effects of social drinking and therapeutic doses of dextropropoxyphene is very limited. Patients should be warned that dextropropoxyphene can cause drowsiness and this may be exaggerated to some extent by alcohol. They should be cautioned about driving or handling potentially hazardous machinery.

Reference

1 Kiplinger G F, Sokol G and Rodda B E. Effects of combined alcohol and propoxyphene on human performance. *Arch int Pharmacodyn* (1974) **212**, 175.

Alcohol + dimethylformamide

Summary

A disulfiram-like reaction can occur in those who drink alcohol after being exposed to dimethylforamamide (DMF) vapour.

Interaction

A maintenance fitter who worked on a repair under a reaction vessel containing dimethylformamide (DMF) and who was exposed to low concentrations of the vapour (10–30 ppm) for about 4 h (he may also have had some on his skin as well), developed a tightness of the chest and a red blotchy face when he later drank half a pint of beer. The symptoms cleared after about 2 h, but recurred on two other occasions over the next 2 days following the ingestion of beer. A second exposure to DMF 3 months later produced the same response after drinking beer.[1]

Two further cases of this reaction with DMF and alcohol are described in another report.[2]

Mechanism

Uncertain. It is postulated that the mechanism may be similar to the disulfiram/alcohol interaction which is discussed on page 25.

Importance and management

Information appears to be limited to these two reports. The incidence is uncertain, but 1 out of the 3 workers exposed to DMF described in the first report[1] experienced this interaction, and 2 out of 3 in the other report.[2] Those who come into contact with DMF, even in very low concentrations, should be warned of this possible interaction with alcohol.

References

1 Chivers C P. Disulfiram effect from inhalation of dimethylformamide. *Lancet* (1978) **i**, 331.
2 Reinl W and Urba H J. Erkrankungen durch dimethylformamid. *Int Arch Gewerbepath Gewerbehyg* (1965) **21**, 333.

Alcohol + disulfiram

Summary

Flushing and fullness of the face and neck, palpitations, giddiness, breathlessness, tachycardia, hypotension, nausea and vomiting can follow the ingestion of alcohol while taking disulfiram. Normally a therapeutically exploited interaction in the treatment of alcoholism

Interaction

A toxic interaction, first observed in 1937 by Dr E. E. Williams amongst workers in the rubber industry manufacturing tetraethylthiuram disulphide.

> 'Beer will cause a flushing of the face and hands, with rapid pulse, and some of the men describe palpitations and a terrible fullness of the face, eyes and head. After a glass of beer (6 ounces) the blood pressure falls about 10 points, the pulse is slightly accelerated and the skin becomes flushed in the face and wrists. In 15 min the blood pressure falls another 10 points, the heart is more rapid, and the patient complains of fullness in the head.'[1]

The later observation[2] by Hald, Jacobsen and Larsen of the same reaction with the ethyl congener (disulfiram) led to its introduction for the treatment of alcoholism. Some patients also experience giddiness, nausea, vomiting, difficulty in breathing and headache. The severity and duration can depend upon the amount of alcohol ingested, but some individuals are extremely sensitive. Respiratory depression, cardiovascular collapse, cardiac arrhythmias, unconsciousness and convulsions may occur. The reaction can be fatal.

Mechanism

Not fully understood. Many of the toxic reactions are due to the inhibition by the disulfiram of the enzyme acetaldehyde dehydrogenase which is concerned with the oxidation of acetaldehyde, the initial metabolite of alcohol. As a consequence the concentrations of acetaldehyde in the body are markedly increased. But not all the symptoms can be reproduced by injecting acetaldehyde, so that some other biochemical changes are also involved.

Importance and management

An extremely well-documented interaction[5] used to deter alcoholics from drinking. Initial treatment should be undertaken under close supervision because an extremely intense reaction may occur in some individuals with even quite small doses of alcohol. Apart from the usual warnings about drinking, patients should also be warned about the unwitting ingestion of alcohol in some pharmaceutical preparations. They should seek informed advice. A disulfiram reaction has been seen following a single dose of an alcohol-containing cough mixture[3] and when alcohol was applied to the skin.

Treatment of severe interactions has included the use of $0 \cdot 5-1 \cdot 0$ g sodium ascorbate by slow intravenous injection, antihistamines, and non-specific supportive measures such as oxygen and the intravenous administration of solute and colloid.

References

1 Williams E E. Effects of alcohol on workers with carbon disulfide. *J Amer med Ass* (1937) **109**, 1472.
2 Hald J, Jacobssen E and Larsen V. The sensitizing effects of tetraethylthiuram disulphide (Antabuse) to ethyl alcohol. *Acta Pharmacol* (1948) **4**, 285.
3 Koff R S, Popadimas I and Honig E. Alcohol in cough medicines: hazards to the disulfiram user. *J Amer med Ass* (1971) **215**, 1988.
4 Garber R S and Bennett R E. Unusual reaction with antabuse: report of three cases. *J Med Soc NJ* (1950) **47**, 168.
5 Kwentus J and Major L F. Disulfiram in the treatment of alcoholism. A review. *J Stud Alc* (1979) **40**, 428.

Alcohol + flupenthixol or haloperidol

Summary

The deleterious effects of alcohol on the performance of skills related to driving are enhanced by flupenthixol. Whether a similarly serious interaction occurs with haloperidol is uncertain.

Interaction

A double-blind study in a number of subjects treated with either 0·5 mg flupenthixol, three times a day for 2 weeks, or single doses of halperidol, 0·5 mg, either alone or with 0·5 g/kg alcohol, showed that the combination of flupenthixol with alcohol impaired the performance of a number of tests (choice reaction, coordination and attention) to such an extent that driving or handling machinery could be dangerous. No interaction of importance was seen with haloperidol.[1,2]

Mechanism

Uncertain. Additive CNS depression?

Importance and management

The documentation is limited and not totally conclusive. The tests with alcohol and flupen-thixol taken chronically indicate that the skills needed to drive a car safely can be seriously impaired. The test with haloperidol was, however, with single doses and the results may not be a reliable indicator of the situation when haloperidol is taken chronically. Caution would be advisable until more information is available.

References

1 Linnoila M. Effects of diazepam, chlordiazepoxide, thioridazine, haloperidol, flupenthixol and alcohol on psychomotor skills related to driving. *Ann Med Exp Biol Fenn* (1973) 51, 125.
2 Linnoila M, Saario I, Olkonieme J, Liljequist R, Himberg J J and Mäki M. Effect of two weeks' treatment with chlordiazepoxide or flupenthixol, alone or in combination with alcohol, on psychomotor skills related to driving. *Arzneim-Forsch (Drug Res)* (1975) 25, 1088.

Alcohol + glutethimide

Summary

The sedative effects of glutethimide are enhanced by alcohol and the performance of psychomotor skills is impaired. Changes in blood-alcohol and glutethimide levels have also been described.

Interaction

A double-blind study on normal subjects who were given glutethimide, 250 mg, alone or with alcohol, 0·5 g/kg, showed that concurrent use subjectively and objectively impaired the performance of a number of psychomotor skill tests (choice reaction, coordination, divided attention).[1]

In a previous study it was reported that during concurrent use the blood alcohol levels were increased 11–30%, but blood-glutethimide levels were reduced.[2] This has not been confirmed.[1] It was also claimed that the effects of glutethimide and alcohol were antagonistic rather than additive.[2]

Mechanism

Both are central nervous depressants which appear to have additive effects.

Importance and management

The documentation is limited and somewhat contradictory; nevertheless patients should be warned about the probable results of taking glutethimide and alcohol together. Handling machinery, driving a car or undertaking any complex task requiring alertness and full coordination is likely to be made more hazardous. There is no evidence of a 'hangover' effect which can result in an interaction with alcohol the next day.[1]

References

1 Saario I and Linnoila M. Effect of subacute treatment with hypnotics, alone or in combination with alcohol, on psychomotor skills related to driving. *Acta pharmacol et toxicol* (1976) 38, 382.
2 Mould G P, Curry S H and Binns T B. Interactions of glutethimide and phenobarbitone with ethanol in man. *J Pharm Pharmac* (1972) 24, 894.

Alcohol + griseofulvin

Summary

Enhancement of the effects of alcohol have been reported to occur in a very small number of patients. A disulfiram-like reaction has also been described in one patient.

Interaction

The descriptions of the griseofulvin–alcohol interactions are very brief. One report describes a man who had '. . . decreased tolerance to alcohol and emotional instability manifested by crying and nervousness so severe that the drug was stopped'.[1] Another states that '. . . a possible potentiation of the effects of alcohol has been noted in a very small number of patients . . .'.[2] I am also personally aware of a man who experienced a marked enhancement of the effects of alcohol while taking griseofulvin. A single case of tachycardia and flushing attributed to concurrent use has also been described.[2]

Mechanism

Not understood.

Importance and management

The documentation is extremely sparse but it would appear to indicate that interactions between alcohol and griseofuvin are uncommon. There seems to be little reason for normally avoiding concurrent use.

References

1 Drowns B V, Fuhrman D L and Dennie C C. Use, abuse and limitations of griseofulvin. *Missouri Med* (1960) **57**, 1473.
2 Simon H J and Rantz L A. Reactions to antimicrobial agents. *Ann Rev Med* (1961) **12**, 119.

Alcohol + indomethacin

Summary

The psychomotor skills related to driving are impaired by indomethacin, but to some extent this effect is antagonized by alcohol.

Interaction, mechanism, importance and management

A study on a large number of volunteers showed that indomethacin, 50 mg, impaired the performance of a number of psychomotor skills related to driving, but when taken with alcohol (0·5 g/kg) the performance improved to some extent.[1] The reasons are not understood. This reaction is in contrast to the phenylbutazone/alcohol interaction.

Reference

1 Linnoila M, Seppälä T and Mattila M J. Acute effects of antipyretic analgesics, alone or in combination with alcohol, on human psychomotor skills related to driving. *Br J clin Pharmac* (1974) **1**, 477.

Alcohol + isoniazid

Summary

Isoniazid increases the hazards of driving after drinking alcohol.

Interaction, mechanism, importance and management

The effects of 750 mg isoniazid (about 10 mg/kg) with about 0·5 g/kg alcohol were examined in 100 volunteers given various psychomotor tests and using a driving simulator. No major interaction was observed in the psychomotor tests, but the number of drivers who 'drove off the road' on the simulator was increased. There may therefore be some extra risks for patients on isoniazid who drink and drive, but the effect does not appear to be large.[1,2]

References

1 Linnoila M and Mattila M J. Effects of isoniazid on psychomotor skills related to driving. *J Clin Pharmacol* (1973) **13**, 343.
2 Linnoila M and Mattila M J. Interaction of alcohol and drugs on psychomotor skills as demonstrated by a driving simulator. *Br J Pharmacol* (1973) **47**, 671. P.

Alcohol + lithium carbonate

Summary
Lithium carbonate alone and combined with alcohol may make car driving more hazardous.

Interaction, mechanism, importance and management
Data on this interaction are very limited. A study[1] on 20 normal subjects given lithium carbonate to achieve blood levels of 0·75 meq/l and 0·5 g/kg alcohol, and who were subjected to various tests (choice reaction, coordination, attention) to assess any impairment of psychomotor skills related to driving indicated that lithium alone and with alcohol may increase the risk of accident.

Reference
1 Linnoila M, Saario I and Maki M. Effects of treatment with diazepam or lithium and alcohol on psychomotor skills related to driving. *Europ J clin Pharmacol* (1974) 7, 337.

Alcohol + meprobamate

Summary
The intoxicant effects of alcohol can be considerably enhanced by the presence of normal daily doses of meprobamate.

Interaction
A study on 24 subjects who were treated with 400 mg meprobamate four times a day for a week, alone or with sufficient alcohol to produce average blood concentration of 50 mg%, showed that concurrent use impaired the performance of a number of psychological tests designed to evaluate coordination and judgement much more than with either drug alone. Some of the subjects were quite obviously drunk while taking both drugs and showed '. . . marked muscular incoordination and little or no concern for the social proprieties . . .'. Two could not walk without assistance. 'Nothing approaching this was seen with alcohol alone'.[1]

Other studies confirm this interaction although the effects described appeared to be less pronounced.[2-7]

Mechanism
Additive depression of the central nervous system. There is also evidence that alcohol may inhibit or induce meprobamate metabolism, depending on whether it is taken acute or chronically, but the contribution of this to the extent of enhanced CNS depression is uncertain.[8,9]

Importance and management
A well-documented and potentially serious interaction. Normal daily dosages of meprobamate, in association with blood alcohol concentrations well within the UK legal limit for driving, can result in potentially dangerous intoxication. Patients should be warned of the hazards.

References
1 Zirkle G A, McAtee O B, King P D and Van Dyke R. Meprobamate and small amounts of alcohol. Effects on human ability, coordination, and judgment. *J Amer med Ass* (1960) 173, 1823.
2 Reisby N and Theilgaard A. The interaction of alcohol and meprobamate in man. *Acta Psychiatr Scand* (1969) Suppl 208, 192.
3 Forney R B and Hughes F W. Meprobamate, ethanol or meprobamate–ethanol combinations on performance of human subjects under delayed audiofeedback (DAF) *J Psychol* (1964) 57, 431.
4 Goldberg L. Behavioural and physiological effects of alcohol on man. *Psychosom Med* (1966) 28, 570.
5 Ashford J R and Cobby J M. Drug interactions. The effects of alcohol and meprobamate applied singly and jointly in human subjects. IV. *J Stud Alc* (1975) Suppl 7, 140.
6 Cobby J M and Ashford J R. Drug Interactions. The effects of alcohol and meprobamate applied singly and jointly in human subjects. V. *J Stud Alc* (1975) Suppl 7, 162.
7 Ashford J R and Carpenter J A. Drug Interactions. The effects of alcohol and meprobamate applied singly and jointly in human subjects. VI. *J Stud Alc* (1975) Suppl 7, 177.
8 Misra P S, Lefèvre A, Ishi H, Rubin E and Lieber C S. Increase of ethanol, meprobamate and pentobarbital metabolism after chronic ethanol administration in man and in rats. *Am J med* (1971) 51, 346.
9 Rubin E, Gang H, Misra P S and Lieber C S. Inhibition of drug metabolism by acute ethanol intoxication. A hepatic microsomal mechanism. *Am J med* (1970) 49, 801.

Alcohol + methaqualone-diphenhydramine (*Mandrax*)

Summary

The mental sedation and impairment of cognitive skills caused by *Mandrax* are enhanced by alcohol. Residual *Mandrax* continues to interact even 3 days later.

Interaction

A double-blind study on 12 normal subjects who were given two *Mandrax* tablets (methaqualone 250 mg + diphenhydramine 25 mg) with and without alcohol (0·5 g/kg) showed that mental and physical sedation, and a reduction in cognitive skills, were enhanced by the concurrent ingestion of alcohol. Residual amounts of *Mandrax* continued to interact as long as 72 h after a single dose. Methaqualone blood levels are also raised by regular moderate amounts of alcohol.[1]

Enhanced effects were observed in another study, but no hangover effects.[2]

Mechanism

Both are central nervous depressants which appear to have additive effects.

Importance and management

The diphenhydramine/alcohol interaction is well documented and discussed elsewhere (see alcohol + antihistamines, page 16) but data about the *Mandrax* alcohol interaction is much more limited. Nevertheless patients on *Mandrax* should be warned about the long 'hangover' effects and the potential serious consequences. Handling machinery, driving a car or undertaking any complex task requiring alertness and full coordination is likely to be made more hazardous. Nitrazepam might be a safer alternative.

References

1 Roden S, Harvey P and Mitchard M. The effect of ethanol on residual plasma concentrations and behaviour in volunteers who have taken Mandrax. *Br J clin Pharmac* (1977) **4**, 245.
2 Saario I and Linnoila M. Effect of subacute treatment with hypnotics, alone or in combination with alcohol, on psychomotor skills related to driving. *Acta pharmacol et toxicol* (1976) **38**, 3382.

Alcohol + metronidazole

Summary

A disulfiram-like reaction has been described in at least two patients taking metronidazole who drank alcohol. Alcohol may also taste unpleasant.

Interaction

A man who had been in a drunken stupor for 3 days was given two metronidazole tablets (a total of 500 mg) one hour apart by his wife in the belief that they would sober him up. Twenty minutes after the first tablet he was awake and complaining that he had been given disulfiram (which he had experienced some months before). Immediately after the second tablet he took another drink and developed a classic disulfiram-like reaction: flushing of the face and neck, blood pressure of 138/92 mmHg, pulse 78, nausea and epigastric discomfort.[1]

There is at least one other report of this reaction.[2] It has also been reported that alcohol tastes badly[1] or is less pleasurable[2] while taking metronidazole.

Mechanism

Uncertain. It is generally believed that the reaction occurs because metronidazole can, like disulfiram, inhibit the activity of acetaldehyde dehydrogenase.[3] See alcohol/disulfiram interaction on page 25.

Importance and management

It appears to be a relatively uncommon reaction. Only 1 out of 50 patients experienced it in a trial of metronidazole for alcoholism.[2] The reaction is more unpleasant than serious but patients should be warned of the possibilities. The manufacturers actually advise against drinking while taking metronidazole.

References

1 Taylor J A T. Metronidazole—a new agent for combined somatic and psychic therapy for alcoholism. *Bull Los Angeles Neurol Soc* (1964) **29**, 158.
2 Penick S. B, Carrier R N and Sheldon J R. Metronidazole in the treatment of alcoholism. *Amer J Psychiat* (1969) **125**, 1063.
3 Fried R and Fried L. The effect of Flagyl on xanthine oxidase and alcohol dehydrogenase. *Biochem Pharmacol* (1966) **15**, 1890.

Alcohol + mianserin

Summary

The effects of alcohol and other CNS depressants may be enhanced by the concurrent use of mianserin.

Interaction, mechanism, importance and management

Drowsiness is a frequently reported side-effect of mianserin, particularly during the first few days of treatment, and additive CNS depression may occur during concurrent treatment with other CNS depressants such as hypnotics, sedatives, tranquillizers, barbiturates etc. Studies on the effects of alcohol with mianserin have shown that they appear to act additively on the CNS to impair psychomotor skills and this would make driving or handling machinery more hazardous.[1,2]

References

1 Matilla M J, Liljequist R and Seppälä T. Effects of amitriptyline and mianserin on psychomotor skills and memory in man. *Br J clin Pharmac* (1978) **5**, 53S.
2 Seppälä T. Psychomotor skills during acute and two-week treatment with mianserin (Org GB 94) and amitriptyline and their combined effects with alcohol. *Ann Clin Res* (1977) **9**, 66.

Alcohol + milk

Summary

The effects of alcohol are reduced by milk.

Interaction, mechanism, importance and management

A study in subjects given alcohol with either water or milk showed that the intoxicant effects of alcohol, as judged by the subjects themselves, were reduced by the presence of the milk. The urinary excretion of alcohol was also found to be depressed.[1] These findings would appear to confirm a long and widely held belief among drinkers. Whether this interaction can be regarded as advantageous or undesirable is a moot point.

Reference

1 Miller D S, Stirling J L and Yudkin J. Effect of ingestion of milk on concentrations of blood alcohol. *Nature* (1966) **212**, 1051.

Alcohol + monosulfiram

Summary

A disulfiram-like reaction is reported in a patient when alcohol was taken following the external use of monosulfiram for scabies.

Interaction

A patient who was being treated with a solution of monsulfiram for scabies developed skin swelling, flushing, sweating, severe tachycardia and nausea when he drank alcohol on each of two occasions.[1]

Mechanism

Monosulfiram (tetraethylthiuram monosulphide) is closely chemically related to disulfiram (tetraethylthiuram disulphide) and it would be reasonable to surmise that the reaction has a similar pharmacological basis to the alcohol/disulfiram reaction (p. 25). This requires confirmation. One presumes that the monosulfiram was absorbed through the skin.

Importance and management
The documentation appears to be limited to this single report. It would seem advisable to warn patients under treatment with monosulfiram of the possibility of this reaction.

Reference
1 Gold S. A skinful of alcohol. *Lancet* (1966) **ii**, 1417.

Alcohol + mushrooms

Summary
A disulfiram-like reaction has been described after eating *Coprinus atramentarius* and drinking alcohol.

Interaction, mechanism, importance and management
A disulfiram-like reaction to alcohol has been described in four patients who ate *Coprinus atramentarius* and who subsequently drank some alcohol.[1] A similar reaction has been described in previous reports.[2,3] This is not the common European field mushroom. Some workers have claimed to have isolated tetraethylthiuram disulphide (disulfiram) from *C. atramentarius* but this has not been confirmed.[4] If this mushroom does in fact contain disulfiram, the reactions described are explained.

References
1 Reynold W A and Lowe F H. Mushrooms and a toxic reaction to alcohol. Report of four cases. *New Eng J Med* (1965) **189**, 630.
2 Buck R. Cited as personal communication in [1].
3 List P H. Cited by Buck.[2]
4 Simandl J and Frane J. Isolation of tetraethylthiuram disulfide from *Coprinus atramentarius*. *Chem Listy* (1956) **50**, 1862.

Alcohol + paraldehyde

Summary
Alcohol and paraldehyde have additive CNS depressant effects. Concurrent use in the treatment of acute intoxication can have a fatal outcome.

Interaction, mechanism, importance and management
A study describes 8 patients who died suddenly and unexpectedly following treatment for acute alcoholic intoxication with 30–60 ml paraldehyde (normal dose range 3–30 ml; fatal dose 120 ml or more).[1] Both drugs are CNS depressants and may therefore be expected to have additive effects.

Reference
1 Kaye S and Haag H B. Study of death due to combined action of alcohol and paraldehyde in man. *Toxical Appl Pharmacol* (1964) **6**, 316.

Alcohol + phenylbutazone

Summary
The psychomotor skills related to driving are impaired by phenylbutazone and further impaired by drinking alcohol.

Interaction

A study on a large number of volunteer students who were given phenylbutazone, 200 mg, alone or with 0·5 g/kg alcohol showed that various psychomotor skills related to driving (choice reaction, coordination and divided attention tests) were impaired by phenylbutazone, and further impaired by the concurrent ingestion of alcohol.[1]

Mechanism

Uncertain. There seems to be additive depression of the central nervous system by both drugs. Phenylbutazone can adversely affect driving skills without the patient being aware of his impaired performance. Changes in blood alcohol levels in the presence of phenylbutazone are probably too small to be important.[1]

Importance and management

The documentation is very limited but this interaction would appear to be well established. Since the patient is likely to remain subjectively unaware that the phenylbutazone is adversely affecting his driving performance, it is important to point out to patients the potential hazards of this drug, whether or not alcohol is taken.

Reference

1 Linnoila M, Seppälä T and Mattila M J. Acute effect of antipyretic analgesics, alone or in combination with alcohol, on human psychomotor skills related to driving. *Br J clin Pharmac* (1974) 1, 477.

Alcohol + procarbazine

Summary

A flush syndrome has been described in patients on procarbazine who ingested alcohol. The manufacturers also state that intolerance to alcohol may occur.

Interaction, mechanism, importance and management

Five patients on procarbazine are described in one report whose faces became very red and hot when they drank wine.[1] Another report states that flushing occurred in three patients on procarbazine after drinking beer.[2] Whether this is related to the alcohol/disulfiram reaction (see page 25) is not known. Intolerance to alcohol is also listed by the manufacturers of procarbazine among the 'contraindications and warnings' which probably refers to the combined CNS depressant effects of procarbazine and alcohol.

References

1 Mathé G, Berumen L, Schweisguth O, Brule G, Schneider M, Cattan A, Amiel J L and Schwarzenberg L. Methyl-hydrazine in the treatment of Hodgkin's disease and various forms of haematosarcoma and leukaemia. *Lancet* (1963) ii, 1077.
2 Dawson W B. Ibenzmethyzin in the management of late Hodgkin's disease. In *Natulan, Ibenzmethyzin*. Report of the proceedings of a symposium, Downing College, Cambridge, June 1965, p. 31. Edited by Jelliffe A M and Marks J (eds). (1965). John Wright, Bristol.

Alcohol + salicylates

Summary

A small increase in the gastrointestinal blood loss caused by aspirin may occur with alcohol, but it is usually of little importance in normal individuals. Buffered aspirin or paracetamol (acetaminophen) do not have this effect.

Interaction

Alcohol + unbuffered aspirin

In one investigation 13 healthy males were given seven tablets of soluble unbuffered aspirin (*Disprin*, 300 mg) daily and 180 ml Australian whisky (31·8% w/v ethanol). The mean blood loss rose from 0·4 ml daily without medication to 3·2 ml a day on aspirin alone, and to 5·3 ml with aspirin and alcohol. Alcohol alone did not cause gastrointestinal bleeding.[1]

An epidemiological survey of a large number of patients with gastrointestinal haemorrhage admitted to hospital showed that there was a statistical association between bleeding and the ingestion of aspirin on its own or with alcohol, but no such association with alcohol alone.[2]

Alcohol + buffered aspirin

A study on 22 normal males who were given three double whiskies (equivalent to 142 ml 40% ethanol) and 728 g sodium acetylsalicylate showed that no increase in gastrointestinal bleeding took place.[3]

Mechanism

Both unbuffered aspirin and alcohol can damage the normal gastric mucosal lining of the stomach, one measure of the injury being a fall in the gastric potential difference. An additive fall has been described with unbuffered aspirin and alcohol, whereas an increase has been described with buffered aspirin.[4] Once the protective mucosal barrier as breached, exfoliation of the mucosal cells occurs and damage to the capillaries follows. The total picture is complex.

Importance and management

The ingestion of salicylates causes some blood loss in most people. 3 g a day for a period of 3–6 days induces an average loss of about 5 ml so.[5] Some increased blood loss undoubtedly occurs with alcohol, but it seems to be quite small and there is no evidence to suggest that it is usually of much importance in normal individuals.

References
1 Goulston K and Cooke A R. Alcohol, aspirin and gastrointestinal bleeding. *Brit Med J* (1968) 4, 664.
2 Needham C D, Kyle J, Jones P F, Johnstone S J and Kerridge D F. Aspirin and alcohol in gastrointestinal haemorrhage. *Gut* (1971) 12, 819.
3 Bouchier I A D and Williams H S. Determination of faecal blood-loss after combined alcohol and sodium acetylsalicylate intake. *Lancet* (1969) i, 178.
4 Murray H S, Strottman M P and Cooke A R. Effect of several drugs on gastric potential differences in man. *Brit Med J* (1974) 1, 19.
5 Woodbury D M. Analgesic-antipyretics, anti-inflammatory agents and inhibitors of uric acid synthesis. In *The Pharmacological Basis of Therapeutics* 4th edn, p. 314. Goodman L S and Gilman A (eds) (1970). Macmillan, New York.

Alcohol + sodium cromoglycate

Summary
Sodium cromoglycate does not interact with alcohol.

Interaction, mechanism, importance and management

A double-blind cross over trial on 17 volunteers showed that 40 mg sodium cromoglycate (*Intal*) had little or no effect on the performance of a number of tests on human perceptual, cognitive and motor skills, alone or with alcohol (0·75 g/kg). Nor did it affect the blood levels of alcohol.[1]

This lack of evidence for an interaction between alcohol and sodium cromoglycate is in line with the common experience of patients on long-term treatment, and no special precautions seem to be necessary.

Reference
1 Crawford W A, Frank H M, Hensley V R, Hensley W J, Starmer G A and Teo R C K. The effect of disodium cromoglycate on human performance alone and in combination with ethanol. *Med J Aust* (1976) 2, 997.

Alcohol + sulpiride or thioridazine

Summary
No marked interaction normally occurs but the effects of alcohol may be expected to be slightly or moderately enhanced by these two drugs.

Interaction

A double-blind crossover study on 37 normal subjects of the effects of sulpiride (150 mg daily) or thioridazine (30–60 mg daily), administered over a 2 week period, showed that the performance of choice reaction, coordination and attention tests was not markedly affected by either of these two drugs, with or without alcohol. The interaction with sulpiride was mild, while thioridazine has some additive effects with alcohol and some moderate deleterious effects on attention.[1,2]

Mechanism

Importance and management

Information is limited but it appears to be a reliably established interaction. No marked effects occur in the doses used, but it would nevertheless be prudent to warn patients that the effects of alcohol may be enhanced to some extent by these two drugs.

References

1 Seppälä T, Saario I and Mattila M J. Two weeks' treatment with chlorpromazine, thioridazine, sulpiride, or bromazepam: actions and interactions with alcohol on psychomotor skills related to driving. *Mod Probl Pharmacopsych* (1976) 11, 85.
2 Linnoila M. Effects of diazepam, chlordiazepoxide, thioridazine, halperidol, flupenthixole and alcohol on psychomotor skills related to driving. *Ann Med Exp Biol Fenn* (1973) 51, 125.

Alcohol + trichloroethylene

Summary

A disulfiram-like reaction can occur in those exposed to trichloroethylene who drink alcohol.

Interaction

A mechanical engineer developed a disulfiram-like reaction to alcohol characterized by facial flushing, a sensation of increased pressure in the head, lacrymation, tachypnoea and blurred vision. It occurred within 12 min of drinking 3 oz. bourbon whisky. The most likely cause was the presence of trichloroethylene used as a degreasing agent in the plant where the man worked because after a week's vacation and following the removal of the trichloroethylene from the plant the reaction ceased to occur.[1]

Other workers in the same plant are reported to have experienced this reaction.[1]

Mechanism

Uncertain. Suggested mechanisms are a disulfiram-like inhibition of acetaldehyde metabolism by trichloroethylene (see the alcohol/disulfiram reaction, page 25) or an increase in the sensitivity of the heart to circulating catecholamines.[1]

Importance and management

The documentation is very limited but the interaction seems to be reasonably well established. The reaction would seem to be more unpleasant and socially disagreeable than serious. Whether this interaction can also occur in those who regularly handle trichloroethylene as an anaesthetic is uncertain. So far there appears to be no reports of this.

Reference

1 Pardys S and Brotman M. Trichloroethylene and alcohol: a straight flush. *J Amer med Ass* (1974) 229, 521.

Alcohol + tricyclic antidepressants

Summary

Impairment by alcohol of the ability to drive or carry out other complex psychomotor skills is increased by amitriptyline, and probably by doxepin, particularly during the first few days of treatment. Nortriptyline and clomipramine appear to interact minimally. Information about other tricyclic antidepressants appears to be lacking.

Interaction

Alcohol + amitriptyline

Three motor skill tests related to driving ability carried out by 21 volunteers with blood-alcohol levels of about 80 mg%, and with amitriptyline in doses of 0·8 mg/kg (about 50 mg in a 10 stone man), demonstrated that the antidepressant added to the effects of alcohol and further impaired the performance of the tests.[1]

Similar results have been described in other reports[2,4,5] using a variety of psychomotor skill tests, the interaction being most marked during the first few days of treatment, but tending to wane as treatment continues.[1,2,4] One somewhat discordant report stated that after 5 days' treatment no significant interaction occurred.[3] There is, in addition, limited evidence from animal studies[9] that amitriptyline can enhance the fatty changes induced in the liver by alcohol, and both compounds can inhibit gastrointestinal motility.[10] A brief report describes two fatalities attributed to amitriptyline with alcohol but the precise cause of death was not given.[11]

Alcohol + doxepin

In a double-blind crossover trial on 21 subjects given various combinations of alcohol and either doxepin (30 or 60 mg) or a placebo, it was found that with blood-alcohol levels of between about 40 and 50 mg%, choice reaction test times were prolonged and the number of mistakes increased. Coordination was obviously impaired after 7 days' treatment with doxepin but not after 14 days.[4]

In an earlier study doxepin appeared to cancel out the deleterious effects of alcohol on the performance of a stimulated driving test.[6]

Alcohol + nortriptyline or chlorimipramine

Other studies in subjects with blood-alcohol levels of 40–50 mg% showed that nortriptyline and chlorimipramine had only slight or no effect on various choice reaction, coordination, learning and memory tests.[4,7,8]

Mechanism

The most likely explanation is that both compounds have central nervous depressant activity. Amitriptyline certainly has sedative properties and causes drowsiness and this is also true of some of the other tricyclics although the extent of the sedation varies considerably. Whether this is the only mechanism involved is not clear.

Importance and management

The amitriptyline–alcohol interaction is well documented and important. Patients should be warned that driving or handling other hazardous machinery may be dangerous, particularly during the first few days of treatment.

The alcohol–doxepin interaction is less well documented and the information is conflicting; nevertheless, to be on the safe side a similar warning should be given. Nortriptyline and chlorimipramine appear to interact minimally with alcohol.

Data about other tricyclic antidepressants appear to be lacking, nevertheless it would be prudent to issue a general caution about any tricyclic antidepressant and alcohol, so that patients are alerted to the possibility of an interaction.

References

1 Landauer A A, Milner G and Patman J. Alcohol and amitriptyline effects on skills related to driving behaviour. *Science* (1969) 163, 1467.
2 Seppälä T. Psychomotor skills during acute and two-week treatment with mianserin (ORG GB 94) and amitriptyline and their combined effects with alcohol. *Ann Clin Res* (1977) 9, 66.
3 Patman J, Landauer A A and Milner G. The combined effect of alcohol and amitriptyline on skills similar to motor car driving. *Med J Aust* (1969) 8, 946.
4 Seppälä T, Linnoila M, Elonen E, Matilla M J and Maki M. Effect of tricyclic antidepressants and alcohol on psychomotor skills related to driving. *Clin Pharmacol Ther* (1975) 17, 515.
5 Matilla M J, Liljequist R and Seppälä T. Effects of amitriptyline and mianserin on psychomotor skills and memory in man. *Br J clin Pharmacol* (1978) 5, 53S.
6 Milner G and Landauer A A. The effects of doxepin, alone and together with alcohol in relation to driving safety. *Med J Aust* (1978) 1, 837.
7 Hughes F W and Forney R B. Delayed audiofeedback (DAF) for induction of anxiety. Effect of nortriptyline, ethanol or nortriptyline–ethanol combinations on performance with DAF. *J Amer med Ass* (1963) 185, 556.
8 Liljequist R, Linnoila M and Mattila M. Effect of two weeks' treatment with chlorimipramine and nortriptyline, alone or in combination with alcohol on learning and memory. *Psychopharmacology* (1974) 39, 181.
9 Milner G and Kakulas K. The potentiation by amitriptyline of liver changes induced by ethanol in mice. *Pathology* (1969) 1, 113.
10 Milner G. Gastrointestinal side-effects and psychotropic drugs. *Med J Aust* (1969) 2, 153.
11 Locket M E and Milner G. Combining the antidepressant drugs. *Brit Med J* (1965) 1, 921.

CHAPTER 3. ANALGESIC, ANTIRHEUMATIC AND URICOSURIC DRUG INTERACTIONS

These drugs are categorized together in this chapter because there is an overlap between the therapeutic applications of some of them, although there are others which bear no relationship at all. There are also drugs listed in Table 3.1, with their proprietary names, for the sake of completeness, but the interactions in which they are involved may not necessarily be dealt with here. Reference should be made to the Index.

Allopurinol + ampicillin

Summary
The incidence of skin rashes among those taking both ampicillin and allopurinol is increased.

Interaction
A retrospective search through the records of 1324 patients, 67 of who were taking allopurinol and ampicillin showed that 15 of them (22%) developed a skin rash compared with 94 (7·5%) of the rest.[1]

Mechanism
Not understood. It was suggested in the study that either the allopurinol or the induced hyperuricaemia was responsible.[1]

Importance and management
There would seem to be no strong reasons for avoiding concurrent use, but prescribers should recognize that the development of a rash is by no means unusual. Whether this reaction also occurs with other penicillins is uncertain.

Reference
1 Boston Collaborative Drug Surveillance Programme. Excess of ampicillin rashes associated with allopurinol or hyperuri-caemia. *New Eng J Med* (1972) **286**, 505.

Allopurinol + iron

Summary
No adverse interaction occurs if iron and allopurinol are administered concurrently.

Interaction, mechanism, importance and management
Some early studies with animals suggested that allopurinol might have an inhibitory effect on the metabolism of iron. This led the manufacturers of allopurinol in some countries to issue a warning

about their concurrent use.[1,2] However it would now seem that no special precautions are necessary if they are administered together.[3]

References

1 Emmerson B T. Effects of allopurinol on iron metabolism in man. *Ann rheum Dis* (1966) **25** 700.
2 Davis P S and Deller D J. Effect of a xanthine–oxidase inhibitor (allopurinol) on radioiron absorption in man. *Lancet* (1966) **ii**, 470.
3 Ascione F J. Allopurinol and iron. *J Amer Med Ass* (1975) **232**, 1010.

Table 3.1. Analgesic, anti-rheumatic and uricosuric agents

Non-proprietary names	Proprietary names
Non-steroidal anti-inflammatory agents (analgesics, antirheumatics, antipyretics)	
Alclofenac	*Prinalgin, Mervan, Neostan, Zumaril*
Azapropazone	*Rheumox*
Diclofenac	*Voltarol*
Fenoprofen	*Fenopron, Progesic*
Flufenamic acid	*Arlef, Ansatin, Flufacid, Lanceat, Meralen, Surika, Orpyrin*
Indomethacin	*Indocid, Imbrilon, Inacid, Infrocin, Metindol, Confortid Indomee, Mezolin, Tannex*
Ibuprofen	*Brufen, Motrin*
Mefenamic acid	*Ponstan, Coslan, Parkemed, Ponstel, Ponstyl*
Naproxen	*Naprosyn, Naxen, Proxen, Synflex*
Oxyphenbutazone	*Tanderil, Butapirone, Iridil, Oxalid, Rheumapax, Tandearil*
Penicillamine	*Cuprimine, Distamine*
Phenylbutazone	*Butazolidin, Butacote, Ethibute, Flexazone, Parazolidin and many others*
Salicylates	
Aspirin	
Aloxiprin	*Palprin, Paloxin*
Benorylate	*Benoral*
Sodium salicylate	
Sulindac	*Clinoril*
Tolmetin	*Tolectin*
Analgesics	
Dextropropoxyphene (propoxyphene)	*Depronal, Distalgesic Doloxene*
Diflusinal	*Dolobid*
Paracetamol (acetaminophen)	
Phenazone (antipyrine)	
Narcotic Analgesics	
Codeine	
Methadone	*Physeptone, Dolophine, Westalone, L-Polamidon*
Morphine	
Pentazocine	*Fortagesic, Fortral, Sosegon, Talwin, Fortal*
Pethidine (meperidine)	
Uricosuric agents & related drugs	
Allopurinol	*Zyloric, Zyloprim, Bloxanth, Epidropal, Foligan, Urosin*
Probenecid	*Benemid, Panuric, Benacen, Proben, Probexin, Colbenemid*
Sulphinpyrazone	*Anturan*

Allopurinol + probenecid

Summary

The theoretical possibility of an adverse interaction between allopurinol and probenecid appears not to be realized in practice.

Interaction, mechanism, importance and management

Uric acid is produced by the stepwise conversion of hypoxanthine→xanthine→uric acid catalysed by xanthine oxidase. By inhibiting this enzyme allopurinol favours the urinary excretion of the more soluble hypoxanthine and xanthine and thus the plasma levels of uric acid fall. However, two interrelated interaction mechanisms are thought possibly to interfere with this. One is that probenecid appears to increase the renal excretion of allopurinol or its active metabolite (oxypurinol, oralloxanthine);[1] the other is that allopurinol is thought to inhibit the metabolism of probenecid, and certainly a considerable extension of the probenecid half-life has been described in one study.[2] All this might be expected to lead to an increased uric acid excretion with the possibility of uric acid precipitation in the kidney.

In practice, there seem to be no serious problems. One report describes the treatment of patients with $0 \cdot 2 - 0 \cdot 6$ g allopurinol and $0 \cdot 5 - 1 \cdot 0$ g probenecid daily who showed an approximately 50% increase in the half-life of allopurinol.[3] The possibility of precipitation of uric acid or its precursors in the kidney can be minimized by alkalinization of the urine and an increased daily fluid intake.

References

1 Elion G B, Yü T-F, Gutman A B and Hitchings G H. Renal clearance of Oxipurinol, the chief metabolite of Allopurinol. *Amer J Med* (1968) **45**, 69.
2 Horwitz D, Thorgeirsson S S and Mitchell J R. The influence of allopurinol and size of dose on the metabolism of phenylbutazone in patients with gout. *Europ J clin Pharmacol* (1977) **12**, 133.
3 Yu T-F and Gutman A B. Effect of Allopurinol (4-Hydroxypyrazolo(3,4-d) pyrimidine) on serum and urinary uric acid in primary and secondary gout. *Amer J Med* (1964) **37**, 885.

Allopurinol + thiazide diuretics

Summary

Severe allergic reactions to allopurinol have been described in a few patients, tentatively attributed to renal failure and the use of thiazide diuretics.

Interaction, mechanism, importance and management

Four patients have been described who developed a hypersensitivity vasculitis while taking allopurinol. The predisposing factors may have been severe renal disease and the use of thiazide diuretics.[1] Other studies have shown that the effects of allopurinol on pyrimidine metabolism are enhanced by the concurrent use of thiazides.[2] Some caution has been suggested if allopurinol is used for thiazide-induced hyperuricaemia when renal function is abnormal.[1] More study is needed.

References

1 Young J L, Boswell R B and Nies A S. Severe allopurinol sensitivity. Association with thiazides and prior renal comprise. *Arch Int Med* (1974) **134**, 553.
2 Wood M H, O'Sullivan W J, Wilson M and Tiller D J. Potentiation of an effect of allopurinol on pyrimidine metabolism by chlorothiazide in man. *Clin Exp Pharmacol Physiol* (1974) **1**, 53.

Azapropazone + antacids or laxatives

Summary
Dihydroxy-aluminium sodium carbonate, magnesium aluminium silicate, bisacodyl and anthraquinone laxatives do not interact significantly with azapropazone

Interaction, mechanism, importance and management
A study on 15 patients taking three 300 mg doses of azapropazone daily showed that the simultaneous administration of any of these antacids or laxatives caused only a minor reduction (5–6%) in the serum levels of azapropazone, indicating that there is no reason to avoid concurrent use.

Information about other antacids and laxatives is lacking.[1]

Reference
1 Von Faust-Tinnefeldt G, Geissler H E and Mutschler E. Azapropazon-Plasmaspiegel unter Begleitmedikation mit einem Antacidum oder Laxans. *Arzneim-Forsch (Drug Res)* (1977) **27**, 2411.

Azapropazone + chloroquine

Summary
Chloroquine does not significantly affect serum azapropazone levels

Interaction, mechanism, importance and management
A study on 12 subjects taking azapropazone, 300 mg three times a day, showed that the concurrent use of chloroquine, 250 mg daily for 7 days, had no effect on the serum levels of azapropazone measured 4 h after administration. Serum azapropazone levels before and during chloroquine treatment were $78 \cdot 4$ and $77 \cdot 5$ $\mu g/ml$ respectively.[1]

Reference
1 Faust-Tinnefeldt G and Geissler H E. Azapropazone und rheumatologische Basistherapie mit Chloroquin unter dem Aspekt der Arzneimittelinteraktion. *Arzneim-Forsch (Drug Res)* (1977) **27**, 2170.

Dextropropoxyphene + orphenadrine

Summary
An alleged adverse interaction (mental confusion, anxiety and tremors) between dextropropoxyphene and orphenadrine would seem to be very rare, if indeed it ever occurs.

Interaction, mechanism
The evidence for an interaction is extremely tenuous. Riker, the manufacturers of orphenadrine, used to state in their package insert that 'mental confusion, anxiety and tremors have been reported in patients receiving orphenadrine and propoxyphene concurrently'. Eli Lilley, the manufacturers of propoxyphene, issued a similar warning. However, in correspondence with both manufacturers, two investigators of this interaction (Pearson and Salter[1]), were informed that the basis of these statements consisted of either

anecdotal reports from clinicians, or cases where patients had received twice the recommended dose of orphenadrine, in all a total of 13 cases. In every case the adverse reactions observed were similar to those reported with either drug alone. A brief report on 5 patients given both drugs to investigate this interaction failed to reveal an adverse interaction.[2]

Importance and management
The documentation is extremely vague and no case of interaction has been firmly established. The investigators cited[1] calculated that the two drugs were probably being used together on 3 000 000 prescriptions a year and at that time (1970), a maximum of 13 doubtful cases had been reported. There seems little reason for avoiding concurrent use, although prescribers should be aware that the advisability of using the two drugs together has been the subject of some debate.

References
1 Pearson R E and Salter F J. Drug interaction?—Orphenadrine with propoxyphene. *New Eng J Med* (1970) **282**, 1215.
2 Puckett W H and Visconti J A. Orphenadrine and propoxyphene (cont.). *New Eng J Med* (1970) **283**, 544.

Dextropropoxyphene + tobacco

Summary
Dextropropoxyphene is less effective as an analgesic in those who smoke than in those who do not.

Interaction
A comprehensive study on a total of 835 patients who were given propoxyphene hydrochloride for mild or moderate pain, or headache, showed that its efficacy as an analgesic was decreased by smoking. The drug was rated as ineffective by the attendant physicians in 10·1% of 335 non-smokers, 15% of 347 patients who smoked 20 cigarettes a day or less, and 20·3% of 153 patients who smoked more than 20 a day.[1]

Mechanism
It is suggested that the components of tobacco smoke induce the liver enzymes concerned with the metabolism of the propoxyphene, thereby increasing its loss from the body and diminishing its effectiveness as an analgesic.[1]

Importance and management
The interaction appears to be well-established. Prescribers should be aware that dextropropoxyphene is twice as likely to be ineffective (1 in 5) in those who smoke 20 cigarettes a day as in those who do not smoke (1 in 10).

Reference
1 Boston Collaborative Drug Surveillance Program. Decreased clinical efficacy of propoxyphene in cigarette smokers. *Clin Pharmacol Ther* (1973) **14**, 259.

Diflusinal + aluminium hydroxide

Summary
The absorption of diflusinal is reduced by the concurrent use of aluminium hydroxide. The importance of this is uncertain.

Interaction, mechanism, importance and management
A study carried out on 4 normal subjects given single 500 mg oral doses of diflusinal showed that the concurrent administration of 45 ml *Aludrox* (2520 mg aluminium hydroxide) taken in three 15 ml doses—2 h before, together with, and 2 h after the diflusinal—reduced the absorption of the diflusinal by about 40%.[1] This, presumably, reduces the therapeutic efficacy of the diflusinal

proportionately but the general importance of this is uncertain. Further study is needed.

Reference
1 Veerbeek R, Tjandramaga T B, Mullie A, Verbesselt R and De Schepper P J. Effect of aluminium hydroxide on diflusinal absorption. *Br J clin Pharmac* (1979) 7, 519.

Diflusinal + aspirin, indomethacin or naproxen

Summary

Aspirin can reduce diflusinal serum levels. Diflusinal can raise indomethacin serum levels, but not those of naproxen. The clinical importance of these interactions is uncertain.

Interaction, mechanism, importance and management

The concurrent administration of diflusinal 500 mg and aspirin 2400 mg daily resulted in a 15% fall in plasma diflusinal levels.[2] The same amounts of diflusinal with 75 mg indomethacin increased the plasma indomethacin levels by 30–35%,[3] but had no effect on naproxen in daily doses of 500 mg.[4] The clinical importance of these observations is uncertain.

References
1 Tempero K F, Cirillo V J and Steelman S L. Diflusinal: a review of pharmacokinetic and pharmacodynamic properties, drug interactions and special tolerability studies in humans. *Br J clin Pharmac* (1977) 4, 315.
2 Perrier C V. Unpublished observations quoted in ref. 1.
3 De Schepper P. Unpublished observations quoted in ref. 1.
4 Dresse A, Gerard M A, Quiraux N, Fischer P and Gerardy J. Effect of diflusinal on the human plasma levels and on the urinary excretion of naproxen. *Arch int Pharmacodyn* (1978) 236, 276.

Flufenamic acid, mefenamic acid, oxyphenbutazone or phenylbutazone + antacids

Summary

In-vitro studies suggest that mefenamic and flufenamic acid may be adsorbed by some antacids which may reduce their bio-availability. Oxyphenbutazone and phenylbutazone seem to be little affected. This requires clinical confirmation.

Interaction, mechanism, importance and management

Table 3.2 summarizes some adsorption studies undertaken with a number of anti-rheumatic drugs and commonly used antacids. These results suggest that recognition should be given to the effects of some antacids during treatment with mefenamic and flufenamic acids, but there appears to be little problem with oxyphenbutazone or phenylbutazone. Clinical confirmation of the importance of these interactions is required.

Reference
1 Naggar V F, Khalil S A and Daabis N A. The in-vitro adsorption of some antirheumatics on antacids. *Pharmazie* (1976) 31, 461.

Table 3.2. Percentage of drug adsorbed per gram of adsorbent, and the percentage eluted using 0·01 N HCl or 0·014 N NaHCO$_3$ (second figure). The eluted percentages are in brackets

	Magnesium trisilicate	Magnesium oxide	Aluminium hydroxide	Bismuth oxycarbonate	Calcium carbonate	Kaolin
Flufenamic acid	0	90 (26, —)	10	79	37	44
Mefenamic acid	0	95 (40, —)	69	26	2	90
Oxyphenbutazone	0	24 (100, —)	27	0	0	0
Phenylbutazone	0	12 (100, 100)	0	0	0	0

Taken from ref. 1.

Flufenamic acid or mefenamic acid + cholestyramine

Summary

Animal studies show that the absorption of both flufenamic and mefenamic acid is markedly reduced by cholestyramine. Whether this is an interaction of importance in man is uncertain.

Interaction, mechanism, importance and management

In-vitro studies with physiological concentrations of bile salt anions showed that cholestyramine binds to both flufenamic and mefenamic acid. Other in-vivo studies in rats showed that a 60–70% reduction in gastrointestinal absorption occurs which suggests that this may possibly be an important interaction in man, but so far clinical data are lacking.[1]

Reference

1 Rosenberg H A and Bates T R. Inhibitory effect of cholestyramine on the absorption of flufenamic and mefenamic acids in rats. *Proc Soc Exp Biol Med* (1974) **145**, 93.

Indomethacin + antacids

Summary

Serum levels of indomethacin can be reduced to some extent by the concurrent use of antacids. This is probably not of great importance.

Interaction, mechanism, importance and management

In-vitro studies[1] carried out with various antacids (magnesium trisilicate, magnesium oxide, aluminium hydroxide, bismuth oxycarbonate, calcium carbonate and kaolin) indicate that indomethacin is adsorbed onto these compounds. Other studies in man[2] comparing the serum levels and amounts of indomethacin absorbed by the gut when single oral doses of indomethacin were taken alone or with *Mergel* (a tableted antacid formulation of aluminium hydroxide, magnesium carbonate and magnesium hydroxide) showed quite clearly that antacids reduce the amounts absorbed due, it would seem, to the adsorption of the indomethacin onto the antacids, although other mechanisms may also be involved. The total amount of indomethacin absorbed after 50 mg oral doses was reduced by 35% when taken with 80% *Mergel*, the peak serum concentrations being proportionately reduced. However, results like these should be interpreted with some caution because in-vitro and single dose studies in healthy volunteers are not necessarily reliable predictors of what may happen in patients on chronic therapy, although some reduction in clinical response would seem to be a probability.

Despite this evidence, the manufacturers of indomethacin make the firm recommendation that it should be taken with either an antacid or food to minimize gastrointestinal disturbances, although they point out that *Indocid* suspension should not be mixed with an antacid, but taken separately, because indomethacin is unstable in an alkaline medium.[3]

References
1 Naggar V F, Khalil S A and Daabis N A. The in-vitro adsorption of some anti-rheumatics on anticids. *Pharmazie* (1976) **31**, 461.
2 Galeazzi R L. The effect of an antacid on the bioavailability of indomethacin. *Europ J clin Pharmacol* (1977) **12**, 65.
3 ABPI. *Data Sheet Compendium 1979–80* p. 655. Pharmind Publications Ltd (1979).

Indomethacin + food

Summary
If indomethacin is taken with food to avoid gastric upset, no interaction of importance takes place.

Interaction, mechanism, importance and management
Studies[1] carried out on patients and healthy subjects given single or multiple oral doses of indomethacin showed that the concurrent ingestion of food caused marked and complex changes in the immediate serum indomethacin concentrations—the mean peak serum levels being delayed and altered—but fluctuations in the serum concentrations were somewhat ironed out. Moreover, a study[2] which compared the indomethacin concentrations in serum and synovial fluid showed that they were about the same 5–9 h after taking indomethacin, so that the alterations which go on during the first 5 h are probably far less important than overall serum levels. Quite apart from the advantages of taking indomethacin at mealtimes to reduce gastrointestinal disturbances (a manufacturer's recommendation) there seems to be little likelihood of an undesirable interaction.

Reference
1 Emori H W, Paulus H, Bluestone R, Champion G D and Pearson C. Indomethacin serum concentrations in man. Effects of dosage, food and antacid. *Ann rheum Dis* (1976) **35**, 333.
2 Emori H W, Champion G D, Bluestone R and Paulus H E. The simultaneous pharmacokinetics of indomethacin in serum and synovial fluid. *Ann rheum Dis* (1973) **32**, 433.

Indomethacin or salicylates + mazindol

Summary
Mazindol is reported not to interact adversely with indomethacin, salicylates or other antirheumatic agents.

Interaction, mechanism, importance and management
A double-blind study of mazindol or a placebo was carried out on 26 obese arthritics, 15 of whom were on salicylates, 11 on indomethacin and 1 on propoxyphene with paracetamol. Additional antirheumatic drugs used were ibuprofen (4 patients), phenylbutazone (1 patient), propoxyphene (7 patients), paracetamol (3 patients) and prednisone (9 patients). No adverse interactions were demonstrated.

Reference
Thorpe P C, Isaac P F and Rodgers J. A controlled trial of mazindol (Sanjorex, Teronac) in the management of obese rheumatic patients. *Curr Ther Res* (1975) **17**, 149.

Indomethacin + probenecid

Summary

The concurrent use of probenecid and indomethacin can double the indomethacin serum levels resulting in clinical improvement in patients with arthritic diseases and, in some cases, to indomethacin toxicity. The uricosuric effects of probenecid are not affected.

Interaction

A study on 6 subjects, 3 of whom were healthy volunteers and 3 were patients with hyperuricaemia and gout, showed that when they were administered 4 g probenecid on the day before and 2 g on each of the 2 days after taking 100 mg indomethacin, the peak serum indomethacin levels at 4 h were raised about 50%, and over the next 48 h remained at least 100% higher than when probenecid was absent.[1]

A later study on 28 patients with osteoarthritis taking indomethacin, orally or rectally, in daily doses of 50–150 mg showed that the concurrent administration of 0·5–1·0 g probenecid daily improved the relief of morning stiffness and joint tenderness, and raised the grip strength indices. The serum indomethacin levels were found to be roughly doubled which paralleled the increased effectiveness of the indomethacin. Four patients demonstrated indomethacin toxicity.[2]

Similar results have been reported in other studies.[3,4]

Mechanism

One explanation which would account for this interaction is that competition takes place in the kidney tubules between probenecid and indomethacin for secretion by a common tubular mechanism which leads to a decrease in indomethacin excretion and a rise in serum levels. This is consistent with the observation that the renal excretion is reduced.[1] But in a later study[4] it has been claimed that a reduction in non-renal excretion accounts for the raised serum levels in a similar way to that shown in animals where it has been demonstrated that probenecid reduces biliary excretion.[5] So a total explanation of the way this interaction takes place is still not available.

Importance and management

The clinical improvement which has been associated with the concurrent use of probenecid and indomethacin[1] would seem to be due to the considerable increases in the serum indomethacin levels. This is not necessarily an unmixed blessing because, as already described,[2] some patients can manifest indomethacin toxicity (headache, dizziness, light-headedness etc.) as a result. Caution is therefore necessary if these two drugs are used together and some reduction in the dosage of indomethacin may be required. It has been shown that the uricosuric effects of probenecid are not affected by indomethacin.[1]

References

1 Skeith M D, Simkin P A and Healey L A. The renal excretion of indomethacin and its inhibition by probenecid. *Clin Pharmacol Ther* (1968) **9**, 89.
2 Brooks P M, Bell M A, Sturrock R D, Famaey J P and Dick W C. The clinical significance of indomethacin–probenecid interaction. *Br J clin Pharmac* (1974) **1**, 287.
3 Emori W, Paulus H E, Bluestone R and Pearson C M. The pharmacokinetics of indomethacin in serum. *Clin Pharmacol Ther* (1973) **14**, 134.
4 Baber N, Halliday L, Littler T, Orme M L'E and Sibeon R. Clinical studies of the interaction between indomethacin and probenecid. *Br J Clin Pharmac* (1978) **5**, 364. P.
5 Duggan D E, Hooke K F, White J D, Noll R M and Stevenson C R. The effects of probenecid upon the individual components of indomethacin elimination. *J Pharmac exp Ther* (1977) **201**, 463.

Indomethacin + salicylates

Summary

It has not been clearly established whether salicylates affect the serum levels of indomethacin or change its therapeutic effectiveness to an extent which is clinically important.

Interaction

The overall picture is confusing and contradictory. Some studies report that aspirin reduces serum indomethacin levels.[1,2,3] Others claim that no interaction occurs[4,5,6] and no changes in clinical effectiveness take place.[6,7] Yet other studies using buffered aspirin claim that the use of buffered aspirin increases the absorption of indomethacin and is associated with an increase in side-effects.[8,9]

Mechanism

Not resolved. Changes in rates of absorption and renal clearance have been proposed.

Importance and management

Although extensively studied, there seems to be no clear and unequivocal evidence to show that concurrent use adversely affects the therapeutic effectiveness of these drugs. However, if both drugs are given concurrently it would be prudent to be on the alert for changes in the response and in the incidence of side effects.

References

1 Rubin A, Rodda B E, Warrick P, Gruber C M and Ridolfo A S. Interactions of aspirin with nonsteroidal antiinflammatory drugs in man. *Arth Rheum* (1973) **16**, 635.
2 Kaldestad E, Hansen T and Brath H K. Interaction of indomethacin and acetylsalicylic acid as shown by the serum concentrations of indomethacin and salicylate. *Europ J clin Pharmacol* (1975) **9**, 199.
3 Jeremy R and Towson J. Interaction between aspirin and indomethacin in the treatment of rheumatoid arthritis. *Med J Aust* (1970) **2**, 127.
4 Champion D, Mongan E, Paulus H, Sarkissian E, Okun R and Pearson C. Effect of concurrent aspirin (ASA) administration on serum concentrations of indomethacin (I). *Arth Rheum* (1971) **14**, 375.
5 Lindquist B, Jensen K M, Johansson H and Hansen T. Effect of concurrent administration of aspirin and indomethacin on serum concentrations. *Clin Pharmacol Ther* (1974) **15**, 247.
6 Brooks P M, Walker J J, Bell M A, Buchanan W W and Rhymer A R. Indomethacin–aspirin interaction: a clinical appraisal. *Brit Med J* (1975) **2**, 69.
7 The Cooperating Clinics Committee of the American Rheumatism Association. A three-month trial of indomethacin in rheumatoid arthritis, with special reference to analysis and inference. *Clin Pharmacol Ther* (1967) **8**, 11.
8 Turner P and Garnham J C. Indomethacin–aspirin interaction. *Brit Med J* (1975) **2**, 368.
9 Garnham J C, Raymond K, Shotton E and Turner P. The effect of buffered aspirin on plasma indomethacin. *Europ J clin Pharmacol* (1975) **8**, 107.

Indomethacin + vaccines

Summary

The anti-inflammatory action of indomethacin alters the response of the body to infection and may cause a severe reaction to vaccination.

Interaction, mechanism, importance and management

The response of the body to infection may be adversely affected by the use of indomethacin. The manufacturers (MSD) state that it 'may mask the signs and symptoms of infection, and antibiotic therapy should be initiated promptly if an infection occurs during therapy with Indocid. It should be used cautiously in patients with existing but controlled infection'.[1] A particularly severe reaction has been described in a man given smallpox vaccination,[2] and severe reactions have been reported in children where the indomethacin appeared to have masked the symptoms of infection.[3,4] Although the information is sparse, there is enough to indicate that immunization with live vaccines should be undertaken with particular care.

References

1 Data Sheet Compendium 1979/80. Pharmind Publications, (1979) London p. 656.
2 Maddocks A C. Indomethacin and vaccination. *Lancet* (1973) **ii**, 210.
3 Rodriguez R S and Barbabosa E. Hemorrhagic chicken pox after indomethacin. *New Eng J Med* (1971) **285**, 690.
4 Chapman R A. Suspected adverse reactions to indomethacin. *Can med Ass J* (1966) 1156.

Methadone + phenytoin

Summary

A single case report indicates that the effects of methadone can be antagonized by the concurrent use of phenytoin.

Interaction, mechanism, importance and management

A patient under treatment with methadone demonstrated methadone withdrawal symptoms shortly after starting to take phenytoin. The symptoms vanished when the phenytoin was discontinued but reappeared when the phenytoin was restarted. The reasons are not known for certain, but the response is consistent with the liver enzyme-inducing characteristics of phenytoin which might be expected to cause an increase in the rate of metabolism of the methadone. The documentation is extremely limited, but it indicates that an increase in the dosage of methadone may be required during concurrent treatment.[1]

Reference

1 Finelli P F. Phenytoin and methadone tolerance. *New Eng J Med* (1976) **294**, 227.

Methadone + rifampicin

Summary

The effects of methadone are reduced by the concurrent use of rifampicin. Patients on methadone maintenance treatment can develop withdrawal symptoms.

Interaction

Because several former heroin addicts on methadone maintenance treatment complained of the onset of withdrawal symptoms when they were given rifampicin for tuberculosis, a study was undertaken to investigate this interaction.

Out of a total of 30 patients being given methadone, 21 of them developed withdrawal symptoms within 1–33 days of starting to take 600–900 mg rifampicin daily. They were also treated with 300 mg isoniazid daily. Seven of the most severely affected developed the symptoms within a week. The symptoms abated when the rifampicin was withdrawn. None of 56 other patients on methadone maintenance and other anti-tubercular therapy (which included isoniazid but not rifampicin) showed withdrawal symptoms.[1-3]

Two other cases of this interaction have been reported.[4]

Mechanism

Studies carried out on 6 of the 7 patients who had experienced severe withdrawal symptoms showed that the serum methadone concentrations were significantly decreased (33–68%) when rifampicin was administered. The urinary excretion of the major metabolite of methadone rose consistently by a mean value of 250%, but there were no consistent alterations in apparent plasma half-lives of methadone. In fact reduced, prolonged, and unchanged terminal half-lives were observed.

Rifampicin is a known enzyme-inducing agent and some of the effects seen may be due to an enhancement of the metabolism of methadone, but this is certainly not the whole explanation and it is possible that rifampicin may also mediate some of the effects seen by changes in drug disposition.

Importance and management

An established interaction. Twenty-one of the total of 30 patients studied developed this interaction, 14 of whom were able with the support of counselling to tolerate the relatively mild symptoms so that there is certainly no contraindication to the use of these two drugs in combination.

When the interaction does develop fully, ethambutol has been found[1,4] to be an effective non-interacting substitute for rifampicin. Isoniazid does not interact either and, from the study described, it would appear that none of the other unnamed antitubercular agents interacts adversely with methadone.

References

1 Kreek M J, Garfield J N, Gutjahr C L and Giusti L M. Rifampcin-induced methadone withdrawal. *New Eng J Med* (1976) **294**, 1104.
2 Kreek M J, Garfield J W, Gutjahr C L, Bowen D, Field F and Rothschild M. Rifampin–methadone relationship. 2. Rifampin effects on plasma concentration, metabolism and excretion of methadone. *Am Rev Resp Dis* (1975) **111**, 926.
3 Garfield J W, Kreek M J and Giusti L. Rifampin–methadone relationship. 1. The clinical effects of Rifampin–methadone interaction. *Am Rev Resp Dis* (1975) **111**, 926.
4 Anon. Surprising side effect of rifampin. *Med World News* (1975) **16**, 60.

Methadone + urinary acidifiers or alkalinizers

Summary
The loss of methadone in the urine is increased by urinary acidifiers and reduced by urinary alkalinizers.

Interaction, mechanisms, importance and management

Although methadone is metabolized to a considerable extent by the liver, a substantial proportion is excreted unchanged in the urine. Since it is a weak base (pKa 8·4), its renal clearance is pH-dependent. In alkaline solution most of the drug exists in the un-ionized form which is readily absorbed by the kidney tubules so that little is lost in the urine. In acid solution, little of the drug is in the un-ionized form so that little can be reabsorbed, and much is lost in the urine. A fuller explanation of this interaction mechanism is to be found on page 9. Alkalinization of the urine with acetazolamide or sodium bicarbonate, or acidification with ammonium chloride may therefore be expected to have an influence on the response to methadone.[1,2,3]

References
1 Inturrisi C E and Verebeley K. Disposition of methadone in man after a single oral dose. *Clin Pharmacol Ther* (1972) **13**, 923.
2 Baselt R C and Casarett L J. Urinary excretion of methadone in man. *Clin Pharmacol Ther* (1972) **13**, 64.
3 Bellward G D, Warren D M, Howald W, Axelson J E and Abbott F S. Methadone maintenance: effect of urinary pH on renal clearance in chronic high and low doses. *Clin Pharmacol Ther* (1977) **22**, 92.

Morphine + neuromuscular blockers

Summary
A single case of hypertension and tachycardia has been described in a patient given pancuronium bromide after induction of anaesthesia with morphine.

Interaction, mechanism, importance and management

A woman about to receive an aortocoronary saphenous-vein by-pass graft was premedicated with morphine and scopolamine. Morphine, 1 mg/kg, was then slowly infused while the patient was ventilated with 50% nitrous oxide and oxygen. With the onset of muscular relaxation with pancuronium, the blood pressure rose sharply from 120/60 to 200/110 mmHg and the pulse increased from 54 to 96. This persisted for several minutes but restabilized when 1% halothane was added.[1] It is suggested that the pancuronium can antagonize the vagal tone (heart slowing) induced by the morphine, thus allowing the blood pressure and heart rate to rise. The authors of the report point out the undesirability of this interaction in those with coronary heart disease.

Reference
1 Grossman E and Jacobi A M. Hemodynamic interaction between pancuronium and morphine. *Anesthesiology* (1974) **40**, 299.

Naproxen + antacids

Summary
The absorption of naproxen can be altered by the use of some antacids, but the importance is uncertain. Some unconfirmed evidence indicates that magnesium oxide may inhibit absorption, but not *Maalox*.

Interaction

A study in 14 normal subjects who were given 300 mg naproxen with various antacids (700 or 1400 mg sodium bicarbonate, 700 mg magnesium carbonate or oxide, or 700 mg aluminium hydroxide) showed that the absorption was affected by their concurrent use. The sodium bicarbonate increased the absorption, whereas magnesium oxide reduced it by about 50%. A subsequent study with *Maalox* (magnesium and aluminium hydroxides) showed that the absorption was slightly increased.[1]

Mechanism

Uncertain. Naproxen becomes more soluble as the pH rises, which may account for the increased absorption with sodium bicarbonate, whereas magnesium and aluminium may form less soluble complexes.[2]

Importance and management

Single dose, short-term (3 h) studies of this kind[1] are not always reliable predictors of what may happen in practice. Much more information is needed. It might, however, be prudent to avoid magnesium oxide, but *Maalox* appears not to interact adversely.

References

1 Segre E J, Sevelius H and Varady J. Effects of antacids on naproxen absorption. *New Eng J Med* (1974) **291**, 582.
2 Segre E J. Drug interactions with naproxen. *Europ J Rheumatol Inflamm* (1979) **2**, 12.

Naproxen + probenecid

Summary

Serum levels of naproxen are raised by the concurrent use of probenecid. The clinical importance is uncertain.

Interaction

A study carried out on 6 healthy volunteers who were taking 250 mg naproxen twice daily showed that the concurrent use of probenecid, 500 mg twice daily, increased the serum naproxen levels by 50%.[1]

Mechanism

Virtually all the naproxen is cleared from the body by renal excretion either unchanged (12%), conjugated (50%) or as 6-O-desmethyl naproxen (37%).[1-3] In the presence of probenecid the half-life of naproxen is prolonged from 14 to 37 h and the urine is found to contain less unchanged naproxen (5%), less conjugated naproxen (15%) but twice as much of the desmethylated compound (79%). A suggested explanation for this is that the probenecid inhibits the clearance of the unchanged and conjugated naproxen so that a larger fraction (but not a larger amount) of the desmethylated form is seen in the urine. Thus unchanged naproxen accumulates in the body and serum levels rise.[1]

Importance and management

An established interaction. No adverse clinical effects have been reported but prescribers should be aware that naproxen serum levels will be raised during concurrent use.

References

1 Runkel R, Mroszczak E, Chaplin M, Sevelius H and Segre E. Naproxen–probenecid interaction. *Clin Pharmacol Ther* (1978) **24**, 706.
2 Runkel R, Forschielli E, Boost G, Chaplin M, Hill R, Sevelius H, Thompson G and Segre E. Naproxen metabolism, excretion and comparative pharmacokinetics. *Scand J Rheumatol* (1973) **2**, 29.
3 Runkel R, Chaplin M D, Sevelius H, Ortega E. and Segre E. Pharmacokinetics of naproxen overdoses. *Clin Pharmacol Ther* (1976) **20**, 269.

Naproxen + salicylates

Summary

Aspirin causes a small reduction in serum naproxen levels, but it appears to be of little or no practical importance. Some evidence suggests that concurrent use may be an effective form of treatment for rheumatoid arthritis.

Interaction

A study on 6 volunteers who were given 1200 mg naproxen alone or with 500 mg aspirin showed that the plasma naproxen levels were slightly depressed by the presence of the aspirin. The total area under the curve was reduced by 16%.[1,2]

The authors of a double-blind study on patients with rheumatoid arthritis claimed that concurrent treatment was more effective than aspirin alone, but the effects of aspirin on serum naproxen levels were not measured.[3]

Mechanism

Not fully resolved. Salicylates displace naproxen from its plasma protein binding sites, and appears to increase its renal clearance.

Importance and management

The data are limited but it would appear from the clinical trial cited[3] that concurrent treatment need not be avoided, and it may in fact be therapeutically advantageous.

References

1 Segre E J, Chaplin M, Forchielli E, Runkel R. and Sevelius H. Naproxen–aspirin interactions in man. *Clin Pharmacol Ther* (1974) **15**, 374.
2 Segre E, Sevelius H, Chaplin M, Forchielli E, Runkel R and Rooks W. Interaction of naproxen and aspirin in the rat and in man. *Scand J Rheumatol* (1973) *Suppl* **2**, 37.
3 Willkens R F and Segre E J. Combination therapy with naproxen and aspirin in rheumatoid arthritis. *Arth Rheum* (1976) **19**, 677.

Oxyphenbutazone + anabolic steroids

Summary

The serum levels of oxyphenbutazone can be raised (about 50%) by the concurrent use of methandrostenolone. The importance of this is uncertain. Phenylbutazone appears not to interact.

Interaction

A study in six subjects who were taking oxphenbutazone, 300–400 mg daily, for periods of 2–5 weeks, and who were additionally given methandrostenolone, 5 or 10 mg/kg daily, showed that plasma levels of oxyphenbutazone were raised by an average of 43% (range 5–100%). Prednisone, 5 mg daily, and dexamethasone, 1·5 mg daily, were found not to affect oxyphenbutazone serum levels.[1]

Two other studies[2,3] confirm the interaction between methandrostenolone and oxyphenbutazone. One of them[2] found no interaction with phenybutazone.

Mechanism

Not understood. One suggestion is that the anabolic steroids alter the distribution of oxyphenbutazone between the tissues and plasma so that more remains in the circulation.[1] The failure of phenylbutazone to interact may be because the phenylbutazone displaces oxyphenbutazone (its normal metabolite) from plasma protein binding sites, thereby raising the levels of unbound oxyphenbutazone and obliterating the effect of the steroid.

Importance and management

The documentation is limited but the interaction seems to be well established. Its importance is uncertain. There appear to be no reports of toxicity arising from concurrent use but the possibility should be borne in mind if both drugs are given together. Phenylbutazone is reported not to interact. Information about other anabolic steroids appears to be lacking. The corticosteroids prednisone and dexamethasone do not, according to the study cited,[1] interact with oxyphenbutazone.

References

1 Weiner M, Siddiqui A A, Shahani R T and Dayton P G. Effect of steroids on disposition of oxyphenbutazone in man. *Proc Soc Exp Biol Med* (1967) **124**, 1170.
2 Hvidberg E, Dayton P G, Read J M and Wilson C H. Studies of the interaction of phenylbutazone, oxyphenbutazone and methandrostenolone in man. *Proc Soc Exp Biol Med* (1968) **129**, 438.
3 Weiner M, Siddiqui A A, Bostanci N and Dayton P G. Drug interactions. The effect of combined administration on the half-life of coumarin and pyrazolone drugs in man. *Fed Proc* (1965) **24**, 153.

Paracetamol + alcohol

Summary
Severe liver damage, in one case with a fatal outcome, has been attributed to the use of therapeutic doses of paracetamol (acetaminophen) by alcoholic patients.

Interaction

Three chronic alcoholic patients developed severe liver damage after taking therapeutic doses of paracetamol (acetaminophen). They demonstrated SGOT levels of 5000–10 000 *i.u.* Two of them had taken only 10 g paracetamol over the two days prior to admission (normal dosage is up to 4 g daily). One of them died in hepatic coma and a post mortem revealed typical paracetamol hepatotoxicity. The other patient had taken 50 g paracetamol. Two of them also developed renal failure.[1]

In subsequent laboratory studies it was shown that the toxicity of paracetamol was increased in mice which had been pretreated for 3 weeks with 10% alcohol in their drinking water (the LD_{50} was reduced from 876 to 518 mg/kg). Liver samples showed central necrosis typical of paracetamol toxicity.[1]

There are other isolated reports where liver toxicity appeared to have resulted from the concurrent use of alcohol and paracetamol X.[2-4]

Mechanism

Not understood. One possibility is that chronic alcohol abuse induces the liver microsomal enzymes, so that large amounts of a highly hepatotoxic metabolite of paracetamol is produced. If there is insufficient glutathione present (alcoholics often have an inadequate dietary intake of protein) to detoxify this metabolite, it becomes bound covalently to hepatic macromolecules and causes damage.

Importance and management

Although not firmly established, there is enough evidence from both human and animal studies to indicate that the use of paracetamol, even in quite small doses, may be a hazard to chronic alcoholics. An editorial in the *Journal of the American Medical Association* discussing the paper cited[1] suggests that '. . . patients should probably be warned that the coadministration of alcohol and acetaminophen (paracetamol), at least in high therapeutic doses, may be harmful . . .'.[5]

References
1 McClain C J, Kromhout J P, Peterson F J and Holtzman J L. Potentiation of acetaminophen hepatotoxicity by alcohol. *J Amer med Ass* (1980) **244**, 251.
2 Goldfinger R, Ahmed K S, Pitchumoni C S. Concomitant alcohol and drug abuse enhancing acetaminophen toxicity. *Am J Gastroenterol* (1978) **70**, 385.
3 Emby D J and Fraser B N. Hepatotoxicity of paracetamol enhanced by ingestion of alcohol. *S Afr med J* (1977) **51**, 208.
4 Barker J D, de Carle D J and Anuras S. Chronic excessive acetaminophen use and liver damage. *Ann Int Med* (1977) **87**, 299.
5 Craig R M. How safe is acetaminophen? *J Amer med Ass* (1980) **244**, 272.

Penicillamine + iron preparations

Summary
There is evidence suggesting that the therapeutic effects of penicillamine may be diminished by the concurrent use of iron salts.

Interaction, mechanism, importance and management

Although iron supplements are sometimes required during treatment with penicillamine, a chemical complex can be formed between the two compounds which may reduce the effects of the penicillamine. In an experimental study in 5 normal subjects administered penicillamine, it was shown that during concurrent treatment with iron, the urinary excretion of copper was reduced suggesting that the absorption and the effects of the penicillamine were depressed.[1] Information on this interaction is very limited, but until more is known it would seem sensible to separate the administration of the two compounds as much as possible to prevent their admixture in the gut. Further study is required.

Reference
1 Lyle W H. Penicillamine and iron. *Lancet* (1976) **ii**, 240.

Pethidine (meperidine) + barbiturates

Summary

A single case report describes greatly enhanced sedation with severe CNS toxicity in a woman given pethidine after receiving phenobarbitone for a fortnight. It has been suggested that reduced analgesia may also occur.

Interaction

A woman patient, whose pain had been satisfactorily controlled with pethidine (meperidine) without particular CNS depression, showed prolonged sedation with severe CNS toxicity when she was later given pethidine, after being treated with 120 mg phenobarbitone daily for a fortnight as prophylactic anticonvulsant therapy.[1]

Mechanism

A thorough analysis[1] of the kinetics and metabolism of pethidine (meperidine) in the patient described, in four other patients and in 2 normal volunteers showed that pretreatment with phenobarbitone greatly increased the production of norpethidine (normeperidine) which is a metabolic product of pethidine and much more toxic than the parent compound. It is presumed that in man, as in animals,[2] the phenobarbitone stimulates the hepatic microsomal enzymes concerned with the N-demethylation of pethidine so that increased amounts of this the more toxic compound are formed. It is not clear how much, if any, the inherent sedative effects of the barbiturate also had some part to play in the severe sedative effects seen in the patient described.

Importance and management

The data is very limited indeed, but it indicates that the toxic potentialities of pethidine may be increased by phenobarbitone. Whether other barbiturates will behave similarly is not certain, but it would seem possible. It has been pointed out[1] that since the metabolic product of pethidine is a less effective analgesic than the parent compound, the depth of analgesia may be reduced. This requires confirmation. In addition, if the pethidine is continued but the phenobarbitone suddenly withdrawn, the toxic concentrations of the norpethidine might lead to convulsions in the absence of the anticonvulsant. This too requires confirmation.

References

1 Stambaugh J E, Wainer I W, Hemphill D M and Schwartz I. A potentially toxic drug interaction between pethidine (meperidine) and phenobarbitone. *Lancet* (1977) **i**, 398.
2 Pantuck E, Conney A H and Kuntzman R. Effect of phenobarbital on the metabolism of pentobarbital and meperidine in foetal rabbits and rats. *Biochem Pharmacol* (1968) **17**, 1441.

Pethidine (meperidine) + furazolidone

Summary

On the basis of animal experiments it has been suggested that pethidine (meperidine) may induce a serious hyperpyrexic reaction in man in the presence of furazolidone, similar to the interaction with the antidepressant MAOI. This has yet to be confirmed.

Interaction, mechanism, importance and management

Studies in rabbits have shown that fatal hyperpyrexia follows the injection of pethidine into animals pretreated orally for 4 days with furazolidone.[1] There is no direct evidence of an adverse interaction between pethidine and furazolidone in man, but on the basis of this serious interaction in rabbits,[1] the known MAO-inhibitory properties of furazolidone in man,[2] and the well-documented adverse MAOI–pethidine interaction in man (see p. 365), there would seem to be the possibility of some risk if these two drugs are used together. More study is required.

References

1 Eltayeb I B and Osman O H. Furazolidone–pethidine interaction in rabbits. *Br J Pharmac* (1975) **55**, 497.
2 Pettinger W A, Soyangio F G and Oates J A. Monoamine-oxidase inhibition by furazolidone in man. *Clin. Res.* (1966) **14**, 258.

Phenazone (antipyrine) + barbiturates

Summary
The metabolism and rate of clearance of phenazone from the body is increased by the concurrent use of barbiturates.

Interaction, mechanism, importance and management
Studies on the changes in phenazone half-life caused by other drugs have become a time-honoured way of finding out if the drugs have any effects on the activity of liver microsomal enzymes. Barbiturates demonstrably induce liver enzymes in man [1,2] and reduce the phenazone half-life (one study[1] with amylobarbitone showed a 42% reduction) but to what extent this is likely to have a significant effect on the analgesic and antipyretic effects of phenazone is uncertain. Some diminution in the response would seem probable.

References
1 O'Malley K, Browning M, Stevenson I and Turnbull M J. Stimulation of drug metabolism in man by tricycle antidepressants. *Europ J clin Pharmacol* (1973) **6**, 102.
2 Vesell E S and Page J G. Genetic control of the phenobarbital-induced shortening of plasma antipyrine half-lives in man. *J Clin Invest* (1969) **48**, 220.

Phenylbutazone + allopurinol

Summary
Allopurinol appears to have no significant effect on phenylbutazone when taken concurrently.

Interaction
The daily[1] administration of 300 mg allopurinol to 6 volunteers for a month was shown in one study to have had no effect on the elimination of phenylbutazone (200 mg daily dose), and similarly had no effect on the steady-state phenylbutazone concentration in 3 patients taking 200 or 300 mg daily.

Another study[2] on 6 patients with acute gouty arthritis showed that the administration of 300 mg allopurinol daily produced small but clinically unimportant effects on the half-life of phenylbutazone being given in dosages within the usual therapeutic range (6 mg/kg).

Mechanism
None.

Importance and management
There is no evidence from either of these studies that the dosage of phenylbutazone requires any alteration in patients taking allopurinol.

References
1 Rawlins M D and Smith S E. Influence of allopurinol on drug metabolism in man. *Br J Pharmac* (1973) **48**, 693.
2 Horwitz D, Thorgeirsson S S and Mitchell J R. The influence of allopurinol and size of dose on the metabolism of phenylbutazone in patients with gout. *Europ J Clin Pharmacol* (1977) **12**, 133.

Phenylbutazone + chlorinated pesticides

Summary
Chronic exposure to lindane and other chlorinated pesticides can increase the rate of metabolism of phenylbutazone.

A study[1] showed that the plasma half-life of phenylbutazone in a group of men who regularly used chlorinated insecticide sprays (mainly lindane) as part of their work was shorter (51 h) than that of a control group (64 h) due, it is believed, to the enzyme-inductive effects of the sprays. This is of doubtful direct clinical importance, but it illustrates the changed metabolism which can occur in those exposed to common environmental chemical agents.

Reference
1 Kolomodin-Hedman B. Decreased plasma half-life of phenylbutazone in workers exposed to chlorinated pesticides. *Europ J clin Pharmacol* (1973) **5**, 195.

Phenylbutazone + indomethacin

Summary
An isolated report describes transient deterioration in renal function during recovery from phenylbutazone-induced renal failure when indomethacin was given concurrently.

Interaction, mechanism, importance
and management
A patient recovering from phenylbutazone-induced renal failure showed a transient deterioration in renal function when concurrently treated with 25 mg indomethacin three times a day.[1] It was suggested that possibly other drugs which inhibit prostaglandin synthesis should be used with caution in those who show this reaction to phenylbutazone.[1] It is interesting to note that indomethacin can competitively inhibit the binding of phenylbutazone to human plasma albumin,[2] and it could be postulated that the transient renal deterioration might have been due to the displacement of the residual phenylbutazone by the indomethacin from its binding sites.

No general conclusions about the advisability or otherwise of using phenylbutazone and indomethacin together or sequentially should be drawn from this single case.

References
1 Kimberly R P and Branstetter R D. Exacerbation of phenylbutazone-related renal failure by indomethacin. *Arch Intern Med* (1978) **138**, 1711.
2 Solomon H M, Schrogie J J and Williams D. The displacement of phenylbutazone-^{14}C and warfarin-^{14}C from human albumin by various drugs and fatty acids. *Biochem Pharmacol* (1968) **17**, 143.

Phenylbutazone + methylphenidate

Summary
Serum levels of phenylbutazone can be raised by the concurrent use of methylphenidate.

Interaction, mechanism, importance
and management
Single dose as well as chronic studies in man using normal daily doses of phenylbutazone, 200–400 mg, and methylphenidate, have shown that the serum levels of phenylbutazone are increased significantly in most individuals.[1] This may be due to inhibition of the metabolism of the phenylbutazone by the methylphenidate. The clinical importance of this interaction is uncertain.

Reference
1 Dayton P G, Johnson L D and Wilson C H. Inhibition of the metabolism of phenylbutazone by methylphenidate in man. *Pharmacologist* (1969) **11**, 272.

Phenylbutazone + phenobarbitone

Summary
Some reduction in the serum levels of phenylbutazone may be expected during concurrent treatment with phenobarbitone, but the practical importance of this has not been determined.

Interaction
Studies carried out in man showed that the half-life of phenylbutazone was reduced from 78 to 57 h by concurrent treatment with 90 mg phenobarbitone.[1]

Other studies on very large numbers of individuals similarly demonstrated a reduction in phenylbutazone half-life after pretreatment with 1·2 mg/kg phenobarbitone nightly for 3 nights.[2]

Mechanism
Barbiturates such as phenobarbitone are potent liver enzyme inducers and it is believed that the reduced half-life of phenylbutazone comes about because its rate of metabolism is increased.[2]

Importance and management
Evidence for this interaction is very limited and its importance has not been determined; nevertheless since it has been shown that subjective improvement in rheumatoid arthritis is more frequent in patients with serum phenylbutazone levels above 50 μg/ml than below this level,[3] an interaction which results in a reduction in serum concentrations might be expected to be important in some cases. If therefore phenobarbitone or any barbiturate is added to established treatment with phenylbutazone, the prescriber should be aware that a deterioration in response is a possibility, although its probability is unknown. Considerable patient variation may be expected.[2]

References
1 Levi A J, Sherlock S and Walker D. Phenylbutazone and isoniazid metabolism in patients with liver disease in relation to previous drug therapy. *Lancet* (1968) i, 1275.
2 Whittaker J A and Price Evans D A. Genetic control of phenylbutazone metabolism in man. *Br. Med J* (1970) 3, 323.
3 Bruck E, Fearnley M E, Meanock I and Patley H. Phenylbutazone therapy. Relation between the toxic and therapeutic effects and the blood level. *Lancet* (1954) i, 225.

Phenylbutazone + salicylates

Summary
The uricosuric effects of phenylbutazone and aspirin are antagonized by concurrent use.

Interaction
A study carried out on 4 patients without gout showed that small doses of aspirin had little effect on the excretion of uric acid in the urine, but when the dose was raised to 5 g daily, marked uricosuria occurred. When phenylbutazone was additonally given in increasing doses (200, 400 and then 600 mg daily over 3 days) the uricosuria was inhibited and this persisted for 24 h after withdrawal of both drugs. The serum levels of uric acid rose from an average of 4 mg to 6 mg%. The interaction was confirmed in a patient with tophaceous gout. Retention of uric acid also occurred if the phenylbutazone is given first.[1]

Mechanism
Not resolved. It is almost certainly mediated by some interference with the mechanisms of uric acid secretion by the kidney tubules.

Importance and management
Information is very limited but it appears to be an established interaction. If serum urate measurements are taken for diagnostic purposes this interaction needs to be taken into account. The potential problems arising from this interaction should also be recognized in patients treated with both drugs.

Reference
1 Oyer J H, Wagner S L and Schmid F R. Suppression of salicylate-induced uricosuria by phenylbutazone. *Amer J Med Sci* (1966) 225, 1.

Phenylbutazone or oxyphenbutazone + tricyclic antidepressants

Summary
The antirheumatic effects of phenylbutazone and oxyphenbutazone are probably not affected by the concurrent use of tricyclic antidepressants, although there is evidence that their absorption may be delayed.

Interaction
A study on 4 depressed women showed that during concurrent treatment with desipramine, 25 mg three times a day, the absorption of phenylbutazone was considerably delayed, but the total amount absorbed, as measured by the urinary excretion of oxyphenbutazone, appeared to be unaltered.[1]

A clinical study on 5 depressed women chronically treated for 2 months with desipramine and nortriptyline, 75 mg daily, demonstrated that these tricyclics had no effect upon the half-life of oxyphenbutazone.[2]

Mechanism
Studies in animals confirm that the tricyclic antidepressants can delay the absorption of phenylbutazone and oxyphenbutazone, probably due to their anticholinergic effects which reduce the motility of the gut.[3,4]

Importance and management
The information is very limited, and the importance of this interaction is uncertain. It seems doubtful if desipramine or nortriptyline are likely to have a significant effect on the total absorption of either oxyphenbutazone or phenylbutazone, but there seem to be no clinical studies which definitely confirm that the antirheumatic effects of these drugs are not reduced. Whether other tricyclic antidepressants interact similarly is not known.

References
1 Consolo S, Morselli, Zaccala M and Garattini S. Delayed absorption of phenylbutazone caused by desmethylimipramine in humans. *Europ J Pharmacol* (1970) 10, 239.
2 Hammer W, Martens S and Sjoqvist F. A comparative study of the metabolism of desmethylimipramine, nortriptyline, and oxyphenbutazone in man. *Clin Pharmacol Ther* (1969) 10, 44.
3 Consolo S. An interaction between desipramine and phenylbutazone. *J Pharm Pharmac* (1968) 20, 574.
4 Consolo S and Garattini S. Effect of desipramine on intestinal absorption of phenylbutazone and other drugs. *Europ J Pharmacol* (1969) 6, 322.

Probenecid + salicylates

Summary
The uricosuric effects of probenecid and the salicylates are mutually antagonistic.

Interaction
In one case investigated, the urinary uric acid excretion in mg/average 24 h was found to be 673 mg with a single 3 gm daily dose of probenecid, 909 mg with a 6 g daily dose of sodium salicylate, but only 114 mg when both drugs were used concurrently.[1]

Similar antagonism has been described in other studies with patients given 2·6–5·2 g aspirin daily.[2,3]

Mechanism
Not understood. It would seem almost certain that the interference occurs at the site of renal tubular secretion.

Importance and management
A well-established interaction. Patients on probenecid should not be given salicylates in substantial amounts if this antagonism is to be avoided, although it seems probable that small analgesic doses may not have a marked effect.

References
1 Seegmiller J E and Grayzel A I. Use of the newer uricosuric agents in the management of gout. *J Amer med Ass* (1960) 173, 1076.
2 Pascale L R, Dubin A and Hoffman W S. Therapeutic value of probenecid (Benemid) in gout. *J Amer med Ass* (1952) 149, 1188.
3 Gutman A B and Yü T F. Benemid (p-di-n-propylsulfamylbenzoic acid) as uricosuric agent in chronic gout arthritis. *Trans Ass Amer Phys* (1951) 64, 279.

Probenecid + sulphinpyrazone

Summary
Probenecid reduces the renal clearance of sulphinpyrazone but the uricosuria remains unaffected.

Interaction, mechanism, importance and management

A study in 8 patients with gout showed that while probenecid was able to inhibit the renal tubular excretion of sulphinpyrazone, reducing it by about 75%, the maximal uric acid clearance observed with each drug alone remained unaltered.[1] There would seem to be little reason for using these two drugs together. Whether the toxic effects of sulphinpyrazone might be increased is not known.

Reference
1 Perel J M, Dayton P G, McMillan Snell M, Yü T F and Gutman A B. Studies of interactions among drugs in man at the renal level: probenecid and sulfinpyrazone. *Clin Pharmacol Ther* (1969) 10, 834.

Salicylates + antacids

Summary
Serum salicylate concentrations can be reduced to sub-therapeutic levels by the concurrent use of some antacids.

Interaction

A study in 13 normal subjects given 4 g aspirin daily for a week showed that during the concurrent use of sodium bicarbonate, 4 g daily, the serum salicylate levels fell from 27 to 15 mg/100 ml. This reflected a rise in the urinary pH from a range of 5·6–6·1 to 6·2–6·9.[1]

A child with rheumatic fever being given 0·6 g aspirin five times a day with 30 ml *Maalox* (aluminium–magnesium hydroxide suspension) demonstrated serum salicylate concentrations between 8·2 and 11·8 mg/100 ml. When the *Maalox* was discontinued, the urinary pH fell from a range of 7/8, to 5·0/6·4, and the serum salicylate concentration rose to about 38 mg/100 ml, calling for a reduction in the dosage.[1]

Similar changes have been reported in other studies.[3, 5]

Mechanism

Aspirin and other salicylates are acidic compounds which are excreted by the kidney tubules and are ionized in solution. In alkaline solution, much of the drug exists in the ionized form which is not readily reabsorbed and is therefore lost in the urine. If the urine is made acid, much more of the drug exists in the un-ionized form which is readily reabsorbed so that less is lost in the urine, and the drug is retained in the body. A more detailed and illustrated account of this interaction mechanism is given on page 9. Magnesium oxide also adsorbs aspirin and sodium salicylate strongly.[4]

Importance and management

A well-established and important interaction for those on chronic treatment with large doses of salicylates. Serum salicylate concentrations can be reduced to sub-therapeutic levels by the use of both 'systemic' antacids (eg. sodium bicarbonate) as well as some 'non-systemic' antacids (eg. magnesium–aluminium hydroxide). Magnesium hydroxide and calcium carbonate glycine have all been shown capable of raising the urinary pH significantly[1] but some very limited evidence suggests that some aluminium-containing antacids (aluminium hydroxide–*Amphojel*, and dihydroxy-aluminium aminoacetate—*Robalate*) may have minimal effects.[1,2] Care should be taken to monitor serum salicylate levels if antacids are added or withdrawn in patients where control of the salicylate levels is critical.

References
1 Levy C. Interactions of salicylates with antacids. Clinical implications with respect to gastrointestinal bleeding and anti-inflammatory activity. *Frontiers of Internal Medicine 1974.*

12th Int Congr Intern Med. Tel Aviv 1974, p. 404 (1975) Karger, Basel.

2 Muirden K R, and Barraclough D R E. Drug interaction in the management of rheumatoid arthritis. *Aust NZ J Med* (1976) 6, (*Suppl 1*) 14.

3 Levy G, Lampman T, Kamath B L and Garrettson L K. Decreased serum salicylate concentrations in children with rheumatic fever treated with antacid. *New Eng J med* (1975) 293, 323.

4 Naggar V F, Khalil S A and Daabis N A. The in-vitro adsorption of some anti-rheumatics on antacids. *Pharmazie* (1976) 31, 461.

5 Hansten P D and Hayton W L. Effect of antacid and ascorbic acid on serum salicylate concentration. *J Clin Pharmacol* (1980) 24, 326.

Salicylates + corticosteroids

Summary

A marked rise in serum salicylate levels can occur during corticosteroid withdrawal following concurrent therapy if the dosage of the salicylate remains unaltered. One case of salicylate intoxication has been reported. Whether the incidence of gastrointestinal ulceration is increased during concurrent use is uncertain.

Interaction

The renal clearance of salicylates from the body can be reduced by the concurrent use of corticosteroids.

A 4-year-old boy with rheumatoid arthritis was treated with at least 20 mg prednisone a day for some time. After admission to hospital he was additionally given 3·6 g choline salicylate daily and the prednisone gradually tapered off to 2 mg a day over a 3 month period. Severe salicylate intoxication developed and, in a retrospective investigation of the cause using frozen serum samples drawn for other purposes, it was found that the serum salicylate had climbed from about 10 to 90 mg% during the withdrawal of the corticosteroid.[1]

Subsequent studies in 3 other patients on choline salicylate or aspirin, and either prednisone or another unnamed corticosteroid, demonstrated similar but less spectacular rises (about three-fold) during corticosteroid withdrawal.[1]

A serum salicylate rise of similar proportions has been described in a patient on aloxiprin during withdrawal of prednisolone.[2]

Mechanism

The mechanism of this interaction is not known, but based on the results of the study already cited[1] it has been suggested that during corticosteroid treatment the rate of clearance of the salicylate is increased and this parallels a general increase in glomerular filtration rate. There was no evidence that the salicylate metabolism was altered. When the corticosteroid is withdrawn, the salicylate returns to its normal clearance rate and thus accumulates within the body. Studies in mice have shown that cortisone similarly protects them from the development of salicylism.[3]

Importance and management

Concurrent treatment with corticosteroids and salicylates is quite common. For example, to quote one of the reports already cited[2], out of 88 consecutive rheumatic arthritic patients referred to the Royal Melbourne Hospital, 51 were taking two or more antirheumatic drugs and of the total group 85% were on aspirin and 50% on corticosteroids. There is certainly no contraindication to their combined use but it should be borne in mind that the salicylates can cause gastrointestinal ulceration and it is generally believed that this is also true of the corticosteroids. Whether in fact concurrent use increases the incidence of ulceration has not been confirmed.

Only one case of salicylism has been described during withdrawal of the corticosteroid, although considerable rises in serum salicylate levels have been seen in a number of other patients and described elsewhere as a '. . . fairly regular occurrence'.[2] Prescribers should be aware of this response.

Only a few of the corticosteroids have been directly implicated in this interaction (prednisone, prednisolone, hydrocortisone) but it may be expected to occur with the others. The interaction has been observed with aspirin, aloxiprin, sodium salicylate and choline salicylate.

References

1 Klinenberg J R and Miller F. Effect of corticosteroids on blood salicylate concentration. *J Amer med Ass* (1965) 194, 601.

2 Muirden K D and Barraclough D R E. Drug interactions in the management of rheumatoid arthritis. *Aust NZ J Med* (1976) 6 (*Suppl 1*) 14.

3 Montuori E. Acción de la cortisona sobre le toxicidad del salicilato di sodio. *Rev Soc Argent Biol* (1954) 30, 44.

Salicylates + levamisole

Summary
A rise in serum salicylate levels in a patient when concurrently treated with levamisole and aspirin was not confirmed in subsequent controlled studies.

Interaction, mechanism, importance and management
A preliminary report[1] of a patient who showed an increase in serum salicylate levels when levamisole was given with aspirin prompted a study of this possible interaction. Nine healthy adults were given 3·9 g of sustained-release aspirin a day in two divided doses for a period of 3 weeks, and during this period they were also given 50 mg levamisole three times a day for a week, each subject acting as his own control. No significant changes in serum salicylate levels were found.[2]

References
1 Laidlaw D A. Rheumatoid arthritis improved by treatment with levamisole and L-histidine. Med J Aust (1976) 2, 382.
2 Rumble R H, Brooks P M and Roberts M S. Interaction between levamisole and aspirin. Br J clin Pharmac (1979) 7, 631.

Salicylates, diazepam, phenobarbitone, propoxyphene, codeine, pentazocine, indomethacin or hydroxyzine + neofam

Summary
The intensity and incidence of side-effects are reported to be increased when neofam is administered with codeine, pentazocine or propoxyphene, but not with the other drugs listed.

Interaction, mechanism, importance and management
A controlled clinical trial was carried out on 45 healthy subjects divided into nine groups of five, each of whom was given 60 mg neofam daily for a period of 3 days with either aspirin 650 mg, diazepam 5 mg, phenobarbitone 60 mg, propoxyphene 65 mg, codeine 60 mg, pentazocine 50 mg, indomethacin 25 mg or hydroxyzine pamoate 50 mg. The subjects were monitored for changes in the intensity and incidence of side-effects, bio-availability of neofam, and changes in vital signs or on various laboratory tests. The only alterations seen were a possibly additive increase in the intensity and incidence of side-effects with neofam and codeine, pentazocine or propoxyphene, the overall conclusion being that there was no good evidence against using neofam with these drugs for short periods.

Reference
1 Lasseter K C, Cohen A and Back E L. Neofam HCl interaction study with eight other drugs. J Int Med Res (1976) 4, 195.

Salicylates + sulphinpyrazone

Summary
The uricosuric effects of sulphinpyrazone and the salicylates are antagonized by the presence of the other drug. Concurrent use should be avoided.

Interaction

Each drug suppresses the uricosuric effects of the other

> 6 g sodium salicylate with 600 mg sulphinpyrazone daily caused a urinary uric acid excretion in one patient of only 30 mg/av. 24 h, whereas when each drug was used by itself in the same doses the excretion was 281 and 527 mg/av. 24 h respectively.[1]
>
> A study carried out on 5 men with gout who were infused with sulphinpyrazone (300 mg to prime followed by 10 mg/min) for about an hour showed that when they were additionally infused with sodium salicylate (3 g to prime followed by 10–20 mg/min) the uricosuria was virtually completely abolished. When the drugs were given in the reverse order to three other patients the same result was seen.[2]

Mechanism

By no means fully understood. Both drugs compete for plasma protein binding sites but the major site for interaction would seem to be the urinary tubule. Sulphinpyrazone competes successfully with salicylate for tubular secretion and salicylate excretion is reduced, but the salicylate blocks the inhibitory effect of sulphinpyrazone on the tubular reabsorption of uric acid so that the uric acid accumulates within the body.[2]

Importance and management

Although the evidence appears to be limited to these two reports, there is enough information to indicate that salicylates should be avoided by patients taking sulphinpyrazone for uricosuria. Small doses of salicylate probably have only a small effect. Virtually all the salicylates except salicylamide are metabolized to salicylic acid and may be expected to interact similarly.

References

1 Seegmiller J E and Grayzel A I. Use of the newer uricosuric agents in the management of gout. *J Amer med Ass* (1960) **173**, 1076.
2 Yü T F, Dayton P G and Gutman A B. Mutual suppression of the uricosuric effects of sulphinpyrazone and salicylate: a study in interactions between drugs. *J Clin Invest* (1963) **42**,

CHAPTER 4. ANTIARRHYTHMIC DRUG INTERACTIONS

The antiarrhythmic agents which can interact with other drugs and which are dealt with in this book are listed in Table 4.1. Some of the interactions are discussed in this chapter. Others are to be found either in chapters devoted to specific groups of drugs (Digitalis Glycosides, Beta-Adrenergic Blockers, Anticonvulsants) or dealt with individually in other chapters where the antiarrhythmic agent is the affecting agent rather than the drug whose activity is altered.

Table 4.1. Antiarrhythmic agents

Non-proprietary names	Proprietary names
Amiodarone	*Cordarone*
Bretylium	*Bretylate, Darenthin*
Digitalis glycosides	—
Disopyramide	*Norpace, Rythmodan*
Lignocaine (lidocaine)	*Xylocaine*
Phenytoin	*Epanutin, Garoin, Dilantin etc.*
Procainamide	*Novacamid, Procapan, Pronestyl*
Propranolol	*Avlocardyl, Dociton, Herzul, Inderal, Kemi, Sumial*
Quinidine	—
Verapamil	*Cordilox, Isoptin, Vasolan*

Amiodarone + beta-blockers

Summary
A case of asystole and another of ventricular fibrillation have been tentatively attributed to the concurrent use of amiodarone and propranolol.

Interaction, mechanism, importance and management
Although amiodarone and practolol have been used together uneventfully in a number of patients (more marked bradycardia and some ECG changes were seen),[1] another report describes two cases of cardiac arrest in patients on amiodarone shortly after starting to take propranolol.[2] One patient developed ventricular fibrillation, and the other asystole. It is not certain that these responses were due to the concurrent use of these drugs, but prescribers should be aware of this possible interaction.

References
1 Antonelli G, Cristallo E, Cesario S and Calabrese P. Modificazioni elettrocardiografiche indotte dalla somministrazione de amiodarone associato a practolol. *Boll Soc Ital Cardiol* (1973) 18, 236.
2 Derrida J P, Ollagnier J, Benaim R, Haiat R and Chiche P. Amiodarone et propranolol: une association dangereuse? *Nouv Pressé med* (1979) 8, 1429.

Bretylium + quinidine

Summary
Animal studies suggest that bretylium may fail to control arrhythmias if given after quinidine-like agents because of antagonism between the drugs.

Interaction, mechanism, importance and management

A study using isolated rabbit hearts demonstrated antagonism between bretylium tosylate and quinidine on the duration of action potential and the refractory period in ventricular fibres.[1] This confirms other studies which have shown that other antiarrhythmic agents antagonized the clinical effects of bretylium when given at the same time, or previously.[2] The effects on A–V conduction are somewhat discordant. The animal study suggested that additive depressant effects occurred, whereas some clinical studies describe improved A–V conduction.[3] Further study is required.

References
1 De Azevedo R M, Watanabe Y and Dreifus L S. Electrophysiologic antagonism of quinidine and bretylium tosylate. *Amer J Cardiol* (1974) **33**, 633.
2 Bernstein J G and Koch-Weser J. Effectiveness of bretylium tosylate against refractory ventricular arrhythmias. *Circulation* (1972) **45**, 1024.
3 Bacaner M. Experimental and clinical effects of bretylium tosylate on ventricular fibrillation, arrhythmias and heart block. *Geriatrics* (1971) **26**, 132.

Disopyramide + anticholinergic agents

Summary
On theoretical grounds, the anticholinergic side-effects of disopyramide and other drugs with anticholinergic activity may be expected to be additive.

Interaction, mechanism, importance and management

There appear to be no case reports or studies of this potential interaction, but because disopyramide has anticholinergic side-effects it seems not unlikely that additive anticholinergic side-effects could develop if used concurrently with other drugs possessing this type of activity. In one study of disopyramide on 24 patients, 8 of them complained of dry mouth, 1 of disturbance of accommodation, and 1 of dysuria.[1] In another study of 17 patients, 4 of them experienced a dry mouth and 1 had difficulty in urinating.[2]

Additive anticholinergic side-effects can certainly occur when two or more drugs with this activity are used together (tricyclic antidepressants, antiparkinson agents, antihistamines, antiemetics, phenothiazines, butyrophenones and thioxanthenes, see page 244) so that it would not be unreasonable to be on the alert for an increased incidence of this type of side-effect if disopyramide is used with drugs of this kind.

References
1 Härtel G, Louhija A and Konttinen A. Disopyramide in the prevention of recurrence of atrial fibrillation after electroconversion. *Clin Pharmacol Ther* (1974) **15**, 551.
2 Vismara L A, Mason D T and Amsterdam E A. Disopyramide phosphate. Clinical efficacy of a new oral anti-arrhythmic agent. *Clin Pharmacol Ther* (1974) **16**, 330.

Disopyramide + beta-blocker

Summary
Two cases of severe bradycardia, one of them having a fatal outcome, followed the intravenous injection of practolol and then disopyramide in the treatment of supraventricular tachycardia.

Interaction, mechanism, importance and management

Two cases have been reported of patients with supraventricular tachycardia (180 beats/min) which was treated firstly with intravenous practolol (20 mg and 10 mg respectively) and then 20 min later with disopyramide (150 and 80 mg respectively). The first patient rapidly developed sinus bradycardia of 25 beats/min, lost consciousness and became profoundly hypotensive. He failed to respond to atropine but reacted favourably to the subsequent insertion of a temporary pacemaker and other treatment. The other patient also showed severe sinus bradycardia which failed to respond to atropine. He was resuscitated with adrenaline but died 5 h later.

The authors of the report suspect an adverse interaction and suggest that intravenous disopyramide should not be given after practolol. There appear to be no other reports of this interaction and the mechanism is not known.

Reference
1 Cumming A D and Robertson C. Interaction between disopyramide and practolol. *Brit Med J* (1979) 3, 1264.

Lignocaine + barbiturates

Summary
Animal studies indicate that serious additive depression of respiration may occur during concurrent use. Whether this can also occur in man is not known.

Interaction, mechanism, importance and management

In a controlled study, 4 out of 6 dogs receiving lignocaine in therapeutic doses died from respiratory arrest when concurrently given 30 mg/kg pentobarbitone. The other two showed apnoea.[1] The reasons are not understood, but it seems possible that was simply due to the additive depressant effects of the two drugs on the respiratory centre. It is not known whether this interaction is of clinical importance, but it should be borne in mind if these or other drugs which can seriously depress respiration are used together.

Reference
1 LeLorier J. Lidocaine and pentobarbital: a potentially lethal drug–drug interaction. *Toxicol Appl Pharmacol* (1978) 44, 657.

Lignocaine + beta-blockers

Summary
Studies in man and in animals indicate that propranolol can prolong the half-life of lignocaine, but the clinical significance in man has not been demonstrated as yet.

Interaction, mechanism, importance and management

In a study in dogs[1] it was found that during treatment with propranolol the half-life of lignocaine was prolonged from 91 to 135 min, the serum concentrations rose from 3·9 to 5·3 μg/ml and the clearance was reduced from 433 to 332 ml/min. Both single dose and continuous infusion studies in man showed similar results. When 7 normal subjects were treated with 80 mg propranolol three times a day, the mean serum levels of lidocaine during the continuous infusion of 2 mg/min were raised by 30% (from 3·02 to 3·93 μg/ml).[2] The reason for this, it is suggested, is that the propranolol decreases the cardiac output and the flow of blood through the liver, so that the amount of lignocaine arriving at the liver for metabolic clearance is decreased. Whether this interaction has any importance in man is unknown, but it seems probable since the therapeutic index of lignocaine is narrow.

References
1 Branch R A, Shand D G, Wilkinson G R and Nies A S. The reduction of lidocaine clearance by dl-propranolol: an example of hemodynamic drug interaction. *J Pharmacol Exp Ther* (1973) **184**, 515.
2 Ochs H R, Carstens G and Greenblatt D J. Reduction in lidocaine clearance during continuous infusion and by co-administration of propranolol. *New Eng J Med* (1980) **303**, 373.

Lignocaine + phenytoin

Summary
A single case report describes sinoatrial arrest following the concurrent intravenous infusion of phenytoin and lignocaine. Another study reported that no changes in the plasma levels of either drug occur but the incidence of central toxic side-effects is increased.

Interaction

A study of 5 patients in a coronary care unit who had received 0·5–3·0 mg/min lignocaine by intravenous infusion for at least 24 h, and who were then additionally given intravenous infusions of phenytoin, showed that no changes in plasma concentrations of either drug occurred, but the incidence of side-effects (vertigo, nausea, nystagmus, diplopia, impaired hearing) was unusually high, although plasma levels were normal. Comparable results were found in parallel studies in dogs.[1]

Sinoatrial arrest occurred in a man following a suspected myocardial infarction with heart block, after receiving 1 mg/kg lignocaine infused intravenously in 1 min, followed 3 min later by 250 mg phenytoin over 5 min. The patient lost consciousness and his blood pressure could not be measured, but he responded to 200 μg isoprenaline.[2]

Mechanism
The increase in side-effects described in the first report[1] is not understood. The sinoatrial arrest in the second report[2] would appear to result from the additive depressant effects of the two drugs on the heart.

Importance and management
Concurrent use is clearly not contraindicated, but considerable caution is necessary when using any two drugs both of which have depressant effects on automatic tissue and where normal doses may prove to be excessive.

References
1 Karlsson E, Collste P and Rawlins M L. Plasma levels of lidocaine during combined treatment with phenytoin and procainamide. *Europ J clin Pharmacol* (1974) **7**, 455.
2 Wood R A. Sinoatrial arrest: an interaction between phenytoin and lignocaine. *Brit Med J* (1971) **1**, 645.

Lignocaine + procainamide

Summary
A single case of delerium has been described during the concurrent use of lignocaine and procainamide.

Interaction, mechanism, importance and management
A single case report describes a man with paroxysmal tachycardia, under treatment with increasing doses of lignocaine by intravenous infusion and procainamide orally who, when given a further intravenous dose of procainamide, became restless, noisy and delerious.[1] Other studies in patients have shown that lignocaine plasma levels are unaffected by procainamide.[2]

The reasons for the adverse reaction described are not understood. One suggestion is that the CNS effects of the two drugs may have been additive.

References
1 Ilyas M, Owens D and Kvasnicka G. Delerium induced by a combination of anti-arrhythmic drugs. *Lancet* (1969) **ii**, 1368.
2 Karlsson E, Collste P and Rawlins M D. Plasma levels of lidocaine during combined treatment with phenytoin and procainamide. *Europ J clin Pharmacol* (1974) **7**, 455.

Quinidine + anthraquinone-containing laxative or metoclopramide

Summary

Quinidine serum levels can be reduced by the concurrent use of a laxative and raised by metoclopramide.

Interaction, mechanism, importance and management

Studies carried out on patients with heart arrhythmias taking 500 mg quinidine bisulphate every 12 h showed that concurrent treatment with an anthraquinone-containing laxative (*Liquidepur*, Fa. Natterman, Cologne) reduced the quinidine serum levels measured 12 h after the last dose of quinidine by about 25%. In cases where the serum levels are already barely adequate to control the arrhythmia any reduction is clearly undesirable.

On the other hand metoclopramide in daily doses of 30 mg increased the mean serum quinidine levels measured $3\frac{1}{2}$ h after the last dose of quinidine by almost 20% (from 1·6 to 1·9 μg/ml) and at 12 h by about 16% (from 2·4 to 2·8 μg/ml).[1]

Reference
1 Guckenbiehl W, Gilfrich H J and Just H. Einfluss von Laxantien und Metoclopramid auf die Chindin-Plasmakonzentration wahrend Langzeittherapie bei Patienten mit Herzrhythmusstorungen. *Med Welt* (1976) **27**, 1273.

Quinidine + barbiturates, phenytoin or primidone

Summary

Serum levels of quinidine can be reduced by the concurrent use of primidone, phenobarbitone or phenytoin. The addition of these anticonvulsants may lead to the loss of arrhythmia control. Withdrawal could result in quinidine intoxication.

Interaction

The metabolism and clearance of quinidine from the body can be increased by primidone, phenytoin or phenobarbitone.

The observation in two patients that phenytoin and phenobarbitone (given as primidone) appeared to increase the clearance of quinidine from the body prompted an investigation on 4 normal subjects. After 2 weeks' treatment with either phenobarbitone or phenytoin in dosages adjusted to given serum levels of 10–20 μg/ml, the elimination half-life of a single 300 mg dose of quinidine was reduced by about 50%, and the total area under the plasma level/time curve by about 60%.[1]

Changes in serum quinidine levels due to pentobarbitone have been described in another report.[2]

Mechanism

The evidence suggests that both phenytoin and phenobarbitone (both known enzyme-inducing agents) increase the metabolism by the liver of the quinidine and increase its loss from the body.[1]

Importance and management

By no means extensively documented, but the available evidence is strong. The pharmacokinetic data suggest that concurrent use of these anticonvulsants can lead to a two- to three-fold change in serum quinidine levels. This is large enough to cause a patient controlled on quinidine to develop quinidine intoxication if the anticonvulsants are withdrawn, or to lose control of cardiac arrhythmias if the anticonvulsants are added. Quinidine serum levels should therefore be monitored if enzyme-inducing agents are added or withdrawn.

Barbiturates other than phenobarbitone and pentobarbitone may be expected to interact similarly, but this awaits confirmation. A 'double' interaction involving quinidine, pentobarbitone and digoxin is described on page 309.

References
1 Data J L, Wilkinson G R and Nies A S. Interaction of quinidine with anticonvulsant drugs. *New Eng J Med* (1976) **294**, 699.
2 Chapron D J, Mumford D and Pitegoff G J. Apparent quinidine-induced digoxin toxicity after withdrawal of pentobarbital. A case of sequential drug interactions. *Arch Int Med* (1979) **139**, 363.

Quinidine + beta-blockers

Summary

An advantageous interaction: relatively modest doses of propranolol and quinidine can be an effective treatment for atrial fibrillation in patients resistant to high doses of quinidine.

Interaction

A man with atrial fibrillation of 10 years' duration which had proved to be totally resistant to large doses of quinidine, returned to sinus rhythm after treatment with 80 mg propranolol daily for 10 days, to which was then added 0·2 g quinidine thee times a day. He was later maintained on the same dose of quinidine with only 20 mg propranolol daily.[1]

Similar successes with this combined treatment have been described elsewhere. Nine out of ten responded favourably in one study,[2] 34 out of 48 in another[3]; and 13 out of 17 in yet another.[4]

Mechanism

The mechanism is by no means fully understood but these two drugs share some pharmacological characteristics (they increase the refractory period and reduce the conduction velocity of the heart muscle) which together appear to be more beneficial than quinidine in higher dosage on its own. An adrenergic blocking action has been attributed to quinidine.[5] Propanolol does not affect the absorption or the kinetics of quinidine.[6]

Importance and management

This is an advantageous, not an adverse interaction. Combined use can be exploited in the treatment of atrial fibrillation.

References
1 Stern S. Synergistic action of propranolol with quinidine. *Am Heart J* (1962) **72**, 569.
2 Stern S and Borman J B. Early conversion of atrial fibrillation after open-heart surgery by combined propranolol and quinidine treatment. *Isr J med Sci* (1969) **5**, 102.
3 Fors W J, Vanderark C R and Reynolds J W. Evaluation of propranolol and quinidine in the treatment of quinidine-resistant arrhythmias. *Amer J Cardiol* (1971) **27**, 190.
4 Stern S. Conversion of chronic atrial fibrillation to sinus rhythm with combined propranolol and quindine treatment. *Amer Heart J* (1967) **74**, 170.
5 Dreifus L S, Rabbino M D and Watanbe Y. Newer agents in the treatment of cardiac arrhythmias. *Med Clin North America* (1964) **48**, 371.
6 Kates R E and Blanford M F. Disposition kinetics of oral quinidine when administered concurrently with propranolol. *J Clin Pharmacol* (1979). **24**, 378.

Quinidine + lignocaine

Summary

A single case of sinoatrial arrest has been described in a patient taking quinidine who was also given lignocaine.

Interaction, mechanism, importance and management

A man with Parkinson's disease was given quinidine, 300 mg 6-hourly, for the control of ventricular ectopic beats. After receiving 600 mg, he was given lignocaine as well, initially a bolus of 80 mg and then an infusion of 4 mg/min because persistent premature ventricular beats developed. Within $2\frac{1}{2}$ h the patient complained of dizziness and weakness and was found to have sinus brady-cardia, SA arrest and atrioventricular escape rhythm. Normal sinus rhythm was resumed once the lignocaine was stopped. The reasons for this reaction are not understood.

Reference
1 Jeresaty R M, Kahn A H and Landry A B. Sinoatrial arrest due to lidocaine in a patient receiving quinidine. *Chest* (1972) **61,** 683.

Quinidine + rifampicin

Summary
The therapeutic effects of quinidine can be markedly reduced by the concurrent use of rifampicin.

Interaction

The observation that a patient whose ventricular dysrhythmia control with quinidine was lost when rifampicin was given, prompted a further study on four volunteers. It was found that concurrent treatment with 600 mg rifampicin daily reduced the mean half-life of the quinidine by almost 60%, and the area under the plasma concentration time curve from 20·1 to 3·4 μg/ml/hr.[1]

Mechanism

The experimental evidence from this study clearly indicated that the rifampicin (a recognized enzyme-inducing agent) increases the metabolism of the quinidine thereby hastening its removal from the body and reducing its effects.

Importance and management

Although the information is very limited, this interaction would seem to be established. The incidence is not known, but the response to quinidine should be closely monitored if rifampicin is given and suitable upwards dosage adjustments made as necessary.

Reference
1 Twum-Barima Y and Carruthers S G. Evaluation of rifampin-quinidine interaction. *Clin Pharmacol Ther* (1980) **27,** 290.

Quinidine + urinary alkalinizers (antacids, diuretics, alkaline salts)

Summary
A large rise in urinary pH due to some antacids, diuretics and alkaline salts can cause retention of quinidine which may lead to quinidine intoxication.

Interaction

Drugs which raise the urinary pH significantly and thereby reduce the excretion of quinidine may cause the development of quinidine toxicity.

A patient being treated with quinidine who took about 8 *Mylanta* tablets each day for a week (aluminium hydroxide gel 200 mg, magnesium hydroxide 200 mg) and large amounts of citrus fruit juice developed quinidine intoxication.[1]

The urinary excretion of quinidine by 4 subjects who were taking 0·2 g by mouth every 6 h was reduced by an average of 50% when the urine was made alkaline by the ingestion of sodium bicarbonate and acetazolamide (0·5 g every 12 h). For urinary pH values of less than 6 the average quinidine concentration was found to be 115 mg/l whereas for urine pH values of more than 7·5 the average concentration fell to 13 mg/l. Further studies on 6 normal subjects showed, as expected, that alkalinization of the urine raised the serum quinidine levels and this was reflected in a prolongation of the Q-T interval. For example raising the urinary pH from about 6 to 7·5 in one subject increased his serum quinidine level from about 1·6 to 2·6 μg/ml.[2]

Various antacids affect urinary pH[3] and their probable effect on quinidine excretion is discussed under 'Importance and management' below.

Mechanism
When the urine is acid, much of the quinidine within the urinary tubule filtrate is in the ionized form (which is lipid-insoluble) and unable to diffuse back into the tubule cells and so is lost in the urine. If the urine is made alkaline, much more of the quinidine is in the un-ionized (lipid-soluble) form so that it is able to diffuse back into the tubule cells and is retained. In this way the urinary pH determines the extent of the loss or retention of the quinidine and governs the serum levels. A more detailed and illustrated account of this type of interaction is described on page 9.

Importance and management
The extent to which different drugs raise the pH will determine whether this interaction reaches significant proportions. *Mylanta* (aluminium and magnesium hydroxide) in normal doses can precipitate quinidine intoxication (case cited). *Maalox* (aluminium and magnesium hydroxide) can raise the pH by 1·0 and may be expected to interact similarly. *Milk of Magnesia* (magnesium hydroxide) and *Titralac* (calcium carbonate–glycine) in normal doses raise the pH by 0·5 so that a smaller response is likely whereas *Amphogel* (aluminium hydroxide) and *Robolate* (dihydroxyaluminium glycinate) have no effect on urinary pH.[3] Acetazolamide and sodium bicarbonate can both raise the urinary pH significantly depending on the dosages used. Patients should be observed closely for any changes in their response to quinidine if these or other drugs which affect urinary pH significantly are added or withdrawn.

References
1 Zinn M B. Quinidine intoxication from alkali ingestion. *Texas med* (1970) **66**, 64.
2 Gerhardt R E, Knouss R F, Thyrium P T, Luchi R J and Morris J J. Quinidine excretion in aciduria and alkaluria. *Ann Int med* (1969) **71**, 927.
3 Gibaldi M. Effect of antacids on pH of urine. *Clin Pharmacol Ther* (1974) **16**, 520.

Verapamil + beta-blockers

Summary
Serious myocardial depression can result from the concurrent use of verapamil and beta-blocking agents in those with impairment of left ventricular function. The manufacturers of verapamil list this drug combination among their contraindications.

Interaction
Verapamil and beta-blocking drugs given together may cause serious myocardial depression.

Two patients with supraventricular tachycardias who had previously been treated with digoxin and practolol, developed ventricular asystole after being administered verapamil.[1]

An examination of the haemodynamic effects of verapamil and practolol administered intravenously alone or together in doses of 0·1 mg/kg to 10 patients, 7 with coronary heart disease and all undergoing cardiac catheterization, showed that each drug had a depressant action on the heart which together was of the order of 10–15%.[2]

Another report of an interaction between verapamil and beta-blockers has been published.[5]

Mechanism
The modes of action of the drugs are different. Verapamil is a 'calcium antagonist' which inhibits the passage of calcium ions into the heart muscle cells and this results in both a reduction in the activity of ATP and in a fall in oxygen consumption. The beta-blockers on the other hand reduce the sympathetic drive to the heart. Both therefore have a negative inotropic effect on the heart which, it would seem, is additive when they are used together. In those with some left

ventricular failure it may be large enough to depress the contraction of the ventricle completely.

Importance and management

Although there are reports of beta-blockers and verapamil having been used together in the treatment of angina,[3] concurrent treatment in those with impaired left ventricular function could be dangerous if, as the study cited above indicates[2], a 10–15% depression in myocardial function takes place.

The manufacturers of verapamil list a number of absolute contraindications to the use of verapamil (the acute stage of myocardial infarction, complete atrioventricular block, cardiogenic shock, overt heart failure), and in addition state, under the heading of 'Relative contraindications to intravenous and high dose oral therapy', that verapamil should not be injected together with a beta-adrenergic blocking agent, or within three times the half-life of that agent. Neither should the beta-blocking agent be administered within three times the half-life of verapamil.[4]

Practolol was the drug used in both reports cited above[1,2] and propranolol in the other,[5] but there is no reason to believe that this interaction is limited to these two beta-blocking drugs.

References

1 Boothby C B, Garrard C S and Pickering D. Verapamil in cardiac arrhythmias. *Br Med J* (1972) **2**, 349.
2 Seabia-Gomes R, Richards A and Sutton R. Hemodynamic effects of verapamil and practolol. *Europ J Cardiol* (1976) **4**, 79.
3 Livesley B, Catley P F, Campbell R C and Oram S. Double-blind evaluation of verapamil, propranolol, and isosorbide dinitrate against a placebo in the treatment of angina pectoris. *Br Med J* (1973) **1**, 375.
4 *Cordilox* (Abbott Laboratories Ltd). ABPI Data Sheet Compendium, p. 2 (1979–80) Abbott Laboratories Ltd.
5 Ljungström A and Åberg H. Interaktion mellan betareceptorblockerare och verapamil. *Lakartidingen* (1973) **70**, 3548.

CHAPTER 5. ANTIBIOTIC AND ANTI-INFECTIVE DRUG INTERACTIONS

The synopses in this chapter are concerned with interactions which either alter the effectiveness of the antimicrobial agent, or have some effect on their toxicity. Interactions where the antimicrobials are the affecting or interacting agent are dealt with elsewhere. A detailed listing is to be found in the Index. Tables 5.3 and 5.4 contain the proprietary and non-proprietary names of the antibiotics and anti-infective drugs in common use.

Antimicrobial agents used in combination

A subject which has been keenly debated for many years is whether or not it is desirable to use antimicrobial agents in combination. Various predictive schemes have been published and two of the well-known ones by Jawetz[1] and Kabins[2] are shown in Tables 5.1 and 5.2.

Table 5.1. The effects of combining antimicrobials

Antimicrobial combination		Result of antimicrobial combination
Group I + (bactericide)	group 1 (bactericide)	Synergism occurred most frequently in this combination
Group I + (bactericide)	group II (bacteriostat)	If group I alone kills rapidly, addition of group II may be antagonistic; if organism was resistant to group I, addition of group II may be synergistic under some circumstances
Group II + (bacteriostat)	group II (bacteriostat)	Synergism rarely occurred in this combination

One of the serious problems with schemes like these is that there is rarely a sufficient correlation between in-vitro and in-vivo studies for the former to give a thoroughly reliable indication of how antimicrobial agents will behave together in clinical practice. Virtually everyone involved in this field is at great pains to emphasize that none of these predictive schemes is any substitute for direct clinical studies.

The arguments for and against combined antimicrobial therapy

Some of the arguments in favour of using antimicrobial agents in combination are as follows. In cases of acute undiagnosed infections the presence of more than one drug

Table 5.2. Guidelines to synergistic and antagonistic antimicrobial combinations

Combination	Interaction	Organisms*	Antimicrobials
Two bactericidal agents†	Synergic	Streptococci	Penicillin and streptomycin
	Additive or indifferent	Most	Most
Two bacteriostatic agents‡	Additive or indifferent	Most	Most
	Synergistic	Many	Sulphonamides and trimethoprim
	Antagonistic	Few Gram-positive and few Gram-negative	Erythromycin and lincomycin; erythromycin and chloramphenicol; lincomycin and chloramphenicol; novobiocin and tetracycline
One bactericidal and one bacteriostatic agent	Antagonistic	Pneumococci	Penicillin and tetracycline
	Additive or indifferent	Most	Most
	Synergistic	Proteus	Polymyxins and sulphonamides
		Brucella cline	Streptomycin and tetracy
		Streptococci	Penicillin and erythromycin
		Salmonella	Ampicillin and chloramphenicol

* Includes only selected examples.

† Penicillins, cephalosporins, aminoglycosides, polymyxins.

‡ Tetracyclines, chloramphenicol, erythromycin, lincomycin, sulphonamides, novobiocin.

increases the chance that at least one effective antimicrobial is present. This may be especially important if the patient is infected by more than one organism. The possibility of the emergence of resistant organisms is decreased by the use of more than one drug, and in some cases two drugs acting at different sites may be more effective than one drug alone. It may also be that two drugs administered below their toxic thresholds may be as effective and less toxic than one drug at a higher concentration.

In contrast there are other arguments against using antimicrobials together. One serious objection is that two drugs may actually be less effective than one on its own. In theory this could arise if a bactericidal drug, which requires actively dividing cells for it to be effective, were used with a bacteriostatic drug. However, in practice this seems to be less important than might be supposed and there are relatively few well-authenticated clinical examples. Another objection is that some broad-spectrum drugs may be suboptimal for particular organisms and may inadequately control the infection. Toxic side-effects may possibly also be increased by the use of more than one drug.

The general consensus of informed opinion is that the advantages of combined antimicrobial treatment are balanced by a number of clear disadvantages, and that usually one drug alone, properly chosen, is likely to be equally effective.[3]

References

1 Jawetz E. The use of combinations of antimicrobial drugs. *Ann Rev Pharmacol* (1968) **8**, 151.

2 Kabins S A. Interactions among antibiotics and other drugs. *J Amer med Ass* (1972) **219**, 206.

3 Cohen N S. Combinations of antibiotics—an introductory review. In *Clinical use of combinations of antibiotics*, p. 1. J Klastersky (*ed*) (1975) Hodder & Stoughton, Sevenoaks.

Table 5.3. Antibiotics

Non-proprietary names	Proprietary names
Aminoglycosides	
Amikacin	*Amikin*
Dihydrostreptomycin	*Guanimycin*
Framycetin	*Soframycin*
Gentamicin	*Cidomycin, Garamycin, Genticin*
Kanamycin	*Kannasyn, Kantex*
Neomycin	
Paromomycin	*Humatin, Gabbromycin*
Sisomicin	
Streptomycin	*Crystamycin*
Tobramycin	*Nebcin*
Antifungals	
Amphotericin B	*Fungizone, Mysteclin*
Griseofulvin	*Fulcin, Grisovin*
Miconazole	
Cephalosporins	
Cefaclor	*Distaclor*
Cefamandole	*Kefadol*
Cefoxitin	*Mefoxin*
Cephalexin	*Ceporex, Keflex*
Cephacetrile	*Celospor*
Cephaloridine	*Ceporin*
Cephradine	*Eskacef, Anspor, Sefril*
Cephaloglycin	*Kafocin*
Cephalothin	*Keflin*
Cephazolin	*Kefzol*
Chloramphenicol	*Chloromycetin*
Macrolides	
Erythromycin	*Erythrocin, Erythromid, Erythroped, Ilotycin*
Triacetyloleandomycin	*Cyclamycin, Tao*
Penicillins	
Ampicillin	*Penbritin*
Carbenicillin	*Pyopen, Microcillin*
Benzylpenicillin	*Crystapen*
Phenoxymethylpenicillin (penicillin V)	*Crystapen V, V-Cil-K*
Polypeptides	
Bacitracin	*Baciguent*
Colistin	*Colomycin*
Polymyxin B	*Aerosporin*
Tetracyclines	
Chlortetracycline	*Aureomycin*
Demeclocycline	*Ledermycin, Declomycin*
Doxycycline	*Vibramycin*
Methacycline	*Rondomycin*
Oxytetracycline	*Terramycin*
Rolitetracycline	*Bristacin, Syntetrin*
Tetracycline	*Achromycin, Totomycin*
Miscellaneous	
Lincomycin	*Lincocin*
Clindamycin	*Dalacin C*
Rifampicin	*Rifadin, Rimactane*

Table 5.4. Some non-antibiotic anti-infective agents

Non-proprietary names	Proprietary names
8-Aminoquinolines	
Pamaquine	
Primaquine	
Co-trimoxazole (trimethoprim + sulphamethoxazole)	*Bactrim, Septrin*
Dapsone	*Avlosulfon*
Ethambutol	*Dexambutol, Etibi, Myambutol, Mynah*
Ethionamide	*Trescatyl, Trescator, Tubenamide*
Furazolidone	*Furoxone*
Hexamine (methenamine)	*Mandelamine*
8-Hydroxyquinoline	
Isoniazid	*INH, Isocid, Niconyl, Nydrazid, Panazid*
	Isotamine, Isotinyl etc.
Mepacrine (quinacrine)	*Atabrine, Tenicridine*
Naldixic acid	*Negram*
Nitrofurantoin	*Furadantin, Macrodantin, Cyantin, Parfuran*
	Trantoin, Furanex
p-Aminosalicyclic acid (PAS)	
Proguanil	*Paludrine, Paludrinol*
Pyrimethamine	*Daraprim, Fansidar, Maloprim, Chlorodin*
	Erbaprelina, Malocide
Quinine	
Sulphasalazine	*Salazopyrin*
Sulphonamides	
Sulphadiazine	*Adiazine, Soludiazine*
Sulphadimethoxine	*Madribon*
Sulphadimidine (-methazine, -merazine)	*Diminsul, Sulfadine*
Sulphafurazole (sulfisoxazole)	*Gantrisin*
Sulphamerazine	*Solumedine*
Sulphamethizole	*Urolucosil, Methisul*
Sulphamethoxazole (ingredient of cotrimoxazole)	
Sulphamethoxypyridazine	*Lederkyn, Midicel*
Sulphametopyrazine	*Dalysep, Kelfizin*
Sulphaphenazole	*Orisulf, Sulfabid*
Sulphasomidine	*Aristmid, Elcosine, Pepsilphen*
Sulphathiazole	*Sulfex, Thiazamide*

8-Aminoquinolines + mepacrine

Summary

Concurrent administration is said by some authorities to be contraindicated because the toxicity of the 8-aminoquinolines is increased by mepacrine (quinacrine).

Interaction, mechanism

Studies in man have shown that the toxic effects of pamaquine (methaemoglobinaemia and granulocytic neutropenia) are increased in subjects concurrently or previously treated with mepacrine.[2] Four patients given only 30 mg pamaquine with 300 mg mepacrine daily were found to have pamaquine serum levels 100% higher than other patients taking three times as much pamaquine with quinine.[1] When given 30 mg pamaquine alone the serum levels averaged 40 μg/l, whereas in the presence of 30 mg mepacrine the pamaquine levels were raised to 450 μg/l. Grossly elevated pamaquine levels were also observed as long as 3 months after the mepacrine had been stopped.[1]

Mechanism

Not fully resolved. One suggestion is that the mepacrine inhibits the enzymes concerned with the metabolic clearance of the pamaquine, thereby prolonging its stay in the body. Another idea is that the mepacrine is a persistent and potent occupier of binding sites within the body normally also used by the pamaquine. The latter is, therefore, not able to get at these sites, so the pamaquine serum levels rise sharply, accompanied by the development of toxicity.

Importance and management

Information is limited but it would appear to be an important interaction. The data cited above concern pamaquine (now superseded), but prima-quine (its successor) probably behaves similarly. Some authorities state that concurrent use is contraindicated.[3] It should also be appreciated that the interaction can also take place as long as 3 months after the withdrawal of the mepacrine. More study is needed.

References

1 Zubrod C G, Kennedy T J and Shannon J A. Studies on the chemotherapy of the human malarias. VIII. The physiological disposition of pamaquine. *J Clin Invest* (1948) 27, (*Suppl*) 114.
2 Earle D P, Bigelow F S, Zubrod C G and Kane C A. Studies on the chemotherapy of the human malarias. IX. Effect of pamaquine on the blood cells of man. *J Clin Invest* (1948) 27, (*Suppl*) 121.
3 Rollo I M. Drugs used in the chemotherapy of malaria. *In The Pharmacological Basis of Therapeutics*, 4th ed., p. 1101. Goodman L S and Gilman A. (eds) 4. (1970) Macmillan.

Amphotericin + corticosteroids

Summary

Both amphotericin and the corticosteroids cause potassium loss which can have adverse effects on cardiac function.

Interaction

The potassium loss induced by both amphotericin and the corticosteroids is well recognized and well documented. Their additive effects on potassium depletion, associated with corticosteroid-induced sodium retention were probably the cause of the congestive heart failure and cardiac enlargement described in three patients under concurrent treatment.[1] Close monitoring of electrolyte levels is important if both drugs are used together, particularly in the elderly where cardiac function may already be impaired.

Reference

3 Rollo I M. Drugs used in the chemotherapy of malaria. In *The* during treatment with amphotericin B and hydrocortisone. Report of three cases. *Am Rev Resp Dis* (1971) 103, 831.

Amphotericin + digitalis glycosides

Summary

Amphotericin causes potassium loss which could lead to the development of digitalis toxicity.

Interaction

Among the well-recognized adverse side-effects of amphotericin treatment is increased potassium loss. In one report the serum potassium levels of a patient fell to 2·8 mEq/l accompanied by classical ECG changes.[1] Another patient showed a serum potassium fall to 0·8 mEq/l.[1] Further reports describe hypokalaemia and ECG changes following the use of amphotericin.[2,3] It would be logical to conclude from this that digitalis toxicity could develop in patients under treatment with both drugs if the potassium levels were allowed to fall unchecked, since hypokalaemia enhances the actions of the digitalis glycosides.

References

1 Sandford W G, Rasch J R and Stonehill A. A therapeutic dilemma. The treatment of disseminated coccidioidomycosis with amphotericin B. *Ann Int Med* (1962) **56**, 553.

2 Holeman C W and Einstein H. The toxic effects of amphotericin B in man. *Californ Med* (1963) **99**, 290.

3 Butler W T, Bennett J E, Hill G J, Szwed C F and Cotlove E. Electrocardiographic and electrolyte abnormalities caused by amphotericin B in dog and man. *Proc Soc Exp biol Med* (1964) **116**, 857.

Amphotericin + miconazole

Summary

A report indicates that miconazole and amphotericin may possibly have antagonistic antifungal effects.

Interaction

Some limited evidence from studies in a few patients and from in-vitro experiments suggests that the antimycotic effects of miconazole and amphotericin (amphotericin B) may be antagonistic.[1] The reasons are not understood. Until more is known it would seem prudent to avoid their concurrent use whenever possible.

Reference

1 Schachter L P, Owellen R J, Rathbun H K and Buchanan B. Antagonism between miconazole and amphotericin B. *Lancet* (1976) **ii**, 318.

Aminoglycosides + amphotericin

Summary

Nephrotoxicity attributed to the concurrent use of gentamicin and amphotericin has been described in four patients.

Interaction, mechanism, importance and management

Four patients under treatment with moderate doses of gentamicin and amphotericin B showed renal deterioration attributed to their concurrent use.[1] Both antibiotics in sufficiently high doses are known to be nephrotoxic and it is suggested that low doses of each may be additive.[1] The documentation of this interaction appears to be limited to this one report. Until more is known it would be prudent to monitor renal function carefully if these two antibiotics are used together.

Reference

1 Churchill D N and Seeley J. Nephrotoxicity associated with combined gentamicin–amphotericin B therapy. *Nephron* (1977) **19**, 176.

Aminoglycosides + cephalexin

Summary

Hypokalaemia has been described in patients treated concurrently with cephalexin and gentamicin.

Interaction, mechanism, importance and management

A report[1] describes 11 patients, most of them taking cytotoxic drugs for leukaemia, 9 of whom showed hypokalaemia after treatment with 1 g cephalexin 6-hourly and 80 mg gentamicin 8-hourly. Whether this was due to the gentamicin alone or to the combined effects of all the drugs is not known. It would be prudent to monitor serum potassium levels if these drugs are used together.

Reference

1 Young G P, Sullivan J and Hurley A. Hypokalaemia due to gentamicin/cephalexin in leukaemia. *Lancet* (1973) ii, 855.

Aminoglycosides + cephalothin

Summary

The nephrotoxic effects of gentamicin and tobramycin are increased by the concurrent use of cephalothin. Whether other aminoglycoside/cephalosporin combinations are also nephrotoxic is uncertain.

Interaction

The probability of nephrotoxicity is markedly increased if gentamicin or tobramycin are given with cephalothin.

> A comparative randomized double-blind trial carried out on a large number of patients with sepsis showed that the incidence of definite nephrotoxicity when treated with gentamicin or tobramycin, with either cephalothin or methicillin, was as follows: gentamicin + cephalothin, 30% (7 out of 23); tobramycin + cephalothin, 21% (5 out of 24); gentamicin + methicillin, 10% (2 out of 20); and tobramycin + methicillin, 4% (1 out of 23).[1]

These results support a number of studies and case reports of nephrotoxicity attributed to the concurrent use of gentamicin with cephalothin[3,4,7-14] or tobramycin with cephalothin.[6] A retrospective study of data collected by the Boston Collaborative Drug Surveillance Program showed that rises in blood urea nitrogen (BUN) were 9·3% for those on gentamicin + cephalothin (247 patients), 6·0% for those on gentamicin alone (334 patients) and 2·0% for those on cephalothin alone (492 patients).[2]

Mechanism

Uncertain. The nephrotoxic effects of gentamicin, tobramycin and the cephalosporins are well documented, and it is generally believed that these effects are additive during concurrent use. Doses which are well tolerated separately can be nephrotoxic when given together.[3]

Importance and management

A very well-documented and potentially serious interaction. There are other reports not listed here. Concurrent use is not contraindicated but special attention should be paid to the dosage selection, and kidney function should be closely monitored for evidence of nephrotoxicity. Information about adverse reactions with other aminoglycosides and cephalosporins appears to be lacking. The incidence of nephrotoxicity with combinations of either gentamicin or tobramycin with methicillin is low (cited above[1]). Tobramycin with clindamycin is reported[5] not to be nephrotoxic although the numbers involved in the study were relatively small.

References

1 Wade J C, Smith C R, Petty B G, Lipsky J J, Conrad G, Ellner J and Lietman P S. Cephalothin plus an aminoglycoside is more nephrotoxic than methicillin plus an aminoglycoside. *Lancet* (1978) ii, 604.

2 Fanning W L. Gump D and Jick H. Gentamicin- and Cephalothin-associated rises in blood urea nitrogen. *Antimicrob Ag Chemother* (1976) 10, 80.

3 Tvedgaard E. Interaction between gentamicin and cephalothin as cause of acute renal failure. *Lancet* (1976) ii, 581.

4 Plager J E. Association of renal injury with combined cephalothin–gentamicin therapy among patients severely ill with malignant disease. *Cancer* (1976) 37, 1937.

5 Gillett P, Wise R, Melikian V and Falk R. Tobramycin/cephalothin nephrotoxicity. *Lancet* (1976) i, 547.

6 Tobias J S, Whitehouse J M and Wrigley P F M. Severe renal dysfunction after tobramycin/cephalothin therapy. *Lancet* (1976) i, 425.

7 Cabanillas F, Burgos R C, Rodriguez R C and Baldizón C. Nephrotoxicity of combined cephalothin–gentamicin regimen. *Arch Intern Med* (1975) 135, 850.

8 Ewald U and Jernelius H. Njurinsufficiens vid behandling med antibiotikakombinationen cefalotin-gentamycin. *Lakartid* (1974) 71, 2595.

9 Kleinknecht D, Ganeval D and Droz D. Acute renal failure after high doses of gentamicin and cephalothin. *Lancet* (1973) i, 1129.

10 Fillastre J P, Laumonier R, Humbert G, Dubois D, Metayer J,

Delpech A, Leroy J. and Robert M. Acute renal failure associated with combined gentamicin and cephalothin therapy. *Brit Med J* (1973) 2, 396.

11 Zazgornik J, Schmidt P, Lugscheider R and Kopsa H. Akutes Nierenversagen bei kombinierter Cephaloridin–Gentamycin-Therapie. *Wien klin Wschr* (1973) 85, 839.

12 Bobrow S N, Jaffe E. and Young R C. Anuria and acute

tubular necrosis associated with gentamicin and cephalothin. *J Amer med Ass* (1972) 222, 1546.

13 Noone P, Pattison J R and Shafi M S. Renal failure in combined gentamicin and cephalothin therapy. *Brit Med J* (1973) 2, 777.

14 Stille W. Indikationen und Gefahren der kombinierten Cephalotin–Gentamycin-Therapie. *Adv Clin Pharmacol* (1973) 8, 54.

Aminoglycosides + clindamycin

Summary

Three cases of acute renal failure have been tentatively attributed to the concurrent use of gentamicin and clindamycin.

Interaction

Three patients with normal renal function who were given 3·9–4·8 mg/kg/day gentamicin for 13–18 days with 0·9–1·8 g/day clindamycin for 7–13 days, developed acute renal failure. They recovered within 3–5 days of discontinuing the antibiotics.[1]

Mechanism

Not known. Gentamicin-induced nephrotoxicity is a recognized reaction. It is possible that clindamycin displaces gentamicin from protein binding sites, thereby enhancing effects.[2] Clindamycin has also been shown to produce lysosomal changes in the renal cells of rats which are similar to those produced by gentamicin.[3]

Importance and management

The documentation is limited to this one report. Until more is known it would clearly be prudent to monitor the renal function carefully if these two antibiotics are used together. Tobramycin with clindamycin is reported not to be nephrotoxic.[4]

References

1 Butkus D E, de Torrente A and Terman D S. Renal failure following gentamicin in combination with clindamycin. Gentamicin nephrotoxicity. *Nephron* (1976) 17, 307.

2 Pyke R E. Quoted as personnal communication in[1].

3 Gray J E, Purmalis A, Purmalis B and Mathews J. Ultrastructural studies of the hepatic changes brought about by clindamycin in animals. *Toxicol Appl Pharmacol* (1971) 19, 217.

4 Gillett P, Wise R, Melikian V and Falk R. Tobramycin/cephalothin nephrotoxicity. *Lancet* (1976) i, 547.

Aminoglycosides + dimenhydrinate

Summary

It has been suggested that dimenhydrinate (diphenhydramine) may undesirably mask the otoxic effects of streptomycin and other aminoglycoside antibiotics.

Interaction, mechanism, importance and management

Dimenhydrinate can block the dizziness, nausea and vomiting which can occur during treatment with streptomycin.[1,2] However Searle, the manufacturers of dimenhydrinate warn that '. . . caution should be used when *Dramamine* (dimenhydrinate) is given in conjunction with certain antibiotics which may cause ototoxicity, since *Dramamine* is capable of masking ototoxic symptoms and an irreversible state may be reached.[1,3]

There seems to be no clinical evidence to confirm this, but there would seem to be an obvious hazard in not taking sufficient notice of the warning signs of developing ototoxicity with streptomycin or any other aminoglycoside.

References

1 Titche L L and Nady A. Control of vestibular toxic effects of streptomycin by Dramamine. *Dis Chest* (1950) 18, 386.

2 Cohen A C and Glinsky G C. Hypersensitivity to streptomycin. *J. Allergy* (1951) 22, 63.

3 *Physicians Desk Reference*, p. 1246 (1972). Medical Economics Inc., USA.

Aminoglycosides + ethacrynic acid

Summary

The concurrent use of ethacrynic acid and the aminoglycoside antibiotics should be avoided because their ototoxic effects are additive. Intravenous administration and the existence of renal impairment are additional causative factors. Even sequential administration is not safe.

Interaction

Concurrent and even sequential treatment with ethacrynic acid and aminoglycoside antibiotics increases the incidence of ototoxicity.

Four patients are described in one report[1] all of whom had some renal impairment and who became permanently deaf after treatment with 1·0–1·5 g kanamycin and 50–150 mg ethacrynic acid. One of the patients was given the two drugs 2 h apart and was deaf within 30 min. Another showed deafness which took almost a fortnight to develop. He was given kanamycin on the first and fifth days of treatment and ethacrynic acid on the second.

There are other reports describing partial or total permanent deafness as a result of giving ethacrynic acid with kanamycin,[3] streptomycin,[2] or neomycin.[2]

In some instances the patient was treated with two or even more of the aminoglycoside antibiotics.

Mechanism

Both the aminoglycoside antibiotics and ethacrynic acid given singly can damage the ear and cause deafness. The site of action of the aminoglycosides would seem to be at the hair cell and that of ethacrynic acid at the stria vascularis.[7]

The aminoglycosides damage the outer hair cells in the basal turn of the organ of Corti, and with continuous administration this damage spreads towards the apex and eventually affects all the outer hair cells.[5] Various biochemical and electrophysiological changes accompany this damage.[6] Ethacrynic acid has been shown to cause swelling of the intermediate cell layer of the stria vascularis (in guinea pigs)[8] and to decrease the ability of the cochlear to generate the alternating current cochlear potential.[7]

A study using guinea pigs showed that using concentrations of kanamycin and ethacrynic acid which, on their own, would have had no ototoxic effects (except after prolonged treatment), when given together produced measurable toxic effects on the ear and that the effects seemed to be additive.[5] Permanent hair cell destruction can occur.[9] But the precise details of how this additive toxicity actually occurs has not been elucidated.

Importance and management

An established interaction. The administration of ethacrynic acid to patients on aminoglycoside antibiotics should be avoided because permanent deafness can result. The ototoxic effects of both drugs are additive so that the use of doses which are normally regarded as safe can result in ear damage. Patients with renal damage appear to be particularly at risk, presumably because the drugs are less rapidly cleared and continue to exert their toxic effects. Most of the reports describe deafness after the intravenous administration of ethacrynic acid and the aminoglycosides, but there are reports of damage resulting from the drugs being given orally. There is also evidence that damage can occur not only during simultaneous use of the two drugs, but also if the ethacrynic acid is given after exposure to the antibiotic.[7]

These are all good reasons for avoiding these drugs, but if it is absolutely necessary to use them, their dosages should be kept as low as possible and regular checks on hearing should be carried out.

Not every aminoglycoside has been implicated in this interaction, but their ototoxicity is clearly established and they may be expected to interact in a similar way.

References

1 Johnson A H and Hamilton C A. Kanamycin ototoxicity—possible potentiation by other drugs. S Med J (1970) 63, 511.
2 Mathog R H and Klein W J. Ototoxicity of ethacrynic acid and aminoglycoside antibiotics in uremia. New Eng J Med (1969) 280, 1223.
3 Ng P S, Conley C E and Ing T S. Deafness after ethacrynic acid. Lancet (1969) i, 673.
4 Meriwether W D, Mangi K J and Serpick A A. Deafness following standard intravenous dose of ethacrynic acid. J Amer med Ass (1971) 216, 795.
5 Prazma J, Browder J P and Fischer N D. Ethacrynic acid ototoxicity potentiation by kanamycin. Ann Oto-rhino-laryng (1974) 83, 111.
6 Iinuma T, Mizukoshi O, Daly J F. Possible effects of various ototoxic drugs upon the ATP-hydrolyzing system in the stria vascularis and spiral ligament of the guinea pig. Laryngoscope (1967) 77, 159.

7 Mathog R H and Capps M J. Ototoxic interactions of ethacrynic acid and streptomycin. *Ann Otol Rhinol Laryngol* (1977) **86**, 158.

8 Quick C A and Duvall A J. Early changes in the cochlear duct from ethacrynic acid: an electron microscopic evaluation. *Laryngoscope* (1970) **80**, 954.

9 West B A, Brummett R E and Himes D L. Interaction of kanamycin and ethacrynic acid. *Arch Otolaryngol* (1973) **98**, 32.

Aminoglycosides + frusemide

Summary

The development of ototoxicity may possibly be enhanced by the concurrent use of high doses of frusemide and gentamicin in patients with renal failure.

Interaction

Nineteen patients with acute renal failure were treated with gentamicin (serum levels maintained below 8 μg/ml) and a continuous infusion of frusemide at a dose of 1 g every 8 h. Two of them suffered permanent and severe deafness.[1]

Seven out of a total of 281 patients with chronic renal failure developed otological symptoms which appeared to have resulted from the concurrent use of gentamicin (in normally subtoxic doses) and frusemide (200 mg average dose).[2]

Mechanism

Not known. Ototoxicity has been associated with the use of both drugs used singly. The rapid infusion of frusemide in man in doses of $0 \cdot 5$–$3 \cdot 0$ g has resulted in transient deafness,[3,4] and permanent deafness has also been described.[5] The ototoxicity of the aminoglycosides is very well documented and appears to be dose-related.[1]

One study[6] carried out in man showed that when used together the plasma clearance of gentamicin was reduced about 30% by 10 mg frusemide given intravenously. This would result in a rise in serum gentamicin levels and if the concentrations were already high, might be expected to lead to ototoxic serum levels. A study of this interaction in guinea pigs using another aminoglycoside, kanamycin, with frusemide showed that doses of both which singly had little or not toxic effects caused permanent ear damage when used together.[7]

Importance and management

Not, by any means, extensively documented.

Since both the aminoglycosides and frusemide singly show ototoxicity, the clinical evidence for this interaction is by no means conclusive, but there is enough data to indicate that an increase in the incidence of otoxicity is a distinct possibility if gentamicin and frusemide are used together. It should, however, be emphasized that it has only been seen in those who have grossly impaired renal function and who are receiving relatively high doses of one or both drugs. Whether it also occurs with frusemide and aminoglycosides other than gentamicin is not known, but there are reports of enhanced ototoxicity with another potent diuretic, ethacrynic acid, when combined with kanamycin, streptomycin and neomycin (see p. 77). This should act as a warning.

References

1 Brown C B, Ogg C S, Cameron J S and Bewick M. High dose frusemide in acute reversible intrinsic renal failure. *Scot med. J* (1974) **19**, 35.

2 Thomsen J, Bech P and Szpirt W. Otological symptoms in chronic renal failure. The possible rôle of aminoglycoside–furosemide interaction. *Arch Oto-Rhino-Laryng* (1976) **214**, 71.

3 Schwartz G H, David D S, Riggio R R, Stenzel K H and Rubin A L. Ototoxicity induced by furosemide. *New Eng J Med* (1970) **282**, 1413.

4 Venkateswaran P S. Transient deafness from high doses of frusemide. *Brit Med J* (1971) **4**, 113.

5 Quick C A and Hoppe W. Permanent deafness associated with furosemide administration. *Ann Oto-rhino-laryng* (1975) **84**, 94.

6 Lawson D H, Tilstone W J and Semple P F. Furosemide interactions: studies in normal volunteers. *Clin Res* (1976) **24**, 3.

7 Brummett R E, Traynor J, Brown R and Himes D. Cochlear damage resulting from kanamycin and furosemide. *Acta Otolaryngol* (1975) **80**, 86.

Aminoglycosides + penicillins

Summary

The serum levels of phenoxymethylpenicillin (pencillin V) following oral dosage can be halved by the concurrent use of neomycin. Whether kanamycin interacts similarly is not known.

Interaction

In a study on 5 normal volunteers it was shown that the administration of 12 g neomycin daily reduced the serum concentrations of phenoxymethyl penicillin, following 250 mg oral doses, by 50%, a return to normal not being achieved until 6 days after the withdrawal of the neomycin.[1]

Mechanism

Uncertain, but it would seem probable that it is related to the reversible malabsorption syndrome which can be caused by neomycin.

Importance and management

The documentation is very limited, but the interaction appears to be established. Parenteral administration of the penicillin or an increase in the oral dosage would seem to be a reasonable solution to the problem, but there is no warrant in the literature to confirm that this is effective. Kanamycin can induce a malabsorption state to a lesser extent than neomycin, but it is not certain whether it also interacts with phenoxymethyl-penicillin. Information about other penicillins is lacking.

Reference

1 Cheng S H and White A. Effect of orally administered neomycin on the absorption of penicillin V. *New Eng J Med* (1962) **267**, 1296.

Aminoglycosides + ticarcillin or carbenicillin

Summary

Gentamicin, sisomicin and tobramycin are inactivated if mixed in intravenous fluids with ticarcillin or carbenicillin. Gentamicin serum levels are markedly reduced by these two penicillins in patients with renal failure, but not in those with normal renal function. There is some evidence that amikacin may not interact.

Interaction

(a) Gentamicin, sisomicin and tobramycin are inactivated by carbenicillin or ticarcillin in-vitro, and (b) some inactivation also occurs in vivo in patients with severe renal impairment, but (c) no interaction of importance occurs in vivo in patients with normal renal function.

(a) Aminoglycosides + penicillins in-vitro

In-vitro studies with a solution of gentamicin, 5 μg/ml, and carbenicillin, 200 μg/ml, showed that the gentamicin became inactivated. These studies were undertaken to check on clinical observations of suspected inactivation.[1]

Similar observations of inactivation have been described in other reports concerning carbenicillin with gentamicin,[2-6] sisomicin[5] or tobramycin,[5] and ticarcillin with gentamicin,[5,6] sisomicin[5] or tobramycin.[5]

(b) Aminoglycosides + penicillins in patients with renal failure

A study on 6 patients with severe renal failure who were receiving carbenicillin (1·5–15 g daily), administered in divided doses three to six times daily by rapid intravenous infusion, showed that the presence of the penicillin prevented the achievement of serum gentamicin levels above 4 μg/ml even though large doses were given.[7] A similar interaction was observed with carbenicillin and tobramycin.[7]

Other reports similarly describe the interaction of carbenicillin with gentamicin[2,6] and gentamicin with ticarcillin.[6] A reduction in gentamicin half-life to about a half or one-third has been described as well.[6,9]

(c) Aminoglycosides + penicillins in patients with normal renal function

A patient with normal renal function was given 80 mg gentamicin intravenously, with and without 4 g carbenicillin. The serum concentration profiles in both cases were very similar, with only a fraction depression due to the carbenicillin.[2]

Mechanism

Carbenicillin and ticarcillin interact chemically with these aminoglycoside antibiotics to form biologically inactive amides between the amino groups on the aminoglycosides, and the beta-lactam ring on the penicillins.[8] Thus both antibiotics are inactivated.

Importance and management

A very well-documented interaction of practical importance. Only a selection of the reports has been listed here. Gentamicin, sisomicin and tobramycin should not be mixed with carbenicillin or ticarcillin in infusion fluids before administration because inactivation occurs.

There is no contraindication to their concurrent use in patients with normal renal function because in-vivo inactivation appears not to occur. Moreover there is good clinical evidence that concurrent use is therapeutically useful in the treatment of *Pseudomonas* infections.[2,10]

An adverse interaction occurs in patients with renal failure. Where concurrent use is thought necessary, it has been recommended that the dosage of the pencillin should be adjusted to renal function and the serum levels of both closely monitored.[7] In-vitro evidence indicates that little or no interaction of importance occurs in serum between amikacin and ticarcillin or carbenicillin.[5]

Interactions between other aminoglycosides and pencillins appear not to have been documented, apart from neomycin and phenoxymethylpenicillin (see previous synopsis).

References

1 McLaughlin J E and Reeves D S. Clinical and laboratory evidence for the inactivation of gentamicin by carbenicillin. *Lancet* (1971) i, 261.
2 Eykyn S, Phillips I and Ridley M. Gentamicin plus carbenicillin. *Lancet* (1971) i, 545.
3 Levison M E and Kaye D. Carbenicillin plus gentamicin. *Lancet* (1971) ii, 45.
4 Lynn B. Carbenicillin plus gentamicin. *Lancet* (1971) i, 653.
5 Holt H A, Broughall J M, McCarthy M and Reeves D S. Interactions between aminoglycoside antibiotics and carbenicillin or ticarcillin. *Infection* (1976) 4, 109.
6 Davies M, Morgan J R and Anand C. Interactions of carbenicillin and ticarcillin with gentamicin. *Antimicrob Ag Chemother* (1975) 7, 431.
7 Weibert R, Keane W and Shapiro F. Carbenicillin inactivation of aminoglycosides in patients with severe renal failure. *Trans Amer Soc Artif Int Organs* (1976) 22, 439.
8 Perenyi T, Graber H and Arr M. Uber die Wechselwirkung der Penizilline und Aminoglycosid-Antibiotika. *Int J Clin Pharmacol Therap and Toxicol* (1974) 10, 50.
9 Riff L J and Jackson G G. Laboratory and clinical conditions for gentamicin activation by carbenicillin. *Arch Intern Med* (1972) 130, 887.
10 Kluge R M, Standiford H C, Tatem B, Young V M, Schimpff S C, Greene W H, Calia F M and Hornick R B. The carbenicillin–gentamicin combination against *pseudomonas aeruginosa*. Correlation of effect with gentamicin sensitivity. *Ann Intern Med* (1974) 81, 584.

Cephalosporins + colistin sulphomethate sodium (colistimethate sodium)

Summary

Four cases of renal failure have been attributed to the concurrent use of cephalothin and colistin sulphomethate sodium.

Interaction

Acute renal failure has been described in 4 patients during treatment with colistin sulphomethate sodium. Three of them were given cephalothin concurrently and the fourth had been previously treated with this antibiotic.[1] The reason for this adverse reaction is not known. Information on this interaction is very sparse, but what is available indicates that renal function should be closely checked if concurrent or sequential treatment with these antibiotics is undertaken.[2]

References

1 Adler S and Segel D P. Nonoliguric renal failure secondary to sodium colistimethate. A report of four cases. *Amer J Med Sci* (1971) 262, 109.
2 Koch-Weser J, Sidel V W, Federman E B, Kanarek P, Finer D C, and Eaton A E. Adverse effects of sodium colistimethate. Manifestations and specific reaction rates during 317 courses of therapy. *Ann Intern Med* (1970) 72, 875.

Cephalosporins + frusemide

Summary

The nephrotoxic effects of cephaloridine may be increased by the concurrent use of frusemide. Cefoxitin may be a suitable alternative.

Interaction

A clinical observation was made that out of 36 cases of acute renal failure in patients receiving cephaloridine, 9 had also been treated with a diuretic, and 7 of those had had frusemide. Other factors such as age and dosage may also have been involved, but the authors related their report to previous animal studies which showed that potent diuretics such as frusemide and ethacrynic acid, enhanced the incidence and extent of tubular necrosis.[1,2]

Several other reports describe nephrotoxicity in patients given both drugs.[3,4,6]

Mechanism

Not understood. Cephaloridine alone is nephrotoxic. A study in 14 patients showed that frusemide increased the serum half-life of cephaloridine by about 25%[8] but why this should happen and the extent to which it might influence the increase in nephrotoxicity is not understood. Another study confirmed that the clearance of cephaloridine is reduced by frusemide.[7] One theory is that it might be related in some way to the acute contraction of the extracellular fluid space which is induced by the diuretic, or the rapid rise in plasma renin activity after their administration.[2]

Importance and management

The data are limited, but the interaction appears to be established. It is clearly potentially serious. It would seem wise to avoid concurrent use wherever possible, particularly in those with renal disease and the elderly. If concurrent use is unavoidable, high dosages should be avoided and a frequent check made on renal function. A possible alternative cephalosporin is cefoxitin which, from studies in man, appears to be relatively free of nephrotoxicity alone or in combination with frusemide.[5] Whether frusemide interacts adversely with some of the other cephalosporins is uncertain, but enhanced nephrotoxicity has been described in animal studies using cephalothin and cephacetrile.[9,10]

References

1 Foord R D. Cephaloridine and the kidney. *Proc VIth Int Cong Chemotherap, Tokyo* (1969) **i**, 597.

2 Dodds M G and Foord R D. Enhancement by potent diuretics of renal tubular necrosis induced by cephaloridine. *Brit J Pharmacol* (1970) **40**, 227.

3 Simpson I J. Nephrotoxicity and acute renal failure associated with cephalothin and cephaloridine. *NZ Med J* (1971) **74**, 312.

4 Kleinknecht D, Jungers P and Fillastre J-P. Nephrotoxicity of cephaloridine. *Ann Intern Med* (1974) **80**, 421.

5 Trollfors B. Effects on renal function of treatment with cefoxin alone or in combination with furosemide. *Scand J Inf Dis* (1978) (*Suppl*) **13**, 73.

6 Lawson D H, Macadam R F, Singh H, Gavras H and Linton A L. The nephrotoxicity of cephaloridine. *Postgrad med J* (1970) **46** (*Suppl*) 36.

7 Lawson D H, Tilstone W J and Semple P F. Furosemide interactions; studies in normal volunteers. *Clin Res* (1976) **24**, 3.

8 Norrby R, Stenqvist K and Elgefors B. Interaction between cephaloridine and furosemide in man. *Scand J Inf Dis* (1976) **8**, 209.

9 Lawson D H, Macadam R F, Singh H, Gavras H, Hartz S, Turnbull D and Linton A. Effect of furosemide on antibiotic-induced renal damage in rats. *J Inf Dis* (1972) **126**, 593.

10 Luscombe D K and Nichols P J. Possible interaction between cephacetrile and frusemide in rabbits and rats. *J Antimicrob Chemother* (1972) **i**, 67.

Cephalosporins + probenecid

Summary

Cephalosporin serum levels are markedly raised by probenecid. Possibly an advantageous interaction in the treatment of some conditions, but it may also represent a potentially hazardous interaction with cephaloridine or cephalothin which can be nephrotoxic.

Interaction

A study undertaken with 10 normal subjects who were given single 500 g oral doses of cephradine or cefaclor showed that the concurrent administration of probenecid (500 mg doses taken 25, 13 and 2 h before the antibiotic) markedly raised the serum concentrations of both cephalosporins. Peak concentrations were very roughly doubled.[1]

Probenecid similarly raises the serum levels of cephaloridine,[2] cefazolin[3] cephacetrile,[4] cephradine,[5] cephaloglycin,[6] cephalothin,[7] cefamandole[8] cefoxitin[9] and cephalexin.[10]

Mechanism

Largely, but not totally, understood. Probenecid inhibits the excretion of the cephalosporins by the kidney tubules, as it does penicillin. A fuller explanation of this interaction mechanism is given on page 10. Thus the cephalosporin is retained in the body and the serum levels rise. However, the extent of the rise cannot be fully accounted for by this mechanism and it has been suggested that some change in tissue distribution may also have a part to play.[1]

Importance and management

An extremely well-documented interaction, only some of the representative references being listed here. Serum levels of the cephalosporin will be much higher if probenecid is used. This has been exploited in the treatment of gonorrhoea with cephalexin, for example. However, elevated serum levels of some cephalosporins, in particular cephaloridine and cephalothin, carry the risk of nephrotoxicity.

References

1 Welling P G, Dean S, Selen A, Kendall M J and Wise R. Probenecid: an unexplained effect on cephalosporin pharmacology. *Br J clin Pharmac* (1979) **8**, 491.

2 Kaplan K, Reisberg B E and Weinstein L. Cephaloridine: antimicrobial activity and pharmacologic behaviour. *Amer J Med Sci* (1967) **253**, 667.

3 Duncan W C. Treatment of gonorrhoea with cefazolin plus probenecid. *J Infect Dis* (1974) **120**, 398.

4 Wise R and Reeves D S. Pharmacological studies on cephacetrile in human volunteers. *Curr Med Res Opin* (1974) **2**, 249.

5 Mischler T W, Sugerman A A, Willard S A, Bannick L J and Neiss E S. Influence of probenecid and food on the bioavailability of cephradine in normal male subjects. *J Clin Pharmacol* (1974) **14**, 604.

6 Applestein J M, Crosby E B, Johnson W D and Kaye D. In-vitro antimicrobial activity and human pharmacology of cephaloglycin. *Appl Microbiol* (1968) **16**, 1006.

7 Tuano S B, Brodie J L and Kirby W M M. Cephaloridine versus cephalothin: relation of the kidney to blood level differences after parenteral administration. *Antimicrob Ag Chemother* (1966) **101**.

8 Griffith R S, Black H R, Brier G L and Wolney J D. Effect of probenecid on the blood levels and urinary excretion of cefamandole. *Antimicrob Ag Chemother* (1977) **11**, 809.

9 Bint A J, Reeves D S and Holt H A. Effect of probenecid on serum cefoxitin concentrations. *J Antimicrob Chemotherap* (1977) **3**, 627.

10 Taylor W A and Holloway W J. Cephalexin in the treatment of gonorrhoea. *Int J Clin Pharmacol* (1972) **6**, 7.

Chloramphenicol + paracetamol

Summary

The half-life of chloramphenicol is prolonged by paracetamol (acetaminophen) which might be expected to increase the toxic effects of the antibiotic.

Interaction

Following an initial observation that the half-life of chloramphenicol in children with kwashiorkor was prolonged by paracetamol, a study was carried out on 6 adults who were given 1 g chloramphenicol and 100 mg paracetamol intravenously. The half-life of the chloramphenicol was found to have increased from 3·25 to 15 h.[1]

Mechanism

Not known. The authors of the report suggest that it might be because some competitive metabolism takes place between two compounds.[1]

Importance and management

The results of experimental observations like these cannot be uncritically applied directly to the situation where both drugs are given orally. However, since chloramphenicol can cause a reversible form of marrow depression which is dose-related and takes place when concentrations reach the 25–35 μg/ml range, there would seem to be a potential hazard in using paracetamol. Until more is known, it would seem prudent to avoid using these two drugs together. More study is needed.

Reference

1 Buchanan N and Moodley G P. Interaction between chloramphenicol and paracetamol. *Brit Med J* (1979) **2**, 307.

Chloramphenicol + penicillins

Summary

Antagonism between these antibiotics has been described in a single case of *Staphylococcus aureus* endocarditis, and in experimental pneumococcal meningitis in dogs. In contrast, no antagonism and even additive antibiotic effects have been described in other infections.

Interactions

(a) Antibiotic antagonism

A man with acute *Staphylococcus aureus* endocarditis showed clinical deterioration and positive blood culture when chloramphenicol was added to methicillin. The patient's serum inhibited the infecting organism at a dilution of 1 in 64, but was not bactericidal even at 1 in 2. After withdrawal of the chloramphenicol, methicillin alone was successful. The patient's serum was then still inhibitory at 1 in 64, but had become bactericidal at 1 in 32.[4]

Antagonism has also been described in experimental pneumococcal meningitis in dogs.[1]

(b) Lack of antagonism, and increased antibiotic effects

A report claims that no antagonism was seen in 65 of 66 patients given chloramphenicol and benzylpenicillin for bronchitis or bronchopneumonia[2]; and a further report states that ampicillin with chloramphenicol was more effective than chloramphenicol alone in the treatment of typhoid.[3]

Mechanisms

By no means fully understood. Chloramphenicol inhibits bacterial protein synthesis and can change an actively growing bacterial colony into a static one. Thus the effects of a bactericide, such as penicillin, which interferes with cell wall synthesis, are blunted, and the death of the organism occurs more slowly. This would seem to explain the antagonism seen with some organisms. Chloramphenicol is bactericidal against *Haemophilus influenzae* and meningococci.[5]

Importance and management

Cases of antagonism between chloramphenicol and the penicillins appear to be rare. There is not only inadequate evidence to impose a general prohibition on their concurrent use, but also (depending on the organism) good evidence to suggest that they can sometimes be used together with advantage.

The authors of the report describing antagonism in the treatment of pneumococcal meningitis in dogs[1] point out that, where the diagnosis of the meningitis is still not clear and chloramphenicol may be thought to be necessary because the condition may be due to *H. influenzae* or one of the enterobacteriaceae, it would seem reasonable to use penicillin or other bactericide first of all, withholding treatment with the bacteriostat for at least one hour.

References

1. Wallace J F, Smith R H, Garcia M and Petersdorf R G. Studies on the pathogenesis of meningitis. VI. Antagonism between penicillin and chloramphenicol in experimental pneumococcal meningitis. *J Lab Clin Med* (1967) **70**, 408.
2. Ardalan P. Zur Frage des Antagonismus von Penicillin und Chloramphenicolus Klinischer sicht. *Prax. Pneumol* (1969) **23**, 722.
3. De Ritis F, Giammanco G and Manzillo G. Chloramphenicol combined with ampicillin in the treatment of typhoid. *Brit Med J* (1972) **4**, 17.
4. Percival A. In *Antibiotic Interactions*, p. 26, Williams J D (ed), (1979) Academic Press.

Chloramphenicol + phenobarbitone

Summary

Each can affect the serum levels of the other. Two children treated with the maximum recommended dosage of chloramphenicol showed grossly depressed serum levels during treatment with phenobarbitone. A single case report describes markedly elevated serum phenobarbitone levels during concurrent treatment with chloramphenicol.

Interaction

Each can interfere with the serum concentrations of the other: (a) the serum levels of chloramphenicol can be lowered by phenobarbitone, and (b) the serum levels of phenobarbitone can be raised by chloramphenicol

(b) Effect of phenobarbitone on serum chloramphenicol concentrations

Two children, one of 7 months and the other of 3 months, were given 100 mg/kg/day chloramphenicol, initially intravenously but later orally, for the treatment of *Haemophilus influenzae* meningitis. At the same time they were administered phenobarbitone (10 mg/kg/day) to prevent convulsions. Despite these high doses of chloramphenicol, (the maximum recommended) which would normally maintain peak blood levels within the range 15–25 mg/l, both children showed depressed serum levels within a few days of beginning concurrent treatment. The first child had serum chloramphenicol levels of 5 mg/l or less until the chloramphenicol dosage was doubled when they rose to between 7 and 11 mg/l.[1]

(b) Effect of chloramphenicol on serum phenobarbitone concentrations

A man who had been admitted to hospital on numerous occasions for pulmonary complications associated with cystic fibrosis, had an average serum phenobarbitone concentration of 35 mg/l while taking 200 mg phenobarbitone daily and chloramphenicol. When the antibiotic was withdrawn, his serum phenobarbitone level averaged only 24 mg/l although his dosage had been increased to 300 mg/day. These observations confirmed those previously made on this patient.[4]

Mechanism

The barbiturates, such as phenobarbitone, are known potent enzyme-inducing agents which increase the metabolism by the liver and the clearance from the body of many drugs administered at the same time. An increased glucuronidation of chloramphenicol with a resultant decrease in its activity has been demonstrated in rats[2] treated with phenobarbitone, and it would seem almost certain that this is the explanation for the interaction seen in these two children. The half-life of chloramphenicol in the second child fell from approximately 7 to 3 h between days 3 and 5 of treatment which is consistent with this suggested interaction mechanism.

The most likely explanation of the increased serum phenobarbitone levels is that the chloramphenicol inhibits its metabolism. This has been described in animals.[5]

Importance and management

The documentation is very limited. The two papers cited[1,4] appear to be the only reports of these interactions in man so that their general importance is not clear.

The serum levels of chloramphenicol should be monitored if phenobarbitone is given concurrently. The authors of the first report[1] found it necessary to double the maximum recommended dose of chloramphenicol to ensure that adequate concentrations were maintained. They also suggest that one of the newer anticonvulsants such as sodium valproate, which has little or no enzyme-inducing activity,[3] might prove to be a better choice than phenobarbitone.

In the second report[2], gross sedation, almost certainly due to elevated phenobarbitone levels, was seen in the patient during one admission to hospital in which he was treated with both drugs. Careful monitoring of the phenobarbitone serum levels and dosage adjustments is therefore required.

References

1 Bloxham R A, Durbin G M, Johnson T and Winterborn M H. Chloramphenicol and phenobarbitone—a drug interaction. *Arch Dis Child* (1979) **54**, 76.

2 Bella D D, Ferrari V, Marca G and Bonanomi L. Chloramphenicol metabolism in the phenobarbital-induced liver. Comparison with thiamphenicol. *Biochem Pharmacol* (1968) **17**, 2381.

3 Oxley J, Hedges A, Makki K A , Monks A and Richens A. Lack of hepatic enzyme-inducing effect of sodium valproate. *Br J clin Pharmac* (1979) **8**, 189.

4 Koup J R, Gibaldi M, McNamara P, Hilligoss D M, Colburn W A and Bruck E. Interaction of chloramphenicol with phenytoin and phenobarbital. Case report. *Clin Pharmacol Ther* (1978) **24**, 571.

5 Adams H R. Prolonged barbiturate anaesthesia by chloramphenicol in laboratory animals. *J Am Vet Med Assoc* (1970) **157**, 1908.

Co-trimoxazole + folic acid

Summary
Patients under treatment for megaloblastic anaemia should not be given co-trimoxazole.

Interaction
Four patients failed to respond to their treatment for megaloblastic anaemia when they were concurrently given co-trimoxazole. The expected reticulocyte response failed to occur in 3 of the patients and the fourth showed no clinical improvement until the co-trimoxazole was withdrawn.[1]

Similar responses have been described in other reports.[2,3]

Mechanism
Not understood. In theory neither sulphamethoxazole nor trimethoprim should disturb folate metabolism in man. Along with other mammals we rely on folate in the diet rather than on synthesizing it from PABA. Moreover mammalian dihydrofolate reductase is about 50 000 times less sensitive to trimethoprim than the bacterial enzyme. But in practice haematological changes can occur in man.

Importance and management
The 'antifolate' effects of co-trimoxazole are well documented. In normal individuals the effects are usually mild and relatively unimportant, but in patients with megaloblastic anaemia the effects are serious and co-trimoxazole should not be given.

References
1 Chanarin I and England J M. Toxicity of trimethoprim–sulphamethoxazole in patients with megaloblastic haemopoiesis. *Brit Med J* (1972) **i**, 651.
2 Rooney P J and Housley E. Trimethoprim–sulphamethoxazole in folic acid deficiency. *Brit Med J* (1972) **2**, 656.
3 Hill A V L and Kerr D N S. Toxicity of co-trimoxazole in nutritional haematinic deficiency. *Postgrad Med J* (1973) **49**, 596.

Dapsone + probenecid

Summary
The serum levels of dapsone can be markedly raised by the concurrent use of probenecid.

Interaction
A study in 12 men who were given 500 mg dapsone with 300 mg probenecid, and 3 h later another 500 mg dapsone, showed that dapsone serum levels were raised about 50% when measured at 4 h. The urinary excretion of dapsone and its metabolites were found to be reduced.[1]

Mechanism
Not fully examined. It would seem probable that the probenecid inhibits the renal excretion of dapsone by the kidney.

Importance and management
The documentation is very limited, but it would seem to be an established interaction. It seems almost certain that probenecid will raise the serum levels of dapsone given chronically. The importance is uncertain, but the extent of the rise and the evidence that haematological toxicity of dapsone may be dose related[2] suggests that it may well be important. This requires confirmation.

References
1 Goodwin C S and Sparell G. Inhibition of dapsone excretion by probenecid. *Lancet* (1969) **ii**, 884.
2 Ellard G A. Dapsone acetylation in dermatitis herpetiformis. *Br J Derm* (1974) **90**, 441.

Erythromycin + lincomycin

Summary

In-vitro evidence suggests that antagonism can occur but this has yet to be confirmed clinically.

Interaction, mechanism, importance and management

An in-vitro study showed that antagonism occurred when a strain of staphylococci resistant to erythromycin but sensitive to lincomycin was exposed to both antibiotics together, but whether this is likely to occur in vivo is uncertain.[1]

Reference

1 Griffith L J, Ostrande W E, Mullins C G and Beswick D E. Drug antagonism between lincomycin and erythromycin. *Science* (1964) **147**, 746.

Erythromycin + penicillins

Summary

Some slight antagonism can occur between erythromycin and penicillin in the treatment of scarlatina.

Interaction

A large scale clinical study on the treatment of uncomplicated scarlatina showed that penicillin was more effective than erythromycin, while the two antibiotics together were slightly less effective, judged by the duration of the fever and the disappearance of the haemolytic streptococci.[1]

An in-vitro study on staphylococci confirmed these findings.[2]

Mechanism

It is suggested that the erythromycin can interfere with the bactericidal actions of penicillin.

Importance and management

Information is limited, but the interaction appears to be established. It would seem advisable to avoid combined use in the treatment of this condition. However, the author of the study cited[1] also points out that in the case of double infections with penicillinase-producing staphylococci, combined treatment would seem likely to be more effective. There is also evidence that erythromycin with ampicillin is an effective treatment for pulmonary nocardiosis.[3]

References

1 Strom J. Penicillin and erythromycin singly and in combination in scarlatina therapy and the interference between them. *Antibiot Chemotherap* (1961) **11**, 694.
2 Manten A. Synergism and antagonism between antibiotic mixtures containing erythromycin. *Antibiot Chemotherap* (1954) **4**, 1228.
3 Bach M C, Monaco A P and Finland M. Pulmonary nocardiosis: therapy with minocycline and with erythromycin plus ampicillin. *J Amer Med Ass* (1973) **224**, 1378.

Erythromycin + urinary acidifiers or alkalinizers

Summary

In the treatment of urinary tract infections, the antibacterial activity of erythromycin is maximal in alkaline urine and minimal in acid urine.

Interaction

Urine from 7 volunteers taking 1 g erythromycin, four times a day, was tested for antibacterial activity against five genera of Gram-negative bacilli (*Escherichia coli, Klebsiella pneumoniae, P. mirabilis, Pseudomonas aeruginosa* and *Serrata* sp.) both before and after treatment with acetazolamide or sodium bicarbonate. A direct correlation was found between the activity of the antibiotic and the urinary pH. Normally acid urine had little or no antibacterial activity, whereas alkalinized urine, up to a pH of 8·5, had.[1]

Clinical trials have confirmed the increased antibacterial effectiveness of erythromycin in the treatment of bacteriuria when the urine is made alkaline.[2,3]

Mechanism

The pH of the urine does not apparently affect the way the kidney handles the antibiotic (most of it is excreted actively rather than passively) but it does have a direct influence on the way the antibiotic affects the micro-organisms. Mechanisms suggested include effects on bacterial cell receptors, induction of active transport mechanisms in bacterial cell walls, and changes in ionization of the antibiotic which enables it to enter the bacterial cell more effectively.

Importance and management

An established interaction which can be exploited. The effectiveness of the antibiotic in treating urinary tract infections is maximized by making the urine alkaline (for example with acetazolamide or sodium bicarbonate). Treatment with urinary acidifiers will minimize the activity of erythromycin and should therefore be avoided.

References

1 Sabath L D, Gerstein D A, Loder P B and Finland M. Excretion of erythromycin and its enhanced activity in urine against gram-negative bacilli with alkalinization. *J Lab Clin Med* (1968) **72**, 916.
2 Zinner S H, Sabath L D, Casey J I and Finland M. Erythromycin and alkalinization of the urine in the treatment of urinary tract infections due to gram-negative bacilli. *Lancet* (1971) i, 1267.
3 Zinner S H, Sabath L D, Casey J I and Finland M. Erythromycin plus alkalinization in the treatment of urinary infections. *Antimicrob Ag Chemotherap* (1969) **9**, 413.

Ethambutol + antacids

Summary

Aluminium hydroxide can reduce the absorption of ethambutol in some patients. The importance of this is uncertain.

Interaction

A study on 13 tuberculous patients and 6 normal subjects, given single 50 mg/kg doses of ethambutol, showed that when 1·5 g aluminium hydroxide was given at the same time, and repeated 15 and 30 min later, the serum ethambutol levels were delayed and reduced in the patients but not in the normal subjects. The average total urinary excretion of ethambutol over a 10 h period was reduced about 15%. There were marked individual variations. Some of the patients showed no interaction and others an increase in absorption.[1]

Mechanism

Uncertain. Aluminium hydroxide may affect gastric emptying.

Importance and management

The documentation is very limited but it indicates that some, but by no means all, patients may have reduced serum ethambutol levels if aluminium hydroxide is used concurrently. The extent to which this can affect the treatment of tuberculosis is uncertain, but prescribers should be aware of this interaction. Information about other antacids appears to be lacking.

Reference

1 Mattila M J, Linnoila M, Seppälä T and Koskinen R. Effect of aluminium hydroxide and glycopyrrhonium on the absorption of ethambutol and alcohol in man. *Br J clin Pharmacol* (1978) **5**, 161.

Ethionamide + thyroxine

Summary

The hypothyroidic effects of ethionamide may antagonize the effects of thyroxine.

Interaction, mechanism, importance and management

Hypothyroidism has been described in 2 tuberculous patients receiving ethionamide, and at least two other cases of thyroid enlargement have been reported, although most patients appear not to experience overt thyroid dysfunction.[1,2] Particular care would seem appropriate in patients requiring treatment for hypothyroidism if ethionamide is also given.

References

1 Moulding T and Fraser R. Hypothyroidism related to ethionamide. *Amer Rev Resp Dis* (1970) **101**, 90.
2 Schless J M, Allison R F, Inglis R M, White E F and Topperman S. The use of ethionamide in combined regimens in the re-treatment of isoniazid-resistant pulmonary tuberculosis. *Amer Rev Resp Dis* (1965) **91**, 728.

Griseofulvin + barbiturates

Summary

The serum levels of griseofulvin and its antifungal effects may be reduced by concurrent treatment with phenobarbitone.

Interaction

A comparative study on 8 normal subjects showed that their serum levels of griseofulvin, in response to a single 1 g oral dose, were reduced by about a third after pretreatment for 2 days with phenobarbitone, 30 mg three times a day.

Six normal subjects were given griseofulvin by slow intravenous infusion (0·1 g) or orally (0·5 g) after taking 30 mg phenobarbitone three times a day for at least four days previously. During oral administration the amount of griseofulvin absorbed was reduced by about 45%, and the peak serum levels measured after 8 h were reduced from 1·35 to 0·9 μg/ml.[2]

A patient with a superficial fungal infection which was sensitive to griseofulvin failed to respond to treatment while taking 120 mg phenobarbitone daily for epilepsy.[3]

Mechanism

It was originally thought, based on experiments in rats[4], that the reduced serum griseofulvin levels came about because of the potent enzyme-inducing effects of the phenobarbitone, but later studies in man[2] in which the griseofulvin was given either orally or intravenously showed that the phenobarbitone was having some effect on the absorption of the griseofulvin from the gut. Even now the picture is by no means fully resolved. One theory is that the phenobarbitone stimulates the secretion of bile which in turn stimulates peristalsis. The result is that the griseofulvin passes through the upper part of the gastrointestinal tract (where most of it is normally absorbed) much more quickly than it otherwise would, and less time is available for full absorption.[2]

The alternative idea is that the phenobarbitone interacts physically with the griseofulvin to make an already poorly soluble drug even less soluble.[2] This notion is supported by in-vitro work which shows that some physico–chemical complexation occurs when griseofulvin and phenobarbitone are mixed together.[5]

Importance and management

Only one clear case of an inadequate response to antifungal treatment has been documented,[3] but it is well supported by the other clinical studies cited (griseofulvin serum concentration reductions of 30–45%) so that there is good reason to believe that this interaction may be important. Wherever possible concurrent treatment with griseofulvin and phenobarbitone should be avoided.

It has been suggested in one of the reports cited[2] that where barbiturate treatment must be continued (as, for example, in epilepsy) the griseofulvin should be given in divided doses three times a day to give the drug a better chance of being absorbed in the upper part of the gut. The total daily dosage may also need to be increased although the effects of this have yet to be studied. It has not been established whether other barbiturates interact similarly.

References
1 Busfield D, Child K J, Atkinson R M and Tomich E G. An effect of phenobarbitone on blood levels of griseofulvin in man. *Lancet* (1963) **ii**, 1042.
2 Riegelman S, Rowland M and Epstein W L. Griseofulvin–phenobarbital interaction in man. *J Amer Med Ass* (1970) **213**, 426.
3 Lorenc E. A new factor in griseofulvin treatment failures. *Missouri Med* (1967) **64**, 32.
4 Busfield D, Child K J and Tomich E G. An effect of phenobarbitone on griseofulvin metabolism in the rat. *Brit J Pharmacol* (1964) **22**, 137.
5 Abougela I K A, Bigford D J, McCorquodale I and Grant D J W. Complex formation and other physico-chemical interactions between griseofulvin and phenobarbitone. *J Pharm Pharmac* (1976) **28**, 44P.

Hexamine compounds + sulphonamides

Summary
Crystalluria can occur with some sulphonamides at the urinary pH values necessary for hexamine (methenamine) to be effective.

Interaction, mechanism, importance and management
Hexamine (methenamine) compounds are only effective as urinary antiseptics if the pH is 5 or lower. At these pH values many of the older sulphonamides (sulphapyridine, sulphamethizole etc.) are insoluble and can crystallize out in the kidney tubules causing physical damage.[1]

Although this is much less likely to occur with some of the newer, more soluble sulphonamides, it would seem preferable to avoid the problem by using some other form of treatment.

Reference
1 Lipton J H. Incompatibility between sulfamethizole and methenamine mandelate. *New Eng J Med* (1963) **268**, 92.

Hexamine compounds + urinary acidifiers or alkalinizers

Summary
Compounds which can raise the urinary pH above 5 are contraindicated during treatment with hexamine compounds (methenamine).

Interaction, mechanism, importance and management
Hexamine (methenamine) and hexamine mandelate are only effective as urinary antiseptics in acid urine, the pH of which should be 5 or lower. This is achieved by the administration of urinary acidifiers such as ammonium chloride or sodium acid phosphate. In the case of hexamine hippurate, the acidification of the urine is maintained by the presence of hippuric acid. The use of compounds which raise the urinary pH (e.g. acetazolamide, sodium bicarbonate, potassium citrate etc.) is clearly contraindicated.

8-Hydroxyquinoline + zinc oxide

Summary
The presence of zinc oxide inhibits the therapeutic effects of 8-hydroxyquinoline in ointments.

Incompatibility
The observation that a patient showed an allergic reaction to 8-hydroxyquinoline in ointments with a paraffin base, but not in a zinc oxide base, prompted a further study of the possible incompatibility between these two compounds. A study in 13 patients confirmed that zinc oxide reduces the eczematogenic (allergic) properties of the 8-hydroxyquinoline, but it also inhibits its antibacterial and antimycotic effects as well, and appears to stimulate the growth of *Candida albicans*.[1]

Mechanism
It seems almost certain that the zinc ions form chelates with 8-hydroxyquinoline which have little or no antibacterial properties.[1,2]

Importance and management
The documentation is limited but the reaction appears to be established. There is no point in using zinc oxide to reduce the allergenic properties of the 8-hydroxyquinoline if, at the same time, the therapeutic effects disappear.

References
1 Fischer T. On 8-hydroxyquinoline–zinc oxide incompatibility. *Dermatologica* (1974) **149**, 129.
2 Alberta A, Rubbo S D, Goldacre R J and Balfour B J. The influence of chemical constitution on antibacterial activity. III. A study of 8-hydroxyquinoline (oxine) and related compounds. *Brit J exp Path* (1974) **28**, 69.

Isoniazid + antacids

Summary
The absorption of isoniazid from the gut is reduced by the concurrent use of aluminium hydroxide.

Interaction
The effect of aluminium hydroxide on the gastrointestinal absorption of isoniazid was examined in 10 patients receiving treatment for active tuberculosis.[1] Aluminium hydroxide (*Amphojel*—Wyeth) (45 ml) was taken at 6 am, 7 am and 8 am, followed immediately by all the medications taken by the patients (including rifampicin, folic acid, paracetamol, ethambutol, digoxin, vitamin B6, diphenhydramine, ferrous sulphate, prochlorperazine, propoxyphene, PAS, tetracycline, ampicillin, streptomycin and isoniazid). Blood samples taken 1, 2, 4 and 6 h later showed that the 1 h serum concentrations of isoniazid and the area under the plasma drug concentration curves were depressed. Peak serum concentrations occurring between 1 and 2 h after ingestion were reduced by approximately 16%, or, expressed in µg/ml/mg of isoniazid/kg body weight to allow for different dosages, by 25%.

Mechanism
Aluminium hydroxide has been shown[2,3] in rat and man to delay gastric emptying. A series of experiments on rats, run concurrently with the experiments on the tuberculous patients already described, confirmed that aluminium hydroxide caused retention of the isoniazid in the stomach, and since isoniazid is largely absorbed from the intestine the marked decrease in serum isoniazid concentration would seem to be explained.

Importance and management
Information appears to be limited to this study. It is not known how important this interaction is in practice, although it is recognized that single high doses of isoniazid are more effective in arresting tuberculosis than the same amount of drug in divided doses.[4,5] Peak serum isoniazid concentrations are therefore important. It would seem wise to follow the recommendations made in the study cited to give the isoniazid at least an hour before the administration of the aluminium hydroxide.[1]

References
1 Hurwitz A and Schlozman D L. Effects of antacids on gastrointestinal absorption of isoniazid in rat and man. *Amer Rev Resp Dis* (1974) **109**, 41.
2 Hava M and Hurwitz A. The relaxing effect of aluminium hydroxide on rat and human gastric smooth muscle *in vitro. Europ J Pharmac* (1973) **7**, 156.

3 Vats T S, Hurwitz A, Robinson R G and Herrin W. Effects of antacids on gastric emptying in children. *Pediat Res* (1973) **22**, 340.
4 Fox W. General considerations in intermittent drug therapy of pulmonary tuberculosis. *Postgrad Med J* (1971) **47**, 729.
5 Hudson L D and Sbarbara J A. Twice weekly tuberculosis chemotherapy. *J Amer med Ass* (1973) **223**, 139.

Isoniazid + cheese or fish

Summary

A few cases have been reported of a flushing reaction with headache, tachycardia, and in some instances hypertension, following the ingestion of cheese during treatment with isoniazid. Similar reactions have been described after eating tuna fish, skipjack and *Sardinella* (amblygaster) *sirm.*

Interaction

Within 3 months of starting to take 300 mg isoniazid daily for the treatment of tuberculosis, a woman experienced a series of unpleasant reactions 10–30 min after eating cheese. These reactions included chills, headache (sometimes severe), itching of the face and scalp, slight diarrhoea, flushing of the face and on one occasion of the whole body, variable and mild tachycardia and a bursting sensation in the head. Blood pressure measurements showed only a modest rise from 95/65 mmHg to 110/80 mmHg. No physical or biochemical abnormalities were found.[1]

A man under treatment with daily doses of isoniazid, 300 mg, and rifampicin 600 mg, experienced a flushing reaction within minutes of starting to eat a meal of onions and cooked cheese (described as being a very strong Cheshire). After five or six mouthfuls the man felt sick and hot all over his body. Shortly afterwards his wife noticed that his face, hands and arms were 'fiery red' and his eyes blood-shot. He also developed palpitations and a frontal headache. The flushing abated after 2 h. There was no itching of the skin, vomiting or diarrhoea, but he developed abdominal rumblings.[3]

Similar reactions (one of them included a rise in blood pressure to 200/110 mmHg)[5] have been described in 2 other patients on isoniazid after eating cheese. There are also other reports of a by no means dissimilar reaction in patients on isoniazid after eating tuna fish[6], skipjack (bonito)[4,7] and *Sardinella* (amblygaster) *sirm.*[8]

Mechanism

Not understood. Unlike iproniazid, isoniazid does not inhibit mitochondrial monoamine oxidase[2] so that the reactions seen cannot easily be directly equated with the 'cheese reaction' or hypertensive crisis which can take place with the MAOI and cheese or other tyramine-rich foods (see p. 370), although there are some features in common such as flushing, headache, tachycardia, and hypertension. Whether the fact that isoniazid strongly inhibits MAO in the plasma is relevant is uncertain. One suggestion[3] is that this reaction may have been a reflection of histamine intoxication.

Bacterial degradation of foods can produce histamine from histidine. Isoniazid is a potent inhibitor of histaminase in the body, and the levels of histamine in the samples of cheese and fish taken by these patients may have been high enough to permit intoxication to develop.

Importance and management

There appear to be only four cases of this isoniazid/cheese reaction on record although the numbers of patients who have experienced a similar reaction with fish is greater. Isoniazid has been in use since 1956 and there would seem no need now to introduce any general dietary restrictions for patients taking it, but if adverse reactions similar to those described are experienced by any other patient on isoniazid, it would clearly be worth while to examine their diet and, if some association seems probable, to advise patients to avoid the offending foodstuffs. The Director of Health Services in Sri Lanka, where a number of adverse reactions involving the tropical fish have been recorded, has issued instructions to hospitals to exclude all three types of fish mentioned from the diets of tuberculous patients.

References
1 Smith C K and Durack D T. Isoniazid and cheese reaction. *Ann Int Med* (1978) **88**, 520.

2 Robinson D S, Lovenberg W, Keiser H and Sjoerdsma A. Effect of drugs on human platelet and plasma amine oxidase activity *in vitro* and *in vivo. Biochem Pharmacol* (1968) **17**, 109.
3 Uragoda C G and Lodha S C. Histamine intoxication in a tuberculous patient after ingestion of cheese. *Tubercle* (1979) **60**, 59.
4 Uragoda C G and Kottegoda S R. Adverse reactions to isoniazid on ingestion of fish with a high histamine content. *Tubercle* (1977) **58**, 83.
5 Lejone J L, Gusmini D and Brochard P. Isoniazid and reaction to cheese. *Ann Int Med* (1979) **91**, 793.
6 Uragoda C G. Histamine poisoning in tuberculous patients after ingestion of tuna fish. *Amer Rev Resp Dis* (1980) **121**, 157.
7 Senanayake N, Vyravanthan S and Kanagasuriyama S. Cerebrovascular accident after a 'skipjack' reaction in a patient taking isoniazid. *Brit Med J* (1978) **2**, 1127.
8 Uragoda C G. Histamine poisoning in tuberculosis patients on ingestion of tropical fish. *J Trop Med Hyg* (1978) **81**, 243.

Isoniazid + disulfiram

Summary

A total of 11 patients on isoniazid have been described who experienced difficulties of coordination and changes in affect and behaviour after taking disulfiram concurrently.

Interaction

Seven tuberculous patients who had been taking 0·6–1 g isoniazid daily for not less than 30 days without problems, developed coordination difficulties and changes in affect and behaviour within 2–8 days of additional treatment with 0·5 g disulfiram daily. These patients represented less than one third of the total group under treatment. Among the symptoms seen were dizziness, disorientation, a staggering gait, insomnia, irritable and querulous behaviour, listlessness and lethargy. One patient showed hypomania. Most of them were also taking chlordiazepoxide and other drugs including PAS, streptomycin, and phenobarbitone. The adverse reactions decreased or disappeared when the disulfiram was either reduced to 0·25 g daily, or withdrawn. Four patients who were given only isoniazid and disulfiram also showed drowsiness and depression.[1]

Mechanism

Uncertain. Both isoniazid and disulfiram can produce side-effects like these in high doses on their own, but in the doses actually used neither drug produced any of these symptoms when used alone in these or any other patients. This suggests some kind of synergy between the two. The authors of the report[1] speculate that isoniazid and disulfiram together possibly inhibit two of three biochemical pathways concerned with the metabolism of dopamine. One of these metabolizes dopamine by dopamine beta-hydroxylase to noradrenaline, and then by MAO to 3,4-dihydroxyphenyl acetic acid. This leaves a third pathway open, catalysed by catechol-O-methyltransferase, which produced a number of methylated products of dopamine. These may have been responsible for the mental and physical changes described in the patients. Of the other drugs used, any involvement by chlordiazepoxide seems to be discounted because 4 other patients given just isoniazid and disulfiram became drowsy and depressed, but recovered when the disulfiram was withdrawn.

Importance and management

Information about this interaction seems to be limited to the report cited, and its general importance is uncertain. All of the patients had been given 0·5 g disulfiram for 10–14 days, then reduced to 0·25 g daily. Bearing in mind that disulfiram is relatively slowly eliminated from the body, and the dosage suggested in Martindale's *Extra Pharmacopoeia*[2] is 0·8 g initially, reduced by 0·2 g daily until the lowest effective dose is achieved (usually about 0·1–0·2 g daily), the dosages being taken by these patients were rather high. So while there is certainly no contraindication to the concurrent use of these drugs (more than two thirds of the group failed to show this interaction[1] and no interaction took place in another patient taking both drugs and rifampicin),[3] patients should be monitored carefully for the development of adverse effects, particularly if high doses of disulfiram are used, and if necessary its dosage should be reduced, or it should be withdrawn.

References

1 Whittington H G and Grey L. Possible interaction between disulfiram and isoniazid. *Amer J Psychiat* (1969) **125** 1725.
2 Martindale, *The Extra Pharmacopoeia* 27th edn, p. 539. Wade A (ed.) (1977).
3 Rothstein E. Rifampin with Disulfiram. *J Am Med Ass* (1972) **219**, 1216.

Lincomycin + cyclamates

Summary
The absorption of lincomycin by the gut can be markedly reduced by the presence of cyclamates.

Interaction, mechanism, importance and management
A study in man[1] has shown that '... in the presence of 1 molar equivalent of cyclamate (an amount present in only a portion of a bottle of diet drink) the area under the serum concentration of lincomycin is only about 25% of that area in the absence of cyclamate when 500 mg oral doses of lincomycin are administered in man.' The reasons are not understood. This would seem to be an interaction of importance. It would seem a wise precaution to separate the administration of lincomycin and foods, drinks, or medicaments containing cyclamates as much as possible. Cyclamates are banned in the UK as sweeteners in beverages, but they are still sometimes found in pharmaceuticals.

Reference
1 Wagner J G. Aspects of pharmacokinetics and biopharmaceutics in relation to drug activity. *Amer J Pharm* (1969) **141**, 5.

Lincomycin + kaolin

Summary
The concurrent use of kaolin-containing anti-diarrhoeal preparations markedly reduces the absorption of lincomycin by the gut. Separating the dosages as much as possible can prevent this interaction. Lincomycin-induced diarrhoea is a potential hazard.

Interaction
A four-way crossover study on 8 normal subjects showed that when they were given 0·5 g lincomycin and 3 fl. oz of *Kaopectate* the amount of the antibiotic absorbed was about 10% of that obtained when the antibiotic was administered by itself. Administration of the *Kaopectate* 2 h before the antibiotic had little or no effect on its absorption whereas when given 2 h after the absorption was reduced by about 50%.[1]

This interaction has been described in another report.[3]

Mechanism
Although the mechanism of this interaction is not known for certain, a probable explanation is that the kaolin component of *Kaopectate* not only adsorbs the lincomycin onto its surface,[1,2] thereby reducing the availability of the antibiotic, but also coats the lining of the gut and acts as a physical barrier to absorption.

Importance and management
Information about this interaction seems to be limited to this one study,[1,3] which appears to have been well controlled and there seems little reason to doubt its general applicability or importance. If good absorption and a good antibiotic response are to be achieved, the lincomycin should not be allowed to come into contact with kaolin in the gut. The administration of the two drugs should be separated as much as possible. Two hours before the antibiotic and even longer afterwards is indicated by the study cited.[1]

To obtain optimal absorption, according to the manufacturers of the antibiotic,[4] nothing except water should be given for a period of 1 or 2 h before and after the antibiotic. The design of a three times a day schedule may therefore be possible, but a four times a day schedule may be difficult. In this case an alternative preparation which does not contain kaolin should be used.

Lincomycin itself can cause diarrhoea in a fairly large proportion of patients which, in some cases, has lead to the development of fatal pseudomembranous colitis. Marked diarrhoea, according to the manufacturers,[4] is an indication that the lincomycin should be stopped immediately.

References

1 Wagner J G. Design and data analysis of biopharmaceutical studies in man. *Can J Pharm Sci* (1966) **1**, 55.
2 E L Rowe. Quoted in [1] above.
3 Wagner J G. Pharmacokinetics. 1. Definitions, modeling and reasons for measuring blood levels and urinary excretion. *Drug Intell* (1968) **2**, 38.
4 Data Sheet Compendium 1979–80, p. 1032. (1979) Pharmind Publications. London.

Naldixic acid + probenecid

Summary

Serum naldixic acid levels are markedly increased by the concurrent use of probenecid.

Interaction

Following the observation that a man who had ingested unknown amounts of several drugs, including naldixic acid and probenecid, showed grossly elevated naldixic acid serum levels, the possible interaction between these two drugs was investigated. Two volunteers, acting as their own controls, ingested 0·5 g naldixic acid with and without 0·5 g probenecid. The peak serum levels of naldixic acid were unaffected at 2 h, but at 8 h the levels were increased three-fold by the presence of the probenecid.[1]

Mechanism

This is not known for certain, but it has been suggested that, as with penicillin and many other drugs, the probenecid competes with the naldixic acid for its excretion by the kidney resulting in its retention.[1]

Importance and management

Information seems to be limited to this single report. It appears to be an established interaction, but its importance is uncertain. Prescribers should be aware of this interaction if concurrent use is undertaken.

Reference

1 Dash H and Mills J. Severe metabolic acidosis associated with naldixic acid overdose. *Ann Int Med* (1976) **84**, 570.

Naldixic acid + nitrofurantoin

Summary

In-vitro studies have demonstrated antagonistic antibacterial effects.

Interaction, mechanism, importance and management

It has been demonstrated by in-vitro studies that the antibacterial activity of naldixic acid can be inhibited by sub-inhibitory concentrations of nitrofurantoin. Forty-four out of 53 strains of *Escherichia coli*, *Salmonella* and *Proteus* showed antagonism;[1] another study confirmed these findings.[2] Whether this similarly occurs in vivo is uncertain, but the advice[1] that concurrent use should be avoided when treating urinary tract infections seems sound.

References

1 Stille W and Ostner K H. Antagonismus Nitrofurantoin–Naldixinsäure. *Klin Wschr* (1966) **44**, 155.
2 Piguet D. *In vitro* inhibitive action of nitrofurantoin on the bacteriostatic activity of naldixic acid. *Ann Inst Pasteur (Paris)* (1969) **116**, 43.

Nitrofurantoin + antacids

Summary

Magnesium trisilicate can markedly reduce the gastrointestinal absorption and the urinary concentrations of nitrofurantoin which may be expected to reduce its antibacterial effectiveness. Aluminium hydroxide and calcium carbonate appear not to interact significantly.

Interaction

A cross-over study on 6 healthy subjects given single 100 mg oral doses of nitrofurantoin with 5 g magnesium trisilicate in 150 ml water showed that the absorption was reduced by more than 50%. The amount of time during which the concentration of nitrofurantoin in the urine was at, or above, the minimal antibacterial inhibitory concentration of 32 μg/ml was also reduced.[1]

In-vitro tests with other antacids showed that the amounts of nitrofurantoin adsorbed were as follows: magnesium trisilicate and charcoal (99%), bismuth oxycarbonate and talc (50–53%), kaolin (31%), magnesium oxide (27%) aluminium hydroxide (2·5%) and calcium carbonate (0%).[1]

Mechanism

To a greater of lesser extent these antacids adsorb nitrofurantoin onto their surfaces. As a result the amount available for absorption by the gut and for excretion by the kidney is considerably reduced.[1]

Importance and management

Information appears to be limited to this report.

Although there is no direct clinical evidence that the concurrent use of magnesium trisilicate has been responsible for the failure of nitrofurantoin to clear up a urinary tract infection, and single-dose studies are not necessarily as reliable a guide as those which are long term, the evidence from the study cited indicates that a clinically important interaction can probably take place between nitrofurantoin and magnesium trisilicate. Bismuth oxycarbonate, charcoal, talc and magnesium oxide appear to interact to a lesser extent and should probably be avoided as well, but aluminium hydroxide and calcium carbonate seem unlikely to interact and could be used to treat the gastrointestinal irritation caused by nitrofurantoin. Direct clinical studies are required to confirm the results reported.

Reference

1 Naggar V F and Khalil S A. Effect of magnesium trisilicate on nitrofurantoin absorption. *Clin Pharmacol Ther* (1979) **25**, 857.

Nitrofurantoin + anticholinergics

Summary

Anticholinergics such as diphenoxylate and propantheline can markedly increase the absorption of nitrofurantoin.

Interaction, mechanism, importance and management

Studies in man show that anticholinergics such as diphenoxylate and propantheline can approximately double the absorption of nitrofurantoin in some individuals, presumably be reducing the motility of the gut, thus increasing its dissolution.[1,2] The importance of this with nitrofurantoin is uncertain (it would be expected to be accompanied by an increase in the effects and possibly in the incidence of adverse reactions) but it illustrates that anticholinergics can probably influence the bioavailability of other drugs.

References

1 Callahan M, Bullock F J, Braun J and Yesair D W. Pharmacodynamics of drug interactions with diphenoxylate. *Fed Proc* (1974) **33**, 513.
2 Jaffe J M. Effect of propantheline on nitrofurantoin absorption. *J Pharm Sci* (1975) **64**, 1729.

Para-aminosalicylic acid + diphenhydramine

Summary

Diphenhydramine affects the motility of the gut and causes a small reduction in the absorption of para-aminosalicylic acid. The importance of this is unknown.

Interaction, mechanism, importance and management

A study[1] in rats and man on mechanisms of drug interaction showed that diphenhydramine in normal dosages (50 mg) given parenterally decreased the amount of para-aminosalicylic acid absorbed by the gut. The peak serum concentration was reduced about 15% although the reduction in the total amount absorbed was not as large. To what extent the concurrent use of diphenhydramine, or any other anticholinergic drug which alters the motility of the gut, can affect the therapeutic response to long-term treatment with para-aminosalicylic acid is not known, but the possibility of a small reduction should be borne in mind.

Reference

1 Lavigne J-G and Marchand C. Inhibition of the gastrointestinal absorption of p-aminosalicylate (PAS) in rats and humans by diphenhydramine. *Clin Pharmacol Ther* (1973) 14, 404.

Para-aminosalicylic acid + isoniazid

Summary

The concurrent use of para-aminosalicylic acid and isoniazid results in raised serum isoniazid levels. A generally advantageous interaction.

Interaction, mechanism, importance and management

A study in man[1] showed that the simultaneous administration of para-aminosalicylic acid and isoniazid resulted in significantly increased serum concentrations of isoniazid, and in extended half-lives due, it is believed, to the inhibition of isoniazid metabolism by the para-aminosalicylic acid. The effect was most marked among the 'fast' inactivators of isoniazid. This would seem to be an advantageous interaction.

Reference

1 Boman G, Borgå O, Hanngren Å, Malmborg A-S and Sjöqvist F. Pharmacokinetic interactions between the tuberculostatics rifampicin, para-aminosalicylic acid and isoniazid. *Acta Pharmac Toxicol* (1970) 28, (Suppl 1) 15.

Para-aminosalicylic acid + probenecid

Summary

The serum levels of para-aminosalicylic acid can be raised two- to four-fold by the concurrent use of probenecid.

Interaction

A study in man showed that when 0·5 g probenecid was administered 6-hourly, the serum levels of para-aminosalicylic acid following single 4 g doses were increased two- to four-fold.[1]

Similar results are described in another report.[2]

Mechanism

Uncertain. One theory is that the probenecid successfully competes with the para-aminosalicylic acid for active excretion by the kidney tubules resulting in the retention of the para-aminosalicylic acid and its accumulation in the body. The probenecid is passively reabsorbed further along the tubule.

Importance and management
The documentation is limited but the interaction appears to be established. Such large increases in serum levels of para-aminosalicylic acid would seem almost certainly to lead to toxicity, but this requires confirmation. It would seem probable that the dosage of the para-aminosalicylic acid could be reduced without losing the required therapeutic response.

References
1 Boger W P and Pitts F W. Influence of p-(di-N-propylsulfa-myl)-benzoic acid, 'Benemid' on para-aminosalicylic acid (PAS) plasma concentrations. *Amer Rev Tuberc* (1950) **61**, 682.
2 Carr D T, Karlson A G and Bridge E V. Concentration of PAS and tuberculostatic potency of serum after administration of PAS with and without Benemid. *Proc Staff Meet Mayo Clin* (1952) **27**, 209.

Penicillins + sulphinpyrazone

Summary
Sulphinpyrazone can reduce the renal excretion of penicillin.

Interaction, mechanism, importance and management
A study[1] in man has shown that the concurrent use of sulphinpyrazone, 600 mg daily, prolongs the half-life of penicillin from 43 to 70 min, probably by competing with its renal excretion in a similar way to probenecid (see p. 10). This would appear to be a potentially advantageous rather than an adverse interaction.

Reference
1 Kampmann J, Hansen J M, Siersboek-Nielsen K and Laursen H. Effect of some drugs on penicillin half-life in blood. *Clin Pharmacol Ther* (1972) **13**, 516.

Penicillins + tetracyclines

Summary
Tetracyclines can antagonize the effectiveness of penicillin in the treatment of pneumococcal meningitis, but the importance of this interaction with other infections is uncertain. It may possibly only be important with infections where a rapid kill is essential.

Interaction
A study on patients with pneumococcal meningitis showed that penicillin alone (1 million units every 2 h) was more effective than penicillin with chlortetra-cycline (0·5 g every 6 h). Out of 14 patients given penicillin alone, 70% recovered compared with only 20% of another group of essentially similar patients who had received both antibiotics.[1]

Another report on the treatment of pneumococcal meningitis with penicillin and tetracyclines confirmed these findings.[2] No difference was seen in initial response to concurrent treatment for scarlet fever, but spontaneous re-infection occurred much less frequently in those who had only received penicillin.[3]

Mechanism
The generally accepted explanation is that bactericides, such as penicillin which inhibits bacterial cell wall synthesis, require cells to be actively growing and dividing to be maximally effective, a situation which will not occur in the presence of bacteriostatic antibiotics such as the tetracyclines.

Importance and management

An important, established and serious interaction in the treatment of pneumococcal meningitis. Penicillin and tetracylines should not be given together. The importance of this interaction with other infections is uncertain, but it demonstrably does not occur in, for example, pneumoccal pneumonia.[4] It has been suggested that anta gonism, if it occurs, may only be significant when it is essential to kill bacteria rapidly.[4]

References

1 Lepper M H and Dowling H F. Treatment of pneumococcic meningitis with penicillin compared with penicillin plus aureomycin: studies including observations on an apparent antagonism between penicillin and aureomycin. *Arch Int Med* (1951) **88**, 489.

2 Olsson R A, Kirby J C and Romansky M J. Pneumococcal meningitis in the adult. Clinical, therapeutic and prognostic aspects in forty-three patients. *Ann Int Med* (1961) **55**, 545.

3 Strom J. The question of antagonism between penicillin and chlortetracycline illustrated by therapeutical experiments in Scarlatina. *Antibiot Med* (1955) 1, 6.

4 Ahern J J and Kirby W M M. Lack of interference of aureomycin in treatment of pneumococcal pneumonia. *Arch Int Med* (1953) **91**, 197.

Pyrimethamine + co-trimoxazole or sulphonamides

Summary

Serious pancytopenia and megaloblastic anaemia have been described in patients under treatment with co-trimoxazole or sulphonamides and pyrimethamine.

Interaction

A woman taking pyrimethamine, 50 mg a week, as malarial prophylaxis, developed petechial haemorrhages and widespread bruising within 10 days of beginning concurrent therapy with co-trimoxazole (320 mg trimethoprim, 800 mg sulphamethoxazole daily) and was found to have gross megaloblastic changes and pancytopenia in addition to being obviously pale and ill. After withdrawal of the two drugs she responded rapidly to hydroxycobalamine and folic acid, with chloroquine as malarial prophylactic cover.[1]

Another woman taking 50 mg pyrimethamine weekly as malarial prophylaxis who in addition took a 14-day course of co-trimoxazole at 'standard dosage', developed a megaloblastic anaemia which responded promptly to withdrawal of the pyrimethamine and treatment with B_{12} and folate.[2]

Similar cases have been described in other patients taking pyrimethamine with co-trimoxazole[4–6] or sulphafurazole.[3] Another case has been referred to elsewhere involving a sulphonamide.[7]

Mechanism

Not known for certain, but a reasonable supposition can be made on the known pharmacology of the drugs concerned.

Pyrimethamine and trimethoprim are closely related compounds (both are 2:4 diamino–pyrimidines) and both selectively inhibit the actions of the enzyme dihydrofolate reductase which is concerned with the eventual synthesis, among other compounds, of the nucleic acids required for the production of new cells. The sulphonamides inhibit another part of the same synthetic chain. The haematological symptoms of the patients referred to would seem therefore to reflect a gross depression of the normal folate metabolism caused by the combined actions of both drugs. In theory this should not occur (see co-trimoxazole + folic acid, p. 85) but in practice it clearly does.

Importance and management

Information is limited and the general importance is uncertain. The incidence is also not known. Megaloblastic anaemia and pancytopenia are among the recognized adverse reactions of both pyrimethamine and, more rarely, of co-trimoxazole taken on their own. There is no obvious contraindication to their concurrent use but it has been suggested by the authors of one of the reports cited[1] that co-trimoxazole should be prescribed '. . . with caution and haematological cover' to patients taking either pyrimethamine or proguanil as prophylactic cover against malaria, and '. . . further caution . . .' in the tropics because of the folate deficiency associated with pregnancy and malnutrition in children. The manufacturers of co-trimoxazole similarly advise that if the

98

dosage of pyrimethamine is high (as was the case in one of the reports cited), the blood picture should be monitored regularly.

References

1 Fleming A F, Warrell D A and Dickmeiss H. Co-trimoxazole and the blood. *Lancet* (1974) **ii**, 284.
2 Andsell V E, Wright S G and Hutchinson D B A. Megaloblastic anaemia associated with combined pyrimethamine and co-trimoxazole administration. *Lancet* (1976) **ii**, 1257.
3 Waxman S and Herbert V. Mechanism of pyrimethamine-induced megaloblastosis in human bone marrow. *New Eng J Med* (1969) **280**, 1316.
4 Malfatti S and Piccini A. Anemia megaloblastica pancitopenica in corso di trattamento con pirimetamina, trimethoprim e sulfametossazolo. *Haematologica* (1976) **61**, 349.
5 Borgstein A and Tozer R A. Infectious mononucleosis and megaloblastic anaemia associated with Daraprim and Bactrim. *Centr Afr J Med* (1974) **20**, 185.
6 Whitman E N. Effects in man of prolonged administration of trimethoprim and sulfisoxazole. *Postgrad Med J* (1969) **45**, (Suppl) 46.
7 Weissbach G. *Zeitschrift fur Aerztliche Fortbild* (1965) **59**, 10.

Quinine + barbiturates

Summary

It is doubtful if an important interaction occurs if phenobarbitone and quinine are used concurrently.

Interaction, mechanism, importance and management

Although animal data indicate that phenobarbitone increases the metabolism and clearance of quinine, some limited evidence suggests that no interaction of importance occurs in man.[1]

Reference

1 Saggers V H, Hariratnajothi N and McLean A E. The effect of diet and phenobarbitone on quinine metabolism in the rat and in man. *Biochem Pharmacol* (1970) **19**, 499.

Quinine + urinary alkalinizers, antacids, diuretics or alkaline salts

Summary

No adverse interactions have been reported between quinine and these other drugs, but there is the theoretical possibility that some changes in serum quinine levels may occur during concurrent use.

Interaction

There is no direct evidence of an adverse interaction in man, but raising the urinary pH can reduce the excretion of quinine in man, and some antacids can lower the gastrointestinal absorption of quinine in rats.

The urinary excretion of quinine in man is virtually halved (from 17 down to 9%) if the urine is made alkaline.[1]

Pretreatment with magnesium and aluminium hydroxide gel depressed the gastrointestinal absorption of quinine in rats and reduced the blood quinine levels by 50–75%.[2]

Mechanism

Urinary alkalinization can increase the amount of un-ionized (lipid-soluble) quinine in the kidney tubule filtrate and allow greater reabsorption. A more detailed account of this mechanism of interaction is to be found on page 9. Aluminium hydroxide, by slowing gastric emptying, reduces the gastrointestinal absorption of quinine. Magnesium hydroxide forms an insoluble quinine precipitate and this too reduces absorption.[2] But to what extent they can also raise quinine serum levels by altering urinary pH is not clear.

Importance and management

There are no reports of adverse interaction between quinine and these other drugs, but prescribers should be aware that there is the theoretical possibility of an interaction: an increased response if the urinary pH rises significantly (acetazolamide, sodium bicarbonate); a reduced response if the absorption from the gut is markedly reduced (some antacids).

References

1 Haag H B, Larson P S, Schwartz J J. The effect of urinary pH on the elimination of quinine in man. *J Pharmacol Exp Ther* (1943) 79, 136.
2 Hurwitz A. The effects of antacids on gastrointestinal drug absorption. II. Effect on sulfadiazine and quinine. *J Pharmacol Exp Ther* (1971) 179, 485.

Rifampicin + isoniazid

Summary

It has been suggested that concurrent use may increase the incidence of hepatotoxicity

Interaction, mechanism, importance and management

Studies in man have shown that the concentrations and half-lives of both drugs are unaffected during combined use.[1] The question of whether concurrent use increases the incidence of hepatotoxicity has been extensively discussed but no definite conclusions have been reached.[2] It would, however, seem prudent to be on the watch for signs of liver damage if both drugs are administered together.

References

1 Boman G. Serum concentration and half-life of rifampicin after simultaneous oral administration of aminosalicylic acid or isoniazid. *Europ J clin Pharmacol* (1974) 7, 217.
2 Pessayre D, Bentata M, Degott C, Nonel O, Miguet J-P, Rueff B and Benhamou J-P. Isoniazid–rifampin fulminant hepatitis. A possible consequence of the enhancement of isoniazid hepatotoxicity by enzyme induction. *Gastroenterology* (1977) 72, 284.

Rifampicin + para-aminosalicylic acid (PAS)

Summary

Serum levels of rifampicin are reduced 50% by the concurrent use of para-aminosalicylic acid granules which contain bentonite.

Interaction

The bentonite excipient in the granules of para-aminosalicylic acid can markedly reduce the gastrointestinal absorption of rifampicin.

> A study in 30 tuberculous patients showed that the serum concentration of rifampicin following 10 mg/kg oral doses were reduced at 2 h more than 50% (from 6·06 to 2·91 µg/ml) by the concurrent use of para-aminosalicylic acid.[1] The preparation used was *PAS-Granulate* (Ferrosan). Subsequent studies by the same workers on normal subjects showed that this was not due to the para-aminosalicylic acid itself but to the bentonite which was the main excipient of the granules.[2]

Other studies confirm the marked reduction in rifampicin serum levels in the presence of para-aminosalicylic acid granules.[3,4]

Mechanism

There is good evidence to show that bentonite in the para-aminosalicylate granules adsorbs the rifampicin, thereby preventing its absorption by the gut and resulting in reduced serum rifampicin levels.[2]

Importance and management

Well documented and important. Separating the

administration of the two drugs by 8–12 h to prevent their mixing in the gut has been suggested as an effective way of preventing this interaction.[1]

References
1 Boman G, Hanngren Å, Malmborg A-S, Borgå O and Sjöqvist F. Drug interaction: decreased serum concentrations of rifampicin when given with PAS. *Lancet* (1971) **i**, 800.
2 Boman G, Lundgren P and Stjernström G. Mechanism of the inhibitory effect of PAS granules on the absorption of rifampicin: absorption of rifampicin by an excipient, bentonite. *Europ J clin Pharmacol* (1975) **8**, 293.
3 Boman G. Serum concentration and half-life of rifampicin after simultaneous oral administration of aminosalicylic acid or isoniazid. *Europ J clin Pharmacol* (1974) **7**, 217.
4 Boman G, Borgå O, Hanngren Å, Malmborg A-S and Sjöqvist F. Pharmacokinetic interactions between the tuberculostatics rifampicin, para-aminosalicylic acid and isoniazid. *Acta Pharmac Toxicol* (1970) **28**, (Suppl 1) 15.

Rifampicin + probenecid

Summary
There is conflicting evidence showing that the serum levels of rifampicin may or may not be increased by the concurrent use of probenecid. This interaction is of doubtful importance.

Interaction
An early report[1] suggested that rifampicin serum levels were raised by probenecid when taken concurrently, but this has not been confirmed in later studies.[2,3]

> A study on 5 healthy volunteers who were given doses of probenecid both before and after taking single 300 mg doses of rifampicin, showed that the mean peak serum–rifampicin levels were raised by 86%, and at 4, 6 and 9 h the percentage increases were 118, 90 and 102 respectively.[1]
>
> Subsequent comparative studies, in patients taking either 600 mg rifampicin or 300 mg rifampicin plus 2 g probenecid taken 30 min before, showed that the latter group had serum rifampicin levels which were only about half those achieved by patients on 600 mg rifampicin.[2]

Similar results were found in a study with patients given 450 mg rifampicin.[3]

Mechanism
Not known.

Importance and management
Rifampicin is an effective antitubercular drug, but expensive, so the idea of giving smaller doses but with probenecid to raise the serum levels was attractive because costs could be reduced. However, the response of patients is clearly so inconsistent and unpredictable that probenecid cannot be used routinely for this purpose, although it should be borne in mind that some patients who are given the two drugs together may show elevated rifampicin levels.

References
1 Kenwright S and Levi A J. Impairment of hepatic uptake of rifamycin antibiotics by probenecid, and its therapeutic implications. *Lancet* (1973) **ii**, 1401.
2 Fallon R J, Lees A W, Allan G W, Smith J and Tyrrell W F. Probenecid and rifampicin serum levels. *Lancet* (1975) **ii**, 792.
3 Allen B W, Ellard G A, Mitchison D A, Hatfield A R W, Kenwright S and Levi A J. Probenecid and serum-rifampicin. *Lancet* (1975) **ii**, 1309.

Sodium fusidate + cholestyramine

Summary
Animal studies indicate that cholestyramine can reduce the gastrointestinal absorption of sodium fusidate. Confirmation of this interaction in man is required.

Interaction, mechanism, importance and management

Both in-vitro and in-vivo studies using rats have shown that cholestyramine can bind with sodium fusidate within the gut, thereby reducing the amount available for absorption. It seems highly likely that a similar interaction will occur in man, resulting in a reduction in the antimicrobial effects of the sodium fusidate. Confirmation of this is as yet lacking. If concurrent use is considered necessary, it would be prudent to separate the administration of the two compounds as much as possible to prevent their admixture in the gut. This has proved to be effective with other drugs which bind to cholestyramine.

Reference

1 Johns W E and Bates T R. Drug–cholestyramine interactions. I. Physicochemical factors affecting in vitro binding of sodium fusidate to cholestyramine. *J Pharm Sci* (1972) **61**, 730.

Sulphasalazine + cholestyramine

Summary

Animal studies indicate that cholestyramine can markedly reduce the activity of sulphasalazine but confirmation of this interaction in man is, as yet, lacking.

Interaction, mechanism, importance and management

Sulphasalazine is believed to be metabolized by bacterial azo-enzymes in the gut to form sulphapyridine and 5-aminosalicylic acid. These two metabolites are thought to be the active substances in the treatment of ulcerative colitis. It has been shown that sulphasalazine can bind with cholestyramine and, when bound, the azo-bond is protected against attack by the bacterial enzymes so that the active metabolites are not released.

A study in rats showed that the concurrent use of cholestyramine and sulphasalazine resulted in a 30-fold increase in the faecal excretion of intact sulphasalazine. It seems probable therefore that concurrent use could seriously reduce the therapeutic efficacy of the sulphasalazine in man, but this requires direct clinical confirmation.

Reference

1 Pieniaszek H J and Bates T R. Cholestyramine-induced inhibition of salicylazosulfapyridine (sulfasalazine) metabolism by rat intestinal microflora. *J Pharmacol Exp Ther* (1976) **198**, 240.

Sulphasalazine + folic acid

Summary

Sulphasalazine can impair the absorption of folic acid by the gut.

Interaction, mechanism, importance and management

Studies in rats have shown that the absorption of folic acid is inhibited by the presence of sulphasalazine. Folic acid absorption is also impaired in patients with inflammatory bowel disease (ulcerative colitis and granulomatous colitis) leading to folic acid deficiency, and the absorption is further impaired if sulphasalazine is used concurrently.[1] The reasons are not understood. The importance of this interaction awaits clinical study.

Reference

1 Franklin J L and Rosenberg I H. Impaired folic acid absorption in inflammatory disease: effects of salicylazosulfapyridine (Azulfidine). *Gastroenterology* (1973) **64**, 517.

Sulphasalazine + iron salts

Summary
Sulphasalazine can impair the absorption of iron.

Interaction, mechanism, importance and management

A study[1] has shown that the concurrent use of sulphasalazine and ferrous sulphate can result in a reduction in the serum levels of sulphasalazine. It has been suggested that this may be because the sulphasalazine chelates with the iron which interferes with its absorption. To what extent this interaction might affect the therapeutic response to either compound is uncertain.

Reference
1 Das K M and Eastwood M A. Effect of iron and calcium on salicylazosulphapyridine metabolism. *Scott Med J* (1973) 18, 45.

Sulphonamides + barbiturates

Summary
The anaesthetic effects of thiopentone are enhanced but shortened by pretreatment with sulphafurazole (sulfisoxazole). Phenobarbitone appears not to interact significantly with sulphasalazine, sulphafurazole or sulphasomidine. Information about other sulphonamide/barbiturate interactions in man appears to be lacking.

Interaction

A study on a large number of patients showed that the prior intravenous administration of 40 mg/kg sulphafurazole reduced the required anaesthetic dosage of thiopentone (thiopental) by 40% but the awakening time was shortened.[1]

This interaction is confirmed by animal experiments.[2] Other studies involving phenobarbital with sulphafurazole,[3] sulphasomidine[3] and sulphasalazine[4] indicate that no interaction of importance occurs with these sulphonamides.

Mechanism

It is suggested that the sulphafurazole successfully competes with the thiopentone for the plasma protein binding sites,[5] the result being that more free and active barbiturate molecules remain in circulation to exert their anaesthetic effects and a smaller dose is therefore required.[1] Changes in the metabolism of some of the barbiturates cited can occur in the presence of phenobarbitone but their importance is doubtful.[3,4]

Importance and management

The evidence for the sulphafurazole/thiopentone interaction is limited but it appears to be strong. Less thiopentone than usual may be required to achieve adequate anaesthesia but since the awakening time is shortened repeat doses may be required. Information about other sulphonamide/barbiturate interactions is also very limited, but none so far reported seems to be of clinical importance.

Reference
1 Csogor S I and Kerek S F. Enhancement of thiopentone anaesthesia by sulphafurazole. *Brit J Anaesth* (1970) 42, 988.
2 Csogor S I, Palfy B and Fetzt G. Influence du sulfathiazol sur l'effet narcotique du thiopentonal et de l'hexobarbital. *Rev Roum Physiol* (1971) 8, 81.
3 Krauer B. Comparative investigations of elimination kinetics of two sulphonamides in children with and without phenobarbital administration. *Schweiz Med Wschr* (1971) 101, 668.
4 Schroder H, Lewkonia R M and Evans D A P. Metabolism of salicylazosulfapyridine in healthy subjects and in patients with ulcerative colitis. Effects of colectomy and of phenobarbital. *Clin Pharmacol Ther* (1973) 14, 802.
5 Csogor S I and Papp J. Competition between sulphonamides and thiopental for the binding sites on plasma proteins. *Arzneim-Forsch.* (1970) 20, 1925.

Sulphonamides + local anaesthetics

Summary

The p-aminobenzoic acid (PABA) derived from certain local anaesthetics can antagonize the effects of sulphonamides and allow the development of local and even generalized infections.

Interaction

Four clinical cases have been described in which local infections occurred in areas where procaine had been injected prior to diagnostic taps in meningitis, or draining procedures in empyema. Extensive cellulitis of the lumbar region occurred in one case, and the patient died of meningitis despite continued therapy with sulphadiazine.[1]

A study[2] in man demonstrated that the amount of procaine in pleural fluid after anaesthesia for thoracentesis was sufficient to inhibit the antibacterial activity of 5% sulphapyridine against type III pneumococci. Other studies in animals have confirmed that antagonism can occur both in vivo[3,4,5] and in vitro[6] with local anaesthetics which are hydrolysed to PABA.

Mechanism

The ester type of local anaesthetic is hydrolysed within the body to produce PABA. This compound can antagonize the effects of the sulphonamides by competitive inhibition. A fuller explanation of the PABA/sulphonamide interaction is given in the synopsis below.

Importance and management

The documentation of this interaction is mostly indirect, but it appears to be established. It is clearly of importance. Local anaesthetics of the ester type which are hydrolysed to PABA (e.g. amethocaine, tetracaine, cocaine, procaine, amylocaine) should be avoided in patients using sulphonamides. The amide type of local anaesthetic which is not hydrolysed to PABA includes bupivacaine, cinchocaine (dibucaine), lignocaine (lidocaine), mepivacaine and prilocaine. These do not interact adversely.

Reference

1 Peterson O L and Finland M. Sulfonamide inhibiting action of procaine. *Amer J Med Sci* (1944) **207**, 166.
2 Boroff D A, Cooper A and Bullowa J G M. Inhibition of sulfapyridine by procaine in chest fluids after procaine anaesthesia. *Proc Soc Exp Biol Med* (1941) **47**, 182.
3 Pfeiffer C C and Grant C W. The procaine–sulfonamide antagonism; an evaluation of local anesthetics for use with sulfonamide therapy. *Anesthesiology* (1944) **5**, 605.
4 Casten D, Fried J J and Hallman F A. Inhibitory effect of procaine on bacteriostatic activity of sulfathiazole. *Surg Gyn Obst* (1943) **76**, 726.
5 Powell H M, Krahl M E and Clowes G H A. Inhibition of chemotherapeutic action of sulfapyridine by local anesthetics. *J Indiana Med Ass* (1942) **35**, 62.
6 Walker B S and Derow M A. The antagonism of local anesthetics against the sulfonamides. *Amer J Med Sci* (1945) **210**, 585.

Sulphonamides + para-aminobenzoic acid (PABA)

Summary

The antibacterial effects of the sulphonamides are antagonized by PABA.

Interaction, mechanism

Many micro-organisms can synthesize their own folate if provided with PABA. Man on the other hand requires folate preformed in his diet. The molecular structure of the sulphonamides is sufficiently similar to PABA for micro-organisms to incorporate the sulphonamide into the synthetic biochemical pathways concerned with making folate, but still sufficiently dissimilar to prevent the synthesis being brought to completion. Starved of folate, the organism ceases to grow and multiply, and it is in this way that the sulphonamides act as bacteriostatic agents.

The term 'competitive antagonist' is used to describe this situation because PABA and the sulphonamide compete with one another to take part in the synthetic reactions, the relative concentrations of each type of molecule being among the factors which determine the 'winner', hence the importance of achieving adequate concentrations of the sulphonamide and of avoiding the introduction of additional PABA molecules.

Importance and management
The interaction between PABA and the sulphonamides has been extensively studied and is very well documented. PABA should not be given to patients receiving sulphonamides.

Tetracyclines + alcohol

Summary
The serum levels of doxycycline may fall below minimal therapeutic concentrations in alcoholic patients, but tetracycline itself is not affected and it seems likely that the other tetracyclines are also unaffected. There is nothing to suggest that moderate amounts of alcohol will affect doxycycline or any other tetracycline in normal subjects.

Interaction
In a comparative study the half-life of doxycycline was found to be 10·5 h in 6 alcoholic subjects compared with 14·7 h in 6 normal healthy volunteers. The half-life of tetracycline was found to be the same in both groups. All of them were given 100 mg doxycycline a day after a 200 mg loading dose, and 500 mg tetracycline twice a day after an initial 750 mg loading dose.[1]

Mechanism
Heavy drinkers can metabolize some drugs much more quickly than non-drinkers due to the enzyme-inducing effects of alcohol,[2] and this interaction with doxycycline would seem to be due to this effect.

Importance and control
Information on this interaction is limited. The shortened half-life of doxycycline in alcoholics is important because, in 2 of the 6 patients described in the study cited, the serum concentrations were seen to fall well below what is generally accepted as the minimum therapeutic concentration. Moreover, since the 6 subjects drank no alcohol at all during the study and the effects of enzyme-inducing agents wane after their withdrawal, the half-life of doxycycline might, while drinking, be even shorter. So it might be better to dose twice a day with doxycycline instead of only once. Alternatively tetracycline could be used because it appears not to be affected.

There is no direct evidence about the effects of drinking on the other tetracycline antibiotics, but based on the lack of effects of some other known enzyme-inducing agents on the tetracyclines it seems possible that they may be unaffected.[3] This needs confirmation.

There is no evidence to suggest that moderate amounts of alcohol interact with any of the tetracyclines in non-alcoholic subjects.

References
1 Neuvonen P J, Penttila O, Roos M and Tirkkonen J. Effect of long-term alcohol consumption on the half-life of tetracycline and doxycycline in man. *Int J Clin Pharmacol* (1976) **14**, 303.
2 Misra P S, Leférre A, Ishii H, Rubin E and Lieber C S. Increase of ethanol, meprobamate and pentobarbital metabolism after chronic ethanol administration in man and rats. *Amer J Med* (1971) **571**, 346.
3 Neuvonen P J, Penttila O, Lehtovaara K and Aho K. Effect of antiepileptic drugs on the elimination of various tetracycline derivatives. *Europ J Clin Pharmacol* (1975) **9**, 147.

Tetracyclines + antacids

Summary
The serum levels, and as a consequence, the therapeutic effectiveness of the tetracycline antibiotics, can be markedly reduced by the concurrent use of alu-

minium-containing antacids due to the formation of less-soluble tetracycline–aluminium chelates. This is almost certainly true for magnesium-, calcium- and bismuth-containing antacids as well. Other antacids such as sodium bicarbonate which raise the gastric pH may also reduce the bioavailability of some tetracycline preparations.

Interaction

The absorption of the tetracycline antibiotics from the gut and the subsequent serum concentration attained can be considerably reduced by the concurrent use of aluminium-containing antacids. This is almost certainly true for the calcium-containing antacids, but not so certainly for those containing magnesium or bismuth.

(a) Aluminium-containing antacids

A study, carried out on 5 patients and 6 normal subjects taking 500 mg chlortetracycline orally every 6 h, showed that when they were given two tablespoons of aluminium hydroxide gel (Amphogel) at the same time, within 48 h the serum chlortetracycline levels had fallen by between 80 and 90%. One of the patients had a recurrence of her urinary tract infection which subsided when the antacid was withdrawn.[1]

An approximately 80% fall in serum chlortetracycline levels due to the concurrent use of aluminium hydroxide was confirmed in another study.[2]

Other studies in man showed that 30 ml aluminium hydroxide gel reduced the serum levels of oxytetracycline by more than 50%;[3] 20 ml aluminium hydroxide caused a 75% reduction in demeclocycline serum levels;[4] 15 ml aluminium hydroxide gel caused a 100% reduction in doxycycline serum levels;[5] and 30 ml magnesium–aluminium hydroxide (Maalox) caused a 90% reduction in tetracycline.

(b) Calcium, magnesium and bismuth-containing antacids

The evidence of an interaction with these antacids is less direct.

An in-vitro study with calcium carbonate[9] and clinical studies on the effects of the presence of calcium ions in the form of milk (see p. 111) or as dicalcium phosphate[7] and as an excipient in tetracycline capsules[8] indicate that an interaction with calcium-containing antacids is a virtual certainty, but no direct clinical studies using an actual antacid appear to have been published.

Magnesium in the form of the sulphate interacts with tetracycline, but in the clinical study on record[8] the dose of magnesium was much higher than would normally be found in the usual dose of antacid. An in-vitro study indicates that magnesium as the oxide may interact.[9]

Bismuth carbonate has been shown to interact with the tetracyclines in vitro, but no clinical studies appear to have been published.[9]

(c) Sodium-containing antacids

A study on eight subjects showed that when they were given a 250 mg capsule of tetracycline hydrochloride with 2 g sodium bicarbonate, the mean absorption of the tetracycline was reduced by 50%. If, however, the tetracycline was dissolved before administration, the absorption was unaffected by the sodium bicarbonate.[10]

Another study stated that 2 g sodium bicarbonate had an insignificant effect on the tetracycline absorption.[12]

Mechanism

The work of Albert and Rees[11] in the mid-fifties demonstrated that the tetracyclines chelate with the metallic ions of aluminium, magnesium, calcium, bismuth and others to form compounds which are much less soluble, and therefore much less readily absorbed by the gut. This provides one explanation for the reduced serum levels which are attained if antacids containing these ions are administered with the tetracyclines.

It has also been shown[10] that the solubility of tetracyclines in the pH range 1–3 is a hundred times greater than at pH 5–6. An antacid which can raise the gastric pH above about 4 for 20–30 min or so, will prevent the full dissolution of the tetracycline, thus allowing a considerable proportion (up to 50%) of the undissolved drug to be emptied into the duodenum. The pH there (5–6) is also unfavourable to the full dissolution of the drug, so that if the antibiotic fails to be fully dissolved in the stomach it is unlikely ever to reach completion in the alkaline intestinal fluids. Thus a good proportion of the drug may remain undissolved and unavailable for absorption. This is an additional reason why these antacids may prevent the full absorption of the tetracycline antibiotics and on its own accounts for the interaction with sodium bicarbonate.

Importance and management

These interactions are established and important.

The reduction in the antibacterial effects will clearly depend on how much the serum levels are lowered, and on the susceptibility of the organisms; but using normal amounts of antacids the reductions cited above (50–100%) are so large that many organisms will not be exposed to serum levels above the minimum inhibitory concentration (MIC). As a general rule, therefore, none of the aluminium, magnesium, calcium or bismuth-containing antacids, or others such as sodium bicarbonate which can markedly change the gastric pH, should be given at the same time as the tetracycline antibiotics. If they must be used, separating the dosage by as long a time interval as possible would seem to be a reasonable way to prevent their mixing in the gut.

Antacids such as sodium bicarbonate and others which only affect bioavailability by altering gastric pH will only interact with tetracycline preparations which are not already dissolved before ingestion (e.g. those in capsule form).

It is usually recommended that the tetracyclines should be taken before food to overcome their gastric irritant effects, but it is not entirely clear how much this affects their bioavailability. One study with demeclocycline demonstrated that it reduced the absorption[4] whereas another claimed that it did not.[5]

References
1 Waisbren B A, and Hueckel J S Reduced absorption of Aureomycin caused by Aluminium Hydroxide gel (Amphojel). *Proc Soc Exp Biol Med NY* (1950) **73**, 73
2 Seed J C and Wilson C E. The effect of aluminium hydroxide on serum aureomycin concentrations after simultaneous oral administration. *Bull Johns Hopkins Hosp* (1950) **86**, 415.
3 Michel J C, Sayer R J and Kirby W M M. Effect of food and antacids on blood levels of Aureomycin and Terramycin. *J Lab Clin Med* (1950) **36**, 632.
4 Scheiner J and Altemeier W A. Experimental study of factors inhibiting absorption and effective therapeutic levels of declomycin. *Surg Gynec Obstet* (1962) **114**, 9.
5 Rosenblatt J E, Barrett J E, Brodie J L and Kirby W M M. Comparison of in vitro activity and clinical pharmacology of doxycycline with other tetracyclines. *Antimicrob Ag Chemother* (1966) **134**.
6 Harcourt R S and Hamburger M. The effect of magnesium sulphate in lowering tetracycline blood levels. *J Lab Clin Med* (1957) **50**, 464.
7 Boger W P and Gavin J J. An evaluation of tetracycline preparations. *New Eng J Med* (1959) **261**, 827.
8 Sweeney W M, Hardy S M, Dornbush A C and Ruegsegger J M. Absorption of tetracycline in human beings as affected by certain excipients. *Antibiol Med Clin Ther* (1957) **4**, 642.
9 Christensen E K J, Kerckhoffs H P M and Huizinga T. De invloed van antacida op de afgifte in vitro van tetracycline-hydrochloride. *Pharm Weckblad* (1967) **102**, 463.
10 Barr W H, Adir J and Garrettson L. Decrease of tetracycline absorption in man by sodium bicarbonate. *Clin Pharmacol Ther* (1971) **12**, 779.
11 Albert A and Rees C W. Avidity of the tetracyclines for the cations of metals. *Nature* (1956) **177**, 433.
12 Garty M and Hurwitz A. Effect of cimetidine and antacids on gastrointestinal absorption of tetracycline. *Clin Pharmacol Ther* (1980) **28**, 203.

Tetracyclines + anticonvulsants

Summary
The serum concentrations of doxycycline are reduced and can fall below the accepted therapeutic minimum in patients on long-term treatment with barbiturates, phenytoin or carbamazepine. Other tetracyclines appear to be unaffected.

Interaction
A study on 14 patients on antiepileptic therapy showed that during treatment with phenytoin (200–500 mg daily) the half-life of doxycycline was 7·1 h (5 patients); with phenytoin (300–350 mg daily) and carbamazepine (800 mg daily) the doxycycline half-life was 7·4 h (4 patients); and with carbamazepine (300–1000 mg daily) the doxycycline half-life was 8·4 h (5 patients). These values are all significantly shorter than the mean doxycycline half-life of 15·1 h observed in 9 control patients receiving no other medication.[1]

An investigation on 16 epileptic patients on long-term anticonvulsant therapy with phenobarbiton, phenytoin and carbamazepine showed that the serum half-life of doxycycline was 7·1 h compared with 13·3 h in healthy volunteers taking only the antibiotic. Doxycycline serum levels in the patients were also found to have fallen below 0·5 μg/ml in almost all of them during the 12–24 h period following their last dose of doxycycline. Tetracycline, methacycline, oxytetracycline, demethyltetracycline and chlortetracycline are not significantly affected by the use of these anticonvulsants.[2]

These two detailed studies confirm the original observations[3] made in a crossover study on 10 patients given doxycycline who were also taking barbiturates either for epilepsy or, in one case, as a hypnotic (amylobarbitone) over an extended period of time. They are also in line with another study involving phenobarbitone and doxycycline.[4]

Mechanism

Not fully established. Phenytoin and the barbiturates are known enzyme-inducing agents and it has been suggested that the shortening of the half-life of doxycycline comes about because its metabolism is accelerated by these anticonvulsants. Preliminary results indicate that displacement of the doxycycline from plasma proteins by phenytoin is not a likely alternative explanation.[3]

Importance and management

An established and important interaction. A fall in serum doxycycline concentrations to below 0·5 μg/ml between 12 and 24 h after the last dose (100 mg) of the antibiotic means that levels have fallen below what is generally accepted as the minimum therapeutic concentration. It has been suggested that this can be accommodated by giving the antibiotic twice a day, or possibly by increasing the dosage.[2] Alternatively, another tetracycline antibiotic could be used such as tetracycline, methacycline, oxytetracycline, demethyltetracycline or chlortetracycline which are reported not to be affected by the concurrent use of the anticonvulsants mentioned.[2]

References
1 Penttila O, Neuvonen P J, Aho K and Lehtovaara R. Interaction between doxycycline and some antiepileptic drugs. *Brit Med J* (1974) **2**, 470.
2 Neuvonen P J, Penttila O, Lehtovaara R and Aho K. Effect of antiepileptic drugs on the elimination of various tetracycline derivatives. *Europ J clin Pharmacol* (1975) **9**, 147.
3 Neuvonen P J and Pentilla O. Interaction between doxycycline and barbiturates. *Brit Med J* (1974) **1**, 535.
4 Alestig K. Studies on the intestinal excretion of doxycycline. *Scand J infect Dis.* (1974) **6**, 265.

Tetracyclines + cimetidine

Summary

There is some disagreement about whether cimetidine does or does not reduce the absorption of tetracycline administered in capsule form.

Interaction

There are two reports describing studies of this interaction. One indicates that a significant reduction in tetracycline absorption occurs, whereas the other states that no significant interaction takes place.

A randomized cross-over study on 5 volunteers who were given two 250 mg capsules of tetracycline hydrochloride showed that during concurrent treatment with cimetidine (200 mg three times a day and 400 mg at bedtime) the absorption of the tetracycline was considerably reduced. The cumulative amount of tetracycline excreted up to 72 h was reduced by about 30% (from 241 to 172 mg). This compares with a statistically insignificant reduction (from 264 to 236 mg) when the tetracycline was given in solution.[1]

In another randomized cross-over study 5 normal subjects were given a 250 mg tetracycline hydrochloride capsule with either 200 ml of water, or 200 ml water plus 300 mg cimetidine. The area under the serum concentration time curve for 24 h with the water was 28·9 μg/ml/h, and with cimetidine was 26·7 μg/ml/h. The authors of the report state quite positively that '. . . we have demonstrated that cimetidine does not affect tetracycline absorption . . .'. However, the serum concentration time curves illustrated in the text showed that at 4 h the tetracycline/cimetidine curve was depressed 20% compared with the tetracycline/water curve.[2]

Mechanism

Uncertain. One suggestion has been made to account for the reduced absorption. Dissolution of the tetracycline in capsule form occurs in the stomach and depends upon the gastric acidity. The cimetidine raises gastric pH (the second study cited indicated a rise from pH 2 to 5) and thereby inhibits the tetracycline dissolution to some extent. Some of the tetracycline may therefore still be undissolved when it reaches the small intestine. Further dissolution on the alkaline conditions of the small intestine is unlikely so that bioavailability is reduced. This suggested mechanism requires confirmation.

Importance and management

The evidence appears to be limited to these two discordant reports. More study (in particular longer-term investigations using multiple dosages) is needed to resolve whether this interaction is important or not. In the meantime it would seem prudent to be on the alert for a reduction in the therapeutic response to tetracycline during concurrent use if given in capsule form. Tetracycline in liquid form does not, according to the first report, interact. Information about other tetracyclines is as yet lacking.

References
1 Cole J J, Charles B G and Ravenscroft P J. Interaction of cimetidine with tetracycline absorption. *Lancet* (1980) **ii**, 536.
2 Garty M and Hurwitz A. Effect of cimetidine and antacids on gastrointestinal absorption of tetracycline. *Clin Pharmacol Ther* (1980) **28**, 203.

Tetracyclines + diuretics

Summary

The concurrent use of tetracyclines and diuretics is associated with rises in blood urea nitrogen levels.

Interaction, mechanism, importance and management

A retrospective study of patient records showed that there was a strong association between tetracycline administration with diuretics (not named) and rises in blood urea nitrogen (BUN) levels. The reasons are not understood. It was concluded that tetracyclines should be avoided in patients on diuretics when alternative antibiotics could be substituted.[1]

References
1 Boston Collaborative Drug Surveillance Program. Tetracycline and drug-attributed rises in blood urea nitrogen. *J Amer med Ass* (1972) **220**, 377.

Tetracyclines + iron preparations

Summary

The absorption by the gut of both the tetracycline antibiotics and of iron salts is markedly reduced by concurrent administration, leading to depressed serum levels and diminished therapeutic effectiveness. If it is necessary to give both drugs, their administration should be separated as much as possible.

Interaction

(a) The effect of iron on tetracycline serum levels

An investigation on 10 healthy adults, who were given single oral doses of tetracycline antibiotics (200–500 mg according to the normal dose recommendations), showed that when they were also given 200 mg ferrous sulphate the average decrease in the serum antibiotic level of tetracycline was 40–50%; of oxytetracycline, 50–60%; and of methacycline and doxycycline, 80–90%.[1] (See illustration on page 3.)

Similar results have been described in other reports[2–5] showing that in some instances the serum levels are reduced below minimal bacterial inhibitory concentrations.

A study undertaken to find out if separating the dosages of the tetracycline and iron could overcome this interaction showed that if the iron was given 3 h before or 2 h after the tetracycline, the serum levels were not significantly depressed.[2,3]

Another investigation with doxycycline showed that even when the iron was given up to 11 h after the doxycycline, the serum concentrations were still lowered 20–45%.[4]

(b) The effect of tetracyclines on the absorption of iron

An investigation of this interaction showed that when 50 mg Fe^{2+} (equivalent to 250 mg ferrous sulphate) was given with 500 mg tetracycline, the absorption of iron in normal subjects was reduced 32–78% and in those with depleted iron stores 40–65%.[8,9]

Mechanisms

The tetracyclines have an affinity for the cations of several metals, including iron, and can form tetracycline-iron chelates.[6,7] These' chelates are much less soluble than the tetracycline itself and therefore much less readily absorbed from the gastrointestinal tract. Thus, the serum levels achieved are considerably reduced.

Separating the dosage of the iron and tetracycline can go a long way towards preventing the two becoming mixed together in the gut so that the physicochemical interaction does not take place.[2,3] However, in the case of doxycycline, some of the antibiotic is secreted back into the gut in the bile after absorption which tends to thwart any attempt to keep the iron and antibiotic apart.[4]

The different extent to which the iron salts interact with the tetracyclines appears to be a reflection of their ability to liberate ferrous and ferric ions which are free to combine with the tetracycline.[5]

The reduction in the absorption of iron also comes about because it is chelated with the tetracycline, as already described, and is therefore not available for absorption.

Importance and management

Well-studied and well-established interactions. Reductions in the serum tetracycline levels of the order of 30–90% due to the presence of iron salts are so large that, as is well demonstrated in one of the studies listed,[3] serum tetracycline levels can fall below concentrations which will inhibit bacterial growth (MIC). The importance of this interaction is clear.

The extent of the reduction in serum antibiotic levels depends on a number of factors: (a) the particular tetracycline used, tetracycline itself in the study cited above[1] was affected the least; (b) the time interval between the administration of the two drugs: giving the iron 3 h before or 2 h after the antibiotic was found to be quite satisfactory with tetracycline itself[2] but a time interval of as long as 11 h was inadequate for doxycycline because it can be absorbed and resecreted in the bile and so comes to be mixed with residual iron. (c) The particular iron preparation used: with

tetracycline the reduction in serum levels with ferrous sulphate was found to be 80–90%; with ferrous fumarate, succinate and gluconate 70–80%; with ferrous tartrate 50%, and with ferrous sodium edetate 30%.[5]

While therefore, it would seem sensible to avoid concurrent use whenever possible, it if is absolutely necessary to continue to give both drugs together, their administration should be separated by as long a time interval as possible, and one of the iron preparations causing the minimum interference should be used.

One suggestion which has been put forward[9] is a schedule in which 500 mg tetracycline is given 30–60 min before breakfast and dinner (total daily dose of 1 g), and 50 mg Fe^{2+} 1 h before lunch and 2 h after dinner. This would provide the patient with tetracycline serum concentrations of about 3–5 μg/ml and a daily iron absorption of 25 mg, sufficient to allow optimal haemoglobin regeneration values of 0·2–0·3 g%/day.

Only tetracycline, oxytetracycline, methacycline and doxycycline have so far been shown to interact with iron, but it seems reasonable to assume that the others will behave in a similar manner. This requires confirmation.

References

1 Neuvonen P J, Gothoni G, Hackman R and af Bjorksten K. Interference of iron with the absorption of tetracyclines in man. *Brit Med J* (1970) 4, 532.

2 Mattila M J, Neuronen P J, Gothoni G and Hackman C R. Interference of iron preparations and milk with the absorption of tetracyclines. *Excerpta Medica Int Congr Ser* no. 254 (1972). Toxicological problems of drug combinations, 128.

3 Gothoni G, Neuronen P J, Matilla M and Hackman R. Iron–tetracycline interaction: effect of time interval between the drugs. *Acta Med Scand* (1972) 191, 409.

4 Neuvonen P J and Penttila O. Effect of oral ferrous sulphate on the half-life of doxycycline in man. *Europ J Clin Pharmacol* (1974) 7, 361.

5 Neuvonen P J and Pentilla O. Inhibitory effect of various iron salts on the absorption of tetracycline in man. *Europ J clin Pharmacol* (1974) 7, 357.

6 Albert A and Rees C W. Avidity of the tetracyclines for the cations of metals. *Nature* (1956) 177, 433.

7 Albert A and Rees C W. Incompatibility of aluminium hydroxide and certain antibiotics. *Brit Med J* (1955) 2, 1027.

8 Heinrich H C, Oppitz K H and Gabbe E E. Hemmung der Eisenabsorption beim Menschen durch Tetracyclin. *Klin Wschr* (1974) 52, 493.

9 Heinrich H C and Oppitz K H. Tetracycline inhibits iron absorption in man. *Naturwissenschaften* (1973) 60, 524.

Tetracyclines + milk and dairy products

Summary

The serum levels and, as a consequence, the therapeutic effectiveness of the tetracycline antibiotics can be markedly reduced if they are allowed to come into contact in the gut with milk or other dairy products due to the formation of less soluble tetracycline–calcium chelates. Doxycycline is the least affected.

Interaction

(a) Demeclocycline + milk, butter milk or cottage cheese

Twelve normal volunteers were given a single 300 mg oral dose of demeclocycline with either 8 oz of fresh pasteurized milk, 8 oz of fresh pasteurized buttermilk (rather less than half a pint) or 4 oz of cottage cheese. Their serum demeclocycline levels were reduced by 70–80% compared with four subjects who had taken the same amount of antibiotic with a meal containing no dairy products.[1]

(b) Tetracycline, methacycline, oxytetracycline or doxycycline + milk

A study on healthy volunteers who were given single oral doses of the antibiotics (300–500 mg) showed that when they drank 300 ml (about half a pint) of milk at the same time the serum antibiotic levels of tetracycline, methacycline and oxytetracycline were reduced by about 50% whereas doxycycline remained unaffected.[2]

Similar results have been obtained from other studies[3,4] with the exception that doxycycline has in fact been found to be affected but to a much lesser extent than most of the other tetracyclines. The maximum serum levels of doxycycline 2 h after a single 100 mg oral dose were found to be reduced by about 20% (from $1 \cdot 79$ to $1 \cdot 45$ μg/ml) after drinking a glass (240 ml) of skimmed milk.[3]

Mechanism

Experiments in the 1950s[5,6] very adequately demonstrated the high affinity which the tetracyclines have for the cations of metals such as calcium which are found in abundance in milk and dairy products. The tetracycline–calcium chelate which forms, if the two are mixed, is much less soluble and therefore much less readily absorbed from the gastrointestinal tract so that the serum levels achieved are considerably lower. Doxycycline has a slightly lesser tendency to form chelates[7] than the other tetracyclines which explains why the serum levels are reduced to a smaller extent. It has also been shown that *in vitro*[8] the tetracycline chelates have a very much reduced antibacterial activity, but what part this

plays in the total interaction in man is not known.

Importance and management

These interactions are very well established and important. Reductions in the serum tetracycline levels of 50–80% due to the presence of milk or milk products are so large that the antibacterial effects of the tetracyclines may be minimal, or even nil. For this reason the tetracyclines should not be taken with milk or meals containing substantial amounts of dairy products such as cheese or yoghourt. As long a time interval as possible should be left between taking the antibiotic and having a meal containing milk products so that the chance of mixing within the gastrointestinal tract is minimized. Doxycycline appears to be affected by food or milk much less than the other tetracyclines and in this respect has an advantage over the others.

The manufacturers of tetracycline as the phosphate (*Tetrex*) claim that the phosphate combines with calcium leaving more free tetracycline available for absorption, so that this particular form of the antibiotic also appears to have advantages.[10]

It is common practice to recommend that the tetracyclines should be taken before food to overcome their gastric irritant effects, but it is not entirely clear whether, or how much, this affects their bioavailability. One study with demeclocycline demonstrated that food reduced the absorption[1] whereas another claimed that it did not.[3]

References

1 Scheiner J and Altemeier W A. Experimental study of factors inhibiting absorption and effective therapeutic levels of declomycin. *Surg Gynec Obstet* (1962) **114**, 9.
2 Neuvonen P, Matilla M, Gothoni G and Hackman R. Interference of iron and milk with absorption of tetracycline. *Scand J Clin Lab Invest* (1971) **116** (Suppl 27) 76.
3 Rosenblatt J E, Barrett J E, Brodie J L and Kirby W M M. Comparison of in vitro activity and clinical pharmacology of doxycycline with other tetracyclines. *Antimicrob Ag Chemother* (1966), 134.
4 Matilla M J, Neuvonen P J, Gothoni G and Hackman C R. Interference of iron preparations and milk with the absorption of tetracyclines. *Excerpta Medica Int Congr Ser* (1971) **254**, 128.
5 Albert A and Rees C W. Avidity of the tetracyclines for the cations of metals. *Nature* (1956) **177**, 433.

6 Albert A and Rees C W. Incompatibility of aluminium hydroxide and certain antibiotics. *Brit Med J* (1955) **2**, 1027.

7 Schach von Wittenau M. Some pharmacokinetic aspects of doxycycline metabolism in man. *Chemotherapy* (1968) **13** (*Suppl*), 41.

8 Weinberg E D. The mutual effects of antimicrobial compounds and metallic ions. *Bacteriol Rev* (1957) **21**, 46.

9 ABPI Data Sheet Compendium, 1979–80, p. 179 (1979) Pharmind Publications, London.

Tetracyclines + zinc sulphate

Summary

The absorption of tetracycline from the gut and the subsequent antibiotic serum concentration achieved can be reduced if zinc sulphate is taken concurrently. Separating their administration as much as possible minimizes the effects of this interaction. Doxycycline interacts minimally with zinc.

Interaction

A study in which 7 subjects were administered 500 mg tetracycline, either alone or with zinc sulphate (200 mg containing 45 mg Zn^{2+}), showed that the serum concentrations of the tetracycline were reduced by 30–40% by the presence of the zinc.[1] The areas under the curves were similarly reduced.

These results were confirmed in another study in which the serum tetracycline concentrations were reduced by over 50%.[2] The reduction in serum zinc concentrations were found to be minimal.[2]

Mechanism

Zinc (like iron, calcium and aluminium) forms a relatively stable and poorly absorbed chelate with tetracycline within the gut which results in a reduction in the amount of antibiotic available for absorption.[3,4]

Importance and management

The documentation is not great, but it is an established interaction. The administration of tetracycline and zinc sulphate should be separated by at least 3 h so that the two compounds come into minimal contact within the gut. This has been shown to be effective with iron salts which chelate with tetracycline in a similar way.[5] An alternative is to use doxycycline which has been shown to interact minimally with zinc.[1] It is not certain whether other tetracyclines behave in the same way as tetracycline, but it would be reasonable to assume that they do. Confirmation of this is required.

The authors of studies in which the effects of this interaction on zinc absorption were studied[2,6] suggest that the reduction in serum zinc concentrations is likely to be of little practical importance.

References

1 Penttila O, Hurme H and Neuvonen P J. Effect of zinc sulphate on the absorption of tetracycline and doxycycline in man. *Europ J Clin Pharmacol* (1975) **9**, 131.

2 Andersson K-E, Bratt L, Dencker H, Kamure C and Lanner E. Inhibition of tetracycline absorption by zinc. *Europ J Clin Pharmacol* (1976) **10**, 59.

3 Albert A and Rees C W. Avidity of the tetracyclines for cations of metals. *Nature* (Lond) (1956) **177**, 433.

4 Doluisio J T and Martin A N. Metal complexation of the tetracycline hydrochlorides. *J Med Chem* (1963) **16**, 16.

5 Gothoni G, Neuvonen P J, Mattila M and Hackman R. Iron–tetracycline interaction: effect of time interval between drugs. *Acta med Scand* (1972) **191**, 409.

6 Andersson K-E, Bratt L, Dencker H and Lanner E. Some aspects of the intestinal absorption of zinc in man. *Europ J clin Pharmacol* (1975) **9**, 423.

CHAPTER 6. ANTICOAGULANT DRUG INTERACTIONS

The blood clotting process

When blood is shed, or clotting initiated in some other way, a highly complex chain or cascade of biochemical reactions is set in motion which ends in the formation of a network or clot of insoluble protein threads enmeshing the blood cells. These threads are produced by the polymerization of the molecules of fibrinogen (a soluble protein present in the plasma) into threads of insoluble fibrin. The penultimate step in the chain of reactions requires the presence of an enzyme, thrombin, which is produced from its precursor, prothrombin, already present in the plasma. Figure 6.1 is a highly simplified diagram to illustrate the final stages of this cascade of reactions.

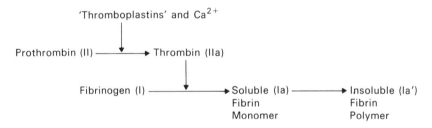

Fig. 6.1. A highly simplified flow diagram to illustrate the final stages in the blood clotting process.

Mode of action of the oral anticoagulants

The oral anticoagulants extend the time taken for blood to clot and, it is believed, also inhibit the pathological formation of blood clots within the blood vessels by reducing the concentrations within the plasma of a number of components necessary for the cascade to proceed, namely factors VII, IX, X and II (prothrombin). The parts played by three of these four are not shown in the schema illustrated but they are essential for the production of the so-called 'thromboplastins'.

The synthesis of normal amounts of these four factors takes place within the liver, with vitamin K as one of the essential ingredients, but, in the presence of an oral anticoagulant, the rate of synthesis of all four is retarded. One of the early theories to explain why this happens was based on the observed resemblance between the molecular shapes of vitamin K and the oral anticoagulants. It was suggested that the molecules were sufficiently similar for the anticoagulant actually to take part in the biochemical reactions by which all four factors are synthesized, but sufficiently dissimilar to prevent the completion of the reactions. The term 'competitive antagonist' is used for this kind of situation because vitamin K and the oral anticoagulants compete with one another to take part in the reactions, their relative concentrations being among the factors which determine 'winner'. Certainly a glance at Fig. 6.2 will show that there is some superficial resemblance between the molecules of vitamin K and the two main types of anticoagulant. This theory is, however, almost certainly too simple and a number of alternative ideas have now been put forward; nevertheless the basic practical principles of a concentration competition between the two types of molecule remains perfectly valid. A reduction in the concentrations and activity of all four factors, VII, IX, X and II (prothrombin) by the oral anticoagulants is embraced by the portmanteau term 'hypoprothrombinaemia'.

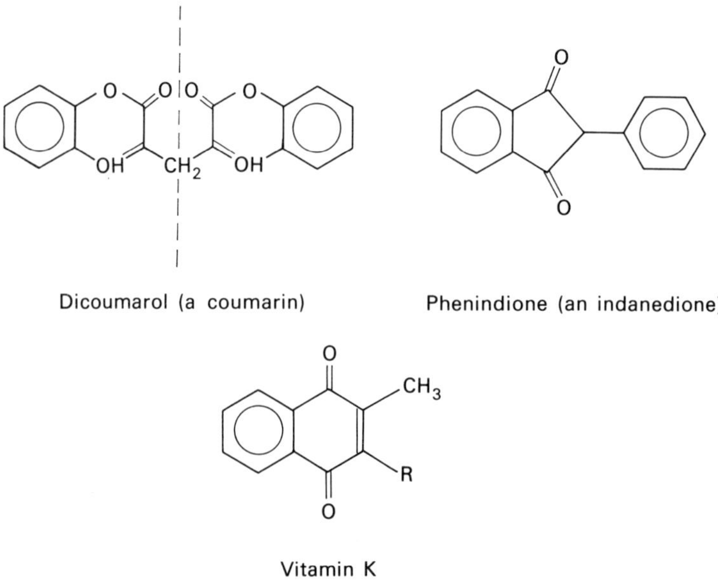

Dicoumarol (a coumarin)   Phenindione (an indanedione)

Vitamin K

Fig. 6.2. A comparison between the molecules of vitamin K, and coumarin and indanedione anticoagulants.

The therapeutic use of the oral anticoagulants

During anticoagulant therapy it is usual to depress the levels of prothrombin and factors VII, IX and X to those which are believed to give protection against intravascular clotting, without running the risk of excessive depression which leads to spontaneous bruising and haemorrhage from the urinary and gastrointestinal tracts. To achieve this each patient is individually 'titrated' with doses of anticoagulant until the desired response has been attained, a procedure which normally takes several days because the oral anticoagulants do not act directly on the blood clotting factors already in circulation, but on the rate of synthesis of new factors by the liver. The 'end-point' of the titration can be determined by one of a number of different but closely related laboratory in-vitro tests which measure the extension in the time taken for the blood to clot (e.g. the so-called 'one-stage prothrombin time'), although the result of the test may be expressed, not in seconds, but as a ratio or a percentage of normal values.

The normal plasma clotting time, using the Quick one-stage prothrombin time test, is about 12 s, a $2-2\frac{1}{2}$ times extension to about 24–30 s or so is usually regarded as adequate in anticoagulant therapy. Other tests include the thrombotest and the prothrombin–proconvertin (P–P) test.

Table 6.1. Anticoagulants

Non-proprietary names	Proprietary names
Oral anticoagulants	
Coumarins	
Cyclocoumarol	—
Cumetharol	*Dicoumoxyl*
Dic(o)umarol (bishydroxycoumarin)	*Dufalone AP, Baracoumin*
Ethylidene dicoumarin	*EDC*
Ethyl biscoumacetate	*Tromexan, Stabilène*
Nicoumalone (acenocoumarol)	*Sinthrome, Sintrom*
Phenprocoumon	*Marcoumar, Marcumar, Liquamar*
Warfarin-deanol	*Adoisine*
Warfarin sodium	*Athrombin, Coumadine, Coumadin Sodium, Marevan, Panwarfin, Waran, Warfilone, Warnerin*
Warfarin potassium	*Athrombin-K*
Indanediones	
Anisindione	*Miradon, Unidone*
Bromindione	*Fluidane, fluidemin*
Clorindione (chlorphenadione)	
Diphenadione	*Dipaxin*
Fluorindione	*Previscan*
Phenindione	*Acluton, Danilone, Dindevan, Eridione, Haemopan, Hedulin, Pindione, Theradione*
Parenteral anticoagulants	
Heparin	*Depo-Heparin, Pularin, Disebrin, Heprinar, Hepathrom, Hamocura, Hepalean, Liquemin, Norheparin, Panheprin, Thrombophob, Thrombo-Vetren*

Anticoagulant interactions

Therapeutically desirable prothrombin levels can be upset by a number of factors including diet, disease and the administration of other drugs, so that it is important to monitor the blood coagulability closely. In the case of drugs, either the addition or the withdrawal may upset the balance in a patient already stabilized on an anticoagulant regimen. At one extreme bleeding will occur and, at the other, the patient will be in danger of further spontaneous thromboses. If one believes in the therapeutic benefits of the oral anticoagulants, either situation is serious and may prove to be fatal, although excessive hypoprothrombinaemia manifests itself more obviously and immediately and is usually regarded as the more serious of the two.

In this chapter the interactions which result in a change in the effects of the oral anticoagulants are listed first, followed by those with heparin. Other interactions in which the anticoagulants are the affecting agents are discussed elsewhere. A full listing is to be found in the index.

Anticoagulants + alcohol

Summary

The effects of the oral anticoagulants are unlikely to be affected in patients with normal liver function by the ingestion of small or moderate amounts of alcohol. However, those who drink heavily or who have some liver disease may show considerable fluctuations in their prothrombin times.

Interaction

Moderate amounts of alcohol appear to have little or no effect on the prothrombin times of antico-agulated patients free of liver disease:

In an investigation[1] on a number of subjects or patients, all of whom were anticoagulated with phenprocoumon, 5 of then drank 250 ml of gin (80 g ethanol) and 8 drank 180–200 ml medicinal brandy over the course of an hour. The very small changes in the thromboplastin times which were seen were not statistically significant.

In another investigation[2] only 1 patient out of 10 on warfarin who drank 8 oz vodka (40% ethanol) a day for 2 weeks showed a significant change in prothrombin times. Since this patient was also taking digoxin, chlorothiazide and ethacrynic acid for congestive heart failure and hepatomegaly, the changes seen were not necessarily due solely to the consumption of alcohol.

Twenty oz (1 pint or 56·4 g ethanol) of a Californian white table wine a day, given over a 3 week period at mealtimes to 8 normal subjects anticoagulated with warfarin, were found to have had no significant effects on either the serum levels of warfarin or on their anticoagulant response.[9]

The situation with those who habitually drink large amounts of alcohol or who have liver impairment is different:

In a study[3] on 15 alcoholics administered a single dose of warfarin who had been drinking heavily (250 g ethanol or more a day) for at least 3 months, the results of a previous investigation[4] were con-firmed that the half-life of warfarin was reduced from 40·1 to 26·5 h but, surprisingly, a comparison of their prothrombin times with those of normal sub-jects showed no differences.

The prothrombin times of an anticoagulated patient[2] with early cirrhosis were found to have risen markedly each Monday morning after week-ends during which he habitually drank 2 quarts of vodka.

A man anticoagulated with warfarin and with some liver dysfunction who drank 50 ml whisky after a period of abstinence, spontaneously haemor-rhaged (epistaxis) several days later and was found to have serum warfarin levels which were elevated compared with his period of abstinence. When he stopped drinking his warfarin serum levels and prothrombin times restabilized.[5]

Mechanism

The most probable explanation of the reduced warfarin half-life found in the alcoholic patients described is that, as in rats[6], the alcohol stimulates the hepatic enzymes concerned with the metabo-lism of warfarin, leading to its more rapid elimina-tion.[3] However, despite this, the prothrombin times were not reduced as might be expected because, it has been surmised, the alcohol may additionally act as a suppressor of prothrombin synthesis so that prothrombin times stay about the same. There is experimental evidence support-ing this which shows that alcohol first raises and then lowers the serum levels of prothrombin and factors VII and X.[7]

It is also not known just why heavy drinking should have altered the prothrombin times of the two patients with liver dysfunction described [2, 5], but a possible explanation is that the alcohol exacerbates the general malfunction of the liver. This is reflected in a biochemical disturbance of the blood clotting mechanism, although the authors of one of the reports[5] suggest that the alcohol may be acting as a liver enzyme inhibitor in this situation.

Importance and management

Although a number of physicians are not in favour of their anticoagulated patients continuing to drink, the results of a few well-controlled trials have not confirmed that there is a general need to deny moderate amounts of alcohol to those on anticoagulant therapy. One investigator of this interaction concluded that '... socially acceptable amounts of alcohol do not interfere with anticoagulant control in patients who eat regularly and who are free of obvious hepatic disease....'[2] The definition of 'socially acceptable amounts' is obviously imprecise, but an advisory booklet[8] commonly given to patients in the UK cautiously suggests 1 pint of beer or 1 sherry per day. However, the results of the investigations cited above suggest that very much less conservative amounts—up to 8 oz/250 ml spirits—do not necessarily create problems with anticoagulant control so that there appears to be a good margin of safety even for the less than abstemious.

For those who drink heavily it may possibly be found necessary to administer above-average doses of the anticoagulant to obtain full control, and it should be borne in mind that some patients in this category may also have some degree of liver damage.

Those with liver damage who continue to drink even moderate amounts, may experience marked fluctuations in their prothrombin times so that an attempt to limit their intake of alcohol is desirable from this as well as from other points of view.

References

1 Waris E. Effect of ethyl alcohol on some coagulation factors in man during anticoagulant therapy. *Ann Med Exp Biol Fenn* (1965) **115**, 53.
2 Udall J A. Drug interference with warfarin therapy. *Clin Med* (1970) **77**, 20.
3 Kater RMH, Roggin G, Tobon F, Zieve P and Iber F L. Increased rate of clearance of drugs from the circulation of alcoholics. *Amer J med Sci* (1969) **258**, 35.
4 Kater R M, Carruli N and Iber F L. Differences in the rate of ethanol metabolism in recently drinking alcoholic and non-alcoholic subjects. *Amer J Clin Nutrition* (1969) **14**, 21.
5 Breckenridge A and Orme M. Clinical implications of enzyme induction. *Ann NY Acad Sci* (1971) **179**, 421.
6 Rubin E, Hutterev F and Lieber C S. Ethanol increases hepatic smooth endoplasmic reticulum and drug metabolizing enzymes. *Science* (1968) **159**, 1469.
7 Riedler G. Einfluss des Alkohols auf die anticoagulantien therapie. *Thromb Diath Haemorr.* (1966) **16**, 613.
8 *The Handbook for Patients taking Anticoagulants.* 1979. Duncan Flockhart, London.
9 O'Reilly R A. Warfarin and wine. *Clin Res* (1978) **26**, 145A.

Anticoagulants + allopurinol

Summary

Most patients treated with oral anticoagulants and allopurinol do not develop an adverse interaction, but because excessive hypoprothrombinaemia and bleeding occurs quite unpredictably in a few individuals it is important to monitor the anticoagulant response in all patients taking both drugs.

Interaction

There are a few reports of individual patients who have shown excessive hypoprothrombinaemia and bleeding during concurrent treatment with anticoagulants and allopurinol, but most of the evidence from studies of this interaction in man indicates that this response is the exception rather than the rule.

When 6 healthy subjects were given 2·5 mg/kg allopurinol twice daily for 14 days the mean half-life of a single dose of dicoumarol was increased from 51 to 152 h.[1]

Another study showed that only 1 of 6 subjects who took '... usual doses of allopurinol ...' for a month showed a reduction (30%) in the elimination of warfarin. No change was seen in the prothrombin ratios of 2 patients on warfarin who took allopurinol for 3 weeks.[2]

In a study on 3 subjects, only one of them showed an increase in the half-life of dicoumarol from 13·1 to 16·9 during allopurinol treatment and the disposition of warfarin remained unaltered.[4]

Case reports of an enhanced anticoagulant response during allopurinol therapy are as follows.

An 82-year-old woman on digitalis and diuretics (unnamed) and anticoagulated with warfarin showed a sharp increase in her prothrombin times when 300 mg allopurinol and indomethacin were added to her drug regimen.[3]

Two patients on long-term treatment with phenprocoumon showed bleeding after treatment with allopurinol was started.[5]

Mechanism

Laboratory experiments run concurrently with the study in man already cited[1] indicate that allopurinol reduces the activity of the liver microsomal enzymes in the rat thereby prolonging and increasing the activity of the anticoagulant. If this also occurs in man it would account for the extended dicoumarol half-life[1,4] and for the reduction in the elimination of warfarin cited,[2] but there is no obvious reason why this interaction should only be demonstrated by a few individuals, other than to point out that there is a wide individual variability in the effects of allopurinol in drug metabolism in man.[2]

Importance and management

A few individuals may show an enhanced anticoagulant response during concurrent treatment with oral anticoagulants and allopurinol, possibly leading to bleeding, but most will not demonstrate this interaction. However, it is important to monitor the anticoagulant response in all patients because of the unpredictability of this interaction.

Only warfarin, dicoumarol and phenprocoumon have so far been shown to interact with allopurinol, but it would be wise to assume that this interaction is a possibility with any of the other oral anticoagulants.

References

1 Vesell E S, Passananti G T and Greene F F. Impairment of drug metabolism in man by allopurinol and nortriptyline. *New Eng J Med* (1970) **283**, 1484.
2 Rawlins M D and Smith S E. Influence of allopurinol on drug metabolism in man. *Br J Pharmac* (1973) **48**, 693.
3 Self T H, Evans W E and Ferguson T. Drug enhancement of warfarin activity. *Lancet* (1975) **ii**, 557.
4 Pond S M, Graham G G, Wade D N and Sudlow G. The effects of allopurinol and clofibrate on the elimination of coumarin anticoagulants in man. *Aust NZ J Med* (1975) **5**, 324.
5 Jahnchen E, Meinertz T and Gilfrich M J. Interaction of allopurinol with phenprocoumon in man. *Klin Wschr* (1977) **55**, 759.

Anticoagulants + anabolic steroids

Summary

The anticoagulant response to warfarin, phenprocoumon, dicoumarol, bromindione or phenindione is markedly enhanced by the concurrent use of norethandrolone, oxymetholone, methandrostenolone, ethyloestrenol or methyltestosterone. It seems probable that this interaction will also take place with all the other oral anticoagulants in the presence of C17-alkylated anabolic steroids, but not with testosterone.

Interaction

Six patients stabilized on warfarin or phenindione were later also given 15 mg oxymetholone daily. One patient developed extensive subcutaneous bleeding and another had haematuria. After 30 days on oxymetholone all 6 patients had thrombotests of less than 5% which returned to the therapeutic range within a few days of stopping the oxymetholone.[1]

Similarly enhanced anticoagulant effects have been described in studies and case reports of interactions in man on warfarin with oxymetholone[4-6] and methandrostenolone[2,4,7,8]; dicoumarol with norethandrolone[3]; bromindione with methadrostenolone[2,4]; phenindione with ethyloestrenol;[9] phenprocoumon with methyltestosterone;[10] and nicoumalone with oxymetholone.[11]

Mechanism

Not understood. Various theories have been put forward to account for this interaction, but there is as yet no totally satisfactory explanation.

Among the suggestions are that these steroids might increase the metabolic destruction of the blood clotting proteins or impair the ability of the liver to synthesize the vitamin K-dependent clotting factors.[2,3] Another idea is that by reducing the levels of plasma triglycerides these steroids might reduce the amounts of vitamin K available to the liver and hence the effects of the anticoagulants would be increased, but the available evidence would not appear to support this notion.[4,7] Other suggestions are that there is an increase in the concentration of free and active anticoagulant molecules at the receptor site or an increased affinity for the anticoagulant by the receptor induced by the steroid.

Importance and management

A marked reduction in the anticoagulant requirements of patients taking oral anticoagulants should be expected if ethyloestrenol, norethandrolone, methandrostenolone, oxymetholone or methyltestosterone are given concurrently. The dosage of the anticoagulant should be reduced to accommodate this interaction and to prevent bleeding. Similarly, after withdrawal of the steroid, the anticoagulant requirements will be increased.

There is as yet no direct documentary evidence that other 17-alkyl substituted steroids such as fluoxymesterone, oxandrolone and stanozolol interact similarly, but it seems probable that they will. Testosterone which is not a 17-alkyl substituted compound has been shown not to interact with warfarin.[6]

Only warfarin, dicoumarol, phenprocoumon, bromindione and phenindione have been shown to interact with these anabolic steroids, but it seems highly likely that all the other oral anticoagulants will interact similarly.

References
1 Longridge R G M, Gillam P M S and Barton G M G. Decreased anticoagulant tolerance with oxymetholone. *Lancet* (1971) ii, 90.

2 Pyörälä K and Kekki M. Decreased anticoagulant tolerance during methadrostenolone therapy. *Scand J Clin Lab Invest* (1963) 15, 367.

3 Schrogie J J and Solomon H M. The anticoagulant response to bishydroxycoumarin. II. The effect of D-thyroxine, clofibrate and norethandrolone. *Clin. Pharmacol Ther* (1967) 8, 70.

4 Murakami M, Odake K, Matsuda T, Onchi K, Umeda T and Nishuro T. Effects of anabolic steroids on anticoagulant requirements. *Jap Circ J* (1965) 29, 243.

5 Robinson B H B, Hawkins J B, Ellis J E and Moore-Robinson M. Decreased anticoagulant tolerance with oxymetholone. *Lancet* (1971) i, 1356.

6 Edwards M S and Curtis J R. Decreased anticoagulant tolerance with oxymetholone. *Lancet* (1971) ii, 221.

7 Dresdale F C and Hayes J C. Potential dangers in the combined use of methandrostenolone and sodium warfarin. *J Med Soc New Jersey* (1967) 64, 609.

8 McLaughlin G E, McCarty D J and Segal B L. Hemarthrosis complicating anticoagulant therapy. A report of three cases. *J Amer Med Ass* (1966) 196, 1020.

9 Vere D W and Fearnley G R. Suspected interaction between phenindione and ethyloestrenol. *Lancet* (1968) ii, 281.

10 Husted S, Andreasen F and Foged L. Increased sensitivity to phenprocoumon during methyltestosterone therapy. *Europ J clin Pharmacol* (1976) 10, 209.

11 De Oya J C, del Rio A, Noya M and Villaneuva A. Decreased anticoagulant tolerance with oxymetholone in paroxysmal nocturnal haemoglobinuria. *Lancet* (1971) ii, 259.

Anticoagulants + aminoglycoside antibiotics

Summary
If the intake of vitamin K is normal, only a small and clinically unimportant increase in the response to oral anticoagulants takes place during concurrent treatment with neomycin, kanamycin or paromomycin. No interaction of any importance is likely with the other aminoglycoside antibiotics administered by injection.

Interaction
The aminoglycoside antibiotics can cause a small but unimportant increase in the response to oral anticoagulant therapy in a few patients, but many show no changes at all. The documentary evidence about the results of using these two groups of drugs together is very sparse.

In one study[1] 6 out of 10 patients on warfarin who were also taking 2 g neomycin/day over a period of 3 weeks showed a gradual increase in their prothrombin times averaging 5·6 s. The author of this report also describes another study on 10 patients taking warfarin with 4 g neomycin/day which produced essentially similar results[2].

In contrast, another report[4] describes 7 patients who were given 1–2 g neomycin daily for 18 weeks which failed to affect their anticoagulant requirements.

A small enhancement of the effects of an unnamed anticoagulant was seen in an investigation on 5 patients taking neomycin with bacitracin, 3 patients on 1 g streptomycin/day, and 2 patients on 1 g streptomycin with 1 Mu of penicillin/day.[3]

A study on a patient on long-term treatment with dicoumarol, and on a volunteer anticoagulated with warfarin, showed that during concurrent treatment with paromomycin the anticoagulant requirements remained unaltered.[5]

Mechanism
It is not known why the prothrombin time is increased slightly in some individuals, but it seems unlikely to result solely from a reduction in the absorption of vitamin K. Even when the supplies are drastically cut there is usually enough to maintain the blood clotting factors at adequate levels, and more than enough when the diet is normal. Vitamin K is found in a variety of foods and this dietary source, supplemented by an additional source of vitamin K synthesized by the flora of the intestinal tract, supplies our require-

119

ments. Neomycin and kanamycin are known to be able to induce a malabsorption syndrome (they have actually been shown to cause steatorrhoea) which is possibly related to their ability to precipitate bile salts and bilirubin.[6] If these naturally occurring surface-active agents are inactivated in this way, the emulsification and absorption of fats is inhibited and with it the absorption of fat-soluble vitamins such as vitamin K. So the possibility exists that these antibiotics not only decimate the activity of the intestinal flora which synthesize vitamin K, but also lower the absorption of the vitamin.

Despite this, spontaneous haemorrhage attributed to the actions of these antibiotics in association with other factors which limit the absorption of vitamin K has only been reported occasionally[7,8] and there have been no bleeding episodes associated with the concurrent use of the oral anticoagulants.

Importance and management
There seems to be no reason to avoid using the orally administered aminoglycoside antibiotics such as neomycin, kanamycin or paromomycin in patients taking oral anticoagulants who have a normal dietary intake of vitamin K, although a small, relatively unimportant, enhancement of the anticoagulant response may be seen in a few individuals.

There are occasional reports of vitamin K deficiency associated with the prolonged oral administration of gut-sterilizing antibiotics when associated with a totally inadequate diet, starvation or some other condition in which the intake of vitamin K is very limited. The response to the oral anticoagulants would be expected to be increased to a significant extent in these individuals.

There is no evidence to suggest that an adverse interaction occurs between the oral anticoagulants and the aminoglycoside antibiotics which are administered parenterally (amikacin, gentamicin, lividomycin, sis(s)omycin, streptomycin, tobramycin).

References
1 Udall J A. Drug interference with warfarin therapy. *Clin Med* (1970) **77**, 20.
2 Udall J A. Human sources and absorption of vitamin K in relation to anticoagulation stability. *J Amer med Ass* (1965) **194**, 107.
3 Magid E. Tolerance to anticoagulants during antibiotic therapy. *Scand J Clin Lab Invest* (1962) **14**, 565.
4 Schade R W B. A comparative study of the effects of cholestyramine and neomycin in the treatment of type II hyperlipoprotinaemia. *Acta med Scand* (1976) **199**, 175.
5 Messinger W J and Samet C M. The effect of a bowel sterilizing antibiotic on blood coagulation mechanisms. The anticholesterol effect of paromomycin. *Angiology* (1965) **16**, 29.
6 Faloon W W, Paes I C, Woolfolk D, Nankin H, Wallace K and Haro E N. Effect of neomycin and kanamycin upon intestinal absorption. *Ann NY Acad Sci* (1966) **132**, 879.
7 Haden H T. Vitamin K deficiency associated with prolonged antibiotic administration. *Arch Int Med* (1957) **100**, 986.
8 Frick P G, Riedler G and Brögli H. Dose response and minimal daily requirement for vitamin K in man. *J Appl Physiol* (1967) **23**, 387.

Anticoagulants + aminosalicylic acid (PAS)

Summary
A single case has been reported of a patient on warfarin who showed an enhanced anticoagulant response when administered PAS and isoniazid concurrently

Interaction
A patient already receiving digoxin, potassium chloride, dioctyl calcium sulfosuccinate, diazepam and warfarin, was additionally given isoniazid, 300 mg, pyridoxine 100 mg and PAS, 12 g daily. The prothrombin time increased from 17·8 to 130 s over 20 days,[1] but no signs of haemorrhage were seen.

Mechanism
Not known. Studies in dogs showed that PAS can enhance the anticoagulant effects of dicoumarol, but no mechanism of interaction has been established[2]. PAS depresses the formation of prothrombin by the liver in man, but the extent is small, and

whether this can account for the interaction described and why it should only apparently affect one individual is not clear.

Importance and management
Concurrent use need not be avoided but prescribers should be aware of the case described.

References
1 Self T H. Interaction of warfarin and aminosalicylic acid. *J. Amer Med Ass* (1973) **223**, 1285.
2 Eade N. R., McLeod P J and MacLeod S M. Potentiation of bishydroxycoumarin in dogs by isoniazid and p-aminosalicylic acid. *Amer Rev Resp Dis* (1971) **103**, 792.

Anticoagulants + antacids

Summary

The absorption of dicoumarol is considerably increased by the concurrent use of magnesium-containing antacids which, at least in theory, might lead to excessive hypoprothrombinaemia and bleeding. Neither warfarin nor dicoumarol interacts with aluminium hydroxide but the absorption of warfarin may possibly be increased by magnesium trisilicate.

Interaction

The administration of 30 ml doses of *Maalox* (a magnesium and aluminium hydroxide mixture) with a single 40 mg oral dose of warfarin, and four subsequent doses of the antacid given at 2-h intervals, failed to have a significant effect on either the plasma levels of warfarin of 6 normal subjects examined or their anticoagulant response.[1]

Another study on 6 subjects given either *Milk of Magnesia* or *Amphogel* (aluminium hydroxide gel) with warfarin similarly showed that no interaction occurred. Dicoumarol was found not to interact with aluminium hydroxide but when it was given with 15 ml *Milk of Magnesia* and a further dose of *Milk of Magnesia* 3 h later, the peak serum levels of dicoumarol were increased by 75% and the area under the serum level curve by 50%.[2]

In contrast, an in-vitro study suggests that magnesium trisilicate may enhance the absorption of warfarin.[4]

Mechanism

It has been suggested[1,3] that dicoumarol chelates with magnesium to form a more readily absorbed compound than dicoumarol itself so that the extent of the absorption is increased. This chelate given orally (at least in dogs[3]) produces a greater prothrombin time response than the same dose of dicoumarol and would seem therefore to retain the anticoagulant properties of the parent compound. The absorption of warfarin on the other hand is much more rapid and complete than dicoumarol so that it is much less likely to be affected by this kind of chemical interaction.

Importance and management

There appear to be no reports describing an adverse interaction (excessive hypoprothrombinaemia and bleeding) when patients on dicoumarol have taken magnesium-containing antacids, but it is a theoretical possibility and it would seem a sensible precaution to avoid concurrent use if possible. Aluminium hydroxide is reported to be a safe, non-interacting alternative, and warfarin interacts with none of the aluminium or magnesium-containing antacids (*Maalox*, *Amphogel*, *Milk of Magnesia*) described in the two reports cited here, but its absorption may possibly be somewhat increased by magnesium trisilicate. It would seem prudent to monitor the effects of concurrent use.

There appears to be nothing documented about the other anticoagulants and antacids.

References

1 Robinson D S, Benjamin D M and McCormack J J. Interaction of warfarin and nonsystemic gastrointestinal drugs. *Clin Pharmacol Ther.* (1971) **12**, 491.
2 Ambre J J and Fischer L J. Effect of coadministration of aluminium and magnesium hydroxides on absorption of anticoagulants in man. *Clin Pharmacol Ther* (1973) **14**, 231.
3 Akers M A, Lach J L and Fischer L J. Alterations in the absorption of bishydroxycoumarin by various excipient materials. *J Pharm Sci* (1973) **62**, 391.
4 McElnay J C, Harron D W G, D'Arcy P F and Collier P S. Interaction of warfarin with antacid constituents. *Brit Med J* (1978) **2**, 1166.

Anticoagulants + ascorbic acid

Summary

Three controlled studies with large numbers of patients have failed to demonstrate any interaction, although two isolated cases have been reported in which the effects of warfarin were antagonized by ascorbic acid.

Interaction

There are only two case reports[1,2] of a reduced response to anticoagulant therapy due to ascorbic acid.

> The prothrombin time of a woman, stabilized on 7·5 mg warfarin sodium/day, who began to take regular amounts of ascorbic acid (dose not stated), fell steadily from 23 s to 19, 17, and then 14 s with no response to an increase in the dosage of warfarin to 10, 15 and then 20 mg/day. The prothrombin time returned to 28 s within 2 days of discontinuing the ascorbic acid.[1]

> A woman who had been taking 16 g ascorbic acid daily proved to be unusually resistant to the actions of warfarin and required 25 mg/day before a significant increase in prothrombin times was achieved. Ultimately a warfarin maintenance dosage of 10 mg/day was established.[2]

The following studies failed to confirm the existence of this interaction:

> Five patients on warfarin showed no change in their thrombotest percentage when they were given 1 g ascorbic acid every day for a fortnight.[3]

> Eighty-four patients on chronic anticoagulant therapy who were given an unstated amount of ascorbic acid showed no change in their thrombotest values over a 10-week period.[4]

> The effect of ascorbic acid on the prothrombin ratios of 19 patients taking warfarin was examined; 14 of them were given 3 g of ascorbic a day for a week and then 5 g a day for the next week, while the other 5 patients took 10 g of ascorbic acid for a week. No clinically important changes in the prothrombin ratios of any of the patients was seen, although it was noticed that there was a mean fall of 17·5% in the total plasma warfarin concentrations.[5]

Mechanism

None of the animal studies which have been carried out (some of which have shown this interaction[6,7] and others which have not[8,9]) has given any definite clues about why this interaction should occur at all, and in so few individuals. The only really useful observation that has been made is that with high doses of ascorbic acid patients usually experience some degree of diarrhoea. This could account for the decreased absorption of warfarin and the reduced serum levels seen in the last study in man described above.[5] It might also account for the two isolated cases of this interaction as well.

Importance and management control

Despite two reports of this interaction, well-controlled clinical studies with large numbers of patients failed to confirm its existence even when large amounts of ascorbic acid were used. Even so, the possibility of an interaction, however remote, should be borne in mind if patients on anticoagulant therapy are taking very large doses of ascorbic acid.

References

1 Rosenthal G. Interaction of ascorbic acid and warfarin. J Am Med Ass (1971) 215, 1671.
2 Smith E C, Skalski R J, Johnson G C and Rossi G V. Interaction of ascorbic acid and warfarin. J Am Med Ass (1972) 221, 1166.
3 Hume R, Johnstone J M S and Weyers E. Interaction of ascorbic acid and warfarin. J Am Med Ass (1972) 219, 1479.
4 Dedichen J. The effect of ascorbic acid given to patients on chronic anticoagulant therapy. Boll Soc Ital Cardiol (1973) 18, 690.
5 Feetam C L, Leach R H and Meynell M J. Lack of a clinically important interaction between warfarin and ascorbic acid. Toxicol Appl Pharmacol (1975) 31, 544.
6 Sigell L T and Flessa H C. Drug interactions with anticoagulants. J Am med Ass (1970) 214, 2035.
7 Sullivan W R, Gangstad E O. and Link K P. Studies on the haemorrhagic sweet clover disease. J Biol Chem (1943) 151, 477.
8 Weintraub M and Griner P F. Warfarin and ascorbic acid: lack lack of evidence for a drug interaction. Toxicol App Pharmacol (1974) 28, 53.
9 Deckert F W. Ascorbic acid and warfarin. J Am Med Ass (1973) 223, 440.

Anticoagulants + azapropazone

Summary

The anticoagulant effects of warfarin are enhanced by azapropazone. Bleeding can occur.

Interaction

A woman[1] stabilized on warfarin (prothrombin ratio 2·8) who was also taking digoxin, frusemide, spironolactone and allopurinol, showed haematemesis within 4 days of being prescribed 300 mg azapropazone four times a day. On admission to hospital her prothrombin ratio was found to have risen to 15·7 and her prothrombin time to 220 s. Six hours after the azapropazone and warfarin had been withdrawn and 4 u of blood and vitamin K administered, the prothrombin time had fallen to 35 s. Subsequent gastroscopic examination showed a benign ulcer, the presumed site of the bleeding.

Three other patients on warfarin have been described who developed bruising within a few days of starting treatment with azapropazone, and the interaction has been experimentally confirmed in 2 volunteers. [2,3]

Mechanism

In-vitro experiments using pure albumin[3] and human serum[4,5] have shown that azapropazone can displace warfarin from its binding sites on plasma proteins. Moreover, with serum concentrations of azapropazone which would be achievable on a dosage regimen of 300 mg taken three times a day, the amount of free, and therefore pharmacologically active, warfarin increases by 40%, which would be expected to enhance the anticoagulant effects of the warfarin. Whether this on its own fully accounts for the clinical effects reported is doubtful.

Importance and management

Although information is limited, this interaction is established and of importance. Considerable increases in prothrombin times can occur within a few days of starting concurrent treatment. The use of both drugs should be avoided. The manufacturers of azapropazone recommend that if it is essential to give this drug to patients on anticoagulant therapy, it should only be done so when the anticoagulant dosage has been reduced to a very low level, after which daily prothrombin determinations and dosage adjustments should be carried out. Whether azapropazone interacts with other anticoagulants is uncertain, but it would be wise to assume that it does. Alternative non-interacting antirheumatic compounds such as ibuprofen are available (see p. 152).

References

1 Powell-Jackson P R. Interaction between azapropazone and warfarin. *Brit Med J* (1977) **1**, 1193.
2 Green A E, Hort J F, Korn H E T and Leach H. Potentiation of warfarin by azapropazone. *Brit Med J* (1977) **1**, 1532.
3 McElnay J C and D'Arcy P F. Interaction between azapropazone and warfarin. *Brit Med J* (1977) **2**, 773.
4 McElnay J C and D'Arcy P F. The effect of azapropazone on the binding of warfarin to human serum proteins. *J Pharm Pharmac* (1978) **30** (*Suppl*) 73P.
5 McElnay J C and D'Arcy P F. Interaction between azapropazone and warfarin. *Experientia* (1978) **34**, 1320.

Anticoagulants + barbiturates

Summary

The effects of the anticoagulants are reduced by the concurrent administration of barbiturates. Although full anticoagulant control can be re-established by increasing the dosage of the anticoagulant, wherever possible the barbiturate should be replaced by other non-interacting drugs. This avoids the risk of haemorrhage which can occur if the barbiturate is subsequently withdrawn without an appropriate reduction in the dosage of the anticoagulant.

Interaction

The response to the oral anticoagulants is reduced by the concurrent administration of the barbiturates. This interaction is very well documented indeed, only two examples being quoted here.

A study on 16 patients on long-term warfarin therapy showed that when they were also given 2 mg/kg phenobarbitone (-al) daily their average daily warfarin requirements rose over a 4-week period from 5·7 to 7·1 mg/day.[1]

An investigation carried out on 12 patients anticoagulated with either warfarin or phenprocoumon demonstrated that when they were concurrently taking secbutobarbitone (butabarbital) sodium in doses of 60 mg daily for the first week, and 120 mg daily for the next 2 weeks, their anticoagulant requirements increased by 35–60%, reaching a maximum 4–5 weeks after the barbiturate had been withdrawn.[2]

Other reports of this interaction in man have been reported between warfarin and amylobarbitone (-al)[3,4,23], butobarbitone (-al),[5] heptabarbitone (-al),[6,7] phenobarbitone (-al),[8-12] quinalbarbitone (secobarbital)[3,4,12-14] and secbutobarbitone (butabarbital);[2] between dicoumarol and aprobarbitone (-al),[15] heptabarbitone (-al),[16,17] phenobarbitone (-al)[18-20] and vinalbarbitone (-al);[15] between ethylbiscoumacetate and amylobarbitone (amobarbital),[16,21] pentobarbitone (-al)[22] and phenobarbitone (-al);[21] between phenprocoumon and secbutobarbitone (butabarbital);[2] and between nicoumalone (acenocoumarol) and heptabarbitone (-al).[16]

Mechanism

The evidence which has accumulated from the many studies on this interaction carried out in man[4,6,8,11,14] and in animals shows that the barbiturates, which are potent liver enzyme-inducing agents, increase the metabolism and the clearance of the anticoagulants from the body, thereby reducing the anticoagulant response. In addition it has been suggested that in the case of dicoumarol its absorption by the gut may be inhibited by heptabarbitone (-al).[17]

Importance and management

This interaction is very well documented and is of obvious importance because, as the anticoagulant response diminishes under the influence of the barbiturate, so the patient will become exposed to the risk of thrombus formation unless the anticoagulant dosage is stepped up.

A very large number of the anticoagulant/barbiturate combinations have been found to interact and it seems reasonable to assume that all the others will do so. The only known exception is secobarbitone (-al) which in daily doses of 100 mg appears to have little[12] or no[13,24] effect on the response to dicoumarol or warfarin, but in daily doses of 200 mg interacts to the same extent as the other barbiturates.[13]

The reduction in the anticoagulant response begins within a week, sometimes even within 2–4 days, after starting the barbiturate, and reaches a maximum about 3 weeks or so later. It may still be evident up to 6 weeks[2] after withdrawal of the barbiturate, although the rate of onset and the return to normal can vary from patient to patient.

It is difficult to predict how much more anticoagulant will be needed to accommodate this interaction but the available evidence indicates that it is approximately 30–60%.[1,2,10,20] Full and stabilized anticoagulant control can be established in the presence of a barbiturate provided both drugs are taken consistently (this may be necessary in the case of epileptic patients taking phenobarbitone)[23] but it is normally not desirable because if the barbiturate is withdrawn without a suitable reduction in the anticoagulant dosage, the enzyme-inducing effects will diminish and the anticoagulant will be metabolized less rapidly. Haemorrhage from excessive hypoprothrom-

binaemia arising like this has been described.[1,10,23]

Alternative sedative and hypnotic drugs which do not interact with the anticoagulants are to be found among the benzodiazepines (see p. 126).

The hope that the barbiturates might have a much smaller inducing effect on the metabolism of R warfarin than on S has not been realized in practice, so that there is no good case for using the R enantiomer instead of the usual racemic mixture to avoid this interaction.[25]

References

1 Robinson D S and McDonald M G. The effect of phenobarbital administration on the control of coagulation achieved during warfarin therapy in man. *J Pharmacol Exp Ther* (1966) 153, 250.
2 Antlitz A M, Tolentino M and Kosai M F. Effect of butabarbital on orally administered anticoagulants. *Curr Ther Res* (1968) 10, 70.
3 Breckenridge A and Orme M. Clinical implications of enzyme induction. *Ann NY Acad Sci* (1971) 179, 421.
4 Robinson D S and Sylwester D. Interaction of commonly prescribed drugs and warfarin. *Ann Int Med* (1970) 72, 853.
5 MacGregor A G, Petrie J C and Wood R A. Therapeutic conferences. Drug interaction. *Brit med J* (1971) 1, 389.
6 Levy G, O'Reilly R A, Aggeler P M and Keech G M. Pharmacokinetic analysis of the effect of barbiturate on the anticoagulant action of warfarin in man. *Clin Pharmacol Ther* (1970) 11, 372.
7 O'Reilly R A and Aggeler P M. Effect of barbiturates on oral anticoagulants in man. *Clin Res* (1969) 17, 153.
8 MacDonald M G, Robinson D S, Sylwester D and Jaffe J J. The effects of phenobarbital, chloral betaine, and glutethimide administration on warfarin plasma levels and hypoprothrombinemic responses in man. *Clin Pharmacol Ther* (1969) 10, 80.
9 Seiler K and Duckert F. Properties of 3-(1-phenyl-propyl)-4-oxycoumarin (Marcoumar) in the plasma when tested in normal cases and under the influence of drugs. *Thromb Diath Haemorrh* (1968) 19, 89.
10 MacDonald M G and Robinson D S. Clinical observations of possible barbiturate interference with anticoagulation. *J Amer Med Ass* (1968) 204, 97.
11 Corn M. Effect of phenobarbital and glutethimide on biological half-life of warfarin. *Thromb Diath Haemorrh* (1966) 16, 606.
12 Udall J A. Clinical implications of warfarin interactions with five sedatives. *Am J Cardiol* (1975) 35, 67.
13 Feuer D J, Wilson W R and Ambre J J. Duration of effect of secobarbital on the anticoagulant effect and metabolism of warfarin. *The Pharmacologist* (1971) 3, 195.
14 Breckenridge A M, Orme M L'E, Davies L, Thorgeirsson S S and Davies D S. Dose-dependent enzyme induction. *Clin Pharmacol Ther* (1973) 14, 514.
15 Johansson S-A. Apparent resistance to oral anticoagulant therapy and influence of hypnotics on some coagulation factors. *Acta Med Scand* (1968) 184, 297.
16 Dayton P G, Tarcan Y, Chenkin T and Weiner M. The influence of barbiturates on coumarin plasma levels and prothrombin response. *J clin Invest* (1961) 40, 1797.
17 Aggeler P M and O'Reilly R A. Effect of heptabarbital on the response to bishydroxycoumarin in man. *J Lab Clin Med* (1969) 74, 229.
18 Corn M and Rockett J F. Inhibition of bishydroxycoumarin activity by phenobarbital. *Med Ann DC* (1965) 34, 578.
19 Cucinell S A, Conney A H, Sansur M and Burns J J. Drug interactions in man. 1 Lowering effect of phenobarbital on

plasma levels of bishydroxycoumarin (Dicumarol) and diphenylhydantoin (Dilantin). *Clin Pharmacol Ther* (1965) 6, 420.

20 Goss J E and Dickhaus D W. Increased bishydroxycoumarin requirements in patients receiving phenobarbital. *New Eng J Med* (1965) 273, 1094.

21 Avellaneda M. Interferencia de los barbituricos en la accion del Tromexan. *Medicina* (1955) 15, 109.

22 Reverchon F and Sapir M. Constatation clinique d'un

antagonisme entre barbituriques et anticoagulants. *La Presse Med* (1961) 69, 1570.

23 Williams J R B, Griffin J P and Parkins A. Effect of concomitantly administered drugs on the control of long term anticoagulant therapy. *Quart J Med* (1976) 45, 63.

24 Cucinell S A, Odessky L, Weiss M and Dayton P G. The effect of chloral hydrate on bishydroxycoumarin metabolism. A fatal outcome. *J Am Med Ass* (1966) 197, 360.

25 Breckenridge A M. Oral anticoagulants. *Practitioner* (1978) 32, 123.

Anticoagulants + benfluorex

Summary

The anticoagulant effects of phenprocoumon are not affected by the use of benfluorex. Information about other anticoagulants appears to be lacking.

Interaction, mechanism, importance and management

A study carried out on 25 patients anticoagulated with phenprocoumon showed that concurrent treatment with 450 mg benfluorex daily over a 9 week period had no effect upon their prothrombin times when compared with equivalent periods before and after the study when they were not

taking benfluorex.[1] There appears to be no information about the effects of benfluorex on other anticoagulants.

Reference

1 De Witte P and Brems H M. Co-administration of benfluorex with oral anticoagulant therapy. *Curr Med Res Opin* (1980) 6, 478.

Anticoagulants + benziodarone

Summary

The anticoagulant effects of warfarin, nicoumalone, diphenadione and ethylbiscoumacetate are enhanced by benziodarone, whereas phenprocoumon, dicoumarol, phenindione and chlorindione do not interact. Dosage reductions of the interacting anticoagulants are necessary to prevent the occurrence of bleeding.

Interaction

The effects of some, but not all, anticoagulants can be enhanced by benziodarone.

The observation that a patient on warfarin bled when given benziodarone prompted a further investigation of this interaction. Ninety patients taking various anticoagulants were given 200 mg benziodarone three times a day for 2 days, and 100 mg three times a day thereafter. No changes in the anticoagulant response were seen in those taking phenprocoumon (8 patients), dicoumarol (9 patients), phenindione (10 patients) or chlorindione (5 patients), but in order to maintain the PP percentages at a constant value it was necessary to reduce the anticoagulant dosage of those taking warfarin by 46% (15 patients), diphenadione by

42% (8 patients), nicoumalone by 25% (7 patients) and ethylbiscoumacetate by 17% (9 patients). A parallel study on 12 normal subjects also demonstrated an interaction with warfarin.[1]

The absence of an interaction with dicoumarol confirms the results of a previous study.[2]

Mechanism

Not understood. Benziodarone alone has no definite effect on the activity of prothrombin or factors VII, IX or X.

Importance and management

Although there appear to be no other studies of this interaction, the available evidence seems to be strong. No particular precautions would appear necessary with the non-interacting anticoagulants, but the dosages of warfarin, diphenadione, nicoumalone and ethylbiscoumacetate will require a reduction if excessive hypoprothrombinaemia and bleeding are to be avoided. Information about other anticoagulants is lacking.

References
1 Pyörälä K, Ikkala E and Siltanen P. Benziodarone (Amplivix) and anticoagulant therapy. *Acta Med Scand* (1963) **173**, 385.
2 Gillot P. Valeur thérapeutique du L 2329 dans l'angine de poitrine. *Acta Cardiol* (1959) **14**, 494.

Anticoagulants + benzodiazepines

Summary
The anticoagulant effects of warfarin are not affected by the concurrent use of chlordiazepoxide, diazepam, nitrazepam or flurazepam. Phenprocoumon is not affected by nitrazepam or ethylbiscoumacetate by chlordiazepoxide. An interaction between any oral anticoagulant and a benzodiazepine seems unlikely. There are, however, three unexplained and unconfirmed cases of interaction attributed to their concurrent use.

Interaction
The benzodiazepines do not normally interact with the oral anticoagulants although a few cases of interaction have been described.

A study on 12 patients anticoagulated with warfarin showed that the concurrent administration for a 30-day period of 10 mg nitrazepam nightly to 3 patients, of 15 mg diazepam daily to 4 patients, and either 15 or 30 mg chlordiazepoxide daily to 5 patients, had no effect on either the steady-state plasma warfarin concentrations, or on their anticoagulant control.[1]

A number of other studies on a very large number of patients administered the drugs for extended periods have confirmed the lack of an interaction between warfarin and chlordiazepoxide,[2–4,7] diazepam,[4,7] nitrazepam[4,6] and flurazepam;[5] between ethylbiscoumacetate and chlordiazepoxide;[8] and between phenprocoumon and nitrazepam.[9]

In contrast there are three discordant reports. A patient on warfarin showed an enhanced anticoagulant response when given diazepam.[10] A patient on dicoumarol developed multiple ecchymoses and a prothrombin time of 53 s within a fortnight of starting to take 20 mg diazepam daily.[11] And a patient showed a fall in serum warfarin levels and in the anticoagulant response when given chlordiazepoxide.[6]

Mechanism
Just why the 3 patients described exhibited an interaction is not understood. The last of the three may have been the result of enzyme-induction because increases in the urinary excretion of 6 beta-hydroxycortisol (an indicator of enzyme induction) have been described during chlordiazepoxide administration.[1,6]

Importance and management
The weight of evidence shows that the benzodiazepines can be safely given to patients taking anticoagulants. By no means all the anticoagulant/benzodiazepine combinations have been examined, but it seems reasonable to expect them all to behave similarly, although this awaits confirmation. The 3 cases of interaction cited cannot be totally dismissed as unimportant, but they are exceptional and it should be said that it is by no means certain (in the first 2 cases at least) that the benzodiazepine was the cause of the changed anticoagulant response.

References
1 Orme M, Breckenridge A and Brooks R V. Interactions of benzodiazepines with warfarin. *Brit Med J* (1972) **3**, 611.
2 Lackner H and Hunt V E. The effect of librium on hemostasis. *Amer J Med Sci* (1968) **256**, 368.
3 Robinson D S and Sylwester D. Interaction of commonly prescribed drugs and warfarin. *Ann Int Med* (1970) **72**, 853.
4 Breckenridge A and Orme E. Interaction of benzodiazepines with oral anticoagulants. In *The Benzodiazepines*, p. 647. Garattini S, Mussini E and Randall L O (eds) (1973). Raven Press, NY.
5 Robinson D S and Amidon E I. Interaction of benzodiazepines with warfarin in man. In *The Benzodiazepines*, p. 641. Garattini S, Mussini E and Randall L O (eds) (1973). Raven Press, NY.

6 Breckenridge A and Orme M. Clinical implications of enzyme induction. *Ann NY Acad Sci* (1971) **179**, 421.
7 Solomon H M, Barakat M J and Ashley C J. Mechanisms of drug interaction. *J Amer Med Ass* (1971) **216**, 1997.
8 Van Dam F E, and Gribnau-Overkamp M J H. The effect of some sedatives (phenobarbital, glutethimide, chlordiazepoxide, chloral hydrate) on the rate of disappearance of ethyl biscoumacetate from the plasma. *Folia Med Neerl* (1967) **10**, 141.
9 Bieger R, De Jonge H, and Loeliger E A. Influence of nitrazepam on oral anticoagulation with phenprocoumon. *Clin Pharmacol Ther* (1972) **13**, 361.
10 McQueen E G. New Zealand Committee on Adverse Drug Reactions. Ninth Annual Report 1974. *New Zealand Med J* (1974) **85**, 305.
11 Taylor P J. Hemorrhage while on anticoagulant therapy precipitated by drug interaction. *Arizona Med* (1967) **24**, 697.

Anticoagulants + benzydamin

Summary

The anticoagulant effects of phenprocoumon are not affected by concurrent benzydamin treatment. The effect on other anticoagulants is not documented.

Interaction, mechanism, importance and management

Ten patients anticoagulated with phenprocoumon showed no significant changes in their anticoagulant response to phenprocoumon while taking 50 mg benzydamin, three times a day, over a 2-week period, although there was some evidence of a fall in the blood levels of the anticoagulant.[1] No particular precautions would appear to be necessary if benzydamin and phenprocoumon are taken concurrently. There are no data about the effects on other anticoagulants.

Reference
1 Duckert F, Widmer L K and Madar G. Gleichzeitige Behandlung mit oralen Antikoagulantien und Benzydamin. *Schweiz med Wschr* (1974) **104**, 1069.

Anticoagulants + beta-blockers

Summary

The effects of the oral anticoagulants are not normally affected by the concurrent use of beta-blocking agents, although 3 patients on phenindione and propranolol have been described who showed haemorrhagic tendencies.

Interaction, mechanism, importance and management

A study carried out on 12 patients[1] anticoagulated with phenprocoumon showed that concurrent treatment with 15 mg pindolol daily for 6 weeks had no significant effect on their prothrombin times. This finding is in agreement with general clinical experience, virtually the only exception being a report of 3 patients taking phenindione and propranolol who displayed haemorrhagic tendencies, although no changes in the Quick time or any other impairment of coagulation were found.[2]

References
1 Vinazzer H. Effect of the beta-receptor blocking agent Visken on the action of coumarin. *Int J Clin Pharmacol* (1975) **12**, 458.
2 Neilson G H and Seldon W A. Propranolol in angina pectoris. *Med J Aust* (1969) **1**, 856.

Anticoagulants + carbamazepine

Summary

The half-life and serum levels of warfarin, and the anticoagulant response are reduced by the concurrent use of carbamazepine. Information about other anticoagulants is lacking.

Interaction

A study on 3 patients showed that after 3 weeks' treatment with carbamazepine (200 mg daily, week 1; 400 mg daily, week 2; 600 mg daily, week 3) their warfarin half-lives were reduced from 84 to 39 h; from 53 to 47 h; and from 72 to 30 respectively. Two patients taking a constant 5 mg daily dose of warfarin and the same dosage regimen of carbamazepine over a 3-week period showed an approximately 50% fall in serum warfarin levels which was reflected in sharp rises in the prothrombin–proconvertin percentages.[1]

This interaction has been described in another report.[2]

Mechanism

Uncertain. The evidence suggests that carbamazepine increases the metabolism of the warfarin by inducing liver microsomal enzymes thereby hastening its clearance from the body.[1,2]

Importance and management

The evidence is limited to these two reports, but they are a clear indication that a reduced anticoagulant response with warfarin can occur during concurrent carbamazepine treatment. The incidence is uncertain. It would be prudent to watch for a similar interaction with any oral anticoagulant although there is no direct evidence with any anticoagulant but warfarin.

References

1 Hansen J M, Siersboek-Nielsen K and Skovsted L. Carbamazepine-induced acceleration of diphenylhydantoin and warfarin metabolism in man. *Clin Pharmacol Ther* (1971) 12, 539.
2 Ross J R and Beeley L. Interaction between carbamazepine and warfarin. *Brit Med J* (1980) 1, 1415.

Anticoagulants + carbon tetrachloride

Summary

A single case has been reported of an enhanced anticoagulant response to dicoumarol following the accidental ingestion of a small amount of carbon tetrachloride.

Interaction

A patient, well controlled on long-term anticoagulant treatment with dicoumarol, accidentally drank about 0·1 ml carbon tetrachloride. Next day his prothrombin time had climbed to 41 s (a fall in prothrombin activity from 18 to less than 10%). Despite withdrawal of the anticoagulant, it was still virtually the same on the following day and marked hypoprothrombinaemia persisted for another 5 days.[1]

Mechanism

Uncertain. Carbon tetrachloride is very hepatotoxic and the change in the anticoagulant response would seem to be a manifestation of this.

Importance and management

Carbon tetrachloride, once used as an anthelmintic in man, is no longer used in human medicine, but it is still employed as an industrial solvent and degreasing agent. On theoretical grounds it would seem possible for anticoagulated patients exposed to substantial amounts of the vapour to show changes in their anticoagulant response, but there seems to be no direct evidence that this has ever taken place.

Reference

1 Luton E F. Carbon tetrachloride exposure during anticoagulant therapy. Dangerous enhancement of hypoprothrombinemic effect. *J Amer Med Ass* (1966) 194, 120.

Anticoagulants + cephalosporins

Summary

It has been suggested that cephaloridine in the absence of an anticoagulant may occasionally prolong prothrombin times. This has been described with cephazolin. It is not certain whether the effects of the anticoagulants are enhanced.

Interaction, mechanism, importance and management

According to the Council on Drugs of the American Medical Association, cephaloridine can induce an extension in prothrombin times, but no evidence is given.[1] This claim has been made elsewhere.[2] A patient has also been described who, 12 days after starting to take 0·5 g cephazolin 8-hourly, was noted to have increased prothrombin and partial thromboplastin times. These returned to normal within 48 h of withdrawing the cephazolin and recurred 10 days after the antibiotic was restarted[3] There appear to be no reports of a cephalosporin/anticoagulant interaction.

References

1 Council on Drugs. Evaluation of a new antibacterial agent, cephaloridine (Loridine). *J Amer Med Ass* (1968) **206**, 1289.
2 Wade A. Martindale's Extra Pharmacopoeia. 27th edn. p. 1099. (1977) Pharma Press, London.
3 Lerner P I and Lubin A. Coagulopathy with cefazolin in uremia. *New Eng J Med* (1974) **290**, 1324.

Anticoagulants + cimetidine

Summary

The anticoagulant effects of warfarin, nicoumalone (acenocoumarol), phenindione, and probably other oral anticoagulants can be enhanced by the concurrent use of cimetidine.

Interaction

A very brief report, published as a letter from the manufacturers of cimetidine, stated that they were aware of 17 cases worldwide indicating that 1 g cimetidine daily could cause a rise in the prothrombin times and blood clotting ratio of about 20% in those stabilized on warfarin.[1]

A study on 6 anticoagulated patients, 4 of them on warfarin, and the other 2 on nicoumalone or phenindione showed that a total of 1 g cimetidine daily increased their prothrombin times by an average of 12 s (range 5–23 s).[3]

Three other reports describe this interaction with warfarin.[2,4,5]

Mechanism

A study of this interaction on 7 volunteers given warfarin indicated that the increased anticoagulant response was due either to the inhibition of the metabolism of the anticoagulant by the cimetidine which caused it to accumulate, or possibly to a decrease in its apparent volume of distribution.[3] The response when taking acenocoumarol or phenindione was more rapid than with warfarin due, presumably, to the differences in rates of elimination of these anticoagulants.

Importance and management

An established and important interaction. The anticoagulant response should be monitored carefully and suitable dosage adjustments made if cimetidine is added to or withdrawn from an established anticoagulant regimen. Only warfarin, nicoumalone and pheninidone are so far implicated in the reports cited, but it seems possible that this interaction will take place with any coumarin or indandione anticoagulant.

References

1 Fluid A C. Cimetidine and oral anticoagulants. *Lancet* (1978) **ii**, 1054.
2 Silver B A and Bell W R. Cimetidine potentiation of the hypoprothrombinaemic effect of warfarin. *Ann Int Med* (1979) **90**, 348.
3 Serlin M J, Sibeon R G, Mossman S, Breckenridge A M, Williams J R B, Atwood J L and Willoughby J M T. Cimetidine:

interaction with oral anticoagulants in man. *Lancet* (1979) **ii**, 317.

4 Hetzel D, Birkett D and Miners J. Cimetidine interaction with warfarin. *Lancet* (1979) **ii**, 639.

5 Breckenridge A M, Challiner M, Mossman S, Park B K, Serlin M J, Sibeon R G, Williams J R B and Willoughby J M T. Cimetidine increases the action of warfarin in man. *Brit J Clin Pharmac* (1979) **8**, 392. P.

Anticoagulants + cinchophen

Summary

The anticoagulant effects of dicoumarol, ethylbiscoumacetate and phenindione, are markedly enhanced by cinchophen. Bleeding may occur.

Interaction

A diabetic man[1] admitted to hospital with a coronary thrombosis was treated with an unnamed anticoagulant. Twelve days later he was additionally treated with cinchophen for gouty arthritis and over the next 2 days he took a total of 4 g, at the end of which time his prothrombin levels were found to be less than 5%. The following day he had haematemeses, and died. A subsequent clinical investigation carried out on 3 patients who were taking phenindione, ethyl biscoumacetate or dicoumarol, following coronary thromboses, showed that within 2 days of starting to take 4 g cinchophen daily the prothrombin levels of two of them fell sharply from a range of 10–25% to less than 5%, while a smaller fall occurred in the third patient.[1]

Mechanism

The evidence which is available suggests that cinchophen has a direct action on the liver, like the oral anticoagulants, which reduces the synthesis of prothrombin. Cinchophen by itself can reduce prothrombin levels in the blood[2] and these hypoprothrombinaemic effects are reversible by the administration of vitamin K.[3] There is a latent period similar to that of dicoumarol before the hypoprothrombinaemia begins, and a short delay after its withdrawal before the prothrombin levels begin to rise again.[1]

Importance and management

Information is extremely limited but it appears to be an established interaction of importance. The incidence is uncertain. Cinchophen should not be given to patients on dicoumarol, ethylbiscoumacetate or phenindione unless prothrombin times can be monitored daily and dosage adjustments made. It is not certain whether the same response is seen with other oral anticoagulants but it seems highly likely.

References

1 Jarnum S. Cinchophen and acetylsalicylic acid in anticoagulant treatment. *Scand J Lab Invest* (1974) **6**, 91.

2 Hueper W C. Toxicity and detoxication of cinchophen. *Arch Pathol* (1946) **41**, 592.

3 Rawls A. Prevention of cinchophen toxicity by use of vitamin K. *NY State J Med* (1942) **42**, 2021.

Anticoagulants + chloral hydrate

Summary

Despite transient hypoprothrombinaemia, the concurrent use of warfarin and chloral hydrate need not be avoided. Whether other anticoagulants behave similarly is uncertain. Chloral betaine, petrichloral and triclofos may be expected to behave like chloral hydrate.

Interaction

Chloral hydrate causes a transient but clinically unimportant enhancement of the anticoagulant response.

A retrospective study, carried out by the Boston Collaborative Drug Surveillance Program on 32 patients to evaluate the influence of chloral hydrate on the early stages of anticoagulation with warfarin, showed that while the loading doses of warfarin in the control and chloral-treated groups were the same, during the first 4 days of treatment the warfarin requirements of the chloral group fell by about one-third, but rose again to normal by the 5th day.[1]

A study carried out on 10 patients with cardiac disease and 4 normal subjects, all anticoagulated with warfarin and given 1 g chloral at night, showed that there was a minor, clinically unimportant, and short-lived increase in the prothrombin times of 5 of them during the first few days of concurrent treatment, but no change in the overall long-term anticoagulant control was seen.[2]

Similar results have been reported in other studies on large numbers of patients taking warfarin and chloral hydrate[3-5,8,11,12] or triclofos.[7] Chloral betaine appears to behave similarly.[10]

An isolated, and by no means fully explained, case of fatal hypoprothrombinaemia in a patient on dicoumarol who was given chloral for 10 days, later replaced by secobarbital, has been reported.[6] Another patient on dicoumarol and chloral showed a reduction in prothrombin times.[6]

Mechanism

Chloral hydrate is mainly metabolized by alcohol dehydrogenase to trichloroacetic acid (TCA) which then successfully competes with warfarin for some of the binding sites on the plasma proteins.[8] The result is that as the TCA is produced, free and active molecules of warfarin flood into the plasma water by displacement and the effects of the warfarin are enhanced. But this is only transient because as the warfarin molecules become exposed to liver metabolism and elimination, so the warfarin half-life shortens and the hypoprothrombinaemic effects are reduced once again.

In this way the apparently paradoxical situation arises in which a fall in the plasma levels of warfarin can appear to be accompanied, if only briefly, by an increase in the hypoprothrombinaemia. Some of the early investigations[9] of this interaction were directed towards the measurement of only one parameter (e.g., warfarin half-life) using single doses of warfarin, or the anticoagulation parameters were measured at time intervals which were too long to detect short-term changes, so that some erroneous conclusions were reached.

Importance and management

Despite the transient hypoprothrombinaemia which can occur, it is not accompanied by bleeding and there is very good evidence that the concurrent use of warfarin and chloral hydrate need not be avoided.[1-5,8,11,12] No special precautions are necessary. Those who wish to be ultracautious might wish to check their patients' anticoagulant response during the first 4–5 days. Whether other anticoagulants behave like warfarin is uncertain because the evidence is sparse, indirect and inconclusive[6,13,14] but what is known about dicoumarol and nicoumalone seems to fit the same pattern as warfarin.

Triclofos[7] and chloral betain[10] appear to behave like chloral hydrate, and since petrichloral, like chloral betaine, is a variant on chloral hydrate which is decomposed in the stomach to chloral hydrate, it may be expected to behave similarly. Dichloralphenazone on the other hand interacts quite differently (see p. 139). Alternative hypnotics which do not interact with the oral anticoagulants are to be found among the benzodiazepines, such as diazepam or flurazepam (see p. 126).

References

1 Boston Collaborative Drug Surveillance Program. Interaction between chloral hydrate and warfarin. *New Eng J Med* (1972) **286**, 53.

2 Udall J A. Warfarin–chloral hydrate interaction. Pharmacological activity and significance. *Ann Int Med* (1974) **81**, 341.

3 Griner P F, Raisz L G, Rickles F R, Wiesner P J and Odoroff C L. Chloral hydrate and warfarin interaction: clinical significance? *Ann Int Med* (1971) **74**, 540.

4 Udall J A. Clinical implications of warfarin interactions with five sedatives. *Amer J Cardiol* (1975) **35**, 67.

5 Udall J A. Warfarin interactions with chloral hydrate and glutethimide. *Curr Ther Res* (1975) **17**, 67.

6 Cucinell S A, Odessky K. Weiss M and Dayton P G. The effect of chloral hydrate on bishydroxycoumarin metabolism. A fatal outcome. *J Amer med Ass* (1966) **197**, 144.

7 Sellers E M, Lang M and Koch-Weser J. Enhancement of warfarin-induced hypoprothrombinaemia by triclofos. *Clin Pharmacol Ther* (1972) **13**, 911.

8 Sellers E M and Koch-Weser J. Kinetics and clinical importance of displacement of warfarin from albumin by acidic drugs. *Ann NY Acad Sci* (1971) **179**, 213.

9 Sellers E M and Koch-Weser J. Potentiation of warfarin-induced hypoprothrombinaemia by chloral hydrate. *New Eng J Med* (1970) **283**, 827.

10 McDonald M G, Robinson D S, Sylwester D and Jaffe J J. The effects of phenobarbital, chloral betaine and glutethimide administration on warfarin plasma levels and hypoprothrombinaemic responses in man. *Clin Pharmacol Ther* (1969) **10**, 80.

11 Breckenridge A, Orme M L'E. Thorgeirsson S, Davies D S and Brooks R V. Drug interactions with warfarin: studies with dichloralphenazone, chloral hydrate and phenazone (antipyrine). *Clin Sci* (1971) **40**, 351.

12 Breckenridge A and Orme M. Clinical implications of enzyme induction. *Ann NY Acad Sci* (1971) **179**, 421.

13 Dayton P G, Tarcan Y, Chenkin Th and Wiener M. The influence of barbiturates on coumarin plasma levels on prothrombin response. *J Clin Invest* (1961) **40**, 1797.

14 van Dam F E and Gribnau-Overkamp M J H. The effects of some sedatives (phenobarbital, glutethimide, chlordiazepoxide, chloral hydrate) on the rate of disappearance of ethylbiscoumacetate from the plasma. *Folia Med Neerl* (1967) **10**, 141.

Anticoagulants + chloramphenicol

Summary

The anticoagulant response to dicoumarol and nicoumalone (acenocoumarol) can be enhanced by the concurrent use of chloramphenicol. Information about other anticoagulants is lacking.

Interaction

A study on 4 patients showed that the half-life of dicoumarol increased from an average of about 8 h to 25 h when given 2 g chloramphenicol daily for 5–8 days.[1]

Three out of 9 patients given a constant daily dose of an unnamed anticoagulant to maintain approximately constant prothrombin–proconvertin values of 10–30% showed a fall in their PP% to less than 6% when concurrently treated with 1–2 g chloramphenicol for 4–6 days.[2] One patient showed a smaller reduction.

There is another report of an enhanced anticoagulant response involving nicoumalone, and a brief comment implicating, but not confirming, an interaction with dicoumarol and with ethyl biscoumacetate.[3] Hypoprothrombinaemia and haemorrhage have been described in patients on chloramphenicol in the absence of an anticoagulant.[4,5]

Mechanism

Uncertain. One suggestion is that chloramphenicol reduces the metabolism of the anticoagulant by inhibiting the liver microsomal enzymes so that the activity of the anticoagulants is increased and prolonged.[1] Another is that chloramphenicol decimates the 'useful' gut flora thereby decreasing a source of vitamin K, but it is doubtful if in reality these bacteria represent an important source of vitamin K except in exceptional cases where dietary levels are very inadequate.[6] A third suggestion is that chloramphenicol blocks the activity of liver cells and reduces the production of prothrombin.[4]

Importance and management

The documentation is sparse, but it indicates that the effects of dicoumarol and nicoumalone can be enhanced by chloramphenicol. The incidence is uncertain. There appears to be no definite direct evidence of an interaction with any of the other anticoagulants (except possibly ethylbiscoumacetate[7]), but it would be prudent to be on the alert for an interaction.

References

1 Christensen L K and Skovsted L. Inhibition of drug metabolism by chloramphenicol. *Lancet* (1969) ii, 1397.
2 Magid E. Tolerance to anticoagulants during antibiotic therapy. *Scand J Clin Lab Invest* (1962) 14, 565.
3 Johnson R, David A and Chartier Y. Clinical experience with G-23350 (Sintrom). *Canada Med Ass J* (1957) 77, 760.
4 Klippel A P and Pitsinger B. Hypoprothrombinemia secondary to antibiotic therapy and manifested by massive gastrointestinal hemorrhage. *Arch Surg* (1968) 96, 266.
5 Matsniotis N, Messaritakas J and Vlachou C. Hypoprothrombinaemic bleeding in infants associated with diarrhoea and antibiotics. *Arch Dis Child* (1970) 45, 586.
6 Udall J A. Human sources and absorption of vitamin K in relation to anticoagulation stability. *J Amer Med Ass* (1965) 194, 127.
7 Wright I S. Pathogenesis and treatment of thrombosis. *Circulation* (1952) 5, 179.

Anticoagulants + chlorthalidone

Summary

The effects of some anticoagulants are reduced by the concurrent use of chlorthalidone, but the change is small and usually of limited clinical importance.

Interaction

In a study on 6 subjects who were given single 1·5 mg/kg doses of warfarin it was shown that the hypoprothrombinaemia was reduced (from 77 to 58 u) by the concurrent use of 100 mg chlorthalidone daily, although the plasma warfarin levels remained unaltered.[1]

A similarly reduced anticoagulant response has been described in another report involving phenprocoumon and chlorindione but no significant effects were seen on the activity of nicoumalone (acenocoumarol).[2]

Mechanism
It seems probable that the effects described resulted from a loss of plasma water caused by the diuretic which led to a concentration of the blood clotting factors.[1]

Importance and management
There is no clear reason to avoid concurrent use of chlorthalidone and the oral anticoagulants because the changes in response are not large, but it would be prudent to monitor the effects, and to make dosage adjustments where necessary.

References
1 O'Reilly R A, Sahud M A and Aggeler P M. Impact of aspirin and chlorthalidone on the pharmacodynamics of oral anticoagulant drugs in man. *Ann NY Acad Sci* (1971) **179**, 173.
2 Vinazzer H. Die Beeinflussung der Antikoagulantientherapie durch ein Diuretikum. *Wien Z Inn Med Ihre Grenzge* (1963) **44**, 323.

Anticoagulants + cholestyramine

Summary
The anticoagulant effects of warfarin and phenprocoumon can be reduced by concurrent treatment with cholestyramine. The effects of the interaction can be minimized by separating the dosages of the drugs by as long a time interval as possible.

Interaction
Ten normal subjects were treated for 1-week periods with either warfarin alone, warfarin with 8 g cholestyramine given three times a day either 30 min after the warfarin or, as in the 3rd week, given 6 h after the warfarin. With warfarin alone the peak serum warfarin levels reached 5·6 μg/ml and the prothrombin times were prolonged by 11 s. With warfarin and cholestyramine separated by 30 min the serum levels reached 2·7 μg/ml and the prothrombin times were prolonged by 8 s. With the warfarin and cholestyramine separated by 6 h, the peak serum levels reached 4·7 μg/ml and the prothrombin times were again prolonged by 11 s.[1]

Comparable results have been found in other studies in man using single doses of warfarin or phenprocoumon given with cholestyramine either at the same time or separated by time intervals. The clearance of the anticoagulant from the body has also been shown to be increased.[2–5,8,12]

Mechanism
Cholestyramine is a non-absorbable anion-exchange resin which is intended to bind bile acids with the gut, but if molecules of an anticoagulant are also present, it will bind these very strongly as well[2,3,5,6,7] and prevent their absorption from the gastrointestinal tract. As a result the serum levels of the anticoagulant and the resultant anticoagulant response are reduced. There is also good evidence that after absorption both warfarin and phenprocoumon undergo enterohepatic recycling, that is to say they (or some metabolite) are returned to the gut by excretion in the bile and reabsorbed so that continuous further contact with the cholestyramine can take place.[4,8]

Since cholestyramine taken by itself reduces the gastrointestinal absorption of dietary fats and fat-soluble vitamins such as vitamin K, it has a direct hypoprothrombinaemic effect of its own in some individuals[10] which has led to bleeding in one patient.[11] This pharmacological characteristic of cholestyramine may therefore offset to some extent the full effects of the cholestyramine/anticoagulant interaction in a few patients.

Importance and management
If warfarin or phenprocoumon and cholestyramine are given concurrently, the anticoagulant response may be reduced. Other studies, admittedly with animals,[7] show that this interaction can also occur with dicoumarol and ethyl biscoumacetate, but there is no reason to suppose that it will not also occur in man. There is no direct evidence of an interaction with the other anticoagulants, but it seems reasonable to assume that they will behave similarly.

Separating the dosages of the anticoagulant and cholestyramine by intervals of 3–6 h has been shown[1,9] to go a long way towards reducing the

133

effects of this interaction, but even if this precaution is taken the prothrombin times should be monitored closely to ensure that adequate anticoagulation is maintained during concurrent treatment.

References

1 Kventzel W P and Brunk S F. Cholestyramine–warfarin interaction. *Clin Res* (1970) **18**, 594.
2 Robinson D S, Benjamin D M and McCormack J J. Interaction of warfarin and non-systemic gastrointestinal drugs. *Clin Pharmacol Ther* (1971) **12**, 491.
3 Benjamin D, Robinson D S and McCormack J J. Cholestyramine binding of warfarin in man and *in vitro*. *Clin Res* (1970) **18**, 336.
4 Jahnchen E, Meinertz T, Gilfrich H-J, Kersting F. and Groth U. Enhanced elimination of warfarin during treatment with cholestyramine. *Br J clin Pharmac* (1978) **5**, 437.
5 Hahn K J, Eiden W, Schettle M, Hahn M, Walter E and Weber E. Effect of cholestyramine on the gastrointestinal absorption of phenprocoumon and acetylsalicylic acid in man. *Europ J Clin Pharmacol* (1972) **4**, 142.
6 Gallo D G, Bailey K K and Sheffner A L. The interaction between cholestyramine and drugs. *Proc Soc Expl Biol Med* (1965) **120**, 60.
7 Tembo A V and Bates T R. Impairment by cholestyramine of dicumarol and tromexan absorption in rats: a potential drug interaction. *J Pharmacol Exp Ther.* (1974) **191**, 53.
8 Meinertz T, Gilfrich H-J, Groth N, Jonen H G and Jähnchen E. Interruption of the enterohepatic circulation of phenprocoumon by cholestyramine. *Clin Pharmacol Ther* (1977) **21**, 731.
9 Cali T J. Combined therapy with cholestyramine and warfarin. *Am J Pharm* (1975) **147**, 166.
10 Casdorph H R. Safe uses of cholestyramine. *Ann Int Med* (1970) **72**, 759.
11 Gross L and Brotman M. Hypoprothrombinaemia and haemorrhage associated with cholestyramine therapy. *Ann Int Med* (1970) **72**, 95.
12 Meinertz T, Gilfrich H-J, Bork R and Jähninen E. Treatment of phenprocoumon intoxication with cholestyramine. *Brit Med J* (1977) **2**, 439.

Anticoagulants + clofibrate

Summary

The anticoagulant effects of warfarin, phenindione and dicoumarol can be markedly enhanced by the concurrent use of clofibrate. Bleeding can occur. Other anticoagulants may be expected to behave similarly. Most patients will require an anticoagulant dosage reduction of about one third.

Interaction

A combined study, carried out in three hospitals, on a total of 42 patients anticoagulated with either warfarin or phenindione showed that when they were additionally treated with either clofibrate or Atromid (clofibrate with androsterone), their anticoagulant response was considerably increased. Ten out of 15 patients in the Belfast hospital required an anticoagulant dosage reduction by about a quarter, and 5 of them bled. All 9 in Edinburgh needed a reduction by about one third. Fourteen out of 18 in Johannesburg also required an anticoagulant dosage reduction.[1]

This interaction has been confirmed in other studies on a considerable number of patients anticoagulated with warfarin[2–4,7,11] phenindione[5,6,8] or dicoumarol.[9] Bleeding has been described frequently, and death due to haemorrhage has been reported in at least two cases.[7,8]

Mechanism

Uncertain. Clofibrate binds to plasma proteins and can displace warfarin from its binding sites, but it is doubtful if this adequately explains this interaction.[12,13,14] One suggestion is that clofibrate might increase the affinity of the anticoagulant for its receptor sites.[9]

Importance and management

A well-documented and important interaction. The anticoagulant dosage will require reduction of about one third if excessive hypoprothrombinaemia and bleeding are to be avoided. The manufacturers recommend a dosage reduction by a half, later adjusted as necessary. Not every patient will necessarily demonstrate this interaction, the incidence being variously reported as between 20 and 100%.[2] Only warfarin, phenindione and dicoumarol have definitely been reported to interact, but other oral anticoagulants may be expected to behave similarly, although this still requires confirmation.

References

1 Oliver M F, Roberts S D, Hayes D, Pantridge J F, Suzman M M and Bersohn I. Effect of Atromid and ethyl chlorophenoxyisobutyrate on anticoagulant requirements. *Lancet* (1963) i, 143.
2 Udall J A. Drug interference with warfarin therapy. *Clin Med* (1970) **77**, 20.

3 Eastham R D. Warfarin dosage, clofibrate, and age of patient. *Lancet* (1973) **ii**, 554.
4 Roberts S D. and Pantridge J F. Effect of Atromid on requirements of warfarin. *J Atheroscler Res* (1963) **3**, 655.
5 Williams G E O, Meynell M J and Gaddie R. Atromid and anticoagulant therapy. *J Atheroscler Res* (1963) **3**, 658.
6 Rogen A S and Ferguson J C. Clinical observations on patients treated with Atromid and anticoagulants. *J Atheroscler Res* (1963) **3**, 671.
7 Solomon R B and Rosner F. Massive hemorrhage and death during treatment with clofibrate and warfarin. *NY State J Med* (1973) **73**, 2002.
8 Rogen A S and Ferguson J C. Effect of Atromid on anticoagulant requirements. *Lancet* (1963) **i**, 272.
9 Schrogie J J and Solomon H M. The anticoagulant response to bishydroxycoumarin. II. The effect of D-thyroxine, clofibrate and norethandrolone. *Clin Pharmacol Ther* (1967) **8**, 70.

10 Bjornsson T D, Meffin P J and Blaschke T F. Interaction of clofibrate with the optical enantiomorphs of warfarin. *Pharmacologist* (1976) **18**, 207.
11 Counihan T B and Keelan P. Atromid in high cholesterol states. *J Atheroscler Res* (1963) **3**, 580.
12 Solomon H M, Schrogie J J and Williams D. The displacement of phenylbutazone-^{14}C and warfarin-^{14}C from human albumin by various drugs and fatty acids. *Biochem Pharmacol* (1968) **17**, 143.
13 Solomon H M and Schrogie J J. The effect of various drugs on the binding of warfarin-^{14}C to human albumin. *Biochem Pharmacol* (1967) **16**, 1219.
14 Bjornsson T D, Meffin P J, Swezy S and Blaschke T F. Clofibrate displaces warfarin from plasma proteins in man: an example of a pure displacement interaction. *J Pharmacol Exp Ther* (1979) **210**, 316.

Anticoagulants + colestipol

Summary

Single-dose experiments suggest that no interaction occurs between colestipol and phenprocoumon, but the effects of long-term concurrent administration are not known. Other anticoagulants probably behave similarly, but direct information is lacking.

Interaction

A randomized crossover study on 4 normal subjects, given single oral doses of phenprocoumon, showed that the blood concentrations of phenprocoumon and the prothrombin response were unaffected by the simultaneous administration of 8 g colestipol when compared with a placebo of 2 g microcrystalline cellulose.[1]

Mechanism

Colestipol, like cholestyramine, is an anion-exchange resin which binds to bile acids as well as to the oral anticoagulants, but in-vitro tests show that at the pH values encountered in the stomach and duodenum the binding is much less than that which occurs with cholestyramine, and the absorption of the phenprocoumon appears to be unaffected.[1]

Importance and management

Single-dose experiments like these are not necessarily reliable predictors of the response during long-term concurrent treatment, but they suggest that a reduction in the effects of phenprocoumon are less likely than with cholestyramine. Other anticoagulants probably behave similarly but this awaits confirmation.

It would, nevertheless, be prudent to check the anticoagulant response carefully during concurrent treatment. If a significant alteration in the prothrombin response were to occur, separating the administration of the drugs by as long a time interval as possible might prove to be effective.

Reference

1 Harvengt C and Desager J P. Effects of colestipol, a new bile acid sequestrant, on the absorption of phenprocoumon in man. *Europ J clin Pharmacol* (1973) **6**, 19.

Anticoagulants + contraceptives (oral)

Summary

The anticoagulant effects of dicoumarol are reported to be decreased, and of nicoumalone (acenocoumarol) to be increased, by the concurrent use of combined oral contraceptives. A dosage adjustment may be necessary. Information about other anticoagulants is lacking.

Interaction

(a) Anticoagulant effects of dicoumarol decreased.

A study on 4 healthy volunteers who were given single 150 or 200 mg doses of dicoumarol after a 20-day course of *Enovid* (norethynodrel and mestranol) showed that the anticoagulant effects were decreased in 3 of the 4, although the half-life of the dicoumarol remained unaltered.[1]

(b) Anticoagulant effects of nicoumalone increased

A survey on 12 women anticoagulated with nicoumalone, following heart valve replacement or due to mitral valve disease, showed that when they were also taking oral contraceptives, over an overage of almost 2 years, their anticoagulant dosage requirements were reduced by about 20% and even then they were anticoagulated to a higher degree (prothrombin ratio of 1·67 compared with 1·50) than when given the anticoagulant alone. The oral contraceptives used were *Neogynona, Microgynon, Eugynon* (ethinyloestradiol with D-norgestrel) or *Topasel* (intramuscular ampoules of oestradiol enanthate with dihydroxyprogesterone acetophenide).[2]

Mechanism

Not understood, despite the enormous amount of work done on the effects of the oral contraceptives on the factors which take part in blood clotting. The contraceptives increase plasma levels of some factors (particularly factors VII and X) and reduce levels of antithrombin III, but what other changes occur which could explain these inconsistent reports is not known.

Importance and management

Direct data about this interaction seem to be limited to these two reports, but they indicate that concurrent use need not be avoided. Some adjustment in the dosage of the anticoagulant may be necessary: with dicoumarol an increase but with nicoumalone a decrease. Documentation about other anticoagulants is lacking.

A study using a progestogen-only contraceptive suggested that this type may possibly not affect the coagulability of the blood as much as the combined-type, but whether this is reflected in an absence of interaction with the oral contraceptives is not documented.[3]

References

1 Schrogie J J, Solomon H M and Zieve P D. Effect of oral contraceptives on vitamin-K dependent clotting activity. *Clin Pharmacol Ther* (1967) **8**, 670.
2 de Teresa E, Vera A, Ortigosa J, Pulpon L A, Arus A P and de Artaza M. Interaction between anticoagulants and contraceptives: an unsuspected finding. *Brit Med J* (1979) **2**, 1260.
3 Poller L, Thomson J M, Tabiowo A and Priest C M. Progesterone oral contraception and blood coagulation. *Brit Med J* (1969) **1**, 554.

Anticoagulants + corticosteroids or ACTH

Summary

Unpredictable changes–increases or decreases—in the effects of the oral anticoagulants may occur during concurrent treatment with ACTH or the corticosteroids.

Interaction

Conflicting and confusing evidence: some reports state that the anticoagulant effects are increased, others that they are decreased.

(a) Increased anticoagulant effects.

Ten out of 14 patients on long-term treatment with either dicoumarol or phenindione who were concurrently treated with ACTH for 4–9 days showed a small but definite increase in their anticoagulant responses.[1]

In another report a patient is described who, while controlled on ethyl biscoumacetate, began to haemorrhage from the gastrointestinal and urinary tracts within 3 days of starting concurrent treatment with 20 mg ACTH daily.[4]

(b) Decreased anticoagulant effects.

A study on 24 patients anticoagulated for several days with dicoumarol showed that 2 h after the administration of 10 mg prednisone their silicone coagulation time had decreased from 28 to 24 min, and after a further 2 h it was 22 min.[2]

A decrease in the anticoagulant effects of ethyl biscoumacetate in 2 patients due to concurrent treatment with ACTH and cortisone is described in another report.[3]

Mechanism

Unknown. There is good evidence to show that the corticosteroids can increase the coagulability of the blood in the absence of anticoagulants[5,6] which might explain the reduction in the anticoagulant effects described[2,3] if it were not that increased anticoagulant effects have also been observed. Increased effects have also been described in animals.[4]

Importance and management

It is very difficult indeed to assess these conflicting reports. The most constructive thing that can be said is that if ACTH or the corticosteroids and the oral anticoagulants are given concurrently there may be the need to adjust the dosage of the anticoagulant, but whether it is likely to be an upwards or downwards adjustment is, at the moment, impossible to predict. Much more work needs to be done on this interaction.

References
1 Hellem A J and Solem J H. The influence of ACTH on prothrombin–proconvertin values in blood during treatment with dicumarol and phenylindanedione. *Acta med Scand* (1954) **150**, 389.
2 Menczel J and Dreyfuss F. Effect of prednisone on blood coagulation time in patients on dicumarol therapy. *J Lab Clin Med* (1960) **56**, 14.
3 Chatterjea J B and Salomon L. Antagonistic effect of ACTH and cortisone on the anticoagulant activity of ethyl biscoumacetate. *Brit Med J* (1954) **2**, 790.
4 van Cauwenberge H and Jaques L B. Haemorrhagic effects of ACTH with anticoagulants. *Can. Med Ass J* (1958) **79**, 536.
5 Cosgriff S W, Diefenbach A F and Vogt W. Hypercoagulability of the blood associated with ACTH and cortisone therapy. *Amer J Med* (150) **9**, 752.
6 Ozsoylu S, Strauss H S and Diamond L K. Effects of corticosteroids on coagulation of the blood. *Nature* (Lond) (1962) **195**, 1214.

Anticoagulants + co-trimoxazole

Summary

The anticoagulant effects of warfarin can be enhanced by concurrent treatment with co-trimoxazole (trimethoprim + sulphamethoxazole). Bleeding can occur. Phenindione is said not to interact but evidence about other anticoagulants is lacking.

Interaction

Six out of a total of 20 patients anticoagulated with warfarin showed an enhancement of their prothrombin ratios within 2–6 days of starting to take two tablets of co-trimoxazole daily for respiratory or urinary tract infections (each tablet contains 80 mg trimethoprim + 400 mg sulphamethoxazole). One patient bled and required the administration of vitamin K. The anticoagulant was temporarily withdrawn from 4 of the patients and the dosage reduced in the last patient to control the excessive hypoprothrombinaemia.[1]

An increased anticoagulant response to warfarin caused by co-trimoxazole has been described in other reports.[2–4,6]

Mechanism

Uncertain. One study of this interaction in man showed that while the co-trimoxazole markedly increased the one-stage prothrombin times, the warfarin plasma levels and half-life remained unaffected, indicating that changes in warfarin metabolism were not responsible[3] Other in-vitro studies using therapeutic concentrations of both drugs showed that the sulphonamide component can displace warfarin from its protein binding sites—an increase in free warfarin from 20·6 to 23·4%, but this is too small an amount to account for the marked changes seen.[1] Another suggestion is that the affinity of the receptor site for vitamin K, or warfarin, or both, is altered.[3]

Importance and management

If co-trimoxazole is given to patients on warfarin an enhancement of the anticoagulant effects should be expected and appropriate precautions taken to prevent excessive hypoprothrombinaemia and bleeding. The incidence is uncertain. One study[3] stated that all 8 subjects examined demonstrated the interaction, whereas the report cited above described it in only 6 out of 20 patients.[1] There appears to be no documentation about the other anticoagulants with the exception of phenindione which is said not to interact.[5] It would be prudent to monitor the anticoagulant response of all patients on any anticoagulant if co-trimoxazole is added.

References
1 Hassall C, Feetam C L, Leach R H and Meynell M J. Potentiation of warfarin by co-trimoxazole. *Lancet* (1975) ii, 1155.
2 Barnett D B and Hancock B W. Anticoagulant resistance: an unusual case. *Brit Med J* (1975) **1**, 608.

3 O'Reilly R A and Motley C H. Racemic warfarin and trimethoprim–sulfamethoxazole interaction in humans. *Ann Int Med* (1979) **91**, 34.

4 Hassall C, Feetam C L, Leach R H and Meynell M J. Potentiation of warfarin by co-trimoxazole. *Brit Med J* (1975) **2**, 684.

5 De Swiet J Potentiation of warfarin by co-trimoxazole. *Brit Med J* (1975) **3**, 491.

6 Tilstone W J, Gray J M B, Nimmo-Smith R H and Lawson D H. Interaction between warfarin and sulphametnoxazole. *Post-grad med J* (1977) **53**, 388.

Anticoagulants + cyclophosphamide

Summary

A single case has been reported in which cyclophosphamide reduced the anticoagulant response to warfarin.

Interaction

A woman being treated for carcinoma of the lung was given daily treatment with 450 mg cyclophosphamide, 5 mg warfarin, 0·25 mg digoxin and occasionally as required paracetamol, codeine, chlordiazepoxide and flurazepam. When the cyclophosphamide was discontinued, her prothrombin time rose over the next 6 days from 23 to 34 s, and continued to climb even when the warfarin dosage was halved and eventually discontinued, before beginning to fall once again.[1]

Mechanism

Not known. It seems unlikely that any of the other drugs apart from the cyclophosphamide was responsible for the interaction.

Importance and management

There appears to be only one report of this interaction, but it would clearly be prudent to be alert to the possibility of a change in the response to warfarin or to any other anticoagulant if cyclophosphamide is added or withdrawn.

Reference

1 Tashima C K. Cyclophosphamide effect on coumarin anticoagulation. *Southern Med J* (1979) **72**, 633.

Anticoagulants + dextropropoxyphene

Summary

The concurrent use of warfarin and dextropropoxyphene is reported to have led to excessive hypoprothrombinaemia and bleeding in 3 patients. Other patients have failed to show this interaction, but the anticoagulants used were not named.

Interaction

Reports on this interaction are discordant

A man taking 6 mg warfarin daily showed marked haematuria within 6 days of starting to take two tablets of *Distalgesic* (dextropropoxyphene 32·5 mg, paracetamol (acetaminophen) 325 mg per tablet) three times a day. His plasma warfarin levels were found to have risen from 1·8 to 2·4 μg/ml. Another patient controlled for 6 weeks on 7 mg warfarin daily showed gross haematuria within only 5 h of taking 6 tablets of *Distalgesic* over a 6 h period. Her prothrombin time was found to have increased from about 30/40 to 130 s.[1]

This interaction has been observed in another patient on warfarin.[2] Death due to unknown causes in a patient on warfarin and dextropropoxyphene has also been reported.[4] In contrast there is a report describing no interaction.

A double-blind study, carried out on 23 patients anticoagulated on unnamed coumarol derivatives who were concurrently taking 450 mg dextropropoxyphene daily for 15 days, failed to show any change in prothrombin times.[7]

Mechanism

Paracetamol in daily doses of 2600–3250 mg has a small but trivial effect[3,4] on the activity of warfarin (see p. 162) so that it would seem that this interaction is due to the dextropropoxyphene component. In-vitro experiments with human plasma have demonstrated that this is almost certainly not a displacement interaction[5] but animal experiments[6] show that dextropropoxyphene can act as a liver microsomal enzyme inhibitor which, if it also occurs in man, would explain the enhancement of the activity of warfarin. But just why the woman described above[1] reacted in such a short time, and why only a few patients demonstrate this interaction is not clear.

Importance and management
The data are very limited but indicate that only a few patients are likely to show this interaction. The incidence is unknown. There seems to be no strong reason for totally avoiding the concurrent use of warfarin or other anticoagulants and dextropropoxyphene, but it would clearly be prudent to monitor prothrombin times closely to confirm that no interaction is taking place. Gener-

ally it might be easier to use another analgesic which is known not to interact (e.g. paracetamol—acetaminophen).

References
1 Orme M and Breckenridge A. Warfarin and distalgesic interaction. *Brit Med J* (1976) **1**, 200.
2 Jones R V. Warfarin and distalgesic interaction. *Brit Med J* (1976) **1**, 460.
3 Antlitz A M, Mead J A, and Tolentino M A. Potentiation of oral anticoagulant therapy by acetaminophen. *Curr Ther Res* (1968) **10**, 501.
4 Udall J A. Drug interference with warfarin therapy. *Clin Med* (1970) **77**, 20.
5 Toribara T Y, Terepka A R and Dewey P A. The ultrafiltrable calcium of human serum. I. Ultrafiltration methods and normal valves. *J Clin Invest* (1957) **36**, 738.
6 Breckenridge A, Orme M L'E, Thorgeirsson S, Davies D S and Brooks R V. Drug interactions with warfarin: studies with dichloralphenazone, chloral hydrate and phenazone (antipyrine). *Clin Sci* (1971) **40**, 351.
7 Franchimont P and Heyden G. Comparative study of ibuprofen and dextropropoxyphene in scapulo-humeral periarthritis following myocardial infarction. XIII Int Cong Rheumatol 30th Sept–6th Oct 1973 Kyoto, Japan.

Anticoagulants + diazoxide

Summary
The theoretical possibility that the concurrent use of diazoxide might enhance the anticoagulant response has not yet been confirmed in patients.

Interaction, mechanism, importance and management
In-vitro studies have shown that, in clinically occurring concentrations, diazoxide can displace significant amounts of warfarin (as much as 70%) from protein binding sites in the plasma so that, on theoretical grounds, it might be expected to do so *in vivo*; but there appears to be no direct documentary evidence that this causes an enhanced anticoagulant response in patients taking both drugs.

Reference
1 Sellers E M and Koch-Weser J. Displacement of warfarin from human albumin by diazoxide and ethacrynic, mefenamic and naldixic acids. *Clin Pharmacol Ther* (1970) **11**, 524.

Anticoagulants + dichloralphenazone

Summary
The anticoagulant effects of warfarin can be reduced by the administration of dichloralphenazone. It seems possible that other anticoagulants will be similarly affected.

Interaction
Five patients on long-term warfarin therapy who were given regular nightly doses of dichloralphenazone of 1·3 g showed an approximately 50%

reduction (range 20·2–68·5%) in plasma warfarin levels over a 14-day period, and an accompanying reduction in the anticoagulant response. One patient on 4 mg warfarin who took 1·3 g dichloralphenazone a day for 28 days showed a fall in her plasma warfarin concentrations from 4·1 to 1·2 μg/ml and a rise in the thrombotest percentage from 9 to 55%. These values returned to normal when the dichloralphenazone was withdrawn.[2]

Similar results have been described in other reports.[1,3]

Mechanism

The experimental evidence indicates that the phenazone (antipyrine) component of the hypnotic is a potent liver enzyme inducer which increases the metabolism and clearance of the warfarin, thereby reducing the anticoagulant response. The effects of the chloral appear to be minimal (see p. 130). Studies in man and animals show that phenazone reduces the plasma warfarin concentrations, shortens its half-life, and increases the urinary excretion of warfarin metabolites and of 6-betahydroxycortisol, all indicating that the liver microsomal enzymes are induced.[2,3]

Importance and management

The information is limited but the interaction appears to be well established. Dichloralphenazone is not a suitable hypnotic for patients on warfarin or, it seems probable, any other oral anticoagulant. Non-interacting substitutes may be found among the benzodiazepines. If the anticoagulant control has been disturbed by using dichloralphenazone, it is important to appreciate that it may take up to a month to restabilize the anticoagulant dosage because the effects of enzyme induction are by no means immediately reversible.

References

1 Breckenridge A, Orme M L'E, Davies D S, Thorgeirsson S and Dollery C T. Induction of drug metabolising enzymes in man and rat by dichloralphenazone. Fourth International Congress on Pharmacology (1969) Basel.
2 Breckenridge A, Orme M L'E, Thorgeirsson S, Davies D S and Brooks R V. Drug interactions with warfarin: studies with dichloralphenazone, chloral hydrate and phenazone (antipyrine). Clin Sci (1971) 40, 351.
3 Breckenridge A and Orme M. Clinical implications of enzyme induction. NY Acad Sci (1971) 179, 421.

Anticoagulants + diclofenac

Summary

The anticoagulant response to nicoumalone (acenocoumarol) and to phenprocoumon is unaffected by the concurrent use of diclofenac. It seems likely that this is also true for the other oral anticoagulants.

Interaction and mechanism

A crossover study on 32 patients anticoagulated with nicoumalone (acenocoumarol) showed that 100 mg daily doses of diclofenac had no effect on the anticoagulant response. The absence of an interaction has been confirmed in a further 20 patients.[1,2]

Other studies have confirmed the absence of an interaction between nicoumalone and diclofenac,[3] and phenprocoumon and diclofenac[4,5]

Importance and management

No action is necessary if diclofenac is administered to patients anticoagulated with either nicoumalone or phenprocoumon. It seems not unreasonable to assume that this is equally true for the other oral anticoagulants but there is, as yet, no direct confirmation of this.

References

1 Michot F. Bericht uber eine klinische Doppleblindstudie zur Frage der moglichen Interaktion zwischen Voltaren und dem oralen Antikoagulans Acenocoumarol.
2 Michot F, Ajdacic K and Glaus L. A double-blind clinical trial to determine if an interaction exists between diclofenac sodium and the oral anticoagulant acenocoumarol (nicoumalone). J Int Med Res (1975) 3, 153.
3 Wagenhauser F. Research findings with a new, non-steroidal, antirheumatic agent. Scand J Rheum (1975) 4, (Suppl 8) S05-01.
4 Krzywanek H J and Breddin K. Beeinflusst Diclofenac die orale Antikoagulantientherapie und die Plättchenaggregation? Med Welt (1977) 28, 1843.
5 Breddin K (1975) Cited as 'Personal Communication' in 2 above.

Anticoagulants + diflusinal

Summary

Some preliminary evidence suggests that the anticoagulant effects of nicoumalone (acenocoumarol) may be enhanced by diflusinal. No interaction was observed in two patients given diflusinal and phenprocoumon, but a study with warfarin suggests that some changes in the anticoagulant control may occur.

Interactions

Nicoumalone + diflusinal

A brief preliminary report[1,2] states that 3 out of 6 individuals stabilized on nicoumalone experienced clinically significant hypoprothrombinaemia (reduction in the serum levels of factors II, VII and X) after concurrent treatment with 750 mg diflusinal daily, and a prolongation of prothrombin times.

Phenprocoumon + diflusinal

The same report states that in a study on 2 patients given phenprocoumon and diflusinal concurrently, no interaction was observed,[1,3] and in subsequent in-vitro studies diflusinal was found to have only a very minor displacement effect on phenprocoumon from plasma protein binding sites.[4]

Warfarin + diflusinal

Five normal subjects were given sufficient warfarin to reduce the prothrombin complex activity (PCA) from 73·6 to 43·2%. The addition of 500 mg diflusinal twice day for 2 weeks had no effect on the PCA but the plasma warfarin concentration fell from 0·75 to 0·53 μg/ml. When the diflusinal was withdrawn, there was a loss in the anticoagulant effects and the PCA rose from 43·4 to 72·4%. After 12 days the plasma warfarin had risen once more to 0·71 μg/ml, almost its previous value.[6]

Mechanism

Not understood.

Importance and management

These preliminary reports and the manufacturer's published information[5] indicate that some changes in the anticoagulant control should be looked for if diflusinal is added to or withdrawn from an established anticoagulant regimen, but there seems to be little consistency in the ways different anticoagulants behave. There seems to be no information available about any of the anticoagulants other than nicoumalone, phenprocoumon and warfarin.

References

1 Tempero K F, Cirillo V J and Steelman S L. Diflusinal: a review of pharmacokinetic and pharmacodynamic properties, drug interactions, and special tolerability studies in humans. *Br J clin Pharmac* (1977) **4**, 31s.
2 Caruso I *et al.* Unpublished observations, quoted in 1 above.
3 Vermylen J. Unpublished observations, quoted in 1 above.
4 De Schepper P. Unpublished observations, quoted in 1 above.
5 'Dolobid' Diflusinal. Basic Data Booklet p. 9. Thomas Morson Pharmaceuticals (October 1978).
6 Serlin M J, Mossman S, Sibeon R G and Breckenridge A M. The effect of diflusinal on the steady-state pharmacodynamics and pharmacokinetics of warfarin. *Br J clin Pharmac* (1980) **8**, 287. P.

Anticoagulants + dipyridamole

Summary

Bleeding can occur during concurrent treatment with anticoagulants and dipyridamole even though prothrombin values remain stable and well within the therapeutic range.

Interaction

Despite stable prothrombin values within the normal therapeutic range, haemorrhage may occur.

Thirty patients with glomerulonephritis, stabilized on either warfarin (28 patients) or phenindione (2 patients), were concurrently treated with dipyridamole in doses of up to 400 mg daily for a month. No significant changes were seen in their prothrombin times (an average of 22·4 s without, and 21·6 s with dipyridamole) but 3 of the patients showed minor bleeding complications (epistaxis, bruising and haematuria) which resolved when either the dipyridamole or the anticoagulant was withdrawn or the dosage reduced.[1]

Mechanism
Unknown. One suggestion is that it may be due to a reduction in platelet adhesiveness or aggregation induced by the dipyridamole.[1]

Importance and management
Since bleeding can occur even when the prothrombin values are stable, some caution is clearly appropriate during concurrent therapy.

The authors of the study[1] suggest that the prothrombin activity should be maintained at the upper end of the therapeutic range as a precautionary measure. Only warfarin and phenindione are documented but it seems reasonable to expect it to occur with other anticoagulants.

Reference
1 Kalowski S and Kincaid-Smith P. Interaction of dipyridamole with anticoagulants in the treatment of glomerulonephritis. *Med J Aust* (1973) **2**, 164.

Anticoagulants + disopyramide

Summary
A single case has been reported of a patient who showed an increased response to warfarin when disopyramide was withdrawn.

Interaction
A patient receiving warfarin (3 mg daily) and disopyramide (100 mg 6 hourly) with digoxin, frusemide and potassium supplements, following a myocardial infarction, required an incremental doubling of the warfarin dosage to 6 mg daily over a 9-day period to maintain prothrombin times within the normal therapeutic range when the disopyramide was withdrawn.[1]

Mechanism
Unknown.

Importance and management
Although there is only one report of this interaction, prescribers should be alert to the possibility of a changed response to warfarin in the presence of disopyramide. Nothing is documented about other anticoagulants, but it would be prudent to watch for a similar interaction.

Reference
1 Haworth E and Burroughs A K. Disopyramide and warfarin interaction. *Br Med J* (1977) **4**, 866.

Anticoagulants + disulfiram

Summary
The anticoagulant effects of warfarin are enhanced by disulfiram and bleeding can occur. Other anticoagulants probably behave similarly but direct information is lacking. Bad breath (smelling of bad eggs) has been described during concurrent treatment.

Interaction
In order to verify a report of haemorrhage which had occurred in a patient treated concurrently with warfarin and disulfiram,[1] 8 normal subjects anticoagulated with warfarin were given 500 mg disulfiram daily for 21 days. In 7 of the subjects the plasma warfarin levels rose by an average of about 20% and the prothrombin activity fell by about 10%.

Other experiments with single doses of warfarin confirmed these results.[2,3,4]

This interaction with warfarin has been described in another report.[5] Bad breath reminiscent of the smell of bad eggs has also been described in patients on warfarin and disulfiram.[6]

142

Mechanism

The most probable explanation, and one which fits the experimental evidence, is that disulfiram inhibits the liver microsomal enzymes concerned with the metabolism of warfarin, thereby prolonging and enhancing its activity.[2,3,4]

Importance and management

The data are limited to 2 patients and 8 normal subjects but it seems probable that most individuals will demonstrate this interaction. Seven out of the 8 subjects did so. If, therefore, disulfiram is given to patients on warfarin the anticoagulant response should be closely monitored. Nothing seems to have been documented about any of the other anticoagulants but it would be wise to expect them to behave in the same way as warfarin.

References

1 Rothstein E. Warfarin effect enhanced by disulfiram. *J Amer Med Ass* (1968) **206**, 1574.
2 O'Reilly R A. Interaction of sodium warfarin and disulfiram. *Ann Int Med* (1973) **78**, 73.
3 O'Reilly R A. Potentiation of anticoagulant effect by disulfiram. *Clin Res* (1971) **19**, 180.
4 O'Reilly R A. Interaction of warfarin and disulfiram in man. *Fed Proc* (1972) **31**, 248.
5 Rothstein E. Warfarin effect enhanced by disulfiram (Antabuse). *J Amer Med Ass* (1972) **221**, 1052.
6 O'Reilly R A and Mothley C H. Breath odor after disulfiram. *J Amer Med Ass* (1977) **238**, 2600.

Anticoagulants + ditazole

Summary

Ditazole does not alter the anticoagulant effects of nicoumalone.

Interaction, mechanism, importance and management

A study on 50 patients with artifical heart valves taking nicoumalone (acenocoumarol) showed that additional treatment with 800 mg ditazole daily had no effect on their prothrombin times.[1]

There seems to be no information about the effects of ditazole on any of the other oral anticoagulants.

Reference

1 Jacovella G and Milazzotto F. Ricerca di interazioni fra ditazolo e anticoagulanti in portatori di protesi valvolari intracardache. *Clinica Terapeutica* (1977) **80**, 425.

Anticoagulants + erythromycin

Summary

A single case report describes bleeding in a patient on warfarin who was given erythromycin.

Interaction, mechanism, importance and management

A single case report describes an elderly woman on warfarin and taking other drugs (digoxin, hydrochlorothiazide, quinidine) who developed haematuria and bruising within a week of starting to take erythromycin stearate, 500 mg four times a day.[1] The mechanism of this response and the extent to which the other drugs may have contributed towards this apparent interaction is not known. There seem to be no other reports of an interaction between warfarin or any other anticoagulant and erythromycin, but it would now seem prudent to check prothrombin times particularly carefully if erythromycin is given to any patient taking an anticoagulant.

Reference

1 Bartle W R. Possible warfarin–erythromycin interaction. *Arch Intern Med* (1980) **140**, 985.

Anticoagulants + ethacrynic acid

Summary

A single case report describes a marked enhancement of the effects of warfarin by ethacrynic acid.

Interaction

There appear to be only five papers describing this possible interaction, four of them being animal and in-vitro experiments and the fifth a single clinical case report. In 1967 Buu-Hoi and his colleagues[1] described experiments in rats in which 50–100 mg/kg ethacrynic acid was found to enhance the hypoprothrombinaemia induced by ethyl biscoumacetate and warfarin. Later in 1970 and 1971 Sellers and Koch-Weser[2-4] published the results of in-vitro experiments carried out using buffered solutions of human plasma albumins to which clinically occurring concentrations of ethacrynic acid had been added. The decrease in the binding of warfarin to albumin due to the ethacrynic acid was found to be 59·5%. In 1975 Petrick and his colleagues[6] published a clinical case report in which they described the marked increase in the anticoagulant response of a woman to warfarin when doses of ethacrynic acid ranging from 50 to 300 mg were administered orally and intravenously.

Mechanism

The animal and in-vitro studies[1-6] clearly demonstrate that ethacrynic acid can displace warfarin from plasma protein binding sites, thereby briefly increasing its activity, but it seems very doubtful if this mechanism acting alone explains the single clinical report mentioned. Nor is it clear why the interaction has only been described in one individual.

Importance and management

There is no clear reason, on the basis of a single case report, for generally avoiding the concurrent use of warfarin and ethacrynic acid, but it would be prudent to be on the alert for the possible development of this interaction. Information about other anticoagulants is lacking.

References

1 Buu-Hoi N P, Hien D P and Hoi T T. Effets de deux diuretiques, l'hydrochlorthiazide et l'acide ethacrynique, sur la coagulation sanguine chez le rat normal et chez le rat recevant des antivitamines K. CR Acad Sci Paris (1976) Serie D **265**, 2165.
2 Sellers E M and Koch-Weser J. Dispacement of warfarin from human albumin by diazoxide and ethacrynic, mefenamic, and naldixic acids. Clin Pharmacol Therap (1970) **11**, 524–9.
3 Sellers E M and Kock-Weser J. Displacement from albumin and potentiation of warfarin by five acidic drugs. Clin Res (1970) **18**, 344.
4 Sellers E M and Kock-Weser J. Kinetics and clinical importance of displacement of warfarin from albumin by acidic drugs. Ann NY Acac Sci (1971) **179**, 213–25.
5 Ronwin E and Zacchei A G. The binding of ethacrynic acid to bovine serum albumin. Can J Biochem (1967) **45**, 1433.
6 Petrick R J, Kronacher N and Alcena V. Interaction between warfarin and ethacryine acid. JAMA (1975) **231**, 843.

Anticoagulants + ethchlorvynol

Summary

The effects of dicoumarol, warfarin and probably the other anticoagulants as well are antagonized by the concurrent use of ethchlorvynol.

Interaction

In a study on 6 patients anticoagulated with dicoumarol, the Quick index rose from 38 to 55% over an 18-day period whilst taking 1 g of ethchlorvynol each day.[2] Another patient is described who was stabilized on dicoumarol and who twice developed haematuria when the ethchlorvynol was discontinued, once for a period of 4 days and the other for a period of 6 days.

This interaction has also been described with warfarin.[1]

Mechanism

The mechanism of this interaction in man is not known although in dogs and rats it has been shown not to be due to liver enzyme induction.[3]

Importance and control

The two reports cited above appear to be the only ones in the literature describing this interaction so that it is difficult to make any statements about its general importance. It is not known whether anticoagulants other than warfarin and dicoumarol interact similarly. However, it would clearly be prudent to monitor the anticoagulant response whenever ethchlorvynol is added to or withdrawn from a stabilized regimen with any anticoagulant. An alternative non-interacting substitute for ethchlorvynol may be found among the benzodiazepines.

References

1 Cullen S I and Catalano P M. Griseofulvin–warfarin antagonism. *J Amer Med Ass* (1967) **199**, 582.

2 Johansson S A. Apparent resistance to oral anticoagulant therapy and influence of hypnotics on some coagulation factors. *Acta med Scand* (1968) **184**, 297.

3 Martin Y C. The effect of ethchlorvynol on the drug-metabolising enzymes of cats and dogs. *Biochem Pharmacol* (1967) **16**, 2041.

Anticoagulants + fenoprofen

Summary

Despite some in-vitro data, there appears to be no direct evidence that fenoprofen enhances the effects of the oral anticoagulants. Caution has nevertheless been advised because fenoprofen reduces the haemostatic function of the platelets.

Interaction, mechanism, importance and management

Although the manufacturers issue the warning that, because of its affinity for serum albumins, fenoprofen may displace drugs such as the oral anticoagulants and cause a prolongation of the prothrombin time, in-vitro data[1] indicate that the extent of the displacement is likely to be too limited (at least in the case of warfarin) to cause a clinically important interaction. There appears to be no direct evidence that an adverse interaction with the oral anticoagulants has occurred in man.

Some caution may however be appropriate because fenoprofen is a potent inhibitor of platelet aggregation.[2]

References

1 Rubin A, Warrick P, Wolen R L, Chernish S M, Ridolfo A S and Gruber C M. Physiological disposition of fenoprofen in man. III. Metabolism and protein binding of fenoprofen. *J Pharmacol Exp Ther* (1972) **183**, 449.

2 Herrman R G, Marshall W S, Crowe V G, Frank J D, Marlett D L and Lacefield W B. Effect of a new anti-inflammatory drug, fenoprofen, on platelet aggregation and thrombus formation (36183). *Proc Soc Exp Biol Med* (1972) **139**, 548.

Anticoagulants + feprazone

Summary

The anticoagulant effects of warfarin are enhanced by feprazone. This can rapidly lead to bleeding.

Interaction

An investigation[1] carried out on 5 patients on long-term warfarin treatment showed that after 5 days' treatment with 300 mg feprazone daily, the mean prothrombin time rose from 29 to 38 s, during which time the warfarin dosage was reduced from approximately 5 to 3 mg/day. All 5 patients showed this interaction. Four days after withdrawal of the feprazone, the prothrombin times were almost back to pretreatment levels.

Mechanism

Feprazone is about 90% bound to plasma proteins so that it seems probable that some of the interaction may be due to displacement of the warfarin from its plasma protein binding sites.

This would result in a rise in the concentration of free, and biologically active, molecules of warfarin and in an increase in the anticoagulant activity. But it is unlikely that this mechanism alone is responsible for the enhanced activity described.

Importance and management
Although the information is limited to this single study, the interaction would appear to be established. Patients on warfarin should not be given feprazone if bleeding is to be avoided—another non-interacting antirheumatic agent should be substituted. There appears to be no evidence concerning the effects of feprazone on other anticoagulants but it seems highly likely that they will interact in a similar way.

Reference
1 Chierichetti S, Bianchi G and Cerri B. Comparison of feprazone and phenylbutazone interaction with warfarin in man. *Curr Ther Res* (1975) **18**, 568.

Anticoagulants + flurbiprofen

Summary
Flurbiprofen does not usually affect the anticoagulant activity of phenprocoumon to any great extent, but a few individuals may develop bleeding.

Interaction
Nineteen patients[1], anticoagulated with a fixed dosage of phenprocoumon, who were given 150 mg flurbiprofen a day for 2 weeks showed a small but significant fall in prothrombin times and in factor VII and X values, but factor IX values fell only during the first week. Factor II remained unchanged. One patient showed haematuria which stopped a week after flurbiprofen was withdrawn. Another had epistaxis and haemorrhoidal bleeding after a week on flurbiprofen. Bleeding stopped a few days after stopping flurbiprofen. Both patients showed a fall in prothrombin values. Only 1 of the 18 patients who completed the study showed a definitely abnormal bleeding time of 11 min, but he showed neither bleeding nor any other side effects. Three patients showed a fall in prothrombin times below the therapeutic range (15–25%).[1]

Mechanism
The phenprocoumon levels in this study[1] remained constant which would seem to exclude the possibility of inhibition of the coumarin-metabolizing enzymes by flurbiprofen.[1] Similarly a study[2] using serum concentrations of 12 μg/ml (the peak serum levels following 100 mg doses of flurbiprofen) showed that less than 10% of the serum albumin sites are occupied by flurbiprofen so that possible displacement, and therefore enhancement, of the actions of the anticoagulants by this mechanism is unlikely.

Importance and management
On the basis of the very limited evidence available it seems that changes in the anticoagulant effects of phenprocoumon are small and usually of limited clinical importance in most individuals, but some may show haemorrhage. For this reason the effects of concurrent use should be monitored carefully. It is not known whether flurbiprofen similarly affects other oral anticoagulants, but it would seem likely. More study is required.

References
1 Marbet G A, Duckert F, Walter M, Six P and Airenne H. Interaction study between phenprocoumon and flurbiprofen. *Curr Med Res Opin* (1977) **5**, 26.
2 Anon. *Froben. Clinical and Technical Review* p. 39 (1977). The Boots Company Ltd, England.

Anticoagulants + food

Summary
The absorption of dicoumarol is considerably increased by being taken with a meal.

Interaction
Ten healthy volunteers were given a single 250 mg dose of a nonmicronized dicoumarol preparation (AP, Ferrosan, Sweden) either with food or on an

empty stomach, and blood samples collected over the next 72 h. Although there were considerable variations between individuals, the peak serum concentrations of dicoumarol when taken with food were considerably higher than when taken on an empty stomach, the average increase being 85%. Two subjects showed an increase of 242 and 206%.[1]

Mechanism
Unknown. One suggestion[1] is that the prolonged retention of the dicoumarol with the food in the upper part of the gastrointestinal tract, associated with increased tablet dissolution, may be responsible for the increased absorption.

Importance and management
On the basis of the work cited[1] it would seem sensible to take the dicoumarol with meals to increase its bioavailability. Alternatively to avoid marked fluctuations in the day-to-day serum concentrations of dicoumarol, it should be taken either consistently with or without food. Whether this food-drug interaction has clinical importance seems doubtful, but this requires confirmation.

Reference
1 Melander A and Wahlin E. Enhancement of dicoumarol bioavailability by concomitant food intake. *Europ J Clin Pharmacol* (1978) **14**, 441.

Anticoagulants + frusemide or bumetanide

Summary
The anticoagulant effects of warfarin appear to be unaffected by the concurrent use of frusemide or bumetanide.

Interaction
A study on 6 normal subjects showed that warfarin plasma levels, half-lives, and prothrombin times, in response to a 50 mg oral dose, were not significantly altered by the presence of frusemide (80 mg daily). A parallel study on 5 normal subjects similarly showed that bumetanide (2 mg daily) did not interact.[1]

Mechanism
None. An in-vitro study with phenprocoumon suggested that displacement of the anticoagulant by frusemide from plasma protein binding sites can take place.[2]

Importance and management
Direct experimental evidence of the absence of an interaction appears to be limited to this single-dose study and with warfarin only. The results are consistent with what the authors describe as the widely held clinical impression that these drugs can be safely administered to patients on coumarin anticoagulants.[1] However, more study is needed to confirm this absence of an interaction with warfarin and other anticoagulants, particularly since there is some in-vitro evidence (see Mechanism) of displacement by frusemide of phenprocoumon.

References
1 Nilsson C M, Horton E S and Robinson D S. The effect of furosemide and bumetanide on warfarin metabolism and anticoagulant response. *J Clin Pharmacol* (1978) **14**, 91.
2 Foged L, Husted S and Andreasen F. Protein binding of phenprocoumon in the absence and presence of furosemide. *Acta Pharmacol et Toxicol* (1976) **39**, 312.

Anticoagulants + glafenine

Summary
The anticoagulant effects of phenprocoumon can be enhanced by the concurrent use of glafenine. A similar interaction possibly occurs with other anticoagulants.

Interaction
A double-blind study on 20 patients, anticoagulated with phenprocoumon and well stabilized over at least 3 months, showed that when they were concurrently treated with 200 mg glafenine three times a day for a period of 4 weeks, a significant

increase in the thrombotest time was observed during the 2nd and 3rd weeks of the trial.[1]

These results confirm those of another report in which 5 out of 7 patients are described who required an anticoagulant dosage reduction while taking glafenine.[2]

Mechanism
Unknown. No significant changes in the phenprocoumon serum levels could be detected in the study cited,[1] although the levels of factors II, VII and X were reduced. This, it has been suggested,[1] might indicate a direct coumarin-like action of glafenine.

Importance and management
The data appear to be limited to these two reports. The incidence and the extent of this interaction is not established, but what is known indicates that during concurrent use a reduction in the dosage of phenprocoumon may be necessary to avoid excessive hypoprothrombinaemia. A similar interaction with other anticoagulants possibly occurs, but direct evidence is lacking.

References
1 Boeiginga J K and van der Vijgh W J F. Double blind study of the effect of glafenine (Glifanan) on oral anticoagulant therapy with phenprocoumon (Marcumar). *Europ J clin Pharmacol* (1977) **12**, 291.
2 Boeijinga J K, Gan T B, Van der Meer J. De invloed van glafenine (Glifanan) op antistollingsbehandeling met coumarinederivaten. *Ned Tijdschr Geneesk* (1974) **118**, 1895.

Anticoagulants + glucagon

Summary
The anticoagulant response to warfarin is rapidly and markedly enhanced by glucagon in large doses (50 mg or more). Bleeding can occur. Information about other anticoagulants is lacking.

Interaction
Eight out of 9 patients on warfarin who were given glucagon for 2 or more days in a total dose exceeding 50 mg showed a marked enhancement of the anticoagulant response. Excessive hypoprothrombinaemia was seen in all 8 with prothrombin times of 30–50 s or more, even though the warfarin dosage was reduced. Three of the patients bled. One patient showed a prothrombin time rise from 16 to 48 s over a 2-day period while taking 36–48 mg glucagon daily. Eleven other patients given a total glucagon dosage of 30 mg over 1–2 days failed to show this interaction.[1]

Mechanism
Uncertain. A study in guinea pigs showed that the injection of glucagon enhanced their anticoagulant response to nicoumalone (acenocoumarol) but the anticoagulant serum levels remained unaffected suggesting that changes in gastrointestinal absorption and anticoagulant metabolism were not responsible.[2]

Importance and management
The change in the anticoagulant response is rapid. The authors of the report cited[1] recommend that if more than 25 mg glucagon/day is given for more than 1 day the dosage of warfarin should be reduced in anticipation and prothrombin times monitored closely. Excessive hypoprothrombinaemia has been successfully treated with phytonadione. Smaller doses (total 30 mg) are reported not to interact.[1] It would be prudent to expect other anticoagulants to interact similarly but there is no direct evidence that they do so.

References
1 Koch-Weser J. Potentiation by glucagon of the hypoprothrombinemic action of warfarin. *Ann Int Med* (1970) **72**, 331.
2 Weiner M and Moses D. The effect of glucagon and insulin on the prothrombin response to coumarin anticoagulants. *Proc Soc Exp Biol Med* (1968) **127**, 761.

Anticoagulants + glutethimide

Summary

The effects of warfarin, ethyl biscoumacetate, and probably the other oral anticoagulants as well, may be antagonized by the concurrent use of glutethimide. There are some discordant reports.

Interaction

Most reports describe a reduction in the effects of the anticoagulants by glutethimide, but there are some discordant reports.

Reduced anticoagulant effects

A study on 10 subjects, stabilized on warfarin and with prothrombin times within the range 18–22 s, showed that when they were concurrently treated with 500 mg glutethimide daily for 4 weeks their prothrombin times were reduced by an average of about 4 s.[5,6]

Other studies have shown that 750 mg glutethimide daily can reduce the half-life of ethyl biscoumacetate by about a third after 10 days' concurrent use.[2,3] The half-life of warfarin is also reduced by a third to a half after 3 weeks' use of 1 g glutethimide daily.[1,4]

Enhanced anticoagulant effects or no interaction

An investigation undertaken with 25 patients taking ethyl biscoumacetate concluded that the concurrent use of glutethimide had no effect on the anticoagulant therapy.[7]

A man on long-term warfarin therapy developed signs of haemorrhage (grossly swollen right arm and ecchymoses) after taking 3·5 g glutethimide over a 5-day period. In a subsequent clinical study his prothrombin times were shown to be *increased* by the use of glutethimide. He was also taking 10 mg pentaerythritol tetranitrate four times a day and had been doing so for 2 years.[8]

Mechanism

Glutethimide, like the barbiturates, can stimulate the activity of the liver enzymes concerned with the metabolism of the oral anticoagulants thereby accelerating their rate of clearance from the body. This is reflected in reduced half-lives and serum levels of the anticoagulants, and in reduced anticoagulant effects. This interaction has been thoroughly investigated in man[1-6] and in animals. There is no good explanation for the reports of 'no interaction'[7] and of an 'enhanced effect'[8]

already described, nor for the fact that some individuals prove to be non-responders in experiments in which most of the subjects showed the interaction.

Importance and management

An established interaction of moderate importance. The incidence is uncertain but in one study[1] 40% of the subjects failed to show the interaction, and in another[6] one of 10 did not. Changes in the effects of warfarin and ethylbiscoumacetate may be expected if gluethimide is added to or withdrawn from stabilized anticoagulant therapy. It is not certain whether glutethimide affects all the oral anticoagulants but it seems possible. The effects of glutethimide may be expected to occur within a few days of beginning its administration, and may continue for up to 3 weeks after its withdrawal.[4] A non-interacting substitute may be found among the benzodiazepines.

References

1 Corn M. Effect of phenobarbital and glutethimide on the biological half-life of warfarin. *Thromb Diath Haemorrh* (1966) 16, 606.
2 van Dam, F E and Overkamp M J H. The effect of some sedatives (phenobarbital, glutethimide chlordiazepoxide, chloral hydrate) on the rate of disappearance of ethyl biscoumacetate from the plasma. *Folia medica Neerlandica* (1967) 10, 141.
3 van Dam F E, Overkamp M and Haanen C. The interaction of drugs. *Lancet* (1966) ii, 1027.
4 MacDonald M G, Robinson D S, Sylwester D and Jaffe J J. The effects of phenobarbital, chloral betaine and glutethimide administration on warfarin plasma levels and hypoprothrombinaemic responses in man. *Clin Pharmacol Ther* (1969) 10, 80.
5 Udall J A. Clinical implications of warfarin interactions with five sedatives. *Amer J Cardiol* (1975) 35, 67.
6 Udall J A. Warfarin interactions with chloral hydrate and glutethimide. *Curr Ther Res* (1975) 17, 67.
7 Grilli H. Glutethimida y tiempo de prothrombina. Su aplicación en la terapeutica anticoagulante. *Pren méd argent* (1959) 46, 2867.
8 Taylor P J. Haemorrhage while on anticoagulant therapy precipitated by drug interaction. *Arizona Med* (1967) 24, 697.
9 Hunningshake D B and Azarnoff D L. Drug interactions with warfarin. *Arch int med* (1968) 121, 349.

Anticoagulants + griseofulvin

Summary

The anticoagulant effects of warfarin can be reduced and even totally antagonized in some patients by the concurrent use of griseofulvin.

Interaction

Three out of 4 subjects (2 of them patients) showed a marked reduction in their response to warfarin when given 1–2 g microcrystalline griseofulvin daily by mouth. The fourth subject (a volunteer) showed no change in the response to warfarin even when the griseofulvin dosage was raised to 4 g daily for 2 weeks.[1]

In another study, only 4 out of 10 patients anticoagulated with warfarin showed any response to the administration of 1 g griseofulvin daily for 2 weeks. The average reduction in the prothrombin time was 4·2 s.[2]

Another report briefly describes a coagulation defect on a patient on warfarin and griseofulvin.[3]

Mechanism

Not understood. One suggestion[1] is that the griseofulvin might possibly act as an enzyme inducer which would result in an increase in the metabolism of the warfarin. There is as yet no experimental evidence to support this idea.

Importance and management

Griseofulvin can reduce the anticoagulant response to warfarin to a marked extent in some, but not all, individuals so that it is important to monitor the prothrombin times if griseofulvin is given to patients stabilized on warfarin. It would also be prudent to do the same if any other anticoagulant is being used, although there is as yet no direct evidence implicating any other anticoagulant.

References

1 Cullen S I and Catalano P M. Griseofulvin–warfarin antagoni m. *J Am Med Ass* (1967) **199**, 582.
2 Udall J A. Drug interference with warfarin therapy. *Clin Med* (1970) **77**, 20.
3 McQueen E G. New Zealand committee on adverse drug reactions: 14th Annual Report. *NZ med J* (1980) **91**, 226.

Anticoagulants + halofenate

Summary

A single case report describes a marked enhancement of the anticoagulant effects of warfarin by halofenate.

Interaction

A patient, previously controlled on 10 mg warfarin daily, showed a dramatic increase in his prothrombin time to 103 s when 10 mg/kg/day of halofenate was administered. The prothrombin times returned to normal when the warfarin dosage was reduced to 2·5 mg daily.[1]

Mechanism

Studies carried out with dogs[2] have shown that halofenate can affect both the synthesis and destruction of prothrombin, the net effect being to prolong the prothrombin time. A parallel mechanism seems to be in operation in the interaction between dextrothryoxine, another serum lipid lowering agent, and an oral anticoagulant.[3] Changes in the metabolism of warfarin cannot be discounted entirely,[5] but alterations in the binding of warfarin to plasma protein binding sites would appear not be involved.[2,4] The paradoxical resistance to warfarin which may possibly be seen if halofenate is administered first appears to be due to an increase in the synthesis of prothrombin.[2]

Importance and management

Although there is only one recorded case of this interaction, it would be prudent to monitor the prothrombin times of any patient on warfarin or any other anticoagulant who is given halofenate. The manufacturers of halofenate (MSD) are quoted as recommending a 50% reduction in warfarin dosage and close attention to prothrombin times.[2] Animal experiments[2] suggest that a delayed enhancement of the anticoagulant effects may be seen if halofenate is withdrawn, and that paradoxically some resistance to warfarin may be seen if the halofenate is given first.

References

1 McMahon F G, Jain A, Ryan J R and Hague D. Some effects of MK 185 on lipid and uric acid metabolism in man. *Univ Mich Med Centre J* (1970) **36**, 247.
2 Weintraub M and Griner P F. Alterations in the effects of warfarin in dogs by halofenate. An influence upon the kinetics of prothrombin. *Thromb Diath Haemorrh* (1975) **34**, 445.
3 Weintraub M, Breckenridge R T and Griner P F. The effects of dextrothyroxine on the kinetics of prothrombin activity: proposed mechanism of the potentiation of warfarin by D-thyroxine. *J Lab Clin Med* (1973) **81**, 273.
4 Hucker H B, Stauffer S C and White S E. Effect of halofenate on binding of various drugs to human plasma proteins and on the plasma half-life of antipyrine in monkeys. *J Pharmacol Sci* (1972) **61**, 1490.
5 Vessell E S and Passanti G T. Differential effects of chronic halofenate administration on drug metabolism in man. *Fed Proc* (1972) **32**, 538.

Anticoagulants + haloperidol

Summary

A single case has been reported of a patient on phenindione who showed a marked reduction in the anticoagulant response when given haloperidol concurrently.

Interaction

A man maintained on 50 mg phenindione daily was subsequently given haloperidol by injection (5 mg 8-hourly for 24 h) followed by 3 mg orally twice a day. Adequate anticoagulation was not achieved even with an increase in the dose of phenindione to 150 mg daily. When the haloperidol dose was halved the necessary dose of anticoagulant was found to be 100 mg daily, and only when the haloperidol was withdrawn was it possible to return to the original anticoagulant dose of 50 mg/day.[1]

Mechanism

Unknown.

Importance and management

Concurrent use need not be avoided, but prescribers should be aware of the single case described. There is nothing documented about any of the other anticoagulants.

Reference

1 Oakley D P and Lautch H. Haloperidol and anticoagulant treatment. *Lancet* (1963) **ii**, 1229.

Anticoagulants + hydrocodone

Summary

An increase in the anticoagulant effects of warfarin apparently due to the concurrent use of hydrocodone has been described in one patient, and partially confirmed in another subject. Data about other anticoagulants are lacking.

Interaction

A patient, well stabilized over a considerable time on warfarin, and also taking propranolol, spironolactone, clofibrate and digoxin, showed a rise in his prothrombin time from about twice to three times his control value when he began to take *Tussionex* (hydrocodone + phenyltoloxamine) for a chronic cough. When the cough syrup was discontinued, his prothrombin times fell once again. In a subsequent study on a volunteer the equivalent dosage of hydrocodone was found to increase the elimination half-life of warfarin from 30 to 42 h.[1]

Mechanism

Unknown. It has been suggested that the hydrocodone inhibits the metabolism of the warfarin thereby enhancing its effects.[1]

Importance and management

This interaction has been described in one patient only, and partially confirmed in one other subject, so that the documentation is clearly extremely limited. There is no obvious reason to avoid the concurrent use of warfarin and preparations containing hydrocodone, but it would be prudent to watch for any reduction in the warfarin requirements. There is no information about other anticoagulants.

Reference

1 Azarnoff D L. Drug interactions: the potential for adverse effects. *Drug Inf J* (1972) **6**, 19.

Anticoagulants + ibuprofen

Summary

In normal doses ibuprofen does not affect the anticoagulant activity of phenprocoumon or warfarin

Absence of interaction

Ibuprofen + phenprocoumon

A study on 19 patients, anticoagulated on a fixed dosage of phenprocoumon, showed that concurrent treatment with 600 mg ibuprofen a day for 2 weeks had no significant effect on their prothrombin times, on factors II, VII, X, on Ivy bleeding time or on the serum concentrations of phenprocoumon.[1,2]

Another study on 24 patients anticoagulated with phenprocoumon also failed to show any effect on thrombotest percentages when the same dosage of ibuprofen was taken over a 2-week period.[3]

Ibuprofen + warfarin

300 or 600 mg ibuprofen taken four times a day (1200 or 2400 mg) for 14 days by 36 volunteers who were anticoagulated with 7·5 mg warfarin a day had no effect on prothrombin times, or on factors II, VII, IX and X. The plasma warfarin levels also remained unaltered.[4]

Fifty patients anticoagulated with warfarin failed to show any change in their percentage coagulation activity after 7 days' treatment with 600–1200 mg ibuprofen daily, and another 30 volunteers showed no alterations in partial thromboplastin times (PTT) when taking ibuprofen alone.[5]

Mechanism

Ibuprofen has no effect on the half-life of antipyrine in man so that no change in the activity of the liver enzymes concerned with the metabolism of the anticoagulants would be expected.[8] Ibuprofen also does not bind to plasma proteins to any great extent and any displacement of the anticoagulants is of minimal importance.[6,7]

Importance and management

No interaction occurs between phenprocoumon or warfarin and ibuprofen in normal doses. Whether extremely large doses might result in some displacement of the anticoagulant from its binding sites, and in an enhancement of its activity, is uncertain.[7] Information about other anticoagulants appears to be lacking, but it seems probable that they will also not interact with ibuprofen. This requires confirmation.

References

1 Thilo D, Nyman F and Duckert F. A study of the effects of the anti-rheumatic drug ibuprofen (Brufen) on patients being treated with the oral anti-coagulant phenprocoumon (Marcoumar). *J Int Med Res* (1974) **2**, 276.

2 Duckert F. The absence of effect of the antirheumatic drug ibuprofen on oral anticoagulation with phenprocoumon. *Curr Med Res Opin* (1975) **3**, 556.

3 Bockhout-Mussert M J and Loeliger E A. Influence of ibuprofen on oral anti-coagulation with phenprocoumon. *J Mt Med Res* (1974) **2**, 279.

4 Penner J A and Abbrecht P H. Lack of interaction between ibuprofen and warfarin. Curr Ther Res (1975) **18**, 862.

5 Goncalves L. Influence of ibuprofin on haemostasis in patients on anticoagulant therapy. *J Int Med Res* (1973) **1**, 180.

6 Anon. *Brufen Clinical and Technical Review*, p. 30 (1976). The Boots Company Ltd, England.

7 Slattery J T and Levy G. Effect of ibuprofen on protein binding of warfarin in human serum. *J Pharm Sci* (1977) **66**, 1060.

8 Lee P. Bell M A, Webb J, Goh V and Chalmers I M. A study on the effects of ibuprofen on the metabolism of antipyrine in man. *Med J Aust* (1973) **2**, 846.

Anticoagulants + ice-cream

Summary

Ice-cream is said to have antagonized the response to warfarin in an isolated case report.

Interaction

A woman patient with thrombophlebitis who was taking 22·5 mg warfarin in single daily doses failed to produce the expected prolongation of her prothrombin time. It was discovered that she took the warfarin in the evening and she always ate ice-cream before going to bed. When the warfarin dosage was switched to the mornings, the prothrombin time increased.[1]

Mechanism

Not known.

Importance

This appears to be the only documented case of this interaction so that no general conclusions can be drawn. It would be worth while looking into the possibility of a food–drug interaction of this kind if a patient fails to achieve the expected therapeutic response to an anticoagulant.

Reference

1 Simon L S and Likes K E. Hypoprothrombinaemic response due to ice-cream. *Drug Intell Clin Pharm* (1978) *12*, 121.

Anticoagulants + indomethacin

Summary

The anticoagulant effects of warfarin, phenprocoumon, nicoumalone (acenocoumarol) and chlorphenadione are not normally altered by the concurrent use of indomethacin. Some caution is still appropriate because indomethacin can irritate the gut and induce bleeding.

Interaction

In 1967 a letter appeared in the *British Medical Journal*[1] about a patient taking warfarin and indomethacin who, when the indomethacin was replaced by phenylbutazone, showed a marked rise in prothrombin ratios and spontaneous bruising of the trunk and hands. The authors of the letter observed that 'the patient reported here did not develop haemorrhagic complications while taking indomethacin. However, this drug should probably be used with circumspection in patients on coumarin anticoagulants in view of the similarity of its action to that of phenylbutazone in displacing protein-bound molecules'. This cautiously worded warning was the starting point of an intertwined mythology about a supposed interaction between indomethacin and the oral anticoagulants which has been repeated time and time again in numerous review articles, charts and tables. However, there is good clinical evidence that normally no interaction occurs, some

of which had been published before the letter quoted above appeared.

Two studies, one with 14 patients treated with indomethacin (25 mg three times a day for periods of 4–44 days) and either chlorphenadione or phenprocoumon, and the other with 16 patients on the same dose of indomethacin for 3 weeks with phenprocoumon, demonstrated that no interaction occurs.[2,3]

Similar results were found in other clinical studies with indomethacin and phenprocoumon,[4] indomethacin and nicoumalone,[5] and indomethacin and warfarin.[6]

In contrast to this strong clinical evidence, there are a few equivocal reports of a possible interaction resulting in an increased anticoagulant response. In one the patient was also taking allopurinol which is known to interact with the oral anticoagulants (see the synopsis on page 117). In another[7] the patients appeared to be inadequately stabilized on their anticoagulant therapy before the indomethacin was administered. In the third case[8] a single individual is mentioned, but no details are given, whereas the enhanced hypoprothrombinaemia described in a fourth case appears to be the result of an interaction.[10]

Mechanism
Unknown.

Importance and control
There is good clinical evidence to show that normally indomethacin has no effect on the anticoagulant response of patients to coumarins (such as warfarin, phenprocoumon and nicoumalone) or to indanediones (such as chlorphenadione). It is reasonable to assume that the other oral anticoagulants will behave in a similar way. However, some caution may be appropriate not only because indomethacin can cause gastrointestinal ulceration and bleeding, (which in one case is reported to have had a fatal outcome,[9]) but also because enhanced hypoprothrombinaemia, though highly improbable, is not totally impossible.[10]

References
1 Hoffbrand B I and Kininmonth D A. Potentiation of anticoagulants. Brit Med J (1967) 2, 838.
2 Müller G and Zollinger W. The influence of indomethacin on blood coagulation, particularly with regard to the interference with anticoagulant treatment. Die Entzundung-Grundlagen und Pharmakologische Beeinflussung. International Symposium on Inflammation. Freiburg im Breisgau. May 4/6, 1966 Ed. Heister R and Hofmann H F (eds) (1966) Urban & Schwarzenberg, Munich, Berlin, Vienna.
3 Frost H and Hess H. Concomitant administration of indomethacin and anticoagulants. Die Entzundung—Grundlagen und Pharmakologische Beeinflussung. International Symposium on Inflammation. Freiburg im Breisgau. May 4/6, 1966 Ed. Heister R and Hofmann H F (eds) (1966) Urban & Schwarzenberg, Munich, Berlin, Vienna.
4 Muller K H and Heurmann K. Is simultaneous therapy with anticoagulant and indomethacin feasible? Med Welt (1966) 17, 1553.
5 Gaspardy Von G, Balint G, und Gaspardy G. Wirkung der Kombination Indomethacin und Syncumar (acenocoumarol) auf den Prothrombinspiegel im Blutplasma. Z Rheumaforsch (1967) 26, 332.
6 Vesell E S Parssananti G T and Johnson A O. Failure of indomethacin and warfarin to interact in normal human volunteers. J Clin Pharmacol (1975) 19, 486.
7 Odegaard A E. Undersokelse av interaksjon mellom antikoagulantia og indometacin. Tidsskr Norske Laegeforen (1974) 94, 2313.
8 Koch-Weser J. Haemorrhagic reactions and drug interactions in 500 warfarin-treated patients. Clin Pharmacol Therap (1973) 14, 139.
9 McQueen E G. New Zealand Committee on Adverse reactions. NZ Med J (1980) 91, 226.
10 Self T H, Soloway M S and Vaughn D. Possible interaction of indomethacin and warfarin. Drug Intell Clin Pharm (1978) 12, 580.

Anticoagulants + insecticides

Summary
A single case has been reported in which a patient totally failed to respond to warfarin after very heavy exposure to an insecticide.

Interaction
A rancher in the USA who was hospitalized on several occasions because of thrombo-embolic epidoses and therefore treated with warfarin, showed a marked reduction in response to warfarin on two occasions after dusting his sheep with a preparation containing 5% toxaphene and 1% gamma-benzene hexachloride. The dusting was done by putting the insecticide in a sack and hitting the sheep with it in an enclosed barn. Daily doses of 7·5 mg warfarin normally maintained his prothrombin time at 35 s (control 12 s) but after exposure to the insecticide 15 mg warfarin failed to have any effect at all.[1]

Mechanism
Both toxaphene and gamma-benzene texachloride have been reported to induce the microsomal enzymes of rats.[2] It seems not unreasonable,

therefore, to assume that in this case[1] the acute and intense exposure to these insecticides caused the induction of the liver enzymes of this patient so that the warfarin was metabolized much more rapidly than usual, and so failed to exert is normal anticoagulant effects.

Importance and management
Extreme exposure of this kind to chlorinated hydrocarbon insecticides is unusual, but it serves to illustrate the interaction potentialities of these compounds. The intensity of the effect will depend on the degree and length of exposure. This interaction should be borne in mind if farm workers and others who use these insecticides intermittently are treated with anticoagulants.

References
1 Jeffery W H, Ahlin T A, Goren C and Hardy W R. Loss of warfarin effect after occupational insecticide exposure. *J Amer med Ass* (1976) **236**, 2881.

2 Conney A H. Environmental factors influencing drug metabolism. In *Fundamentals of Drug Metabolism and Disposition* p. 253. LaDu, B N, Mandel H G and Way E L (eds) (1971). Williams and Wilkins Co.

Anticoagulants + isoniazid

Summary

An isolated report attributes a bleeding episode in a patient anticoagulated with warfarin to the concurrent use of isoniazid. An enhanced response to dicoumarol has also been described in dogs.

Interaction

A man anticoagulated with warfarin, 10 mg daily, and with a prothrombin time of 28·7 s, was started on a course of 300 mg isoniazid for tuberculosis. Eight days later his prothrombin time was 26·3 s. About a fortnight later (the report does not give the precise details) he accidentally doubled the dosage of isoniazid, and 10 days later he was readmitted to hospital with bleeding gums, haematuria and bilateral flank pain and tenderness. His prothrombin time was found to have risen to 53·3 s. He was later restabilized on 7·5 mg warfarin and 300 mg isoniazid daily. There was no evidence of any other drug intake which might have accounted for the bleeding episode.[3]

An investigation on five dogs anticoagulated with dicoumarol showed that the concurrent administration of isoniazid enhanced the anticoagulant effects.[1] Two patients (not taking anticoagulants) and under treatment with isoniazid, streptomycin and PAS developed haemorrhage attributed to the anticoagulant effects of isoniazid.[2]

Mechanism

Not understood. The authors of the report concerning the interaction in dogs attributed the response described to inhibition by the isoniazid of the liver microsomal enzymes concerned with the metabolism of the dicoumarol, but clear experimental evidence to support this idea has not been presented.[1]

Importance and management

Information is extremely limited and an interaction has not been unequivocally established. It would seem prudent however to monitor the effects if isoniazid is added to an established regimen of warfarin, or any other anticoagulant. More study is required.

References
1 Eade N R, McLeod P J and MacLeod S M. Potentiation of bishydroxycoumarin in dogs by isoniazid and p-aminosalicylic acid. *Am Rev Resp Dis* (1971) **103**, 792.
2 Castell F A. Accion anticoagulante de la isoniazide. *Enfermedades de Torax* (1969) **69**, 153.
3 Rosenthal A R, Self T H, Baker E D and Londen R A. Interaction of isoniazid and warfarin. *J Amer med Ass* (1977) **238**, 2177.

Anticoagulants + laxatives or liquid paraffin

Summary

The theoretical possibility that the concurrent use of laxatives or liquid paraffin might affect the response to oral anticoagulants appears to be unconfirmed.

Interaction, mechanism, importance and management

On theoretical grounds laxatives and liquid paraffin (mineral oil) might be expected to affect the response to oral anticoagulants. Changes in the speed of peristalsis induced by the laxative might alter the absorption of vitamin K and the anticoagulants. Liquid paraffin might also impair the absorption of the lipid-soluble vitamin K. But despite warnings in various books, reviews and lists of drug interactions, there appears to be no direct evidence, as yet, that this is an interaction of practical importance. See also anticoagulants + psyllium (p. 166).

Anticoagulants + meprobamate

Summary

The anticoagulant effects of warfarin are not significantly altered by the concurrent administration of meprobamate.

Interaction

On the evidence from experiments carried out with dogs which showed that the half-life of warfarin was reduced by meprobamate,[1] the suggestion was made that the anticoagulant effects of warfarin in man would be similarly diminished, but clinical studies have failed to demonstrate an interaction of any significance in man:

When 9 men[2] stabilized on log-term warfarin therapy were given 1600 mg meprobamate daily for 14 days, 3 of them showed a small increase in prothrombin times, 5 of them a small decrease, and 1 remained the same.

Ten patients stabilized on warfarin who were given 2400 mg meprobamate daily for 4 weeks showed a small but clinically unimportant reduction in their prothrombin times when compared with a similar control group taking a placebo[3]

Mechanism

Unknown.

Importance and control

The changes in prothrombin times which have been seen[2,3] are too small to be of clinical importance and no special precautions appear to be necessary if meprobamate in normal dosage is given to patients on warfarin. It seems likely that this will equally be true for other anticoagulants as well, but direct confirmation if this is required.

References

1 Hunningshare D B and Azarnoff D L. Drug interactions with warfarin. *Arch Int Med* (1968) **121**, 349.
2 Udall J A. Warfarin therapy not influenced by meprobamate. A controlled study in nine men. *Curr Ther Res* (1970) **12**, 724.
3 Gould I, Michael A, Fisch S and Gomprecht R F. Prothrombin levels maintained with meprobamate and warfarin. A controlled study. *J Amer Med Ass* (1972) **220**, 1460.

Anticoagulants + mefenamic acid

Summary

It seems probable that mefenamic acid does not significantly enhance the effects of warfarin, but the absence of an interaction has yet to be firmly established.

Interaction

A single crossover trial on 12 volunteers taking warfarin sodium and whose prothrombin concentrations were within the 17·5–23·5% range (mean 20·03%) showed that when they were also given 2 g mefenamic acid daily for a week their prothrombin concentrations fell by another 3·49%. Microscopic haematuria were seen in 3 of the subjects, but no overt haemorrhage. Their prothrombin concentrations were 15–25% of normal, well within the accepted anticoagulation range.[1]

Mechanisms

Both mefenamic acid and warfarin bind strongly to plasma proteins. Although mefenamic acid may not actually directly compete with warfarin[2] for the same binding sites, it may be capable of altering the structure of the plasma proteins so that a considerable amount of the warfarin becomes unbound and passes into solution in the plasma water. In-vitro studies using human albumin and an equilibrium dialysis technique have shown that with typical plasma concentrations of mefenamic acid of 20–50 $\mu g/ml$ (representing about 4 g daily) the estimated increase in the free, and biologically active, warfarin concentration is 140–340%.[2,3] This might be expected to lead to a marked increase in the activity of warfarin and to haemorrhage, but in the study already described[1] no bleeding was seen. This would suggest that in practice some other factor normally modifies the extent of this interaction.

Importance and management
The information is very limited and equivocal. The possibility of an increase in the anticoagulant

effects of warfarin should be borne in mind if mefenamic acid is given concurrently, but it should be emphasized that so far there are no clinical reports of an interaction, and some evidence[1] that it does not occur. Information about other anticoagulants is lacking.

References
1 Holmes E L. Pharmacology of the fenamates: IV. Toleration by normal human subjects. *Ann Phys Med* (1966) **9** (*Suppl*) 36.
2 Sellers E M and Koch-Weser J. Displacement of warfarin from human albumin by diazoxide and ethacrynic, mefenamic and naldixic acids. *Clin Pharmacol Therap* (1969) **11**, 524.
3 Sellers E M and Koch-Weser J. Kinetics and clinical importance of displacement of warfarin from albumin by acidic drugs. *Ann NY Acad Sci* (1971) **179**, 213.

Anticoagulants + mercaptopurine

Summary
A single case report describes a reduction in the effects of warfarin during concurrent treatment with 6-mercaptopurine. Information about other anticoagulants is lacking.

Interaction
A patient with chronic granulocytic leukaemia, well stabilized on warfarin, showed a marked reduction in his hypoprothrombinaemic response on each of two occasions when treated with 6-mercaptopurine, which returned to normal when the mercaptopurine was withdrawn.[1]

Mechanism
Uncertain. It was originally suggested[1] that the mercaptopurine might induce the liver microsomal enzymes concerned with the metabolism of the anticoagulant thereby reducing its effects, but more recent data from animal experiments indicate that it may result from changes in synthesis or inactivation of the prothrombin complex.[2]

Importance and management
On the basis of a single case report there seems to be no good reason to avoid concurrent treatment with warfarin and 6-mercaptopurine, but it would be prudent to be on the alert for a change in the anticoagulant requirements if mercaptopurine is given or withdrawn. It is not known whether a similar interaction occurs with other anticoagulants.

References
1 Spiers A S D and Mibashan R S. Increased warfarin requirement during mercaptopurine therapy: a new drug interaction. *Lancet* (1974) **ii**, 221.
2 Martini A and Jahnchen E. Studies in rats on the mechanisms by which 6-mercaptopurine inhibits the anticoagulant effect of warfarin. *J Pharmacol Exp Ther* (1977) **201**, 547.

Anticoagulants + methaqualone

Summary
A small but unimportant reduction in the anticoagulant effects of warfarin can occur during the concurrent use of methaqualone. Information about the other anticoagulants is lacking.

Interaction
Ten patients anticoagulated with warfarin who

were given 0·3 g methaqualone at bedtime for 3 weeks showed a small, but clinically unimportant, fall in their prothrombin times. Their average pro-thrombin times before, during and after concurrent treatment were 20·9, 20·4 and 19·6s respectively.[1]

Another report describes a patient whose war-farin plasma levels were unaffected by methaqua-lone, but who showed some evidence of enzyme induction.[2]

Mechanism

The small change in prothrombin times is prob-ably a reflection of a limited degree of enzyme induction by the methaqualone which results in the metabolism and the clearance of the warfarin being slightly increased. Methaqualone has cer-tainly been shown to have enzyme-inductive properties in man.[2,3]

Importance and management

The documentation of this interaction is limited, but the evidence available indicates that the reduction in the effects of warfarin is likely to be insignificant. Nothing seems to have been reported about the other anticoagulants.

References
1 Udall J A. Clinical implications of warfarin interactions with five sedatives. *Amer J Cardiol* (1975) **35**, 67.
2 Whitfield J B, Moss D W, Neale G, Orme M & Breckenridge A. Changes in plasma α-glutamyl transpeptidase activity asso-ciated with alterations in drug metabolism in man. *Brit Med J* (1973) **1**, 316.
3 Nayak R K, Smyth R D, Chamberlain A P. Methaqualone pharmacokinetics after single and multiple dose adminis-tration in man. *J Pharmacokinet Biopharmaceut* (1974) **2**, 107.

Anticoagulants + methylphenidate

Summary

Limited and conflicting evidence indicates that methylphenidate may or may not enhance the anticoagulant effects of ethylbiscoumacetate. There is no evidence about any of the other anticoagulants.

Interaction

Conflicting evidence indicates that methylpheni-date does or does not prolong the half-life of ethyl biscoumacetate.

A study on 4 normal subjects given ethyl biscoum-acetate (20 mg/kg) showed that after 3–5 days' treatment with methylphenidate (10 mg twice daily) the half-life of the anticoagulant was on average approximately doubled.[1]

A subsequent double-blind study on 12 subjects failed to show any changes in the half-life or the prothrombin times due to ethyl biscoumacetate during concurrent treatment with methylphenidate, 20 mg daily.[2]

Mechanism

Unknown. The authors of the study describing an interaction suggest that methylphenidate inhibits the metabolism of the anticoagulant.[1]

Importance and management

The data are very limited. The second of the two studies (no interaction) was the better controlled and may therefore be the more reliable guide; nevertheless it would be prudent to watch for a change (an enhancement) in the anticoagulant response if these drugs are used together. There are no data about any of the other anticoagulants.

References
1 Garrettson L K, Perel J M and Dayton P G. Methylphenidate interaction with both anticonvulsants and ethyl biscoumace-tate. *J Amer Med Ass* (1969) **207**, 2053.
2 Hague D E, Smith M E Ryan J R and McMahon F G. The interaction of methyophenidate and prolintane with ethyl biscoumacetate metabolism. *Fed Proc* (1971) **30**, 366 (*Abs*).

Anticoagulants + metronidazole

Summary

The anticoagulant effects of warfarin can be markedly enhanced by concurrent treatment with metronidazole. Bleeding can occur. Information about other anticoagulants is lacking.

Interaction

A woman who had been taking warfarin for 6 years, following surgery for the insertion of an artificial mitral valve, showed bruising 10 days after starting a course of metronidazole. After 17 days' concurrent treatment she was hospitalized with severe pain in one leg and was observed to have ecchymoses and haemorrhage of the legs. Her prothrombin time was found to have risen from her normal 17–19 s to 147 s.[1]

Eight normal subjects were given single oral doses of either a racemic warfarin mixture, S(−) warfarin or R(+) warfarin, alone or after 7 days' treatment with 750 mg metronidazole daily, and the effects on their prothrombin responses measured. No change in the response to R(+) warfarin was seen, but the mean response to S(−) warfarin was virtually doubled and the half-life prolonged by about 60%. The half-life of the racemic warfarin mixture was increased by about one third (from 35 to 46 h).[2]

Mechanism

It is suggested that metronidazole inhibits the activity of the enzymes responsible for the ring oxidation of the S(−) warfarin, but does not affect the R(+) warfarin which is metabolized primarily by the reduction of side chains. Thus the racemate which has the more potent hypoprothrombinaemic actions is retained within the body and its activity is enhanced and prolonged, whereas the R(+) racemate remains unaffected.[2]

Importance and management

A marked increase in the anticoagulant response to normal commercially available (racemic mixture) warfarin may be expected during concurrent treatment with metronidazole. Appropriate precautions should be taken to prevent excessive hypoprothrombinaemia and bleeding. Paradoxically 1 of the 8 subjects cited[2] showed a marked interaction with R(+) warfarin so that even if pure R(+) and S(−) warfarin were readily available it would not be possible to guarantee that no interaction would take place with metronidazole. There appears to be no documentation about other anticoagulants.

References

1 Kazmier F J. A significant interaction between metronidazole and warfarin. *Mayo Clin Proc* (1976) **51**, 782.
2 O'Reilly R A. The stereoselective interaction of warfarin and metronidazole in man. *New Eng J Med* (1976) **295**, 354.

Anticoagulants + mianserin

Summary

Clinical evidence shows that the anticoagulant effects of phenprocoumon are unaffected by the concurrent use of mianserin.

Interaction and mechanism

A double-blind randomized study, carried out on 60 subjects anticoagulated with phenprocoumon, showed that the concurrent use of mianserin in 30–60 mg daily doses for 3 weeks had no significant effect on the prothrombin, bleeding or coagulation times.[1]

Importance and control

No special precautions appear to be necessary if mianserin is given to patients anticoagulated with phenprocoumon, but whether this is equally true of the other oral anticoagulants awaits confirmation. One manufacturer of mianserin cautiously advises that while '. . . concurrent anticoagulant therapy of the coumarin type (e.g. warfarin) is permissible, normal monitoring procedures should be undertaken'.[2]

References

1 Kopera H, Schenk H and Stulemeijer S. Phenprocoumon requirement, whole blood coagulation time, bleeding time and plasma γ-GT in patients receiving mianserin. *Europ J clin Pharmacol* (1978) **13**, 351.
2 *Norval* (Bencard). ABPI. Data Sheet Compendium, p. 112 (1979–80).

Anticoagulants + monoamine oxidase inhibitors

Summary

The theoretical possibility that the concurrent use of MAOI might enhance the effects of the oral anticoagulants seems not to have been confirmed in man as yet.

Interaction, mechanism, importance and management

A number of animal studies[1-4] have shown that the monoamine oxidase inhibitors can enhance the effects of some oral anticoagulants, but reports of an altered anticoagulant response in man appear to be lacking.

References

1 Fumarola D and De Rinaldis P. Ricerche sperimentali sugli inibitori della mono-aminossidasi. Influenza della nialamide sulla attivita degli anticoagulanti indiretti. *Haematologica* (1964) **49**, 1263.
2 Reber K and Studer A. Beeinflussung der Wirkung einiger indirekter Antikoagulantien durch Monoaminoxydase-Hemmer. *Thromb Diath Haemorrh* (1965) **14**, 83.
3 De Nicola P, Fumarola D and De Rinaldis P. Beeinflussung der gerinnungshemmenden Wirkung der indirekten Antikoagulantien durch die MAO-Inhibitoren. *Thromb Diath Haemorrh* (1964) **12** (*Suppl*), 125.
4 Hrdina P, Rusnakova M and Kovalcik V. Changes of hypoprothrombinaemic activity of indirect anticoagulants after MAO inhibitors and reserpine. *Biochem Pharmacol* (1953) **12** (*Suppl*), 241.

Anticoagulants + naldixic acid

Summary

An isolated report describes a considerably enhanced anticoagulant response to warfarin during treatment with naldixic acid.

Interaction

A woman satisfactorily anticoagulated over a 9-month period on 11 mg warfarin daily and with a prothrombin ratio of 2·0, developed a purpuric rash on her abdomen and bruising on her left leg and back within 6 days of starting to take 2·0 g naldixic acid daily for a urinary tract infection. Her prothrombin time was found to have risen to 45 s. Both drugs were withdrawn. She was later discharged well with a prothrombin time of 22 s on 10 mg warfarin daily.[1]

Mechanism

In-vitro experiments[2,3] have shown that naldixic acid can displace warfarin from its binding sites on human plasma albumin at concentrations equivalent to those which would be found in man using normal doses of both drugs. The estimated increase in the free (and therefore biologically active) concentration of warfarin is 64–160% which might be expected to enhance the hypoprothrombinaemic actions of warfarin. While this may go some way towards explaining the single case described above, the question which immediately poses itself is why it has apparently only affected this one individual.

Importance and management

This one report, associated with the in-vitro data, indicates that an interaction is possible but its probability is uncertain. It would be prudent to monitor the anticoagulant response closely if naldixic acid is given to any patient on anticoagulant therapy, but there is not enough evidence to prohibit their concurrent use.

References

1 Hoffbrand B I. Interaction of naldixic acid and warfarin. *Br Med J* (1974) **2**, 666.
2 Seller E M and Koch-Wester J. Kinetics and clinical importance of displacement of warfarin from albumin by acidic drugs. *Ann NY Acad Sci* (1971) **179**, 213.
3 Sellers E M and Koch-Weser J. Displacement of warfarin from human albumin by diazoxide and ethacrynic, mefamanic, and naldixic acids. *Clin Pharmacol Ther* (1970) **11**, 524.

Anticoagulants + naproxen

Summary
The anticoagulant response to warfarin is normally unaffected by the concurrent use of naproxen, but the remote possibility of bleeding cannot be entirely discounted. It seems likely that the response with the other oral anticoagulants will be the same.

Interaction
A study carried out on 10 healthy volunteers who were given 750 mg naproxen daily for 17 days showed that it had no significant effect on the total clearance, volume of distribution, half-life or anticoagulant activity of a single 50 mg oral dose of warfarin[1].

Similar results were found in another study.[2]

Mechanism
Although naproxen binds strongly to serum albumins[3,4] and displaces warfarin by about 13%, the effect is demonstrably too small to have a clinically important effect on prothrombin times.[1,2]

Importance and control
Although these studies show quite clearly that the anticoagulant response to warfarin is not altered by naproxen in normal doses, the manufacturers of naproxen have published the warning that '...due to the high plasma protein binding of naproxen, patients simultaneously receiving anticoagulants should be observed for signs of overdosage.'[5] It seems probable that this ultracautious statement stems from an appreciation[6] of the fact that, since there is a *statistically* significant interaction with warfarin (normally too small to matter), it is likely that in someone somewhere it may reach *clinically* significant proportions. Added to which, naproxen, like other antirheumatic agents, interferes with platelet function and prolongs bleeding times[7] so that the potential for bleeding exists and should be recognized if the two drugs are used together. It seems probable that other anticoagulants will behave similarly, but this requires confirmation.

References
1 Slattery J T, Levy G, Jain A and McMahon F G. Effect of naproxen on the kinetics of elimination and anticoagulant activity of a single dose of warfarin. *Clin Pharmacol Ther.* (1979) **25**, 51.
2 Jain A, McMahon F G, Slattery J T and Levy G. Effect of naproxen on the steady-state serum concentration and anticoagulant activity of warfarin. *Clin Pharmacol Ther* (1979) **25**, 61.
3 Mason R W and McQueen E G. Protein binding of indomethacin. Binding of indomethacin to human plasma albumin and its displacement from binding by ibuprofen, phenylbutazone and salicylate *in vitro*. *Pharmacology* (1974) **12**, 12.
4 Yacobi A and Levy G. Effect of naproxen on protein binding of warfarin in human serum. *Res Commun Chem Pathol Pharmacol* (1976) **15**, 369.
5 *Naprosyn*. Syntax Pharmaceuticals. Data Shell Compendium, p. 1016. 1979–80.
6 Segre E J. Drug interactions with naproxen. *Europ. J. Rheumatology Inflammation* (1979) **2**, 12.
7 Nadell J, Bruno J, Varady J and Segre E J. Effect of naproxen and of aspirin on bleeding time and platelet aggregation. *J Clin Pharmacol* (1974) **14**, 176.

Anticoagulants + oxyphenbutazone

Summary
The anticoagulant effects of warfarin are enhanced by oxyphenbutazone and can lead to serious bleeding. A similar interaction may be expected with other oral anticoagulants.

Interaction
A man taking warfarin who began a course of oxyphenbutazone, 400 mg, daily, developed gross haematuria within 9 days and was found to have a prothrombin time of 68 s. A subsequent experiment on him demonstrated quite clearly the marked effect of oxyphenbutazone on the hypoprothrombinaemia due to warfarin.[3]

Two other similar cases have been described.[1,2]

Mechanism

Oxyphenbutazone is the major metabolite of phenylbutazone in the body so that it may be presumed that the general explanation of the anticoagulant/phenylbutazone interaction equally applies to oxyphenbutazone (see p. 164). A clinical investigation with dicoumarol showed that oxyphenbutazone slowed the elimination of the anticoagulant in some subjects, associated with an increased anticoagulant response,[4] so that as with phenylbutazone, a straightforward drug-displacement mechanism is almost certainly not the whole story.

Importance and management

Although there appear to be very few reports of an adverse interaction between oxyphenbutazone and an oral anticoagulant, and all of them involving warfarin, it would be prudent to apply all the precautions described on page 164 to oxyphenbutazone because it is the major metabolic product of phenylbutazone in the body and may be expected to interact in a very similar manner.

References

1 Hobbs C B, Miller A L and Thornley J H. Potentiation of anticoagulant therapy by oxyphenulbutazone. A probable case. *Postgrad Med J* (1965) **41**, 563.
2 Fox S L. Potentiation of anticoagulants caused by pyrazole compounds. *J Amer Med Ass* (1964) **188**, 320.
3 Taylor P J. Haemorrhage while on anticoagulant therapy precipitated by drug interaction. *Arizona Med* (1967) **24**, 697.
4 Weiner M, Siddiqui A A, Bostanci N, and Dayton P G. Drug interactions: the effect of combined administration on the half-life of coumarin and pyrazolone drugs in man. *Fed Proc* (1965) **24**, 153.

Anticoagulants + paracetamol (acetaminophen)

Summary

The anticoagulant effects of warfarin, dicoumarol, anisindione and phenprocoumon are very slightly enhanced by therapeutic doses of paracetamol (acetaminophen). The interaction is of no practical importance.

Interaction

A study[1] on 37 patients taking warfarin, dicoumarol, anisindione or phenprocoumon showed that a daily dose of 2·6 g paracetamol (acetaminophen) for 2 weeks caused an average increase in the prothrombin times of 3·7 s.

A further study[2] on 10 patients maintained on warfarin or phenprocoumon showed that two 650 mg doses of paracetamol (acetaminophen) had no effect on prothrombin times.

Another study[3] on 10 patients taking warfarin and 3·25 g paracetamol (acetaminophen) showed that a small but statistically non-significant 1·2 s rise in the prothrombin time took place.

Mechanism

The mechanism of the small change in the prothrombin times appears not to have been investigated

Importance and management

This interaction is well established, and would appear to be of no practical importance. Patients on warfarin, dicoumarol, anisindione or phenprocoumon who need an analgesic substitute for aspirin may safely use paracetamol. Information about other anticoagulants is lacking but it seems probable that they will behave similarly.

References

1 Antlitz A M, Mead J A, and Tolentino M A. Potentiation of oral anticoagulant therapy by acetaminophen. *Curr Ther Res* (1968) **10**, 501.
2 Antlitz A M and Awalt L F. A double blind study of acetaminophen used in conjunction with oral anticoagulant therapy. *Curr Ther Res* (1969) **11**, 360.
3 Udall J A. Drug interference with warfarin therapy. *Clin Med* (1978) **77**, 20.

Anticoagulants + phenazone (antipyrine)

Summary

The concurrent use of phenazone causes a marked reduction in the anticoagulant effects of warfarin. Other anticoagulants are probably similarly affected.

Interaction

The anticoagulant effects of warfarin are reduced by the concurrent use of phenazone.

A study on 5 patients, anticoagulated with warfarin, showed that concurrent treatment over 50 days with 600 mg phenazone daily caused a significant reduction in the plasma warfarin levels and prothrombin times of all 5. The mean plasma warfarin concentration was halved (from 2·93 to 1·41 $\mu g/ml$) between the beginning and the last 14 days of concurrent treatment. One patient illustrated in the study showed a change in the prothrombin percentage during the period from 5 to 50%. In an associated study, pretreatment for 30 days with 600 mg phenazone daily caused a fall in the warfarin half lives of 2 patients from 47 to 27 h, and from 69 to 39 h.[1-3]

Mechanism

A wealth of evidence (fall in steady-state plasma warfarin levels and an increase in the urinary excretion of 6-beta hydrocortisol in man) indi-

cates that phenazone is a potent inducer of the liver microsomal enzymes. This results in the increased metabolism and clearance of the warfarin from the body, and a fall in its anticoagulant effects.[1-3]

Importance and management

A reduction in the anticoagulant effects of warfarin may be expected if phenazone is administered concurrently. A similar effect seems possible with other anticoagulants.

References

1 Breckenridge A and Orme M. Clinical implication of enzyme induction. *Ann NY Acad Sci* (1971) **179** 421.
2 Breckenridge A, Orme M L'E, Thorgeirsson S, Davies D S and Brooks R V. Drug interactions with warfarin: studies with dichloralphenazone, chloral hydrate and phenazone (Antipyrine). *Clin Sci* (1971) **40**, 351.
3 Breckenridge A, Orme M L'E, Thorgeirsson S and Dollery C T. Induction of drug metabolising enzymes in man and rat by dichloralphenazone. *4th Int Cong Pharmacol* (Basel), p. 182. July 14–18, 1969.

Anticoagulants + phenothiazines

Summary

No interaction of any importance has been reported between chlorpromazine and nicoumalone or any other anticoagulant and a phenothiazine.

Interaction, mechanism, importance and management

Although chlorpromazine in doses of 40–100 mg is said to have '. . . played a slightly sensitizing role. . .' in 2 out of 8 patients on nicoumalone[1] and is reported to enhance the anticoagulant response of this anticoagulant in animals[2], there

is nothing to suggest that special care is necessary during concurrent therapy in man.

References

1 Johnson R, David A and Chartier Y. Clinical experience with G-23350 (Sintrom). *Can Med Ass J* (1957) **77**, 760.
2 Weiner M. Effect of centrally active drugs on the action of coumarin anticoagulants. *Nature* (1966) **212**, 1599.

Anticoagulants + phenylbutazone

Summary

The anticoagulant effects of warfarin, phenprocoumon, nicoumalone (acenocoumarol) and probably most of the other oral anticoagulants can be markedly enhanced by the concurrent use of phenylbutazone. Serious bleeding can occur. Successful concurrent use has been achieved by careful dosage adjustment with some anticoagulants.

Interaction

The effects of most of the oral anticoagulants are

markedly increased by the concurrent use of phenylbutazone and can quickly lead to serious bleeding. This interaction was first described in 1956[1] and has been observed and thoroughly investigated on many occasions since. Two brief case histories involving warfarin as illustrations:

Phenylbutazone added to a stabilized anticoagulant regimen

A man anticoagulated with warfarin, following mitral valve replacement, was subsequently given phenylbutazone by his general practitioner for back pain. On admission to hospital about a week later he had epistaxis, and his face, legs, and arms had begun to swell. He showed extensive bruising of the jaw, elbow and calves, some evidence of gastrointestinal bleeding, and a prothrombin time of 89 s.[2]

Anticoagulant added to treatment with phenylbuta-zone.

A man, hospitalized for myocardial infarction, was given during the course of his treatment a single 600 mg dose of phenylbutazone. Next day, when coagulation studies were carried out, his prothrombin time was 12 s and he was given 40 mg warfarin to initiate anticoagulant therapy. Within 48 h he developed massive gastrointestinal bleeding and was found to have a prothrombin time exceeding 100 s.[3]

There are other reports of this interaction in man involving warfarin,[4-11] phenprocoumon[1] and nicoumalone.[16] There is also a single unconfirmed report of this interaction in 2 patients taking phenindione.[14]

Mechanism

By no means fully understood. The orthodox, and often-repeated explanation, is that it takes place because both phenylbutazone and the anticoagulants are extremely highly bound to plasma proteins and compete for the same binding sites. Displacement has been well demonstrated by in-vitro experiments[4,9,13,17,18]. The 'classic' illustration of this is shown in Fig. 1.3 on page 6. The phenylbutazone displaces large numbers of the free and active anticoagulant molecules into plasma water and this results in an increased hypoprothrombinaemic response by the liver. However, more recent work on warfarin suggests that this explanation on its own is far too simplistic and that the total picture is much more complex.[10,12]

Clinically available warfarin is a racemate, that is to say a mixture of two isomers, R(+) warfarin and S(−) warfarin which do not behave identically. Not only is S warfarin five times more potent that R warfarin, but it has been shown[12] that phenylbutazone inhibits the metabolism of each in man differently, and there is some evidence to suggest that the overall interaction may

also be explained by the inhibition of S warfarin which favours it accumulation. But what part some of the metabolites of phenylbutazone might have in inhibiting or displacing warfarin within an interplay of several different factors is not known.

Importance and management

Because the effects of this interaction can be so serious, a 'blanket' warning advising the use of other non-interacting antirheumatics (e.g. ibuprofen, page 152) instead of phenylbutazone is a wise precaution but a total prohibition with each and every anticoagulant may not always be necessary.

Warfarin + phenylbutazone

An extremely well-documented and serious interaction.[2-11] Haemorrhage can occur rapidly whichever drug is given first, and the evidence indicates that it will affect most if not all patients.[5] Concurrent use should be avoided.

Phenprocoumon + phenylbutazone

Direct evidence of a serious interaction seems to be limited to one report,[1] the first. In contrast there is another[19] in which both drugs were used together in the prophylactic treatment of thromboembolism apparently uneventfully, presumably because the response and the dosage were carefully monitored and controlled.

Nicoumalone (acenocoumarol) + phenylbutazone

In a study on the prophylactic treatment of post-operative thromboembolism, 357 patients were given 600 mg phenylbutazone daily from the operation day, to which was added nicoumalone from day 5 onwards. The anticoagulant dosage was found to about 25% less than that required by a control group on nicoumalone alone,[16] so it is clear that with appropriate precautions these two can be used together.

Other Anticoagulants + phenylbutazone

In-vitro experiments with dicoumarol show that it binds to the same albumin binding sites as warfarin and can be displaced by phenylbutazone.[13] Phenindione and fluorophenindione do not bind to the same sites as phenylbutazone and are not displaced by it[13] but despite this, an early report implicated phenindione in a bleeding interaction in 2 patients.[14] It would seem wise to avoid the use of any of these anticoagulants. There appears to be no other evidence, direct or indirect, about any of the other anticoagulants.

References

1 Sigg A, Pestalozzi H, Clauss A and Koller F. Verstärkung der Antikaogulantienwirkung durch Butazolidin. *Schweiz med Woch* (1956) **86**, 1194.
2 Bull J and Mackinnon J. Phenylbutazone and anticoagulant control. *Practitioner* (1975) **215**, 767.
3 Robinson D S. The application of basic principles of drug interaction to clinical practice. *J Urology* (1975) **113**, 100.
4 Aggeler P M, O'Reilly R A, Leong L and Kowitz P E. Potentiation of anticoagulant effect of warfarin by phenylbutazone. *New Eng J Med* (1967) **276**, 196.
5 Udall J A. Drug interference with warfarin therapy. *Clin Med* (1970) **77**, 20.
6 McLaughlin G E, McCarty D J, and Segal B L. Hemarthrosis complicating anticoagulant therapy: report of three cases. *J Amer med Ass* (1966) **196**, 202.
7 Hoffbrand B I and Kininmonth D A. Potentiation of anticoagulants. *Brit Med J* (1967) **2**, 838.
8 Eisen M J. Combined effect of sodium warfarin and phenylbutazone. *J Amer Med Ass* (1964) **189**, 64.
9 O'Reilly R A. The binding of sodium warfarin to plasma albumin and its displacement by phenylbutazone. *Ann NY Acad Sci* (1973) **226**, 293.
10 Schary W L, Lewis R J and Rowland M. Warfarin–phenylbutazone interaction in man. A long-term multiple-dose study. *Res Comm Chem Pathol Pharmacol* (1975) **10**, 663.
11 Chierichetti S, Bianchi G and Cerri B. Comparison of feprazone and phenylbutazone interaction with warfarin in man. *Curr Ther Res* (1975) **18**, 568.
12 Lewis R J, Trager W F, Chan K K, Breckenridge A, Orme M, Rowland M and Schary W. Warfarin. Stereochemical aspects of its metabolism and the interaction with phenylbutazone. *J Clin Invest* (1974) **53**, 1607.
13 Tillement J-P, Zini R, Mattei C and Singlas E. Effect of phenylbutazone on the binding of vitamin K antagonists to albumin. *Europ J clin Pharmacol* (1973) **6**, 15.
14 Kindermann A. Vasculäres Allergid nach Butalidon und Gefahren Kombinierter Anwendung mit Athrombon (Phenylindandion). *Dermatol Wochenschr.* (1961) **143**, 172.
15 Seiler K and Duckert F. Properties of 3-(1-phenyl-propyl)-4-oxycoumarin (marcoumar) in the plasma when tested in normal cases under the influence of drugs. *Thromb Diath Haemorrh* (1968) **19**, 89.
16 Guggisberg W and Montigel C. Erfahrungen mit kombinierter Butazolidin–Sintrom—Prophylaxe und Butazolidin—prophylaxe thromboembolischer Erkrankungen. *Ther Umsch* (1958) **15**, 227.
17 Solomon H M and Schrogie J J. The effect of various drugs on the binding of warfarin-^{14}C to human albumin. *Biochem Pharmacol* (1967) **16**, 1219.
18 O'Reilly R A. Interaction of several coumarin compounds with human and canine plasma albumin. *Mol Pharmacol* (1970) **7**, 209.
19 Kaufmann P. Vergleich zwischen einer Thromboembolieprophylaxe mit Antikoagulantien und mit Butazolidin. *Schweiz Med Wochenschr* (1957) (*Suppl* 24) **87**, 755.

Anticoagulants + phenyramidol

Summary

The anticoagulant effects of warfarin, dicoumarol and phenindione may be enhanced by the concurrent use of phenyramidol. Bleeding has occurred. Other anticoagulants may be expected to interact similarly.

Interaction

The observation that 2 patients on warfarin showed a marked prolongation of their prothrombin times (one of them bled) when also given phenyramidol (400 mg three or four times a day), prompted the investigation of this interaction in 9 other patients on warfarin, dicoumarol, phenprocoumon or phenindione who were given 800–1600 mg phenyramidol daily. All of them (with the exception of the patient on phenprocoumon who only received the phenyramidiol for 3 days), showed a marked prolongation of their prothrombin times which because apparent in some cases within 3 days, and was well manifested in most of them by the end of a week.[1]

Mechanism

A study of this interaction in man (and observed in mice and rabbits) showed that in the presence of phenyramidol the half-life of dicoumarol was prolonged from 21 to 46 h, and the coagulation activity, 60 h, after taking a single 150 mg dose of the anticoagulant, was reduced from 96 to 45%. From this it is concluded that the phenyramidol inhibits the hepatic metabolism of the anticoagulant, thereby prolonging its stay in the body and its activity.[2]

Importance and management

There appear to be only two studies on this interaction,[1,2] but the evidence is strong. A reduction in the anticoagulant dosage is necessary if excessive hypoprothrombinaemia and bleeding are to be avoided. Only warfarin, dicoumarol and phenindione are definitely implicated, but it may beexpected to occur with any of the other anticoagulants including phenprocoumon. Failure to demonstrate an interaction with phenprocoumon[1] may have been because the phenyramidol was given for such a short time.

References

1 Carter S A. Potentiation of the effect of orally administered anticoagulants by phenyramidol hydrochloride. *New Eng J Med* (1965) **273**, 423.
2 Solomon H M and Schrogie J J. The effect of phenyramidol on the metabolism of bisphydroxycoumarin. *J Pharmacol Exp Therap* (1966) **154**, 660.

Anticoagulants + prolintane

Summary

The anticoagulant effects of ethyl biscoumacetate are not affected by the concurrent use of prolintane. Information about other anticoagulants is lacking.

Interaction

The responses to single 20 mg/kg doses of ethyl biscoumacetate were examined on 12 subjects before and after 4 days' treatment with prolintane, 20 mg daily. The prothrombin times and the mean half-lives of the anticoagulant 1 day before and 1 and 8 days after prolintane treatment were 16·5, 17·0 and 16·8 s, and 2·67, 2·67 and 2·67 h respectively.[1]

Mechanism

None.

Importance and management

The data are extremely limited but it indicates that an interaction is unlikely to occur between ethyl biscoumacetate and prolintane. There appear to be no data about other anticoagulants.

References

1 Hague D E, Smith M E, Ryan J R and McMahon F G. The interaction of methylphenidate and prolintane with ethylbiscoumacetate metabolism. *Fed Proc* (1971) **30**, 336 (*Abs*).

Anticoagulants + psyllium

Summary

Psyllium colloid does not affect the absorption or the anticoagulant effects of warfarin. There is no evidence about the other anticoagulants.

Interaction

A study on 6 subjects showed that when psyllium in the form of a colloid (*Metamucil*, Searle) in a small amount of water was given in four 14 g doses, the first administered with a single 40 mg oral dose of warfarin, and the other three doses at 2 h intervals, the plasma warfarin concentrations over the next 48 h and the mean prothrombin times were not significantly affected.[1]

Mechanism

None

Importance and management

No particular precautions appear to be necessary if warfarin and psyllium are given concurrently. Whether other oral anticoagulants behave similarly is not documented.

Reference

1 Robinson D S, Benjamin D M and McCormack J J. Interaction of warfarin and nonsystemic gastrointestinal drugs. *Clin Pharmacol Ther* (1971) **12**, 491.

Anticoagulants + quinidine

Summary

The anticoagulant effects of warfarin can be enhanced in some but not all patients by the concurrent use of quinidine. Bleeding has been described.

Interaction

The first suggestion that quinidine had hypo-prothrombinaemic actions was made in 1945.[1] An association between the development of bleeding in patients on anticoagulants and quinidine was again suggested in 1955, but no details were given.[2]

> Three patients[3] stabilized on warfarin with prothrombin levels within the range 18–25% began to haemorrhage within 7–10 days of starting to take 800–1400 mg quinidine daily and were found by then to have prothrombin levels of 6–8%. Bleeding ceased when the warfarin was withdrawn.

Another report describes a patient who was difficult to stabilize on warfarin while taking 600 mg quinidine daily.[4] In contrast:

> Ten patients on long-term anticoagulant treatment with warfarin (2·5–12·5 mg daily) showed no significant alteration in their prothrombin times when they were given 800 mg quinidine daily for 2 weeks.[5–7]

Mechanism
The most likely, but as yet unconfirmed, explanation of this interaction is that quinidine, like quinine (see Anticoagulants + quinine, below) has a direct action of its own on the liver and depresses the synthesis of vitamin K-dependent blood clotting factors. One of the 3 patients already described[2] was found to have a prothrombin level of 45% in the absence of warfarin while taking 1200 mg quinidine daily, and the prothrombin level only returned to normal when the quinidine was withdrawn 3 months later. Another patient had a prothrombin level of 50% on daily therapy with 800–1400 mg quinidine, 500 mg gitalin and 300 mg phenytoin but no warfarin. None of the 3 patients in this report[3] showed any deterioration of hepatic function which might be an alternative explanation for what was seen. So the hypoprothrombinaemic actions of quinidine, added to those of warfarin, would account for the markedly reduced prothrombin levels and the bleeding which took place, but just why it should only occur in a few, but not all patients, is not clear.

Importance and management
Since the enhancement of the actions of warfarin occurs in some[2–4] but not all[5–7] patients it would be prudent to monitor the effects of quinidine on prothrombin times carefully, if it is used concurrently, to avoid the possibility of excessive hypoprothrombinaemia and bleeding. Whether this interaction can also take place with other anticoagulants is not known, but it seems not unlikely. An alternative antiarrhythmic agent which appears not to interact with the oral anticoagulants is procainamide.

References
1 Pirk L A and Engelberg R. Hypoprothrombinaemic action of quinine sulfate. *J Am Med Ass* (1945) **128**, 1093.
2 Beaumont J L and Tarrit A. Les accidents haemorrhagiques survenus au cours de 1500 traitments anticoagulants. *Sang* (1955) **26**, 680.
3 Gazzaniga A B, and Stewart D R. Possible quinidine-induced haemorrhage in a patient on warfarin sodium. *New Eng J Med* (1969) **280**, 711.
4 Koch-Weser J. Quinidine-induced hypoprothrombinaemic haemorrhage in patients on chronic warfarin therapy. *Ann Int Med* (1968) **68**, 511.
5 Udall J. Quinidine and hypoprothrombinaemia. *Ann Int Med* (1968) **69**, 403.
6 Udall J. Drug interference with warfarin therapy. *Am J Cardiol* (1969) **23**, 143.
7 Udall J. Drug interference with warfarin therapy. *Clin Med* (1970) **77**, 20.

Anticoagulants + quinine

Summary
In normal doses quinine may cause a very small and probably clinically unimportant enhancement of the effects of the oral anticoagulants.

Interaction
A study[1] undertaken with 5 normal subjects who were given 0·33 g quinine sulphate by mouth (no anticoagulant) for periods of 6–16 days showed that their prothrombin times were increased by 5–11·8 s. When another study[2] failed to confirm these results, the authors of the first study repeated their experiments on another 5 normal subjects, but this time using two different methods of measuring the prothrombin times. Firstly they employed the Page method,[4] originally used in their first study, which entails the use of Russell viper venom as the thromboplastic agent and they found that the prothrombin times were extended by quinine by 9·9–12·6 s. Then using the Quick method (which Quick himself had used when he

failed to demonstrate the interaction and which employs a tissue extract as the thromboplastin) they found that the prothrombin times of their subjects were only extended by 0–2·1 s.

Mechanism
In the studies described[1,3] the extension of the prothrombin times could be completely reversed by the concurrent ingestion of 10 mg vitamin K (menadiol sodium diphosphate) suggesting that quinine is, like the oral anticoagulants, a competitive antagonist of vitamin K within the liver. Moreover, both the increase in prothrombin times due to quinine, and their decrease in response to withdrawal or reversal by vitamin K, was not immediate but took place over several days. This would be consistent with a pharmacological action involving changes in the synthesis by the liver of the blood clotting factors.

Importance and management
It would seem possible for quinine to enhance the effects of the oral anticoagulants, but the extent is very small and almost certainly clinically unimportant, although direct confirmation of this in the literature appears to be lacking. More study is required.

References
1 Pirk L A and Engelberg R. Hypoprothrombinemic action of quinine sulfate. *J Am Med Ass* (1945) **128**, 1093.
2 Quick A J. Effect of synthetic vitamin K and quinine sulphate on the prothrombin level. *J Lab Clin Med* (1946) **31**, 79.
3 Pirk L A and Engelberg R. Hypoprothrombinaemic action of quinine sulfate. *Am J Med Sci* (1947) **213**, 593.
4 Page R C, de Beer E J and Orr M L. Prothrombin studies using Russell viper venom: relation of clotting time to prothrombin concentration in human plasma. *J Lab Clin Med* (1941) **27**, 197.
5 Mandel E H. The anticoagulant properties of chloroquine dihydrochloride (*Aralen*), hydroxychloroquine sulfate (*Plaquenil*) and quinine dihydiochloride. *J Mt Sinai Hosp* (1962) **29**, 71.

Anticoagulants + rifampicin

Summary
The anticoagulant effects of nicoumalone (acenocoumarol), phenprocoumon and warfarin are markedly reduced by concurrent treatment with rifampicin. Information about other anticoagulants is lacking.

Interaction
A study on 18 patients anticoagulated with nicoumalone (acenocoumarol) showed that when they were also treated with rifampicin (450 mg twice a day) for 7 days the dosage of the anticoagulant had to be increased to maintain the Quick value within the therapeutic range.[1]

There are a number of other reports and studies of this interaction in man involving nicoumalone,[6] warfarin[2–5] and phenprocoumon.[7]

Mechanism
Not absolutely certainly established, but studies in man[3,4] indicate that rifampicin may act as a liver enzyme-inducing agent which accelerates the rate of metabolism and clearance from the body of the anticoagulants, thereby reducing their effects. Concurrent use of rifampicin was found in one study to reduce the serum warfarin levels and the prothrombin response by about 50%.[3]

Importance and management
A well-documented interaction and clinically important. A marked reduction in the response to nicoumalone, phenprocoumon and warfarin may be expected about 5–7 days after concurrent treatment begins,[1,2] persisting for about the same length of time after withdrawal of the rifampicin. With warfarin there is evidence[2] that the dosage may need to be approximately doubled, to accommodate the interaction, and reduced by an equivalent amount if the rifampicin is withdrawn. A similar interaction may be expected with other anticoagulants but this awaits confirmation.

References
1 Michot F, Bürgi M and Büttner J. Rimactan (Rifampizin) und Antikoagulantientherapie. *Schweiz med Wschr* (1970) **100**, 583.
2 Romankiewicz J A and Erhman M. Rifampin and warfarin: A drug interaction. *Ann Int Med* (1975) **82**. 224.
3 O'Reilly R A. Interaction of sodium warfarin and rifampin. *Ann Int Med* (1974) **81**, 337.
4 O'Reilly R A. Interaction of rifampicin in man. *Clin Res* (1973) **21**, 207.
5 Self T H and Mann R B. Interaction of rifampicin and warfarin. *Chest* (1975) **67**, 490.
6 Sennwald G. Etude de l'influence de la rifampicine sur l'effet anticoagulant de l'acenocoumarol *Rev medicale Suisse Romande* (1974) **94**, 945.
7 Boekhout-Mussert R J, Bieger R, van Brummelen A and Lemkes H H D. Inhibition by rifampicin of the anticoagulant effect of phenprocoumon. *J Amer Med Ass* (1974) **229**, 1903.

Anticoagulants + *Rowachol*

Summary
The suggestion that *Rowachol* may effect the response to oral anticoagulants has yet to be confirmed.

Interaction, mechanism, importance and management
Rowachol is an orally administered agent used for the treatment of gallstones and contains six cyclical plant monoterpenes (menthol, menthone, pinene, borneal, camphene, cineol and olive oil). Since a number of the cyclic monoterpenes are known potent liver enzyme-inducing agents,[1,2] there is the possibility that the response to concurrent anticoagulant treatment may be reduced. Whether this theoretical problem will prove to be of practical importance awaits confirmation.

References
1 Parke D V and Rahman H. The effects of some terpenoids and other dietary nutrients on hepatic drug-metabolizing enzymes. *Biochem J* (1969) **113**, 12.
2 Jori A, Bianchetti A and Prestini P E. Effect of essential oils on drug metabolism. *Biochem Pharmacol* (1969) **18**, 2081.

Anticoagulants + salicylates

Summary
Aspirin in doses as low as 2 g daily can enhance the effects of oral anticoagulants. These low doses can also damage the stomach wall, induce blood loss and prolong bleeding times. For these reasons anticoagulated patients should avoid the use of aspirin. Paracetamol (acetaminophen) is a safer analgesic substitute.

Interaction
A study was carried out on 17 patients anticoagulated with nicoumalone and receiving an average of 3·1 mg daily. During an experimental period of a week while also taking 2·4 g aspirin daily the anticoagulant requirements of 11 of them fell to 2·2 mg daily (an average reduction of 30%). The other 6 required dosage changes of less than 0·5 mg daily and these were regarded as insignificant.[1]

An investigation was undertaken on 11 normal subjects during the long-term administration of warfarin (9 patients) or dicoumarol (2 patients). While concurrently taking 1·96 g aspirin daily, 4 of them showed a significant reduction in their one-stage prothrombin activity but no haemorrhagic signs, whereas 2 of the others who had had no significant reduction in prothrombin activity demonstrated mild haemorrhagic signs. Four other subjects on warfarin given 3·9 g aspirin daily all showed both a reduction in prothrombin activity and of mild haemorrhage. It was also demonstrated in 6 individuals that 1·95 g aspirin daily increased their bleeding times from 4·0 min to 10·3 min.[2]

Similar results to those cited[2] have been described by one of the same authors in another report.[3]

One investigator was unable to show changes in the prothrombin times of patients on warfarin concurrently treated with 3 g aspirin daily,[4] but others confirm the considerable prolongation in the bleeding times.[8,9]

Mechanism
It has been known for almost 40 years that aspirin on its own has hypoprothrombinaemic effects. Five to six grams daily can prolong the prothrombin times by up to twice their normal values, although there is considerable variation between individuals.[5–7] These effects can be reversed by the administration of vitamin K, from which it is concluded that aspirin acts like the oral anticoagulants as a vitamin K antagonist. The effects of aspirin with the oral anticoagulants in prolonging prothrombin times would seem to be due to simple addition of the effects.

The prolongation of the cutaneous bleeding times by aspirin is complex, but it is associated with an aspirin-induced interference with platelet aggregation.[2]

Importance and management

An established interaction, although the available data is not extensive and is largely confined to warfarin, diocoumarol and nicoumalone (aceno-coumarol). Generally speaking concurrent use should be avoided: (a) because an enhancement of the anticoagulant effects can occur in some patients, even with daily doses of aspirin of 2 g or less, and with larger doses the hypoprothrombinaemia is even further increased; (b) of equal or greater importance is the fact that aspirin damages the stomach lining, induces blood loss and considerably extends the bleeding time. There is no clear evidence to show whether the occasional use of single small doses of aspirin is important or not. Paracetamol (acetaminophen) appears to be a safer analgesic substitute (see p 162).

Patients taking anticoagulants should be warned that a considerable number of proprietary analgesic and antipyretic compounds contain aspirin, and they should seek informed advice before using them. Information about other sali- cylates is sparse but salicylamide is reported to have little effect on prothrombin times.[5]

References

1 Watson R M and Pierson N J. Effect of anticoagulant therapy upon aspirin-induced gastrointestinal bleeding. *Circulation* (1961) **24**, 613.
2 O'Reilly R A. Sahud M A and Aggeler P M. Impact of aspirin and chlorthalidone on the pharmacodynamics of oral anticoagulant drugs in man. *Ann N Y Acad Sci* (1971) **179**, 173.
3 O'Reilly R A and Aggeler P M. Determinants of the response to oral anticoagulants drugs in man. *Pharmacol Rev* (1970) **22**, 35.
4 Udall J A. Drug interference with warfarin therapy. *Am J Cardiol* (1969) **23**, 143.
5 Shapiro S. Studies on prothrombin. VI. The effect of synthetic vitamin K on the prothrombinopenia induced by salicylate in man. *J Amer Med Ass* (1944), **125**, 546.
6 Quick A J and Clesceri L. Influence of acetylsalicylic acid and salicylamide on the coagulation of the blood. *J Pharmac Exp Ther* (1960) **128**, 95.
7 Meyer O O and Howard B. Production of hypoprothrombinaemia and hypocoagulability of the blood with salicylates. *J Pharmac Exp Ther* (1943) **53**, 251.
8 Gast L F. Influence of aspirin on haemostatic parameters. *Ann Rheum Dis* (1964) **23**, 500.
9 Nadell J, Bruno J, Yarady J and Segre E J. Effect of naproxen and of aspirin on bleeding time and platelet aggregation. *J Clin Pharmacol* (1974) **13**, 176.

Anticoagulants + sodium valproate

Summary

No direct evidence of an interaction, but sodium valproate has been reported to reduce plasma fibrinogen levels significantly.

Interaction, mechanism, importance and management

A report on a 16-year-old epileptic patient stated that treatment with 1200 mg sodium valproate daily for 2 months caused a fall in plasma fibrinogen levels from 2·1 g/l to 1·4 g/l and a week later to 1·25 g/l. Normal levels returned when the valproate was withdrawn.[1] Thrombocytopenia, reduced platelet adhesiveness and a prolongation of bleeding time have also been described in children.[1] Whether or not sodium valproate can affect the response of patients to anticoagulants is uncertain, but it would seem prudent to check that no adverse response is occurring during concurrent treatment.

Reference

1 Dale B M. Purdie G H and Rischbieth R H. Fibrinogen depletion with sodium valproate. *Lancet* (1978) i, 1316.

Anticoagulants + spironolactone

Summary

The anticoagulant effects of warfarin can be reduced by the use of spironolactone.

Interaction

A study undertaken with 9 normal subjects who were given single 1·5 mg/kg oral doses of warfarin showed that the concurrent use of 200 mg spironolactone reduced the prothrombin time (expressed as a percentage of the control activity with warfarin alone) from 100% to 76%. The plasma warfarin concentration was unchanged, but the venous haematocrit was increased.[1]

Mechanism
The conclusion drawn from the results of the study was that the spironolactone-induced diuresis concentrated the blood clotting factors, thereby decreasing the anticoagulant effects of the warfarin.[1]

Importance and management
An established interaction, although information appears to be limited to this single report. The extent to which the use of spironolactone affects the anticoagulant control with warfarin in patients during long-term treatment is uncertain, but a reduction in the hypoprothrombinaemia should be expected, and suitable dosage adjustments made. Information about other anticoagulants is lacking, but if the suggested mechanism of interaction is correct, they are likely to be similarly affected.

Reference
1 O'Reilly R A. Spironolactone and warfarin interaction. *Clin Pharmacol Ther* (1980) **27**, 198.

Anticoagulants + sulindac

Summary
Four patients have been described who showed a marked enhancement of the anticoagulant effects of warfarin when concurrently treated with sulindac.

Interaction
A patient taking ferrous sulphate, phenobarbitone, sulphasalazine and on long-term warfarin treatment (6 mg/day) showed a marked prolongation of his prothrombin time more than three times the control value within 5 days of taking 100 mg sulindac twice a day. Both warfarin and sulindac were withdrawn and the patient restabilized a week later on a slightly lower warfarin dosage.[1,2,5]

A man well stabilized on warfarin for 7 years showed a rise in his prothrombin time from 20·3 to 26 s after taking 200 mg sulindac twice a day for 3 weeks. Over the next few weeks his daily warfarin dosage was progressively stepped down from 7·5 mg to less than 5 mg and eventually his prothrombin time restabilized in the presence of the sulindac.[3]

A woman stabilized on 2 mg warfarin daily who took only three 100 mg doses of sulindac passed bright red blood per rectum 4 days later. Her prothrombin times were found to have risen from twice the control value to 4·6 times the control value.

Another case in a man with a renal tubular defect has also been described.[5]

Mechanism
Not understood

Importance and management
Since there are now 4 cases of this interaction on record, the possibility of this interaction should be borne in mind if sulindac is given. The incidence is uncertain, but it seems unlikely to affect every patient because investigations in healthy subjects taking warfarin and sulindac failed to demonstrate this interaction.[5,6] The manufacturers of sulindac advise that while it has a smaller effect on platelet function and bleeding time than aspirin, it is a weak inhibitor of platelet function and patients who may be adversely affected should be observed carefully.[4] It is noteworthy that the second of the 2 patients[3] was restabilized on two-thirds of the dosage of warfarin while taking 400 mg sulindac daily. The first and the third patients had much more extreme reactions[3] which serves to emphasize the variability of the response. Whether sulindac interacts with other anticoagulants is as yet uncertain.

References
1 Beeley L (ed) Bulletin of the West Midlands Adverse Reaction Group University of Birmingham, England. (1978) No 6.
2 Beeley L and Baker S. Personal communication (1978).
3 Carter S A. Potential effect of sulindac response of prothrombin-time to oral anticoagulants. *Lancet* (1979) **ii**, 698.
4 Clinoral (Merck, Sharp and Dohme Ltd). *ABPI Data Sheet Compendium* (1979–80), p. 615.
5 Ross J R Y and Beeley L. Sulindac, prothrombin time and anticoagulants. *Lancet* (1979) **ii**, 1075.
6 Loftin J P and Vesell E S. Interaction between sulindac and warfarin: different results in normal subjects and in an unusual patient with a potassium-losing renal tubular defect. *J Clin Pharmacol* (1979) **11–12**, 733.

Anticoagulants + suloctidil, fenbufen or zomepirac

Summary

Suloctidil has been shown not to interact significantly with phenprocoumon, nor fenbufen or zomepirac with warfarin.

Interaction, mechanism, importance and management

Clinical studies with 8 patients on phenprocoumon taking 300 mg suloctidil three times a day,[1] with 16 subjects on warfarin taking 400 mg fenbufen twice a day[2] and with 16 subjects on warfarin taking 150 mg zomepirac four times a day[3] showed no clinically significant changes in the response to these anticoagulants. Information about other anticoagulants is lacking.

References

1 Verhaeghe R and Vanhoof A. The concomitant use of suloctidil and a long-acting oral anticoagulant. *Acta Clin Belg* (1977) **32**, 1.

2 Savitsky J P, Terzakis T, Bina P, Chiccarelli F and Haynes J. Fenbufen–warfarin interaction in healthy volunteers. *Clin Pharmacol Ther* (1980) **27**, 284.

3 Minn F L and Zinny M A. Zomepirac and warfarin: a clinical study to determine if interaction exists. *J Clin Pharmacol* (1980) **12–13**, 418.

Anticoagulants + sulphinpyrazone

Summary

The anticoagulant effects of warfarin, and possibly other anticoagulants, may be enhanced by the concurrent use of sulphinpyrazone, leading to bleeding. The dosage of the anticoagulant should be reduced appropriately.

Interaction

A patient maintained on 45 mg warfarin a week for 3 years, with stable prothrombin times ranging between 24 and 28 s, showed mild gum bleeding and a prothrombin time of 58 s within 10 days of taking 400 mg sulphinpyrazone daily. When the warfarin dosage was reduced to 30 mg a week, the prothrombin times returned to the therapeutic range.[1]

Severe gastrointestinal haemorrhage in a patient on warfarin has been attributed to the concurrent use of sulphinpyrazone.[2] In another report the maintenance dose of warfarin is said to have been approximately halved in patients taking 600 mg sulphinpyrazone daily.[3] Enhancement of the actions of warfarin have also been described in yet another case report.[6]

Mechanism

At least some of the increase in the effects of warfarin by sulphinpyrazone may be due to a plasma protein binding interaction. In-vitro experiments[3,4] have shown that the addition of 30 μmol of sulphinpyrazone to dilute human serum containing 1·66 μg/ml phenprocoumon increased the proportion of non-bound anticoagulant molecules (which would be biologically active if in circulation) from 1 to 17%. But the total explanation may prove to be as complex as that with phenylbutazone with which sulphinpyrazone has a close chemical relationship (see p. 164).

Importance and management

Although the direct documentary evidence for this interaction is relatively sparse, it is clearly an interaction of clinical importance. If sulphinpyrazone is given to patients on an established warfarin regimen the prothrombin times should be carefully monitored and a suitable reduction made to the warfarin dosage. A 50% reduction has been mentioned in one of the reports cited[3], and in another a two-thirds dosage of warfarin re-established stable prothrombin times.[1] It has been asserted[2] that because the monitoring and precise dosage adjustments are difficult to implement, the use of sulphinpyrazone in patients on anticoagulants who are not hospitalized is contraindicated.

It is not known whether the same interaction takes place with anticoagulants other than warfarin, but it would clearly be prudent to monitor prothrombin times extremely carefully if sulphinpyrazone is given.

References

1 Weiss M. Potentiation of coumarin effect by sulphinpyrazone. *Lancet* (1979) **i**, 609.

2 Mattingley D, Bradley M. and Selley P J. Hazards of sulphinpyrazone. *Br Med J* (1978) **2**, 1786.
3 Tulloch J A and Marr T C K. Sulphinpyrazone and warfarin after myocardial infarction. *Br Med J* (1979) **ii**, 133.
4 Seiler K and Duckert F. Properties of 3-(1-phenyl-propyl)-4-oxycoumarin (Marcoumar) in the plasma when tested in normal cases and under the influence of drugs. *Diath Haemorrh* (1968) **19**, 389.
5 Davis J W and Johns L E. Possible interaction of sulfinpyrazone with coumarins. *New Eng J Med* (1978) **299**, 955.
6 Bailey R R and Reddy J. Potentiation of warfarin action by sulphinpyrazone. *Lancet* (1980) **i**, 254.

Anticoagulants + sulphonamides

Summary

Despite a widely held belief that sulphonamides enhance the effects of the oral anticoagulants, there is no firm clinical evidence to confirm that an interaction of general importance usually occurs.

Interaction, mechanism.

(a) Gut-sterilizing sulphonamides

Succinylsulphathiazole, phthalylsulphathiazole and others in this group can drastically reduce the flora of the intestine and thereby reduce the intestinal bacterial synthesis of vitamin K, but this has not been shown to be an essential or important source of the vitamin unless dietary amounts are exceptionally low.[1] So the vitamin K/anti-coagulant balance is unlikely to be disturbed significantly in most patients.

(b) Long-acting sulphonamides

A study on 16 patients given single oral doses of phenindione (50 mg) with 500 mg sulphaphenazole showed that the prothrombin times measured 24 h later were increased by 16·8 s compared with 10·3 s in 12 other patients who had only had phenindione.[2] These patients almost certainly had some hypoalbuminaemia. This confirms in-vitro data with phenprocoumon and sulphamethoxine[3] and warfarin with sulphaphenazole[4] that these long-acting sulphonamides can cause a significant displacement of the anticoagulants from plasma protein binding sites, but it is not confirmation that a sizable and important enhancement of the anticoagulant-induced hypoprothrombinaemia will occur during concurrent treatment with these drugs.

(c) Short-acting sulphonamides

An isolated case has been described of a man taking digitalis, diuretics, antacids and warfarin who was later given a course of sulphafurazole (sulfisoxazole), 500 mg every 6 h, to treat a urinary tract infection. After 9 days his prothrombin time has risen from 20 to 28 s, and after 14 days haematuria, haemoptysis and gingival bleeding occurred. Two days later his prothrombin time was measured as 60 s.[5]

A study on 2 patients showed that the half-life of warfarin was increased from 65 to 93 h after 1 week's course of sulphamethizole, 1 g four times a day.[6]

Importance and management

Direct evidence of interactions is extremely sparse. Most of the data available come from experimental studies rather than from clinical observations in patients undergoing treatment, and is inconclusive. It would seem that concurrent administration of the oral anticoagulants and most sulphonamides need not be avoided, although it would clearly be prudent to monitor the anticoagulant response because the occasional patient may react unpredictably. In contrast, co-trimoxazole certainly interacts (see p. 137).

References

1 Udall J A. Human sources and absorption of vitamin K in relation to anticoagulation stability. *J Amer med Ass* (1965) **194**, 107.
2 Varma D R, Gupta R K, Gupta S and Sharma K K. Prothrombin response to phenindione during hypoalbuminaemia. *Br J clin Pharmac* (1975) **2**, 467.
3 Seiler K and Duckert F. Properties of 3-(1-phenyl-propyl)-4-oxycoumarin (Marcoumar) in the plasma when tested in normal cases and under the influence of drugs. *Thromb Diath Haemorrh* (1968) **19**, 89.

4 Solomon H M and Schrogie J J. The effect of various drugs on the binding of warfarin C^{14} to human albumin. *Biochem Pharmacol* (1967) **16**, 219.

5 Self T H, Evans W and Ferguson T. Interaction of sulfisoxazole and warfarin. *Circulation* (1975) **52**, 528.

6 Lumholtz B, Siersbaek-Nielsen K, Skovsted L, Kampmann J and Hansen J M. Sulfamethizole-induced inhibition of diphenylhydantoin, tolbutamide, and warfarin metabolism. *Clin Pharmacol Ther* (1976) **17**, 731.

Anticoagulants + tetracyclic antidepressants

Summary

The anticoagulant response to nicoumalone (acenocoumarol) is unaffected by concurrent treatment with maprotiline.

Interaction

A study on 20 patients anticoagulated with nicoumalone (acenocoumarol) over a 4-week period showed that concurrent treatment during weeks 2 and 3 with maprotiline (50 mg three times a day) had no effect on their anticoagulant response.[1]

Mechanism

Unknown.

Importance and management

No particular precautions appear to be necessary if nicoumalone and maprotiline are given concurrently. Nothing seems to be documented about other anticoagulants but it seems likely that they will behave similarly. This awaits confirmation.

Reference
1 Michot F, Glaus K, Jack D B and Theobald W. Antikoagulatorische Wirkung von Sintrom und Konzentration von Ludiomil in Blut bei gleichzeitiger Verabreichung beider Präparate. *Med Klin* (1975) **70**, 626.

Anticoagulants + tetracyclines

Summary

The effects of the anticoagulants are not usually altered by concurrent treatment with tetracyclines although a few isolated cases of enhancement have been described.

Interaction

Nine patients were given constant doses of an unnamed anticoagulant to maintain their PP% between 30 and 10%. When treated concurrently with chlortetracyline (250 mg four times a day) for 4 days, 6 of them showed a PP% fall to less than 6.[1]

A study on the effects of antibiotics on the response to dicoumarol describes 1 patient out of a total of 20 who bled during concurrent treatment with tetracycline. No further details are given.[2]

An enhanced effect is briefly mentioned in other reports.[7,8]

Mechanism

Unknown. There is some evidence that tetracyclines on their own can modify the factors necessary for normal blood clotting in man and reduce prothrombin activity.[3] Hypoprothrombinaemia and bleeding in the absence of anticoagulants apparently caused by tetracyline treatment have been described[4,5] but what part other factors may have played is not certain.

The idea that the tetracylines or any other broad-spectrum anti-infective agent can decimate the intestinal flora of the gut thereby depleting the body of an essential source of vitamin K has been shown to be incorrect, apart from exceptional cases where normal dietary sources of vitamin K are extremely low.[6]

Importance and management

The documentation is extremely limited. It seems unlikely that patients will normally show changes in their response to anticoagulants during concurrent treatment with tetracyclines although it should be appreciated that a few cases have been described.

References

1 Magid E. Tolerance to anticoagulants during antibiotic therapy. *Scand J clin Lab Invest* (1962) **14**, 565.
2 Chiavazza F and Merialdi A. Sulle interferenze fra dicumarolo ed antibiotci. *Minerva Ginecol* (1973) **25**, 630.
3 Searcy R L, Craig R G, Foreman J A and Bergquist L M. Blood clotting anomalies associated with intensive tetracycline therapy. *Clin Res* (1964) **12**, 230.
4 Rios J F. Haemorrhagic diathesis induced by antimicrobials. *J Amer med Ass* (1968) **205**, 142.
5 Klippel A P and Pitsinger B. Hypoprothrombinemia secondary to antibiotic therapy and manifested by massive gastrointestinal haemorrhage. *Arch Surg* (1968) **96**, 266.
6 Udall J A. Human sources and absorption of vitamin K in relation to anticoagulation stability. *J Amer med Ass* (1965) **194**, 107.
7 Wright I S. Pathogenesis and treatment of thrombosis. *Circulation* (1952) **5**, 178.
8 Scarrone L A, Beck D F and Wright I S. Tromexan and dicumarol in thromboembolism. *Circulation* (1952) **6**, 489.

Anticoagulants + thiazides

Summary

The effects of warfarin appear to be unaffected by the concurrent use of chlorothiazide. It seems probable that other thiazides and anticoagulants will similarly not interact, but this awaits confirmation.

Interaction

A randomized study on 8 normal subjects who were given single oral doses of warfarin (40–60 mg) and chlorothiazide showed that the mean half-life of the anticoagulant was increased slightly (from 38·8 to 43·9 h) but the prothrombin time was barely affected (from 18·9 to 18·6 s).[1]

Mechanism

None.

Importance and management

Although this study was on normal subjects rather than on patients requiring diuretic treatment and, moreover, with single oral doses (both of which introduce some doubt into the direct applicability of the results to the clinical situation) it seems probable that the thiazides have little or no effect on the response to warfarin. Information about other thiazides and anticoagulants is lacking, but they probably behave similarly.

Reference

1 Robinson D S and Sylwester D. Interaction of commonly prescribed drugs and warfarin. *Ann Int Med* (1970) **72**, 853.

Anticoagulants + thyroid compounds or anti-thyroid compounds

Summary

The effects of warfarin, dicoumarol, nicoumalone, phenindione and probably the other anticoagulants as well, are increased by the concurrent use of thyroid compounds. A reduction in dosage of the anticoagulant will be necessary if excessive hypoprothrombinaemia and bleeding are to be avoided. A reduction in the effects of the anticoagulants may be expected if antithyroid compounds are used, but this awaits confirmation. Propylthiouracil may paradoxically sometimes cause hypoprothrombinaemia and bleeding.

Interaction

Hypothyroidic patients are resistant to the anticoagulants whereas hyperthyroidic patients are relatively sensitive.[6,8,11] Drug-induced changes in the thyroid status will alter the response to the oral anticoagulants. Euthyroidic patients given

175

d-thyroxine as an antilipaemic agent will also show an enhanced anticoagulant response.

(a) Anticoagulants + thyroid compounds

Hypothyroidic patient given thyroxine replacement treatment:—

> A patient with myxoedema required a gradual reduction in his daily dosage of phenindione from 200 to 75 mg after normal thyroid status was restored by the administration of liothyronine. Another myxoedematous patient on nicoumalone required a reduction from 16 to 5 mg daily.[3]

Euthyroidic patients given d-thyroxine for hypercholesteremia:—

> Seven out of 11 patients anticoagulated with warfarin showed prolongations of their prothrombin times and required reductions in their warfarin dosages by 2·5 to 30 mg weekly during the first 4 weeks of concurrent treatment with 4–8 mg d-thyroxine daily. One patient bled.[1]

Similar responses have been described in other reports and studies involving warfarin,[4,12] dicoumarol[2] and acenocoumarol.[5]

(b) Anticoagulants + antithyroid compounds

See the comments under 'Importance and management' below.

Mechanism

Not completely resolved. The biological disappearance from the blood of the factors concerned with blood clotting (in particular factors II, VII, IX and X) is decreased in myxoedema and increased in thyrotoxicosis.[5] Patients stabilized on anticoagulant therapy who are subsequently given thyroxine (either as replacement therapy or to control hypercholesteraemia) require a decrease in the anticoagulant dosage because, while the anticoagulant reduces the rate of blood clotting synthesis, the thyroxine increases the rate of catabolism, resulting in a greater net reduction than with either alone.

It has also been suggested,[7,4] arising from some studies in which it was shown that the half-life and plasma concentrations of dicoumarol were unaffected by thyroxine (although its effects were increased), that the hormone increases the affinity of the anticoagulants for its receptors in the liver. It might also be because, like other antilipaemic drugs, the thyroxine lowers serum lipid levels and thereby reduces the amounts of vitamin K available to the liver.

Importance and management

A clearly documented and important interaction occurs between the anticoagulants and thyroid compounds. Hypothyroidic patients stabilized on an anticoagulant and who are given thyroxine as replacement therapy, or euthyroidic patients treated with thyroxine for hypercholesteraemia may require a downward adjustment of their anticoagulant dosage if excessive hypoprothrombinaemia and bleeding are to be avoided. Only warfarin, dicoumarol, phenindione and nicoumalone appear to have been implicated in this interaction but it may be expected to occur with the other anticoagulants.

No interaction has been documented between the anticoagulants and the antithyroid drugs such as carbimazole, propylthiouracil etc., used in the treatment of hyperthyroidism, but as the thyroid status returns to normal it would be logical to expect that normally an increase in the anticoagulant dosage would be required. However, very occasionally, propylthiouracil in the absence of an oral anticoagulant has been reported to cause hypoprothrombinaemia and bleeding[9,10] so that sometimes, paradoxically, this drug may have the effect of increasing rather than decreasing the response of patients to anticoagulants.

References

1 Owens J C, Neeley W B, and Owen W R. Effect of sodium dextrothyroxine in patients receiving anticoagulants. *New Eng J med* (1962) **266**, 76.

2 Jones R J and Cohen L. Sodium dextro-thyroxine in coronary disease and hypercholesteremia. *Circulation* (1961) **24**, 164.

3 Walters M B. The relationship between thyroid function and anticoagulant therapy. *Amer J Cardiol* (1963).

4 Solomon H M and Schrogie J J. Change in receptor site affinity: A proposed explanation for the potentiating effect of D-thyroxine on the anticoagulant response to warfarin. *Clin Pharmacol Ther* (1967) **8**, 797.

5 Loeliger E A, van der Esch B, Mattern M J and Hemker H C. The biological disappearance rate of prothrombin, factors VII, IX and X from plasma in hypothyroidism, hyperthyroidism and during fever. *Thromb Diath Haemorrh* (1964) **10**, 267.

6 Vagenakis A G. Enhancement of warfarin-induced hypoprothrombinaemia by thyrotoxicosis. *Johns Hopkins med J* (1972) **131**, 69.

7 Schrogie J J and Solomon H M. The anticoagulant response to bishydroxycoumarin. II. The effect of D-thyroxine, clofibrate and norethandrolone. *Clin Pharmacol Ther* (1967) **8**, 70.

8 Self T H, Straughn A B and Weisburst M R. Effect of hyperthyroidism on hypoprothrombinaemic response to warfarin. *Am J Hosp Pharm* (1976) **33**, 387.

9 D'Angelo G and LeGresley L. Severe hypoprothrombinaemia after propylthiouracil therapy. *Can med Ass J* (1959) **71**, 479.

10 Gotta A W, Sullivan C A, Seaman J and Jean-Giles B. Prolonged intraoperative bleeding caused by propylthiouracil-induced hypoprothrombinemia. *Anesthesiology* (1972) **37**, 562.

11 McIntosh T J. Increased sensitivity to warfarin in thyrotoxicosis. *J Clin Invest* (1970) **49**, 63A.

12 Winters W L and Soloff L A. Observations on sodium d-thyroxine as a hypercholestermic agent in persons with hypercholesteremia with and without ischemic heart disease. *Amer J med Sci* (1962) **103**, 458.

Anticoagulants + tienilic acid

Summary
The anticoagulant effects of ethyl biscoumacetate and nicoumalone (acenocoumarol) can be enhanced by the the concurrent use of tienilic acid (ticrynafen) leading to bleeding.

Interaction
Two patients anticoagulated with ethyl biscoumacetate developed spontaneous bleeding (haematuria, ecchymoses of the legs and gastrointestinal bleeding) following the addition of 250 mg tienilic acid daily to their drug regimen. The thrombotest percentage of one of them was found to have fallen below 10%.[1]

Enhanced anticoagulant effects have been described in other reports when tienilic acid was given to patients on ethylbiscoumacetate, nicoumalone (acenocoumarol)[2,3] or warfarin.[5]

Mechanism
Not understood. A plasma protein binding displacement mechanism has been suggested[1] as a parallel with another potent diuretic, ethacrynic acid, but in-vitro studies using human serum and warfarin have not confirmed this idea.[4]

Importance and management
The documentation of this interaction is very limited, but it is clearly of importance. The incidence is not known. The anticoagulant response should be closely monitored if tienilic acid is added to an established anticoagulant regimen and dosage adjustments made. Only ethyl biscoumacetate, warfarin and nicoumalone have so far been implicated, but it would clearly be prudent to be on the alert for this interaction to take place with any oral anticoagulant.

References
1 Detilleux M, Caquet R and Laroche C. Potentialisation de l'effet des anticoagulants coumariniques par un nouveaux diurétique, l'acide tienilique. *Nouv Presse méd* (1976) **36**, 2395.
2 Portier H, Destaing F and Chavve L. Potentialisation de l'effet des anticoagulantes coumariniques pour l'acide tienilique: un nouvelle observation. *Nouv Presse méd* (1977) **6**, 468.
3 Grand A, Drouin B and Arche G J. Potentialisation de l'action anticoagulante des antivitamines K par l'acide tienilique. *Nouv Presse méd* (1977) **6**, 2691.
4 Slattery J T and Levy G. Ticrynafen effect on warfarin protein binding in human serum. *J Pharm Sci* (1979) **68**, 393.
5 McLain D A, Garriga F J and Kantor O S. Adverse reactions associated with ticrynafen use. *J Amer Med Ass* (1980) **243**, 763.

Anticoagulants + tolmetin

Summary
The anticoagulant effects of phenprocoumon and warfarin, and the bleeding time during nicoumalone (acenocoumarol) treatment are unaffected by concurrent treatment with tolmetin.

Interaction
Phenprocoumon + tolmetin
Fifteen patients on long-term treatment with phenprocoumon were given 200 mg tolmetin four times a day over a 10-day period. No significant changes in any of the parameters of coagulation measured were found although a '. . . clinically irrelevant prolongation of bleeding time. . . ' was seen.[1]

Warfarin + tolmetin
Fifteen subjects anticoagulated with warfarin showed no alterations in their prothrombin times when concurrently taking 1200 mg tolmetin daily over a 3-week period[2]

Nicoumalone (acenocoumarol) + tolmetin
No changes in the bleeding time were observed in normal subjects or patients taking tolmetin, 800 mg daily, over periods of 8 weeks while anticoagulated with nicoumalone.[3]

Mechanism
None.

Importance and management

No special precautions appear to be necessary if tolmetin is given to patients anticoagulated with phenprocoumon, warfarin or nicoumalone. Whether this is equally true for the other oral anticoagulants awaits confirmation.

References

1 Rust O, Biland L, Thilo D, Nyman D and Duckert F. Prufung des Antirheumatikums Tolmetin auf Interaktionen mit oralen Antikoagulantien. *Schweiz med Wschr* (1975) **105**, 752.

2 Whitsett T L, Barry J P, Czerwinski A W, Hall W H, and Hampton J W. Tolmetin and warfarin. A clinical investigation to determine if interaction exists. In *Tolmetin, a New Non-steroidal Anti-Inflammatory Agent*, p. 160. Ward J R (ed). Proceedings of a Symposium. Washington DC. April 1975 *Excerpta Medica*. Amsterdam, New York.

3 Maibach E. Über die Beeinflussung der Blutungszeit durch tolectin. *Schweiz Rundschau Med (Praxis)* (1978) **67**, 161.

Anticoagulants + tricyclic antidepressants

Summary

The anticoagulant response to dicoumarol may be enhanced in some individuals by amitriptyline or nortripytline. There are no data about other anticoagulants and tricyclic antidepressants, except warfarin which appears not to interact.

Interaction

Tricyclic antidepressants may prolong the half-life of dicoumarol in some individuals, but warfarin appears to be unaffected:

> In a study on 6 volunteers, nortriptyline in therapeutic doses (0·2 mg/kg three times a day) administered over 8 days increased the average half-life of dicoumarol from 35 to 106 h. The effect of this on the anticoagulant-induced hypoprothrombinaemia was not determined.[1,2]
>
> An investigation on 12 normal subjects showed that treatment with either nortriptyline, 40 mg daily, or amitryptyline, 25 mg 8-hourly, over a 9-day period had no consistent effect on the half-life of dicoumarol. In some cases the half-life was prolonged, in others it remained the same or was shortened. In parallel experiments these two tricyclics were found to have no effect on the half-life and elimination of warfarin.[3]

Mechanism

Not understood. One suggestion to account for the prolongation of the dicoumarol half-life is that the tricyclic antidepressants inhibit its metabolism[1,2] but this was not confirmed by other studies.[3] There is even evidence that the tricyclics may induce drug metabolism. Animal studies failed to show any effect by desipramine (5–10 mg/kg) on the hypoprothrombinaemia due to nicoumalone.[4]

Another suggestion is that the tricylics slow intestinal motility (they have anticholinergic properties) which may increase the time available for the dissolution and absorption of the dicoumarol and increase its bioavailability.[3]

Importance and management

Data are limited, but there is no clear reason to avoid the concurrent use of dicoumarol and the tricyclic antidepressants. Changes in the anticoagulant dosage requirements may be expected in some individuals. It would be prudent to watch for a similar response with other anticoagulants, although nothing seems to have been documented in man on any except warfarin which appears not to interact.[3]

References

1 Vesell E S, Passananti T and Greene F E. Impairment of drug metabolism in man by allopurinol and nortriptyline. *New Eng J Med* (1970) **283**, 1484.

2 Vessel E S, Passananti G T and Aurori K C. Anomalous results of studies on drug interaction in man. *Pharmacology* (1975) **13**, 101.

3 Pond S M, Graham G G, Birkett D J and Wade D N. Effects of tricyclic antidepressants on drug metabolism. *Clin Pharmacol Ther* (1975) **18**, 191.

4 Weiner M. Effect of centrally active drugs on the action of coumarin anticoagulants. *Nature* (1966) **212**, 1599.

Anticoagulants + vitamin E

Summary

There is some very limited evidence that the effects of warfarin, dicoumarol and probably other anticoagulants may be enhanced by the concurrent use of vitamin E.

Interaction

A patient, anticoagulated with warfarin and treated with digoxin, frusemide, clofibrate, potassium chloride elixir and phenytoin (later substituted by quinidine), developed ecchymoses, haematuria, and possibly gastrointestinal bleeding. He was found to have a prothrombin time of 36 s. Later the patient admitted that he had been taking 1200 IU vitamin E daily over the previous 2 months. A later study showed that his plasma levels of factors II, VII, IX and X could be markedly reduced by the concurrent use of vitamin E and bleeding could be induced.[1]

A study on 3 volunteers given 42 IU vitamin E daily for a month showed that the mean prothrombin activity, in response to a single 150 mg dose of dicoumarol at 36 h, was reduced from 52 to 33%.[2]

Mechanism

Not known. Large doses of vitamin E (2–4 g) alone are reported not to affect the coagulation mechanism in man,[3] but in animals the prothrombin response is prolonged and bleeding can occur.[4] It can be corrected by the use of vitamin K. One suggestion is that it may interfere with the activity of vitamin K in producing the blood clotting factors.[1]

Importance and management

The documentation of this interaction is very limited. There seems to be no clear reason for anticoagulated patients to avoid taking vitamin E supplements but an enhancement of the anticoagulant effects may occur in some individuals.

References

1 Corrigan J J and Marcus F I. Coagulopathy associated with vitamin E ingestion. *J Amer Med Ass* (1974) **230**, 1300.
2 Schrogie J J. Coagulopathy and fat-soluble vitamins. *J Amer Med Ass* (1975) **232**, 341.
3 Hillman R W. Tocopherol excess in man: Creatinuria associated with prolonged ingestion. *Am J Clin Nutr* (1957) **5**, 597.
4 Doisey E A. Nutritional hypoprothrombinemia and metabolism of vitamin K. *Fed Proc* (1961) **20**, 989.

Anticoagulants + vitamin K

Summary

The effects of anticoagulants can be antagonized by the concurrent use of vitamin K. Significant amounts are contained in some proprietary chilblain preparations and health foods.

Interaction

Vitamin K antagonizes the response to the oral anticoagulants and is used as an effective antidote to overdosage, but unintentional and unwanted antagonism can also occur:

A patient with mitral stenosis and atrial fibrillation, who was anticoagulated with nicoumalone, showed a fall in her British corrected anticoagulant response ratio to 1·2 (normal range 1·8–3·0) within 2 days of starting to take an over-the-counter chilblain preparation (*Gon*) which contained, in addition to nicotinamide, 10 mg acetomenaphthone per tablet. The patient took a total of 50 mg vitamin K over 48 h.[1]

Similar antagonism has been described in a woman on warfarin taking a health food (*Ensure*) which was providing about 0·50 mg vitamin K a day.[2] A reduction in the effects of dicoumarol has been attributed in a very brief report to a diet containing particularly large amounts of green vegetables rich in vitamin K.[3]

Mechanism

The oral anticoagulants compete with the normal supply of vitamin K from the gut to reduce the synthesis by the liver of blood clotting factors, (see page 113). If this supply is boosted by an unusually large intake of vitamin K, the competition swings in favour of the vitamin and the synthesis of the blood clotting factors begins to return to normal. In this way the prothrombin time also returns to its usual value.

Importance and management

A very well established interaction although reports of accidental antagonism are few. It may be expected to occur to a greater or lesser extent with all patients on any oral anticoagulant. It is a potentially serious interaction if it accepted that oral anticoagulants are an effective protection against thrombosis. Proprietary compounds containing vitamin K should not be given to patients on oral anticoagulants. Over-the-counter chilblain preparations such as *Gon*, *Amisyn* and *Pernivit* in recommended doses provide 40–60 mg acetomenaphthone daily which is enough to cause antagonism. There may be other health foods apart from the one cited which contain vitamin K in significant amounts. It seems doubtful if green vegetables normally contain enough to disturb the anticoagulant control.

References

1 Heald G E and Poller L. Anticoagulants and treatment for chilblains. *Brit Med J* (1974) **2**, 455.
2 O'Reilly R A and Rytand D A. 'Resistance' to warfarin due to unrecognized vitamin K supplementation. *New Eng J Med* (1980) **303**, 160.
3 Quick A. Leafy vegetables in diet alter prothrombin time in patients taking anticoagulant drugs. *J Amer Med Ass* (1964) **187**, 27.

Heparin + aspirin

Summary

Heparin and aspirin used together as prophylactic treatment for deep-vein thrombosis in those with fractures of the hip can result in serious bleeding complications.

Interaction

A group of 17 patients[1] with fractures of the hip were treated prophylactically for the prevention of deep-vein thrombosis as follows: 5 received conventional treatment with warfarin, their prothrombin times being maintained at approximately 1·5 times the control value. The other 12 were given 5000 u heparin subcutaneously every 12 h and 600 mg aspirin twice daily before and after the operation. Eight of this latter group developed serious bleeding complications, including haematomas of the hip and thigh in 3 patients, bleeding through the wound in 4 patients, and uterine bleeding in the other patient.

Mechanism

Unknown

Importance and management

The question of whether heparin and aspirin should or should not be used together has been the subject of debate and contention for several years.[2] It was dogmatically stated in 1969 that aspirin '. . . should be scrupulously avoided in patients receiving heparin',[3] an assertion based apparently on in-vitro evidence and remaining unconfirmed by the author and his colleagues in a subsequent clinical study published in 1975.[4] However, the results of the report cited above would seem to justify the original cautionary statement.

The number of patients involved in this study[1] was small, nevertheless since two-thirds of the group developed serious bleeding complications of one kind or another, heparin and aspirin when used together in the doses indicated are clearly hazardous. It is also suggested by the authors that these hazards are particularly great in those with intertrochanteric fractures.

References

1 Yett H S, Skillman J J and Salzman E W. The hazards of aspirin plus heparin. *New Eng J Med* (1978) **298**, 1092.
2 Rubenstein J J. Aspirin, heparin and haemorrhage. *New Eng J Med* (1976) **294**, 1122.
3 Deykin D. The use of heparin *New Eng J Med* (1969) **280**, 937.
4 Salzman E W, Deykin D and Shapiro R M. Management of heparin therapy. *New Eng J Med* (1975) **292**, 1046.

Heparin + dextran

Summary
The anticoagulant effects of heparin are increased by dextran. It has been recommended that the heparin dosage should be reduced to one third or a half during concurrent use.

Interaction
A study carried out on 9 patients with peripheral vascular disease showed that the mean clotting time 1 h after the infusion of 10 000 u heparin was increased from 36 to 69 s when given at the same time as 500 ml dextran. The effect persisted for 3 h. Dextran itself had no effect on clotting time, but the mean clotting time after 5000 u heparin with dextran was almost the same as after 10 000 u heparin without dextran. The increase was slight at 2 500 u heparin. There were no demonstrable changes in bleeding time induced by either heparin or dextran at the doses used.[1,2]

This abstract[1] contains some contradictory and confusing typographical errors but the correct text has been confirmed.[2] The study confirms a previous single case report.[3]

Mechanism
Unknown.

Importance and management
The evidence for this interaction is very limited[1-3] but it appears to be strong. It has been recommended[1] that during concurrent use the dosage of heparin should be reduced to a half or one-third.

References
1 Atik M. Potentiation of heparin by dextran and its clinical implication. *Thromb Haemorrh* (1977) **38**, 275.
2 Atik M. Personal communication (1980).
3 Bloom W L and Brewer S S. The independent yet synergistic effects of heparin and dextran. *Acta Chir Scand* (1968) **387**, (*Suppl*) 53.

Heparin + probenecid

Summary
The effects of heparin can be enhanced by probenecid.

Interaction
In 1950 a woman with subacute bacterial endocarditis was treated with oral probenecid and penicillin administered by means of a slowly dripping intravenous infusion, kept open with minimal doses of heparin. After a total of 215 mg heparin (approximately 20,000 iu) had been given over a 3-week period, increasing epistaxes developed and the clotting time was found to be 24 min (normal 5–6). This was controlled with protamine.[1]

Mechanism
Uncertain. Possibly probenecid inhibits the excretion of the heparin.

Importance and management
Information on this interaction is extremely limited, however it has previously been observed[2] that carinamide, the predecessor of probenecid, also markedly prolonged clotting times in the presence of heparin which would suggest that the case cited[1] may not be an isolated phenomenon. A close watch should be kept on the effects of heparin if probenecid is used concurrently.

References
1 Sanchez G. Enhancement of heparin effects by probenecid. *New Eng J Med* (1975) **292**, 48.
2 Sirak H D. McCleery R S and Artz C P. The effect of carinamide with heparin on the coagulation of human blood: a preliminary report. *Surgery* (1948) **24**, 811.

CHAPTER 7. ANTICONVULSANT DRUG INTERACTIONS

The anticonvulsant drugs listed in Table 7.1 find their major application in the treatment of various types of epilepsy, although some of them are also used for other conditions. The list is not exclusive by any means, but it contains the anticonvulsant drugs which are discussed either in this chapter or elsewhere in this book. In addition, some of the barbiturates which are not used as anticonvulsants are also categorized here (see Table 7.1). The index should be consulted for the full list of interactions involving all of these drugs.

Table 7.1. Anticonvulsant drugs

Non-proprietary names	Proprietary names
Acetazolamide	*Diamox, Defiltran, Diuramid, Glaucomide*
Carbamazepine	*Tegretol, Tegretal*
Clonazepam	*B7, Rivotrial, Iktorivil*
Ethosuximide	*Asamid, Atysmal, Capitus, Epilio, Petimal Petnidan, Pyknolesinum, Suxinutin*
Methylphenobarbitone (mephobarbital)	*Prominal*
Pheneturide	*Benuride, Trinuride*
Phenobarbitone (phenobarbital)	*Gardenal, Luminal*
Phenytoin (diphenylhydantoin)	*Cansoin, Cimitol, Dantoin, Dantinal, Epanutin, Epelin, Lepsiral, Fenantoin, Dilantin, Dilobid*
Primidone	*Mysoline, Mylepsin, Elmdone, Midone, Liskantin*
Sodium valproate (dipropylacetate)	*Depakene, Depakine, Epilim, Ergenyl, Urekene*
Sulthiame	*Conadil, Contravil, Elisal, Ospolot, Riker 594*

Anticonvulsant therapy

For many years the mainstay of the treatment of epilepsy has been phenytoin (diphenylhydantoin). It is given in daily doses of 150–600 mg to achieve serum concentrations of about 5–15 μg/ml. The dosage is adjusted for the individual needs of each patient until serum levels are reached which maximally control the frequency of seizures without causing phenytoin intoxication. Intoxication begins at serum levels of about 20 μg/ml and is characterized by nystagmus, ataxia, drowsiness and lethargy. Any disturbance of the serum phenytoin concentrations caused by the interaction of drugs very readily manifests itself, either as an increase in fit frequency (due to a fall in serum phenytoin concentrations), or as intoxication (due to a rise in phenytoin concentrations). Many of the interactions described occur because the metabolism of the phenytoin by the liver is increased or decreased by the presence of another drug. Phenytoin itself is also a potent liver enzyme-inducing agent, and this characteristic accounts for a number of interactions where the activity of other drugs is altered by the presence of this anticonvulsant.

Phenobarbitone and other barbiturates have also been extremely widely used as anticonvulsants for many years in dosages of about 100–400 mg daily. Toxicity manifests itself in the form of excessive drowsiness, ataxia, dizziness and blurred vision. The barbiturates as a group are all potent liver enzyme-inducing agents and they take part in a number of interactions with other drugs.

Barbiturates or carbamazepine + benzodiazepines

Summary

An isolated case of barbiturate intoxication occurred during concurrent treatment with phenobarbitone and chlordiazepoxide. Clonazepam does not affect serum barbiturate, or carbamazepine levels, but carbamazepine can lower serum clonazepam levels.

Interaction, mechanism, importance and management

A man treated concurrently with phenobarbitone and chlordiazepoxide demonstrated drowsiness, unsteadiness, slurred speech, nystagmus, poor memory and hallucinations, all of which disappeared once the phenobarbitone was withdrawn. Substantial doses of chlordiazepoxide were well tolerated.[1]

In another study clonazepam was given in slowly increasing doses up to a maximum dose of 4–6 mg/day to patients on phenobarbitone or carbamazepine, alone or in combination. Over a 6-week period, no alterations in the serum levels of phenobarbitone or carbamazepine were seen.[2]

A study with 7 subjects given 1 mg clonazepam daily showed that the concurrent adminis-tration of 200 mg carbamazepine over a 3-week period reduced the clonazepam half-life and reduced its serum levels.[3]

It would seem from these reports that clonazepam serum levels should be monitored if carbamazepine is given concurrently, but clonazepam does not apparently affect carbamazepine or phenobarbitone serum levels.

References

1 Kane F J and McCurdy R L. An unusual reaction to combined Librium–barbiturate therapy. *Am J Psychiatry* (1964) 120, 816.
2 Johannessen S I, Strandjord R E and Munthe-Kaas A W. Lack of effect of clonazepam on serum levels of diphenylhydantoin, phenobarbital and carbamazepine. *Acta Neurol Scand* (1977) 55, 506.
3 Lai A A, Levy R H and Cutler R E. Time course of interaction between carbamazepine and clonazepam. *Clin Pharmacol Ther* (1978) 24, 316.

Barbiturates + caffeine

Summary

The hypnotic effects of pentobarbital are antagonized by the concurrent use of caffeine. Caffeine-containing drinks should be avoided at bedtime if satisfactory hypnosis is to be achieved.

Interaction

A well-controlled study on 42 medical and surgical patients who were given either a placebo, 250 mg caffeine or 100 mg pentobarbital alone or together, showed that the caffeine totally cancelled out the hypnotic effects of the barbiturate. The effects of the pentobarbital-caffeine combination were indistinguishable from the placebo.[1]

Mechanism

Caffeine stimulates the cerebral cortex and impairs sleep whereas pentobarbital depresses the cortex and promotes sleep. These mutually opposing actions would seem to explain the interaction described.

Importance and management

There appears to be only this one direct study[1] of this interaction, but it is well supported by common experience and the numerous studies of the properties of each of these compounds.

Patients requiring barbiturate hypnotics should avoid caffeine-containing drinks (tea, coffee, Coca-Cola etc.) at bedtime if the hypnotic is to be effective.

Reference
1 Forrest W H, Bellville J W and Brown B W. The interaction of caffeine with pentobarbital as a night-time hypnotic. *Anesthesiology* (1972) **36**, 37.

Barbiturates + promethazine with scopolamine

Summary

A study suggests that the concurrent use of these drugs increases the incidence of operative agitation.

Interaction, mechanism, importance and management

Studies in man indicate that pentobarbitone with scopolamine and promethazine used as pre-anaesthetic medication increase the incidence of pre-operative, operative, and post-operative agitation. It is suggested that this triple combination

of drugs should be avoided.[1] Further study is needed.

Reference
1 Macris S G and Levy L. Preanesthetic medication: untoward effects of certain drug combinations. *Anesthesiology* (1965) **26**, 256.

Barbiturates + rifampicin

Summary

Rifampicin increases the metabolism of hexobarbitone approximately three-fold and its effects may be expected to be reduced accordingly. It is uncertain whether phenobarbitone reduces serum levels of rifampicin. Information about other barbiturates appears to be lacking.

Interaction

Hexobarbitone + rifampicin

A study in 6 healthy volunteers showed that after treatment with 1200 mg rifampicin daily for 8 days, the average elimination half-life of hexobarbitone had decreased from 407 to 171 min, and the metabolic clearance had increased approximately three-fold.[1]

Similar results have been found in other studies in normal subjects[2] and in those with cirrhosis or cholestasis.[3]

Rifampicin + phenobarbitone

The evidence is conflicting. One study showed

that phenobarbitone had no significant effect on the half-life of rifampicin[4] whereas another indicated that the serum levels of rifampicin were reduced.[5]

Mechanism

Rifampicin is a potent liver enzyme inducing agent and accelerates the metabolism of hexobarbitone.[1] Whether phenobarbitone (also a potent enzyme-inducing agent) can affect the metabolism of the rifampicin in a similar way is not clear.

Importance and management

The hexobarbitone/rifampicin interaction is adequately documented. A reduction in the effectiveness of hexobarbitone may be expected during concurrent use. Whether rifampicin affects other barbiturates in a similar way is uncertain. It is also not clear whether phenobarbitone and other barbiturates can reduce serum rifampicin levels, but it would be prudent to be on the alert for both interactions during concurrent use.

References
1 Breimer D D, Zilly W and Richter E. Influence of rifampicin on drug metabolism: differences between hexobarbital and antipyrine. *Clin Pharmacol Ther* (1977) **21**, 470.

2 Zilly W, Breimer D D and Richter E. Induction of drug metabolism in man after rifampicin treatment measured by increased hexobarbital and tolbutamide clearance. *Europ J clin Pharmacol* (1975) **9**, 219.
3 Zilly W, Breimer D D and Richter E. Stimulation of drug metabolism by rifampicin in patients with cirrhosis or cholestasis measured by increased hexobarbital and tolbutamide clearance. *Europ J clin Pharmacol* (1977) **11**, 287.
4 Acocella G, Bonollo L, Mainardi M, Margaroli P and Nicolis F B. Kinetic studies on rifampicin. III. Effect of phenobarbital on the half-life of the antibiotic. *Tijdschrift Gastro-Enterologie* (1974) **17**, 151.
5 De la Roy Y de R, Beauchant G, Breuil K, y Patté F. Diminution de taux sérique de rifampicine par le phénobarbital. *Presse Méd* (1971) **79**, 350.

Barbiturates + sodium valproate

Summary
The addition of sodium valproate to established epileptic treatment with phenobarbitone can lead to an increase in the serum concentrations of phenobarbitone and the development of sedation and lethargy. A one-third to one-half reduction in the phenobarbitone dosage can be safely carried out without loss of seizure control

Interaction
A long-term study over 9 months on 11 epileptic patients showed that when they were treated with sodium valproate (11–42 mg/kg daily) in addition to phenobarbitone (90–400 mg daily), they complained of sedation and, on average, the dosage of phenobarbitone could be reduced to 54% with continued good seizure control.[1] Two other patients given a constant dose of phenobarbitone had significantly increased phenobarbitone levels (12 and 48% respectively).[1]

In another study on 7 patients, sodium valproate in daily doses of 1200 mg daily raised the serum phenobarbitone concentrations by an average of 27% (from 22 to 28 μg/ml).[2]

Similar increases in serum phenobarbitone concentrations or sedation, caused by the presence of sodium valproate have been described in numerous other reports.[3–7, 9–13]

Mechanism
Not known. One suggestion is that it may be related to some sodium valproate-induced decrease in the renal excretion of phenobarbitone because acidification of the urine may occur when valproate is taken.[1, 13]

Importance and management
A well-established and thoroughly examined interaction. An increase in the serum concentrations of phenobarbitone, probably accompanied by the toxic symptoms of sedation and lethargy, is a likely occurrence if sodium valproate is added to an established phenobarbitone regimen. On the basis of the long-term study cited above[1] with sodium valproate using the dosages described, it would seem that the phenobarbitone dosage can be safely reduced by a third to a half (and even more in some cases) with full seizure control.

References
1 Wilder B J, Willmore L J, Bruni J and Villarreal H J. Valproic acid: Interaction with other anticonvulsant drugs. *Neurology* (1978) **28**, 892.
2 Richens A and Ahmad S. Controlled trial of sodium valproate in severe epilepsy. *Br Med J* (1975) **3**, 255.
3 Meinardi H and Bongers E. Analytical data in connection with the clinical use of di-n-propylacetate. In *Clinical Pharmacology of Antiepileptic Drugs*, p. 235. Schneider H, Janz D, Gardner-Thorp G, Meinardi H and Sherwin A L (eds) (1975). Springer-Verlag, NY, Berlin.
4 Schobben F, Van der Kleijn E and Gabreels F J M. Pharmacokinetics of di-n-Propylacetate in epileptic patients. *Europ J clin pharmacol* (1975) **8**, 97.
5 Gram L, Wulff K and Rasmussen K E. Valproate sodium: a controlled clinical trial including monitoring of drug levels. *Epilepsia* (1977) **18**, 141.
6 Jeavons P M and Clark J E. Sodium valproate in treatment of epilepsy. *Br Med J* (1974) **2**, 584.
7 Volzke E and Doose H. Dipropylacetate (Dépakine, Ergenyl) in the treatment of epilepsy. *Epilepsia* (Amst) (1973) **14**, 185.
8 Millet Y, Sainty J M, Galland M C, Sidoine R and Jonglard J. Problèmes posés par l'association thérapeutique phénobar-

bital–dipropylacétate de sodium a propos d'un cas. *Europ J Toxicol* (1976) **9**, 381.

9 Jeavons P M, Clark J E and Maheshwari M C. Treatment of generalized epilepsies of childhood and adolescence with sodium valproate ('Epilim'). *Develop Med Child Neurol* (1977) **19**, 9.

10 Vakil S D, Critchley E M R, Philips J C, Haydock C, Cocks A and Dyer T. The effect of sodium valproate (*Epilim*) on phenytoin and phenobarbitone blood levels. In *Clinical and Pharmacological Aspects of Sodium Valproate (Epilim) in the Treatment of Epilepsy*, p. 75. Proceedings of a Symposium held at the University of Nottingham, September 1975.

11 Richens A, Scoular I T, Ahmad S and Jordan B J. Pharmacokinetics and efficacy of Epilim in patients receiving long-term therapy with other antiepileptic drugs. In *Clinical*

and *Pharmacological Aspects of Sodium Valproate (Epilim) in the Treatment of Epilepsy*, p. 78. Proceedings of a Symposium held at the University of Nottingham, September 1975.

12 Scott D F, Boxer C M and Herzberg J L. A study of the hypnotic effects of Epilim and its possible interaction with phenabarbitone. In *Clinical and Pharmacological Aspects of Sodium Valproate (Epilim) in the Treatment of Epilepsy*, p. 155. Proceedings of a Symposium held at the University of Nottingham, September 1975.

13 Loiseau P, Orgogozo J M, Brachet-Liermain A and Morselli P L. Pharmacokinetic studies on the interaction between phenobarbital and valproic acid. In *Adv. Epileptol. Proc. Cong. Int. League. Epilepsy 13th* p. 261. Meinardi H. and Rowan A. (eds) (1977/78).

Barbiturates + triacetyloleandomycin

Summary

A single case report describes a fall in serum phenobarbitone levels during the concurrent use of triacetyloleandomycin (troleandomycin).

Interaction, mechanism, importance and management

A single case has been reported of a patient on phenobarbitone and carbamazepine who showed a fall in serum phenobarbitone levels (from about 40 to 31 μg/ml) over a 3-day period when treated with triacetyloleandomycin.[1] The general importance of this is uncertain but it would clearly be

prudent to be on the alert for changes in the seizure control during the use of this antibiotic. See also carbamazepine + triacetyloleandomycin (p. 187).

Reference

1 Dravet C, Mesdjian E, Cenraud B and Roger J. Interaction between carbamazepine and triacetyloleandomycin. *Lancet* (1977) **i**, 810.

Carbamazepine + dextropropoxyphene

Summary

Carbamazepine serum levels may be raised, in some cases to toxic levels, by the concurrent use of dextropropoxyphene.

Interaction

The observation that the concurrent use of carbamazepine and dextropropoxyphene resulted in toxicity (headache, dizziness, ataxia, nausea and tiredness) prompted a study of this possible interaction in 7 subjects. The 5 who completed the study and who were given propoxyphene hydrochloride, 65 mg three times a day, showed a mean rise in serum carbamzepine levels of 65% and a mean decrease in plasma clearance of 42%.[1]

Mechanism

Uncertain. It is suggested that the dextropropoxy-

phene inhibits the metabolism of carbamazepine leading to its accumulation in the body.[1]

Importance and management

The evidence is not extensive but it appears to be strong. If dextropropoxyphene is used with carbamazepine, a very close watch should be kept on the anticonvulsant serum levels to prevent intoxication. In most cases it would seem simpler to use an alternative non-interacting analgesic.

Reference

1 Dam M and Christiansen J. Interaction of propoxyphene with carbamazepine. *Lancet* (1977) **ii**, 509.

Carbamazepine + phenobarbitone

Summary

Carbamazepine serum levels are reduced by the concurrent use of phenobarbitone, but seizure control appears to remain unaffected.

Interaction, mechanism, importance and management

A study carried out over four 21-day periods on epileptic patients who were being treated with 1200 mg carbamazepine and 300 mg phenobarbitone daily showed that the serum levels of carbamazepine were reduced by the concurrent treatment, but the seizure control remained unaffected.[1] The same response has been described in other studies.[2,3]

References

1 Cereghino J J, Brock J T, Van Meter J C, Penry J K, Smith L D and White B G. The efficacy of carbamazepine combinations in epilepsy. *Clin Pharmacol Ther* (1975) **18**, 733.
2 Kane A, Höjer B, and Wilson J T. Kinetics of carbamazepine and its 10,11-epoxide metabolite in children. *Clin Pharmacol Ther* (1976) **19**, 276.
3 Christiansen J and Dam M. Influence of phenobarbitol and diphenylhydantoin on plasma carbamazepine levels in patients with epilepsy. *Acta Neurol Scand* (1973) **49**, 543.

Carbamazepine + sodium valproate

Summary

Extremely brief comments in two reports suggest that drowsiness may occur during concurrent use, and carbamazepine serum levels may be slightly reduced.

Interaction, mechanism, importance and management

The information is extremely limited. One report[1] briefly comments that drowsiness occurred in 1 patient which disappeared when the dosage of carbamazepine was reduced. The other report[2] also equally briefly states that 5 patients on both drugs showed unchanged, or slightly lower, carbamazepine serum levels. These reactions appear to be relatively unimportant, but this requires further confirmation.

References

1 Jeavons P M and Clark J E. Sodium valproate in the treatment of epilepsy. *Br Med J* (1974) **2**, 584.
2 Wilder B J. Willmore L J, Bruni J and Villarreal H J. Valproic acid: interaction with other anticonvulsant drugs. *Neurology* (1978) **28**, 892.

Carbamazepine + triacetyloleandomycin

Summary

A report describes 8 cases of carbamazepine intoxication caused by the concurrent use of carbamazepine and triacetyloleandomycin (troleandomycin).

Interaction

Carbamazepine serum levels are increased by triacetyloleandomycin.

Eight epileptic patients, under treatment with carbamazepine, developed signs of intoxication (disturbed balance, nausea, vomiting, excessive drowsiness) within 24 h of starting to take triacetyloleandomycin. The only 2 patients available for examination showed a sharp increase in serum carbamazepine serum levels (a rise in 1 patient from 5 to 28 μg/ml over 3 days) during treatment with the antibiotic, and a rapid fall following withdrawal.[1] The rise in carbamazepine serum levels in one patient also on phenobarbitone was paralleled by a fall in serum phenobarbitone levels (see p. 186).

Mechanism
Unknown. It is suggested that the antibiotic slows the rate of metabolism of the carbamazepine by the liver microsomal enzymes so that the anticonvulsant accumulates within the body.[1]

Importance and management
An important and established interaction although there is only one report. The evidence seems strong. The rapidity of its development (24 h) and the marked rise in serum carbamazepine levels suggest that it would be difficult to control the carbamazepine levels by adjusting its dosage. It would seem prudent to avoid concurrent use.

Reference
1 Dravet C, Mesdjian E, Cenraud B and Roger J. Interaction between carbamazepine and triacetyloleandomycin. *Lancet* (1977), i, 810.

Ethosuximide + carbamazepine, methylphenobarbitone, phenobarbitone, phenytoin, or primidone

Summary
Of these anticonvulsants, only methylphenobarbitone has been found to increase serum ethosuximide levels. Two case reports describe a rise in serum phenytoin levels induced by ethosuximide and phenytoin intoxication has also been seen.

Interaction, mechanism, importance and management
A study[1] on the factors which might influence the plasma concentrations of ethosuximide, carried out on 46 epileptic patients on combined anticonvulsant therapy, indicated that with the exception of methylphenobarbitone, which caused a rise, none of the other anticonvulsants had any effects on the serum levels of ethosuximide. A single case has been reported[2] in which the addition of ethosuximide, in daily doses within the range 1750–2000 mg, to a phenytoin regimen of 200 mg daily appeared to have been responsible for a rise in the serum phenytoin levels of 1 patient from about 15 to 23 μg/ml over a 2-month period. Two other cases where ethosuximide appeared to have contributed to the development of phenytoin toxicity have been described.[4,5] The reason for this is not known. In another study[3] ethosuximide was found not to affect the serum levels of primidone taken concurrently.

References
1 Smith G A, McKauge L, Dubetz D, Tyrer J H and Eadie M J. Factors influencing plasma concentrations of ethosuximide. *Clin Pharmacokinet* (1979) 4, 38.
2 Lander C M, Eadie M J and Tyrer J H. Interactions between anticonvulsants. *Proc Aust Assoc Neurol* (1975) 12, 111.
3 Schmidt D. The effect of phenytoin and ethosuximide on primidone metabolism in patients with epilepsy. *J Neurol* (1975) 209, 115.
4 Dawson G W, Brown H W and Clark B G. Serum phenytoin after ethosuximide. *Ann Neurol* (1978) 4, 583.
5 Frantzen E, Hansen J M and Hansen O E. Phenytoin (Dilantin) intoxication. *Acta Neurol Scand* (1967) 43, 440.

Pheneturide + folic acid

Summary
Is there the possibility of a loss in seizure control during concurrent use?

Interaction, mechanism, importance and management
Serum folate levels are depressed in epileptic patients under treatment with pheneturide.[1] Whether the use of a folate dietary supplements leads to a reduction in serum pheneturide levels

and in some loss of seizure control, as it does with phenytoin (see p. 200), is uncertain, but this possibility should be borne in mind.

Reference
1 Latham A N, Millbank L, Richens A and Rowe D J F. Liver enzyme induction by anticonvulsant drugs, and its relationship to disturbed calcium and folic acid metabolism. *J Clin Pharmacol* (1973) **13**, 337.

Phenytoin, phenobarbitone, or primidone + acetazolamide

Summary

In a very small number of patients the concurrent use of phenytoin, phenobarbitone and primidone with acetazolamide has been associated with (a) the development of severe osteomalacia, or (b) a reduction in serum primidone levels and in seizure control.

Interaction

(a) Osteomalacia

Two young women, taking 750 mg acetazolamide daily with phenytoin or primidone or phenobarbitone for atypical seizures developed severe osteomalacia despite a normal intake of calcium. There was no evidence of malabsorption. When the acetazolamide was withdrawn the hyperchloraemic acidosis, shown by both patients, abated and the high urinary calcium excretion fell by 50%.[1]

(b) Reduced serum primidone levels

An epileptic patient, under treatment with primidone and acetazolamide, showed an increase in seizure frequency associated with a virtual absence of primidone or phenobarbitone in the serum. When the acetazolamide was withdrawn the primidone absorption recommenced. Subsequent studies in two other patients showed that primidone absorption was reduced in one, but not in the other, during acetazolamide treatment.[2]

Mechanism

Unknown. Mild osteomalacia induced by anticonvulsants is a recognized phenomenon[3] but in what way it can be exaggerated by acetazolamide is not understood. Changes in primidone absorption induced by the acetazolamide are also unexplained.

Importance and management

The documentation of both types of interaction is extremely limited and their incidence is uncertain. Concurrent use would not seem to be contraindicated but it is clear that the effects of concurrent use should be closely checked for the possible development of these adverse reactions.

References
1 Mallette L E. Anticonvulsants, acetazolamide and osteomalacia. *New Eng J Med* (1975) **292**, 668.
2 Syversen G B, Morgan J P, Weintraub M and Myers G J. Acetazolamide-induced interference with primidone absorption. *Arch Neurol* (1977) **34**, 80.
3 Anast C S. Anticonvulsant drugs and calcium metabolism. *New Eng J Med* (1975) **292**, 567.

Phenytoin + alcohol

Summary

Chronic heavy drinking can cause a marked reduction in serum phenytoin levels, but occasional drinking has little effect.

Interaction

The chronic ingestion of alcohol increases the rate of metabolism of phenytoin.

A comparative study on 15 drinkers (defined as those who had consumed a minimum of 200 g ethanol daily for at least 3 weeks) and 76 control subjects

189

showed that the mean half-life of the phenytoin (900 mg for 3 days) in the drinkers was 16·3 h, and in the non-drinkers 23·5 h. The blood-phenytoin levels of the drinkers, 24 h after the last dose of phenytoin, was approximately half that of the non-drinkers.[1]

The metabolism of phenytoin is not affected by acute ingestion of alcohol.[4]

Mechanism
Supported by animal data, the evidence suggests that alcohol induces liver microsomal enzymes, thereby increasing the rate of metabolism and clearance of the phenytoin from the body.[1,2,3]

Importance and management
Information on this interaction is very limited but the study cited[1] indicates that phenytoin serum levels are affected by the chronic ingestion of large amounts of alcohol, and phenytoin requirements are increased in those who drink heavily. The effect of moderate drinking seems not to have been determined, but it is probably relatively small. Occasional drinking has no effect.[4]

References
1 Kater R M H, Roggin G, Tobon F, Zieve P and Iber F L. Increased rate of clearance of drugs from the circulation of alcoholics. *Amer J Med Sci* (1969) **258**, 35.
2 Lieber C S and DeCarli L M. Ethanol oxidation by hepatic microsomes: Adaptive increase after ethanol feeding. *Science* (1968) **162**, 197.
3 Rubin E and Lieber C S. Hepatic microsomal enzymes in man and rat: Induction and inhibition by ethanol. *Science* (1968) **162**, 690.
4 Schmidt D. Effect of ethanol intake on phenytoin metabolism in volunteers. *Experientia* (1975) **31**, 1313.

Phenytoin + antacids

Summary
The administration of antacids with phenytoin may have been responsible for the loss of seizure control in a few epileptic patients, but generally no interaction of any importance appears to take place.

Interaction
Three patients[1] taking phenytoin were found to have low serum phenytoin levels (2–4 μg/ml) when they were given phenytoin and unnamed antacids at the same time, but if the antacid administration were delayed 2–3 h the serum levels of the phenytoin rose two- to three-fold.

A controlled study[2] with 6 epileptic patients, taking 300–350 mg phenytoin daily, showed that when they were simultaneously given 15 ml *Gelusil Suspension* (magnesium trisilicate 620 mg/aluminium hydroxide 310 mg in every 5 ml) with every 100 mg phenytoin, their average serum phenytoin levels were reduced by about 12% (from 40 to 35 μmol/l). In a parallel study 30 ml (10 g) calcium carbonate suspension was found to have no significant effect on the phenytoin levels.

Another study[3] on 6 normal volunteers, given 10 ml Aluminium Hydroxide Gel, BP, or 10 ml magnesium hydroxide mixture (550 mg magnesium hydroxide) with single 100 mg oral doses of phenytoin, failed to demonstrate any change in the rate, or extent, of absorption of phenytoin, but in the same report 2 epileptic patients are described who apparently began to show inadequate seizure control with phenytoin which coincided with their ingestion of antacids for dyspepsia.

A study[4] on 2 normal volunteers given multiple doses of either 30 ml of a magnesium and aluminium hydroxide mixture, 30 ml aluminium hydroxide–magnesium trisilicate mixture, or 2 g calcium carbonate, all administered at 2-h intervals starting 4 h before a single 300 mg oral doses of phenytoin and finishing 8 h afterwards, showed that the absorption of the phenytoin remained totally unaffected.

In another study reduced levels of phenytoin were seen in patients given either aluminium hydroxide-magnesium hydroxide or calcium carbonate.[5]

Mechanism
It is not at all clear why only a few patients appear to demonstrate an interaction between phenytoin and antacids, nor is the mechanism of interaction understood.

Importance and control
The reports described indicate that some loss of seizure control can occur in a few patients[1,3] who take phenytoin and antacids concurrently, but generally it would seem that no significant interaction takes place. If there is any hint that an epileptic patient is being affected by the use of an antacid, the separation of the doses by 2–3 h appears to minimize the likelihood of an interaction.[1]

References

1 Pippinger L. Quoted by Kutt H. in 'Interactions of antiepileptic drugs' *Epilepsia* (1975) **16**, 393.
2 Kulshrestha V K, Thomas M, Wadsworth J and Richens A. Interaction between phenytoin and antacids. *Br J Clin Pharmac* (1978) **6**, 177.
3 O'Brien L S, Orme M L'E and Breckenridge A M. Failure of antacids to alter the pharmacokinetics of phenytoin. *Br J Clin Pharmac* (1978) **6**, 176.
4 Chapron D J, Kramer P A, Mariano S L and Hohnadel D C. Effect of calcium and antacids on phenytoin bioavailability. *Arch Neurol* (1979) **36**, 436.
5 Garnett W R, Carter B L and Bellock J M. Biavailability of phenytoin administered with antacids. *Therap Drug Monitoring* (1979) **1**, 435.

Phenytoin + anticoagulants

Summary

Phenytoin can reduce the anticoagulant effects of dicoumarol and increase the effects of warfarin, whereas the effects of phenprocoumon are usually unaltered. The serum levels of phenytoin can be increased by dicoumarol and phenprocoumon, but they are usually unaltered by warfarin and phenindione.

Interactions

There is no consistency about the ways different anticoagulants interact with phenytoin, or are themselves affected by phenytoin, so for the sake of clarity the data presented in this synopsis are divided into two sections and summarized in tabular form under 'Importance and management'.

(a) The effects of phenytoin on the oral anticoagulants:

Dicoumarol + phenytoin

Serum levels of dicoumarol and the anticoagulant effects are reduced by the concurrent use of phenytoin.

A study was carried out on 6 subjects taking constant daily doses of dicoumarol (40–160 mg daily) and who were also given 300 mg phenytoin daily for a week. Five days after starting the phenytoin, the serum dicoumarol levels began to fall from 29 μg/ml, and continued to fall to 21 μg/ml 5 days after the phenytoin had been withdrawn. No significant changes in the prothrombin–proconvertin percentage (PP%) took place until 3 days after withdrawing the phenytoin, when it climbed from 20 to 50%.[1] Four other subjects, given 60 mg daily doses of dicoumarol, showed a fall in serum dicoumarol levels from 20 to 5 μg/ml over a $6\frac{1}{2}$-week period during which they also received 300 mg phenytoin daily for the first week, reduced to 100 mg daily for the remainder of the study. The PP%, after 2 weeks of phenytoin treatment rose from 20 to 70% and only fell to pre-phenytoin treatment levels $5\frac{1}{2}$ weeks after withdrawing the phenytoin.[1]

Phenprocoumon + phenytoin

Serum levels of phenprocoumon and the antico-agulants are usually unaffected by the concurrent use of phenprocoumon.

An investigation with patients on long-term treatment with phenprocoumon showed that, while in the majority of cases phenytoin caused no significant alteration in either the serum phenprocoumon concentrations or in the anticoagulant control, a few patients showed a fall and others a rise in the serum levels of the anticoagulant.[2]

Warfarin + phenytoin

Prothrombin times can be prolonged by the use of phenytoin.

A report describes a patient anticoagulated with warfarin (2·5 mg 5 days of the week and 5 mg on the other 2 days) and with a prothrombin time of 21 s. When concurrently treated with 300 mg phenytoin daily, the prothrombin time within a month had increased to 32 s despite a reduction in the warfarin dosage to 2·5 mg daily. When the warfarin was withdrawn, the patient was restabilized on the former warfarin regimen. Another patient is said to have shown this interaction but no details are given.[8]

(b) The effects of the oral anticoagulants on phenytoin:

Phenytoin + dicoumarol

Serum levels of phenytoin can be increased by the concurrent use of dicoumarol. Intoxication may develop.

A study carried out on 6 subjects taking 300 mg phenytoin daily showed that when they were additionally given dicoumarol (in dosages adjusted to give prothrombin values of about 30%) their serum

191

phenytoin levels rose over a period of 7 days by an average of almost 10 μg/ml (126%).[4] Similar results are described in another study.[7]

A patient anticoagulated with dicoumarol developed phenytoin intoxication within only 6 days of starting additional treatment with 300 mg phenytoin daily.[6]

Phenytoin + phenprocoumon
Serum levels of phenytoin can be increased by the concurrent use of phenprocoumon.

A study on 4 patients taking 300 mg phenytoin daily showed that when they were additionally given phenprocoumon (in dosages adjusted to give PP values within the therapeutic range), their serum phenytoin levels rose from 10 to 14 μg/ml over a period of 7 days. The half-life of the phenytoin was increased from a mean of 9·9 to 14 h.[7]

Phenytoin + warfarin
Serum levels of phenytoin are usually not affected by the concurrent use of warfarin, but a single case report describes an increase:

A study on 2 patients taking 300 mg phenytoin daily showed that when they were additionally given warfarin (in dosages adjusted to give PP values within the therapeutic range), their serum phenytoin levels remained unaltered over a 7 day period.[7] In four other patients it was also confirmed that the half-life of phenytoin remained unaffected.[7]

A patient who had been maintained on 300 mg phenytoin daily for over a year developed signs of phenytoin intoxication within a short time of starting concurrent anticoagulant treatment with warfarin.[5]

Phenytoin + phenindione
Serum levels of phenytoin are usually not affected by the concurrent use of warfarin.

A study on 4 patients taking 300 mg phenytoin daily showed that when they were additionally given phenidione (in dosages adjusted to give PP values within the therapeutic range), their serum phenytoin levels remained virtually unaltered over a 7-day

period. The half-life of the phenytoin in 4 patients showed an insignificant rise (from 13·0 to 13·6 h).[7]

Mechanism
Not fully understood. One postulate to account for the reduction in the serum levels of dicoumarol by phenytoin is that the phenytoin (a known potent enzyme-inducing agent) stimulates the biotransformation of the anticoagulant and increases its rate of clearance. However, there seems to be no clear experimental evidence to confirm this idea. But there is some evidence that phenytoin can, like some of the oral anticoagulants, depress the production of the blood clotting factors, so that some of the changes in the PP% described might be due to this.[3]

The most likely explanation of the effects of the anticoagulants on phenytoin is that they inhibit its biotransformation, causing it to accumulate within the body. This is reflected in the prolonged half-lives seen during the use of dicoumarol and phenprocoumon.[4,7]

Importance and management
None of these interactions has been extensively documented, although some of them have been carefully studied in a few patients and appear to be adequately established. The development of phenytoin intoxication and a loss in anticoagulant control are clearly important. Interacting pairs of drugs should be avoided wherever possible, but with close monitoring and careful dosage adjustments it may be possible to accommodate the interactions. It would seem prudent to monitor the effects of the concurrent use of any anticoagulant and phenytoin carefully to confirm that stable serum levels are being maintained.

References
1 Hansen J M, Siersbæk-Nielsen K, Kristensen M, Skovsted L and Christensen L K. Effect of diphenylhydantoin on the metabolism of dicoumarol in man. *Acta Med Scand* (1971) 189, 15.

Table 7.2. Summary of interactions between phenytoin and anticoaglants

Concurrent treatment with phenytoin and anticoagulants	Effect on serum anticoagulant levels	Effect on serum phenytoin levels
Dicoumarol	Reduced[1]	Markedly increased[6,4,7]
Phenprocoumon	Usually unaltered[2]	Increased[7]
Warfarin	Increased[8]	Usually unaltered[7] single case of increase[5]
Phenindione	Not documented	Usually unaltered[4,7]
Other anticoagulants	Not documented	Not documented

2 Chrishe H W, Tauchert M and Hilger H H. Effect of phenytoin on the metabolism of phenprocoumon. *Eur J Clin Invest* (1974) **4**, 331.
3 Solomon G E, Hilgartner M W and Kutt H. Coagulation defects caused by diphenylhydantoin. *Neurology* (1972) **22**, 1165.
4 Hansen J M, Kristensen M, Skovsted L and Christensen L K. Dicoumarol-induced diphenylhydantoin intoxication. *Lancet* (1966) **ii**, 265.
5 Rothermich N O. Diphenylhydantoin intoxication. *Lancet* (1966) **ii**, 640.

6 Frantzen E, Hansen J M, Hansen O E and Kristensen M. Phenytoin (Dilantin) intoxication. *Acta Neurol Scand* (1967) **43**, 440
7 Skovsted L, Kristensen M, Hansen J M and Siersbaek-Nielsen K. The effect of different oral anticoagulants on diphenylhydantoin (DPH) and tolbutamide metabolism. *Acta med Scand* (1976) **199**, 513.
8 Nappi J M. Warfarin and phenytoin interaction. *Ann Int med* (1979) **90**, 852.

Phenytoin + barbiturates

Summary

Concurrent use is common and usually advantageous. Changes in serum phenytoin levels (often decreases but sometimes increases) can occur if phenobarbitone is added. Seizure control is not usually adversely affected. Phenytoin intoxication following barbiturate withdrawal has been observed. The addition of phenytoin to phenobarbitone treatment may result in elevated phenobarbitone levels and some barbiturate toxicity.

Interaction

(a) Phenytoin treatment to which phenobarbitone is added

A well-controlled clinical study on 12 epileptic patients given phenytoin (3·7–6·8 mg/kg daily), with and without phenobarbitone (1·4–2·5 mg/kg daily), showed that during treatment with both drugs the phenytoin serum levels were depressed. Five patients showed a mean reduction of two thirds (from 15·7 to 5·7 μg/ml) during concurrent treatment. In most cases phenytoin serum levels rose again when the phenobarbitone was withdrawn. In one case this occurred so rapidly and steeply that the patient developed ataxia and a cerebellar syndrome with phenytoin levels up to 60 μg/ml, despite a reduction in the phenytoin dosage.[1]

This interaction has been described in other reports,[2–6] but a rise[4–7] or no alteration[3–6] in serum phenytoin levels have also been described.

(b) Phenobarbitone treatment to which phenytoin is added

A study on 40 epileptic children showed that the addition of phenytoin to established treatment with phenobarbitone resulted in elevated phenobarbitone levels. In 5 patients illustrated the phenobarbitone serum levels were approximately doubled by the presence of the barbiturate. In some case mild ataxia occurred but the relatively high barbiturate levels were well tolerated.[2]

Mechanism

Phenobarbitone can have a dual effect on phenytoin metabolism: it may cause liver enzyme induction which results in a more rapid clearance of the phenytoin from the body, or it may inhibit metabolism by competing for enzyme systems.

The total effect will depend upon a balance between the two. The reason for the elevated serum levels of phenobarbitone is not fully understood.

Importance and management

These interactions are well documented. Concurrent use is common and can be therapeutically advantageous, and in fact some manufacturers market fixed-dose combinations of both drugs (*Epanutin with phenobarbitone, Garoin*). Problems may arise if one or the other drug is added or withdrawn. The response requires close monitoring to ensure that drug intoxication does not occur, or that seizure control does not worsen. Other barbiturates are also enzyme-inducing agents and may be expected to interact similarly.

References

1 Morselli P L, Rizzo M and Garattini S. Interaction between phenobarbital and diphenylhydantoin in animals and in epileptic patients. *Ann NY Acad Sci* (1971) **179**, 88.
2 Cucinell S A, Conney A H, Sansur M and Burns J J. Drug interactions in man. I. Lowering effect of phenobarbital on plasma levels of bishydroxycoumarin (Dicumarol) and diphenylhydantoin (Dilantin). *Clin Pharmacol Ther* (1965) **6**, 420.
3 Buchanan R A, Heffelfinger J C and Weiss C F. The effect of phenobarbital on diphenylhydantoin metabolism in children. *Paediatrics* (1969) **43**, 114.
4 Kutt H, Haynes J, Verebeley K and McDowell F. The effect of phenobarbital on plasma diphenylhydantoin level and meta-

bolism in man and rat liver microsomes. *Neurology* (1969) **19**, 611.
5 Diamond W D and Buchanan R A. A clinical study of the effect of phenobarbital on diphenylhydantoin plasma levels. *J Clin Pharmacol* (1970) **10**, 306.
6 Garrettson L K and Dayton P G. Disappearance of phenobarbi-

tal and diphenylhydantoin from serum of children. *Clin Pharmacol Ther* (1970) **11**, 674.
7 Booker H E, Tormay A and Toussaint J. Concurrent administration of phenobarbital and diphenylhydantoin: Lack of interference effect. *Neurology* (1971) **21**, 383.

Phenytoin + benzodiazepines

Summary

Reports of this interaction are inconsistent. In the presence of benzodiazepines the serum levels of phenytoin may rise (intoxication has been described), fall, or remain unaltered. The serum levels of clonazepam may fall during concurrent treatment with phenytoin.

Interaction

(a) Increased phenytoin serum levels

The observation that the incidence of phenytoin intoxication appeared to be increased among patients receiving, in addition to phenytoin, chlordiazepoxide or diazepam, prompted a more detailed study. Twenty-five patients, administered 300–400 mg phenytoin daily with one of these benzodiazepines, were found to have serum phenytoin levels which were 80–90% higher than those not taking a benzodiazepine, and some individuals demonstrated even greater increases.[1]

Seven out of a total of 37 children taking phenytoin, who were also given clonazepam in doses of 0·03–0·33 mg/kg/day, showed a rise in serum phenytoin levels to toxic concentrations above 20 μg/ml.[2]

Increased phenytoin serum levels and intoxication have also been attributed in other reports to the concurrent use of diazepam,[4,5,11,12] clonazepam,[7,15,16] chlordiazepoxide[3] and possibly, but not certainly, to nitrazepam.[6]

(b) Decreased phenytoin serum levels

A study on 15 epileptic patients taking phenytoin, phenobarbitone and diazepam (an average of 0·3 mg/kg) showed that 7 of them had serum phenytoin levels which were lower than expected. None of the 15 demonstrated elevated serum phenytoin levels.[8]

A double-blind crossover trial of 24 patients on phenytoin who were given 4–6 mg clonazepam showed that over a 2-month period their mean serum phenytoin levels fell by about 18%.[9]

Other studies describe similar findings with diazepam[10] and clonazepam.[13]

(c) Unaltered phenytoin serum levels

Unaltered phenytoin levels have been described in other reports with clonazepam.[13,14]

In addition to all these reports, a study in patients given 250–400 mg phenytoin daily showed that the clonazepam serum levels over a 3-week period were reduced by more than 50% (from 183 to 81 ng/ml).[17]

Mechanism

The inconsistency of these reports is not understood. Benzodiazepine-induced changes in the metabolism of the phenytoin, both enzyme induction and inhibition,[9,10,13] as well as alterations in the apparent volume of distribution, have been discussed. Enzyme induction may possibly account for the fall in serum clonazapam levels.

Importance and management

A confusing picture. The concurrent use of benzodiazepines and phenytoin certainly need not be avoided (and has proved to be successful in many cases), but the serum phenytoin concentrations should be monitored so that undesirable changes can be detected. Only diazepam, chlordiazepoxide, nitrazepam and clonazepam have been implicated, but it would seem possible that the other benzodiazepines may interact similarly.

References

1 Vajda F J E, Prineas R J and Lovell R R H. Interaction between phenytoin and the benzodiazepines. *Lancet* (1971) **i**, 346.
2 Eeg-Oloffson O. Experiences with Rivotril in treatment with epilepsy—particularly minor motor epilepsy—in mentally retarded children. *Acta Neurol Scand* (1973) **49** (Suppl 53), 29.
3 Kutt H and McDowell F J. Management of epilepsy with diphenylhydantoin sodium. *J Amer Med Ass* (1968) **203**, 969.
4 Rogers H J, Haslam R A, Longstreth J and Lietman P S. Diphenylhydantoin–diazepam interaction: a pharmacokinetic analysis. *Pediatr Res* (1975) **9**, 286.

5 Rogers H J, Haslam R A, Longstreth J and Lietman P S. Phenytoin intoxication during concurrent diazepam therapy. *J Neurol Neurosurg Psychiat* (1977) **40**, 890.
6 Treasure T and Toseland P A. Hyperglycaemia due to phenytoin toxicity. *Arch Dis Child* (1971) **46**, 563.
7 Windorfer P. Drug interactions during anticonvulsive therapy. *Int. J Clin Pharmacol* (1976) **14**, 231.
8 Siris J H, Pippenger C E, Werner W L and Masland R L. Anticonvulsant drug–serum levels in psychiatric patients with seizure disorders. *NY State J Med* (1974) **74**, 1554.
9 Edwards V E and Eadie M J. Clonazepam—a clinical study of its effectiveness as an anticonvulsant. *Proc Aus Assoc Neurol* (1973) **10**, 61.
10 Houghton G W and Richens A. The effect of benzodiazepines and pheneturide on phenytoin metabolism in man. *Br J Clin Pharmacol* (1974) **1**, P344.
11 Kaviks J, Berry S W and Wood D. Serum folic acid and phenytoin levels in permanently hospitalized patients receiving anticonvulsant drug therapy. *Med J Aust* (1971) **2**, 369.
12 Shuttleworth E, Wise G and Paulson G. Choreoathetosis and diphenylhydantoin intoxication. *J Amer med Ass* (1974) **230**, 1170.
13 Huang C Y, McLeod J G, Sampson D and Hensley W J. Clonazepam in the treatment of epilepsy. *Med J Aust* (1974) **2**, 5.
14 Johannessen S I, Strandjord E E and Munthe-Kaas A W. Lack of effect of clonazepam on serum levels of diphenylhydantoin, phenobarbital and carbamazepine. *Acta Neurol Scand* (1977) **55**, 506.
15 Janz D and Schneider H. Bericht über *Wodadiboff* II. In 'Antiepileptische Langzeitmedikation' *Biblthea Psychiatr* (1975) **151**, 55 (Karger Verlag, Basel).
16 Windorfer A and Sauer W. Drug interactions during anticonvulsant therapy in childhood: diphenylhydantoin, primidone, phenobarbitone, clonazepam, nitrazepam, carbamazepam and dipropylacetate. *Neuropaediatric* (1977) **8**, 29.
17 Sjö O, Hvidberg E F, Naestroft J and Lund M. Pharmacokinetics and side-effects of clonazepam and its 7-amino metabolite in man. *Europ J Clin Pharmacol* (1975) **8**, 249.

Phenytoin + carbamazepine

Summary

When phenytoin and carbamazine are administered together, the serum concentrations of each may be depressed by the presence of the other.

Interaction

(a) Reduction in serum phenytoin levels caused by carbamazepine

Carbamazepine, in daily doses of 600 mg, was found to have caused a decline in the serum phenytoin levels of 3 out of 7 patients, 4–14 days after its addition to their phenytoin dosage regimen. Their serum phenytoin concentrations fell from 15 to 7 μg/ml, 18 to 12 μg/ml and 16 to 10 μg/ml respectively, but returned to their previous values 10 days after withdrawal of the carbamazepine.[1]

This reduction by carbamazepine of the serum levels of phenytoin has also been described in a number of other reports,[2,3,6] although there is one exception which claims a quantitatively insignificant *rise* instead.[4]

(b) Reduction in serum carbamazepine levels caused by phenytoin

A series of multiple regression analyses carried out on data from a large number of patients (the precise number is not clear from the report), showed that phenytoin had a statistically significant effect in the serum carbamazepine levels, the average reduction being 0·9 μg/ml for each 2 mg/kg of phenytoin taken each day.[4]

Decreased carbamazepine serum levels have been described in another study.[7]

Mechanism

The most likely explanation of the reduced phenytoin serum levels is that the carbamazepine induces the liver microsomal enzymes concerned with the metabolism of the phenytoin, so that it is cleared from the body more quickly. A study associated with the report already cited,[1] observed that after at least 9 days' treatment with carbamazepine, the half-life of phenytoin in 5 epileptics was shortened from 10·6 to 6·4 h. This suggested mechanism remains unconfirmed. Just why some, but not all, patients demonstrate this interaction is not clear.

It has also been suggested that the reduced serum carbamazepine levels may also be accounted for by a similar effect of phenytoin on the metabolism of the carbamazepine.[5]

Importance and management

Although serum levels of each anticonvulsant can fall as a result of concurrent treatment, there seems to be no direct evidence that seizure control is made more difficult as a result. However, the interaction should be borne in mind, particularly when serum levels of the two drugs are monitored during epileptic treatment.

References

1 Hansen J M, Siersboek-Nielsen K and Skovsted L. Carbamazepine-induced acceleration of diphenylhydantoin and warfarin administration in man. *Clin Pharmacol Ther* (1971) **12**, 539.

2 Cereghino J J, van Meter J.C, Brock J T, Penry J K, Smith L D and White B G. Preliminary observations of serum carbamazepine concentration in epileptic patients. *Neurology* (Minneap) (1973) **23**, 357.

3 Hooper W D, Dubetz D K, Eadie M J and Tyrer J H. Preliminary observations on the clinical pharmacology of carbamazepine ('Tegretol'). *Proc Aust Assoc Neurol* (1974) **11**, 189.

4 Lander C M, Eadie M J and Tyrer J H. Interactions between anticonvulsants. *Proc Aust Assoc Neurol* (1975) **12**, 111.

5 Christiansen J and Dam M. Influence of phenobarbital and diphenylhydantoin on plasma carbamazepine levels in patients with epilepsy. *Acta Neurol Scandinav* (1973) **49**, 543.

6 Windorfer A and Sauer W. Drug interactions during anticonvulsant therapy in childhood: diphenylhydantoin, primidone, phenobarbitone, clonazepam, intrazepam, carbamazepine and dipropylacetate. *Neuropädiatrie* (1977) **8**, 29.

7 Cereghino J J, Block J T, van Meter J C, Penry J K, Smith L D and White B G. The efficacy of carbamazepine combinations in epilepsy. *Clin Pharmacol Ther* (1975) **18**, 733.

Phenytoin + chloramphenicol

Summary

The serum levels of phenytoin can be raised by the concurrent use of chloramphenicol to concentrations which, in some cases, may be high enough to manifest toxicity.

Interaction

A study on 5 patients[1] showed that the half-life of phenytoin was more than doubled by the administration of chloramphenicol. The serum phenytoin levels of 1 patient taking 250 mg phenytoin daily rose from about 2 μg/ml to between 7 and 11 μg/ml within 4 days of additionally taking 2 g chloramphenicol a day.

A man taking 400 mg phenytoin a day developed signs of phenytoin toxicity and a serum concentration of 24 μg/ml within a week of beginning treatment with chloramphenicol (four 6-hourly doses of 1 g intravenously initially, followed by 2 g every 6 h). His initial phenytoin serum concentration is not known precisely but it was probably about 7 μg/ml.[2] This case is confused by a number of changes in the treatment being given. See the illustration on p. 8.

This interaction has been described in a number of other reports.[3,4,6]

Mechanism

The most probable explanation of this interaction is that chloramphenicol, a known enzyme-inhibiting drug,[5] inhibits the liver microsomal enzymes concerned with the metabolism of phenytoin, thereby reducing its rate of clearance from the body. If the dosage of the anticonvulsant remains unaltered (as in the cases cited), the phenytoin will accumulate and the serum levels may rise to concentrations at which the toxic effects of the phenytoin will manifest themselves.

Importance and management

The information available indicates that a two- to four-fold rise in serum phenytoin levels can occur within a few days of beginning concurrent treatment with chloramphenicol. Whether or not all patients demonstrate this interaction has yet to be confirmed, but it would be prudent to assume that they will. Chloramphenicol is usually only given to treat serious acute infections for short periods so that the interaction may be accommodated by close monitoring of serum phenytoin levels, and dosage adjustments. An alternative (and probably better) solution is to use a non-interacting antibiotic.

References

1 Christensen L K and Skovsted L. Inhibition of drug metabolism by chloramphenicol. *Lancet* (1969) **ii**, 1397.

2 Ballek R E, Reidenberg M M and Orr L. Inhibition of DPH metabolism by chloramphenicol. *Lancet* (1973) **i**, 150.

3 Houghton G W and Richens A. Inhibition of phenytoin metabolism by other drugs used in epilepsy. *Int J Clin Pharmacol* (1975) **12**, 210.

4 Rose J Q, Choi H K, Schentag J J, Kinkel W R and Jusko W J. Intoxication caused by interaction of chloramphenicol and phenytoin. *J Amer med Ass* (1977) **237**, 2630.

5 Dixon R L, and Fouts J R. Inhibition of microsomal drug metabolic pathway by chloramphenicol. *Biochem Pharmacol* (1962) **11**, 715.

6 Koup J R, Gibaldi M, McNamara P, Hilligoss D M, Colburn W A and Bruck E. Interaction of chloramphenicol with phenytoin and phenobarbital. *Clin Pharmacol Ther* (1978) **24**, 571.

Phenytoin + chlorpheniramine

Summary

Two isolated cases of phenytoin intoxication have been reported in patients concurrently treated with phenytoin and chlorpheniramine.

Interaction

An epileptic woman, taking daily doses of 60 mg phenobarbitone and 300 mg phenytoin, developed phenytoin intoxication a week or so after starting to take 4 mg chlorpheniramine three times a day. Her serum phenytoin levels were found to be about 65 μg/ml. The toxic symptoms disappeared and the plasma levels fell when the chlorpheniramine was withdrawn.[1]

An epileptic woman, on treatment with anticonvulsants including 250 mg phenytoin daily, was given 12–16 mg of chlorpheniramine daily for hay fever. Twelve days later she showed slight grimacing movements of the face and involuntary movements of the jaw, but no speech slurring, ataxia or nystagmus although the serum phenytoin levels were later found to be 30 μg/ml. When the chlorpheniramine was withdrawn, the abnormal movements vanished and the serum phenytoin levels fell to about 16 μg/ml.[2]

Mechanism

Uncertain, but it seems probable that the chlorpheniramine inhibit the liver microsomal enzymes concerned with the phenytoin metabolism, thereby allowing the anticonvulsant to accumulate in the body.

Importance and management

The general importance is uncertain. Only 2 cases of an adverse interaction with an antihistamine phenothiazine have been reported, although there are a few reports involving neuroleptic phenothiazines (see p. 206). Concurrent use is not generally contraindicated, but it would clearly be prudent to be on the alert for the development of phenytoin intoxication if this type of antihistamine is used. There seem to be no reports of interactions with other antihistamines.

References

1 Pugh R N H, Geddes A M and Yeoman W B. Interaction of phenytoin with chlorpheniramine. *Br J clin Pharmac* (1975) 2, 173.
2 Ahmad S, Laidlaw J, Houghton G W and Richens A. Involuntary movements caused by phenytoin intoxication in epileptic patients. *J Neurol Neurosurg Psychiat* (1975) 38, 225.

Phenytoin + cimetidine

Summary

Phenytoin serum levels can be raised by the concurrent use of cimetidine, and mild phenytoin intoxication has been observed. A case of severe neutropenia attributed to concurrent use has been described.

Interaction

A study on 9 patients taking phenytoin showed that concurrent treatment with cimetidine (1 g daily) over a three-week period increased the steady-state serum phenytoin levels by 60% (from 5·7 to 9·1 μg/ml). Two weeks after the cimetidine was withdrawn the serum phenytoin levels had fallen once again to virtually the former levels (5·8 μg/ml).[1]

Smaller rises (13–33% in serum phenytoin levels have been described in another report, and the development of mild phenytoin toxicity in one patient.[3] A single case of severe and life-threatening neutropenia attributed to the concurrent use of high doses of these drugs has also been reported.[2]

Mechanisms

A study run concurrently with the one cited,[1] using antipyrine as a marker of changes in liver enzyme metabolism, indicated that the cimetidine can act as an inhibitor of phenytoin metabolism, thereby prolonging its stay in the body. This is reflected in rise in the serum phenytoin levels.[1]

Both cimetidine and phenytoin are known to be able to depress the activity of the bone marrow in some patients, and some synergistic action may possibly account for the neutropenia described.[2]

Importance and management

Only one case of phenytoin intoxication appears to have been reported and the information seems to be limited to the studies described.[1] It would be prudent to keep a close check on the phenytoin serum levels of patients who are given cimetidine to confirm that concentrations do not rise to toxic proportions. More study is needed to confirm the general importance and incidence of this interaction. It has also been suggested[2] that peripheral blood counts should be monitored carefully if these drugs are used together.

References
1 Neuvonen P J, Riitta A, Tokola R and Kaste M. Cimetidine–phenytoin interaction: effect on serum phenytoin concentration and antipyrine test in man. *Naunyn-Schmied Arch Pharmacol* (1980) **313** (Suppl) R60.
2 Sazie E and Jaffe J P. Severe granulocytopenia with cimetidine and phenytoin. *Ann Int Med* (1980) **93**, 151.
3 Hetzel D J., Bochner F., Hallpike J F., Shearman D J C and Hann C S. Cimetidine interaction with phenytoin. *Brit. Med. J.* (1981) **282**, 1512

Phenytoin + dextropropoxyphene

Summary

Elevated serum phenytoin levels caused by the use of dextropropoxyphene have been described in an isolated report.

Interaction, mechanism, importance and management
An isolated case has been reported of a patient who showed a marked elevation of the serum phenytoin levels while also taking dextropropoxyphene.[1] Concurrent use would not seem to be generally contraindicated, but prescribers should be aware of this interaction.

Reference
1 Kutt H. Biochemical and genetic factors regulating Dilantin metabolism in man. *Ann NY Acad Sci* (1971) **179**, 704.

Phenytoin + diazoxide

Summary

Two reports indicate that phenytoin serum levels can be markedly reduced by the concurrent use of diazoxide. There is some evidence that the effects of diazoxide may also be reduced.

Interaction
Therapeutic serum levels of phenytoin (10–20 μg/ml) were not achieved in 2 children, receiving 17 and 30 mg/kg/day phenytoin respectively, while concurrently taking diazoxide. Once the diazoxide was withdrawn, satisfactory phenytoin serum levels were achieved with phenytoin dosages of only 6·6 and 10 mg/kg/day. When diazoxide was restarted in one of them experimentally, serum phenytoin levels fell to undetectable levels over 3 days and seizures occurred.[1,2]

Another report[3] similarly describes this interaction and, in addition, it would appear that the effects of the diazoxide were also reduced.[3,4]

Mechanism
Clinical and laboratory data obtained from the studies cited[1,2,3] indicate that the diazoxide increases the metabolism of the phenytoin and its clearance from the body. Protein binding displacement may also have some part to play. The half-life of diazoxide is reduced by phenytoin.[4]

Importance and management
An established interaction, but its incidence is not known. Information about this interaction is limited but it is clearly of importance. Increased dosages of phenytoin may be necessary during the concurrent use of diazoxide if seizure control is to be maintained, and reduced dosages following its withdrawal if phenytoin toxicity is to be avoided. There is less information about the effects of phenytoin on diazoxide, but its effects would also seem to be reduced.

References
1 Roe T F, Podosin R L and Blaskovics M E. Drug Interaction. Diazoxide and Diphenylhydantoin. *Pediatr Res* (1975) **9**, 285.
2 Roe T F, Podosin R L and Blaskovics M E. Drug Interaction. Diazoxide and diphenylhydantoin. *J Pediatr* (1975) **87**, 480.
3 Petro D J, Vannucci R C and Kulin H E. Diazoxide-diphenylhydantoin interaction. *J Pediatr* (1975) **89**, 331.
4 Pruitt A W, Dayton P G and Patterson J H. Disposition of Diazoxide in children. *Clin Pharmacol Ther* (1973) **14**, 73.

Phenytoin + dichloralphenazone

Summary

Serum phenytoin levels may be reduced by the concurrent use of dichloralphenazone.

Interaction, mechanism, importance and management

A study in 5 normal subjects showed that the total body clearance of phenytoin administered intravenously was doubled when they were given 1 g dichloralphenazone each night for 13 nights.[1] The phenazone component of the dichloralphenazone is a known enzyme-inducer and the increased clearance of the phenytoin may be due to an enhancement of its metabolism. This requires confirmation. The clinical importance of this interaction is as yet uncertain, but it would seem prudent to be on the alert for some loss in seizure control if dichloralphenazone is added to an established phenytoin regimen.

Reference

1 Riddell J G, Salem S A M and McDevitt D G. Interaction between phenytoin and dichloralphenazone. *Br J Clin Pharmacol* (1980) **9**, 118 P.

Phenytoin + disulfiram

Summary

Serum levels of phenytoin can be markedly and rapidly increased by the concurrent use of disulfiram. Phenytoin intoxication may develop. There is evidence that phenobarbitone is not affected by disulfiram.

Interaction

The phenytoin–disulfiram interaction was first observed in epileptic patients in Dianalund in Denmark.[1,5] It was subsequently thoroughly investigated:

Four patients on long-term treatment with phenytoin were concurrently administered 400 mg disulfiram daily for a period of 9 days. Rises in the serum phenytoin concentrations of 100–500% were seen with no signs of levelling off until the disulfiram was withdrawn. Two of the patients developed mild signs of intoxication. The other drugs being taken by the patients included primidone, carbamazepine, thioridazine, amitryptyline and chlorpromazine.[2] In a follow-up study on 2 patients, 1 of them showed ataxia and a rise in phenytoin serum levels from about 18 to 28 µg/ml within 5 days of starting to take the disulfiram.[3]

An investigation on 10 volunteers showed that within 4 days of beginning to take oral doses of disulfiram (1st day 400 mg three times a day, 2nd day 400 mg, and 3rd and 4th days 200 mg) the half-life of intravenously administered phenytoin increased from 11 to 19 h. No other drugs were given.[4]

There is another case report of this interaction.[6]

Mechanism

The disulfiram inhibits the liver enzymes concerned with the metabolism of the phenytoin, thereby prolonging its stay in the body and resulting in a rise in serum levels (in some instances to toxic concentrations). In the study cited,[4] the half-life of the phenytoin was increased by 70% and its clearance rate reduced by one-third during treatment with disulfiram.

Importance and management

A well-established, important, and potentially serious interaction. Its incidence is not known precisely, but the available evidence indicates that it is high. It develops rapidly, Olesen, who was responsible for the early studies described[2,3] has offered the opinion that the dose of phenytoin '. . . could of course be reduced, but it would be difficult to maintain the very precise balance required . . .'. An alternative would be to use calcium carbimide instead of disulfiram. A study in 4 patients[3] showed that 50 mg daily for a week, followed by 100 mg daily for 2 weeks, had no effect on the serum levels of phenytoin, and signs of phenytoin toxicity were absent. Another solution might be to use another anticonvulsant. The serum concentrations of phenobarbitone were observed in parallel experiments[2,3] to those already discussed to have fluctuated at the most by 10% when disulfiram was taken concurrently. Three of the patients were taking primidone and the other patient phenobarbitone. In the single case mentioned[6] signs of toxicity disappeared when the phenytoin was replaced by carbamazepine.

References

1 Kiorboe E. Phenytoin intoxication during treatment with Antabuse. *Epilepsia* (1966) 7, 246.

2 Olesen O V. Disulfiramum (Antabuse) as inhibitor of phenytoin metabolism. *Acta pharmacol et toxicol* (1966) 24, 317.

3 Olesen O V. The influence of disulfiram and calcium carbimide on the serum diphenylhydantoin excretion of HPPH in the urine. *Arch Neurol* (1967) 16, 642.

4 Svendsen T L, Kristensen M B, Hansen J M and Skovsted L. The influence of disulfiram on the half life and metabolic clearance rate of diphenylhydantoin and tolbutamide in man. *Europ J clin Pharmacol* (1976) 9, 439.

5 Kiorboe E. Antabus som arsag til forgifttning med fenytoin. *Ugeskr laeg* (1966) 128, 1531.

6 Dry J and Pradalier A. Intoxication par la phénytoïn au cours d'une association thérapeutique avec le disulfirame. *Thérapie* (1973) 28, 799.

Phenytoin, Phenobarbitone, or primidone + folic acid

Summary

If folic acid supplements are given to treat anticonvulsant-induced folate deficiency, the serum anticonvulsant levels may be reduced, leading to a decreased seizure control in some patients.

Interaction

Epileptic patients taking phenytoin, and other anticonvulsants, can become folate deficient. The administration of folic acid supplements can result in reduced serum anticonvulsant levels, and lead to a loss in seizure control.

A study over a 1–3 year period on 26 epileptic patients with folic acid deficiency (less than 5 ng/ml) due to anticonvulsant treatment with two or more drugs (phenytoin, phenobarbitone, primidone), showed that when they were also given 15 mg folic acid daily the mental state of 22 of them improved to a variable degree, but the frequency and severity of fits in 13 (50%) increased to such an extent that the vitamin had to be withdrawn.[1]

Another study on 50 folate-deficient epileptics, taking phenytoin with phenobarbitone and primidone, showed that after 1 months' treatment with 5 mg folic acid daily, the serum phenytoin levels of one group (10 patients) fell from 20 to 10 μg/ml, and of the other group taking 15 mg daily, from 14 to 10 μg/ml. Only 1 patient showed a marked increase in fit frequency and severity.[2]

Similar results have been described in other studies and reports.[2,3,8]

Mechanism

Patients taking anticonvulsants not infrequently show subnormal serum folic acid levels. This can be reflected in a depression of their general mental health and even in frank megaloblastic anaemia in some instances.[7] One study,[4] for example, found that out of a total of 149 epileptics taking phenytoin, phenobarbitone and primidone, either singly or in combination, 87 of them (58%) had low serum folic acid levels. Other studies had indicated percentages between 27 and 76.[4]

One theory to account for this is that the enzyme-inducing characteristics of the anticonvulsants, particularly phenytoin, make excessive demands on folate as a co-factor in drug hydroxylation so that serum folate levels become depressed. Ultimately the drug metabolism becomes limited by the lack of folate, and even the production of red cells may suffer.

If, however, a folic acid supplement is given to treat this folate deficiency, the metabolism of the anticonvulsant is no longer held back by the lack of folate and continues again unchecked, resulting in a reduction in serum anticonvulsant levels which, in some instances, may become so low that seizure control is partially or totally lost.

Importance and management

A well-documented and important interaction. If folic acid is given to patients already taking anticonvulsants (and phenytoin in particular) some reduction in serum anticonvulsant levels may occur. Various studies[2,5] describe reductions of 16–50% in serum phenytoin levels after taking 5–15 mg daily doses of folic acid for periods of 2–4 weeks. This could clearly lead to a reduction in seizure control in some patients.

The incidence is not certain. One study[1] claimed that it was as high as 50% (13 out of 26), another[2] only 2% (1 out of 50). Yet another stated that no loss of seizure control was seen (51 patients).[6] Mary Bayliss and her colleagues have suggested that folic acid supplements should only be given to folate-deficient epileptics taking phenytoin or other anticonvulsants when there can be effective monitoring of their serum anticonvulsant concentrations.[2]

References

1 Reynolds E H. Effects of folic acid on the mental state and fit-frequency of drug-treated epileptic patients. *Lancet* (1967) i, 1086.
2 Baylis E M, Crowley J M, Preece J M, Sylvester P E and Marks V. Influence of folic acid on blood-phenytoin levels. *Lancet* (1971) i, 62.
3 Strauss R G and Bernstein R. Folic acid and *Dilantin* antagonism in pregnancy. *Obstet Gynecol* (1974) 44, 345.
4 Davis R E and Woodliff H J. Folic acid deficiency in patients receiving anticonvulsant drugs. *Med J Aust* (1971) 2, 1070.
5 Furlanut M, Benetello P, Avogaro A and Dainese R. Effects of folic acid on phenytoin kinetics in healthy subjects. *Clin Pharmacol Ther* (1978) 24, 294.
6 Grant R H E and Stores O P R. Folic acid in folate-deficient patients with epilepsy. *Br Med J* (1970) 4, 644.
7 Ryan G M S and Forshaw J W B. Megaloblastic anaemia due to phenytoin sodium. *Br Med J* (1955) 11, 242.
8 Latham A N, Millbank L, Richens A and Rowe D J F. Liver enzyme induction by anticonvulsant drugs, and its relationship to disturbed calcium and folic acid metabolism. *J Clin Pharmacol* (1973) 13, 337.

Phenytoin + food

Summary

Because the absorption of phenytoin is accelerated, and possibly increased, if it is taken with food, it should be taken consistently with or without a meal. Those who experience mild transient toxic effects might be advised not to take phenytoin with food.

Interaction

A study, carried out on eight healthy volunteers who were given single 300 mg oral doses of phenytoin as the acid in a micronized form (*Fentoin*, ACO, Sweden), showed that concurrent ingestion with a meal accelerated the absorption of the phenytoin. The peak serum concentrations averaged 40% higher than when taken without food and the areas under the absorption curves were increased by 27%.[1]

Mechanism

Not known. The authors of this report suggest that drug dissolution and dispersion is improved by the prolonged retention of the phenytoin tablet in the upper part of the gastrointestinal tract by the presence of the food and, moreover, food-induced secretion of bile might enhance the dissolution of phenytoin which is lipophilic.[1]

Importance and management

With the particular preparation used in the study described, the total amount of phenytoin absorbed is unlikely to be altered by food,[2,3] but with some other non-micronized preparations it seems probable that the absorption may be far from complete[3] and food intake may, therefore, markedly affect how much is eventually absorbed. It has been suggested[1] that it would be reasonable to take phenytoin either always with, or always without, food to avoid causing unnecessary fluctuations in serum phenytoin levels. Those patients who experience transient toxic effects during the 4–6 h after taking phenytoin with a meal might also benefit from taking it several hours before a meal, so that the peak serum levels are lowered and the absorption prolonged.

References

1 Melander A, Brante G, Johansson Ö and Wåhlin-Boll E. Influence of food on the absorption of phenytoin in man. *Europ J Clin Pharmacol* (1979) 15, 269.
2 Rane A. Personal Communication cited in 1.
3 Lund L. Clinical significance of generic inequivalence of three different pharmaceutical preparations of phenytoin. *Europ J Clin Pharmacol* (1974) 7, 119.

Phenytoin + hypoglycaemic agents

Summary

Large and toxic doses of phenytoin have been observed to cause hyperglycaemia, but normal doses do not usually affect the control of diabetes. A single case has been reported in which tolazamide cause the development of phenytoin intoxication.

Interactions

(a) The effect of phenytoin on the response to hypoglycaemic agents

Although phenytoin has been shown in a number of reports[1-4,7,8] to elevate the blood sugar levels of both diabetic and non-diabetics, in virtually all the cases on record the phenytoin dosage was large or even in the toxic range, and there is no evidence that a hyperglycaemic response to average doses of phenytoin is normally sufficiently large to interfere with the control of diabetes either with diet alone or with conventional hypoglycaemic agents. In a single case[2] involving hyperglycaemia in which both phenytoin and insulin were used concurrently, the situation was complicated by the use of other drugs and by kidney impairment, so that no general conclusions can be drawn.

(b) The effect of a hypoglycaemic agents on the response to phenytoin

A single case has been reported of a man in whom the concurrent administration of phenytoin, 50 mg three times a day, led, after several weeks, to the development of phenytoin intoxication (ataxia, drowsiness etc.), which disappeared when the tolazamide was replaced by insulin.[10]

An investigation in 17 epileptic patients under treatment with phenytoin, 100–400 mg daily, and who were given 500 mg tolbutamide three times a day, showed that although there was a transient rise in the amount of non-protein-bound phenytoin, no signs of phenytoin intoxication appeared.[11]

Mechanisms

Investigations in animals and man[5,6] suggest that the phenytoin-induced hyperglycaemia comes about because the release of insulin from the pancreas is impaired. This implies that no interaction is possible in those without functional pancreatic tissue. The tolazamide/phenytoin interaction remains unexplained.[12]

Importance and management

The evidence suggests that no interaction of importance normally occurs between these drugs. Millichap, one of the investigators of the hyperglycaemic effects of phenytoin, has observed that '... from a practical standpoint a diabetogenic effect is a very unlikely hazard of diphenylhydantoin (phenytoin) therapy. Indeed, in the management of epilepsy in patients with juvenile diabetes, we have observed that diphenylhydantoin is not contraindicated when given in average doses, and the control of seizures with this anticonvulsant generally does not necessitate the use of larger amounts of insulin.'[4]

There is only one case on record of a sulphonylurea/phenytoin interaction, and the evidence suggests that it is unusual.

References

1 Klein J P. Diphenylhydantoin intoxication associated with hyperglycaemia. *J Paediat* (1966) **69**, 463.
2 Goldberg E M and Sanbar S S. Hyperglycaemic, non-ketotic coma following administration of Dilantin (diphenylhydantoin). *Diabetes* (1969) **18**, 101.
3 Peters B H and Samaan N A. Hyperglycaemia with relative hypoinsulinaemia in diphenylhydantoin intoxication. *New Eng J Med* (1969) **281**, 91.
4 Millichap J G. Hyperglycaemic effect of diphenylhydantoin. *New Eng J Med* (1969) **281**, 447.
5 Kizer J S, Cordon-Vargas M, Brendel K and Bressler R. The in-vitro inhibition of insulin secretion by diphenylhydantoin. *J Clin Invest* (1970) **49**, 1942.
6 Levin S R, Booker J, Smith D F and Grodsky M. Inhibition of insulin secretion by diphenylhydantoin in the isolated perfused pancreas. *J Clin Endocrinol Metab* (1970) **30**, 400.
7 Fariss B L and Lutcher C L. Diphenylhydantoin-induced hyperglycaemia and impaired insulin release. *Diabetes* (1971) **46**, 563.
8 Treasure T and Toseland P A. Hyperglycaemia due to phenytoin toxicity. *Arch Dis Childh* (1971) **46**, 563.
9 Malherbe C, Burrill K C, Levin S R, Karam J H and Forsham P H. Effect of diphenylhydantoin on insulin secretion in man. *New Eng J Med* (1972) **286**, 339.
10 Pannekoek J.H. (1969). Cited in 11.
11 Wesseling H and Mols-Thürkow I. Diphenylhydantoin (DPH) and tolbutamide in man. *Europ J clin Pharmacol* (1975) **8**, 75.
12 Wesseling H, Mols-Thürkow I and Mulder G J. Effect of sulphonylureas (tolazamide, tolbutamide and chlorpropamide) on the metabolism of diphenylhydantoin in the rat. *Biochem Pharmacol* (1973) **22**, 3033.

Phenytoin + isoniazid

Summary

The administration of isoniazid to epileptic patients taking phenytoin can result in a rise in serum phenytoin levels. Those who are 'slow' metabolizers of isoniazid (10–25%) may develop phenytoin intoxication if suitable dosage adjustments are not made.

Interaction

The first indication that isoniazid could induce phenytoin intoxication was reported in 1962 when approximately 10% of the 637 patients in a school for epileptics, who were additionally taking phenobarbitone and who were also treated with daily doses of 300 mg or less of isoniazid, developed drowsiness, incoordination and an unsteady gait.[1]

Further studies of this interaction[3,4] showed that it takes place in about 10% of the patients taking normal doses of phenytoin and isoniazid, and that these patients have unusually high serum levels of isoniazid. Phenytoin, in daily doses of 300 mg, was administered to 32 patients who were also taking 300 mg isoniazid and 15 g para-aminosalicylic acid daily. Within a week, 6 of them had phenytoin serum levels which averaged almost 5 μg/ml higher than the rest of the group and, on the following days when the levels climbed above 20 μg/ml, the typical signs of phenytoin toxicity were seen. These 6 all demonstrated unusually high serum isonizid serum levels.

Phenytoin toxicity induced by the concurrent use of isoniazid has been reported on a number of subsequent occasions,[2,5-9,11] one of which describes a fatality. The incidence of this interaction would appear to be between 10 and 25% of those administered both drugs.

Mechanism

Isoniazid inhibits the liver microsomal enzymes concerned with the metabolism of phenytoin, as a result the phenytoin accumulates and its serum levels rise.[3,4] The reason that only a proportion of patients show this interaction to any great extent is because some people are 'fast' and others 'slow' metabolizers of isoniazid, the particular category being genetically determined. Those who are 'slow' isoniazid metabolizers attain blood levels of isoniazid which are sufficiently high to cause considerable inhibition of phenytoin metabolism, whereas the 'fast' metabolizers remove the isoniazid too quickly for this to occur. Some individuals therefore will show a rapid rise in phenytoin levels which will eventually reach toxic levels, whereas others will show only a relatively slow and unimportant rise to a plateau within, or slightly above, the usual therapeutic range.[3,4] It has been confirmed in animal experiments that the degree of inhibition by isoniazid of phenytoin metabolism is in direct proportion to the isoniazid concentrations.[4]

Animal experiments have also shown that cycloserine and para-aminosalicylic acid possess enzyme-inhibitory activity, but isoniazid is by far the most potent of the three.[10] Whether in combined anti-tubercular therapy their actions are additive, or whether they can decrease the rate of acetylation of isoniazid and thereby magnify its inhibitory activity, is not certain.

Importance and management

A well-documented, well-established and potentially serious interaction. About 50% of the population are slow or relatively slow metabolizers of isoniazid, but not all of them are likely to have their serum phenytoin levels increased by isoniazid into the toxic range (beginning at about 20 μg/ml). Different reports indicate that somewhere between 10 and 25% of those given both drugs may demonstrate this interaction.[1,2,3,4,11]

It is important to emphasize that the development of the adverse effects may take only a few days in some patients, but several weeks in others, so that patients taking both drugs should be kept under observation for signs of phenytoin toxicity or, better, their serum phenytoin levels should be monitored closely.

The interaction can be accommodated by suitable dosage reductions of the phenytoin.

References

1 Murray F J. Outbreak of unexpected reactions among epileptics taking isoniazid. *Amer Rev Resp Dis* (1962) **86**, 729.
2 Kutt H, Winters W, McDowell F H. Depression of para-hydroxylation of diphenylhydantoin by antituberculosis chemotherapy. *Neurol* (1966) **16**, 594.
3 Kutt H, Brennan R, Dehejia H and Verebeley K. Diphenylhydantoin intoxication. A complication of isoniazid therapy. *Amer Rev Resp Dis* (1970) **101**, 377.

4 Brennan R W, Dehejia H, Kutt H, Verebeley K and McDowell F. Diphenylhydantoin intoxication attendant to slow inactivation of isomazid. *Neurology* (1970) **20**, 687.

5 Manigand G, Thieblot Ph, and Deparis M. Accidents de la diphénylhydantoïne induits par les traitements antituberculeux. *Presse Med* (1971) **79**, 815.

6 Beauvais P, Mercier D, Hanoteau J. and Brissand H-E. Intoxication a la diphénylhydantoïne induite par l'isoniazide. *Arch Franc Péd* (1973) **30**, 541.

7 Johnson J. Epanutin and isoniazid interaction. *Br Med J* (1975) **1**, 152.

8 Johnson J and Freeman H L. Death due to isoniazid (INH) and phenytoin. *Br J Psychiatr* (1975) **129**, 511.

9 Geering J M, Ruch W and Dettli L. Diphenylhydantoin-Intoxikation durch Diphenylhydantoin–Isoniazid-Interaktion. *Schweiz med Wschr* (1974) **104**, 1224.

10 Kutt H, Verebeley K and McDowell F. Inhibition of diphenylhydantoin metabolism in rats and in rat liver microsomes by anti-tubercular drugs. *Neurology* (1968) **18**, 706.

11 Miller R R, Porter J and Greenblatt D J. Clinical importance of the interaction of phenytoin and isoniazid. A report from the Boston Collaborative Drug Surveilance program. *Chest* (1979) **75**, 356.

Phenytoin + loxapine

Summary

A single case report describes depressed serum phenytoin levels during concurrent treatment with loxapine. This neuroleptic also lowers the convulsive threshold.

Interaction

A single case report states that, during concurrent treatment with loxapine, the serum phenytoin levels of an epileptic patient were depressed, but showed a marked rise when the loxapine was discontinued.[1]

Mechanism

Unknown.

Importance and management

Quite apart from the implications of the single case described, loxapine can lower the convulsive threshold, particularly in epileptic patients. Considerable care should clearly be exercised if these drugs are used concurrently.

Reference

1 Ryan G M and Matthews P A. Phenytoin metabolism stimulated by loxapine. *Drug Intell Clin Pharm* (1977) **11**, 428.

Phenytoin, phenobarbitone or primidone + methylphenidate

Summary

Elevated serum phenytoin levels and phenytoin toxicity have occurred in 2 patients treated with phenytoin and methylphenidate concurrently, but it is an uncommon reaction. One of the patients also showed raised primidone and phenobarbitone serum levels.

Interaction

A hyperkinetic epileptic boy of five, receiving phenytoin (8·9 mg/kg/day) and primidone (17·7 mg/kg/day), developed ataxia without nystagmus when additionally treated with methylphenidate (20–40 mg daily). The serum levels of the anticonvulsants were found to be raised to toxic levels, and only began to fall when the methylphenidate dosage was reduced. Eventually the methylphenidate was withdrawn because the ataxia continued.[1]

In other clinical studies and observations on 3 subjects,[2] 11 patients,[3] and over a hundred patients,[4] this interaction was not seen, but one other patient[2] demonstrated the symptoms of phenytoin intoxication on one occasion when given methylphenidate concurrently, but later failed to do so. No other changes in primidone or phenobarbitone serum levels have been observed.

Mechanism

It has been suggested[1] that methylphenidate acts as an enzyme inhibitor, slowing the metabolism of the phenytoin and leading to its accumulation in the plasma of just those few individuals where the drug-metabolizing system is virtually saturated by the large doses of phenytoin. Certainly the child described was taking large doses.[1]

Importance and management

This is an uncommon interaction, but its possibility should be borne in mind during concurrent treatment, particularly if the dosages of the anticonvulsants are high.

References

1 Garrettson L K, Perel J M and Dayton P G. Methylphenidate interaction with both anticonvulsants and ethyl biscoumacetate. A new action of methylphenidate. *J Amer Med Ass* (1969) 207, 2053.
2 Mirkin B L and Wright F. Drug interactions: Effect of methylphenidate on the disposition of diphenylhydantoin in man. *Neurology* (1971) 21, 1123.
3 Kupferberg H J, Jeffery W and Hunninghake D B. Effect of methylphenidate on plasma anticonvulsant levels. *Clin Pharmacol Ther* (1972) 13, 201.
4 Oettinger L. Interaction of methylphenidate and diphenylhydantoin. *Drug Ther* (1976) 5, 107.

Phenytoin + para-aminosalicylic acid (PAS)

Summary

An interaction has not been established.

Interaction, mechanism, importance and management

Phenytoin toxicity has been described in patients taking isoniazid and PAS, due to inhibition of the liver enzymes concerned with the metabolism of the phenytoin, but it seems doubtful if this interaction takes place in the absence of isoniazid. See also phenytoin + isoniazid, page 203.

Phenytoin + pheneturide

Summary

Phenytoin serum levels can be raised approximately 50% by the concurrent use of phenturide which may lead to phenytoin intoxication in some cases.

Interaction

A study on 9 patients showed that the half-life of phenytoin was prolonged from 32 to 47 h by the concurrent use of pheneturide. The mean serum concentrations were raised by about 50% (from 35 to 53 μM, but fell rapidly once the pheneturide was withdrawn.[1]

This study confirms a previous report of this interaction.[2]

Mechanism

Uncertain. Pheneturide is similar in structure to phenytoin and it may be that the two drugs compete for the same metabolic enzymes, thereby resulting, at least initially, in a reduction in the metabolism of the phenytoin which results in its accumulation.

Importance and management

Although the documentation is limited it would appear to be a reliably established interaction. Rises in serum phenytoin levels should be expected during concurrent use. In patients with already high serum concentrations, phenytoin intoxication may develop. Appropriate precautions should be taken.

References

1 Houghton G W and Richens A. Inhibition of phenytoin metabolism by other drugs used in epilepsy. *Int J Clin Pharmacol* (1975) 12, 210.
2 Huisman J W, van Heycop Ten Ham M W and van Zijl C H W. Influence of ethylphenacemide on serum levels of other anticonvulsant drugs. *Epilepsia* (1970) 11, 207.

Phenytoin + phenothiazines

Summary

A few reports indicate that occasionally the serum levels of phenytoin can be raised or lowered by the concurrent use of chlorpromazine, thioridazine or prochlorperazine.

Interaction

Phenytoin + chlorpromazine or prochlorperazine

A patient under treatment with daily doses of 300 mg phenytoin, 1 g primidone and 400 mg sulthiame, showed a rise in serum phenytoin levels from about $7 \cdot 5\ \mu g/ml$ to $15\ \mu g/ml$ during 1 month's concurrent treatment with 50 mg chlorpromazine daily. Four other patients similarly treated with 50–100 mg chlorpromazine showed no interaction.[1]

In another report[2] on 3 patients, none showed a rise but 1 showed a fall in serum phenytoin levels. Yet another report[3] simply states (without giving any details) that in rare instances chlorpromazine and prochlorperazine have been noted to impair phenytoin metabolism.

Phenytoin + thioridazine

In a study on 6 patients under treatment with phenytoin, phenobarbitone and thioridazine, 1 patient showed an elevated serum phenytoin concentration ($38\ \mu g/ml$) whereas 4 showed depressed levels.[2]

Phenytoin intoxication has been described in two patients concurrently treated with thioridazine.[4]

Mechanism

Uncertain. One suggestion is that since phenytoin metabolism within the liver is a saturable process, if another drug is added which competes for the same metabolic mechanism, total saturation can occur. This results in a reduction in the metabolism of the phenytoin and a rise in the serum levels.

Importance and management

It would clearly be prudent to watch for changes in phenytoin serum levels during concurrent treatment with chlorpromazine, thioridazine or prochlorperazine, but from the very limited data available it would seem that the incidence of this interaction is low. Whether other phenothiazines behave similarly is uncertain, but not improbable. One which certainly does is the antihistamine phenothiazine, chlorpheniramine (see p. 197).

References

1 Houghton G W and Richens A. Inhibition of phenytoin metabolism by other drugs used in epilepsy. *Int J clin Pharmacol* (1975) **12**, 2210.
2 Siris J H, Pippenger C E, Werner W L and Masland R L. Anticonvulsant drug-serum levels in psychiatric patients with seizure disorders. Effects of certain psychotropic drugs. *New York State J Med* (1974) **74**, 1554.
3 Kutt H and McDowell F. Management of epilepsy with diphenylhydantoin sodium. Dosage regulation for problem patients. *J Amer med Ass* (1968) **203**, 969.
4 Vincent F M. Phenothiazine-induced phenytoin intoxication. *Ann Int Med* (1980) **93**, 56.

Phenytoin + phenylbutazone

Summary

Phenytoin serum levels can be increased by the concurrent use of phenylbutazone. Phenytoin intoxication may develop. Oxyphenbutazone possibly interacts similarly, but this requires confirmation.

Interaction

A study was carried out on 6 epileptics, taking 200–350 mg phenytoin daily, and who were also given 300 mg phenylbutazone a day for a fortnight. During the first 3 days the serum phenytoin levels fell from about 15 to 13 $\mu g/ml$, after which they climbed steadily to about 19 $\mu g/ml$ when the study was completed. One of the patients, who was also taking 600 mg carbamazepine daily, had his first seizure for 2 months within 2 days of starting to take phenylbutazone, thereafter he experienced nausea, dizziness and nervousness. During this period his serum phenytoin levels first fell, and then rose from 15·2 to 21·8 μg/ml over a 9-day period. The symptoms disappeared and the serum phenytoin levels returned to normal within a fortnight of withdrawing the phenylbutazone.[1]

Mechanism

Phenylbutazone, which is a highly plasma protein bound drug, can increase the amount of free and unbound phenytoin molecules in the plasma by displacement.[1] This would seem to be related in some way to the transient fall in serum phenytoin levels during the first 3 days of treatment, but the precise association is not clear. After that, the predominant effect of phenylbutazone is to inhibit the activity of the liver microsomal enzymes concerned with the metabolism of the phenytoin, causing it to accumulate, and the serum levels to rise. This was seen from the 3rd day of treatment and accounts for the development of toxicity in the same patient. This inhibitory effect of phenylbutazone on the metabolism of phenytoin has been clearly demonstrated in animals,[3] and in man, in whom the half-life of phenytoin was shown in one study to be increased from 13·7 to 22 h.[4]

Importance and management

An established and potentially serious interaction, although the documentation is limited. Only 1 patient in the study cited[1] actually demonstrated phenytoin toxicity, although it should be emphasized that the investigation only ran for a fortnight, at the end of which the phenytoin serum levels had reached 19 μg/ml and were still climbing steadily with no sign of a plateau having been reached. So, it seems highly likely that if the study had been continued longer, other patients would have similarly developed intoxication once the 20 μg/ml level had been reached.

Patients treated with both drugs should be closely monitored and suitable phenytoin dosage reductions made where necessary. The incidence is uncertain, but there is evidence that some individuals are much more likely to show this interaction than others.[1,4]

There is no direct evidence that oxyphenbutazone interacts like phenylbutazone, but since it is the main metabolic product of phenylbutazone in the body and, in animal experiments, has been shown to prolong the half-life of phenytoin,[5] it would be prudent to expect it to interact similarly.

References

1 Neuvonen P J, Lehtovaara R, Bardy A and Elomaa E. Antipyretic analgesics in patients on antiepileptic drug therapy. *Europ J clin Pharmacol* (1979) **15**, 263.

2 Lunde P K M. Plasma protein binding of diphenylhydantoin in man: Interaction with other drugs and the effect of temperature and plasma dilution. *Clin Pharmacol Ther* (1970) **11**, 846.

3 Shoeman D M and Azarnoff D L. Diphenylhydantoin potency and plasma protein binding. *J Pharmacol Exp Ther* (1975) **195**, 84.

4 Andreasen P B, Frøland A, Skovsted L, Andersen S A and Hauge M. Diphenylhydantoin half-life in man and its inhibition by phenylbutazone: the role of genetic factors. *Acta Med Scand* (1973) **193**, 561.

5 Soda D M and Levy G. Inhibition of drug metabolism by hydroxylated metabolites: cross-inhibition and specificity. *J Pharm Sci* (1975) **64**, 1928.

Phenytoin + phenyramidol

Summary

Serum levels of phenytoin can be approximately doubled by the concurrent use of phenyramidol.

Interaction

The observation that epileptic patients, poorly controlled on phenytoin, improved when also given phenyramidol prompted a more detailed study. Five human volunteers, given 100 mg phenytoin three times a day, showed an average prolongation of the phenytoin half-life from 25 to 55 h when concurrently treated with 400 mg phenyramidol three times a day. Their average plasma phenytoin levels, at 12 h, were approximately doubled (from 6·6 to 12·0 μg/ml).[1]

Mechanism

The evidence suggests that phenyramidol inhibits the activity of the liver enzymes concerned with the metabolism of phenytoin, thereby prolonging its stay in the body and causing the serum levels to rise. The epileptic patients improved presumably because their phenytoin serum levels were increased.

Importance and management

Information is very limited but the interaction would appear to be established. The incidence is uncertain, but all 5 volunteers demonstrated rises in serum phenytoin levels ranging from about 40 to 200%. Phenytoin serum levels should be monitored closely if phenyramidol is given concurrently, and the phenytoin dosage suitably reduced to ensure that intoxication does not occur.

Reference

1 Solomon H M and Schrogie J J. The effect of phenyramidol on the metabolism of diphenylhydantoin. *Clin Pharmacol Ther* (1967) **8**, 554.

Phenytoin + primidone

Summary

Serum *phenobarbitone* levels are markedly increased in patients on primidone who are concurrently treated with phenytoin.

Interaction

A study on 44 patients, taking both primidone and phenytoin, showed that their serum phenobarbitone:primidone ratio was high (4·35) compared with 15 other patients (1·05) who were only taking primidone. Two of the latter patients who had been taking primidone for several years were found to have no detectable amounts of phenobarbitone.[1]

Similar results are described in other studies.[2,3,4]

Mechanism

One suggestion to account for this interaction is that the phenytoin induces the liver enzymes concerned with the oxidation of primidone to phenobarbitone, so that greater than usual amounts are produced.[1,2]

Importance and management

On the whole, this would seem to be an advantageous interaction since the metabolic product of primidone is phenobarbitone, which is itself an active anticonvulsant. At the same time it should be borne in mind that it is possible for the phenobarbitone serum levels to approach toxic concentrations, particularly if a quite small dose of phenobarbitone were to be added.

References

1 Fincham R W, Schottelius D D and Sahs A L. The influence of diphenylhydantoin on primidone metabolism. *Arch Neurol* (1974) **30**, 259.
2 Fincham R W, Schottelius D D and Sahs A L. The influence of diphenylhydantoin on primidone metabolism. *Trans Am Neurol Ass* (1973) **98**, 197.
3 Schmidt D. The effect of phenytoin and ethosuximide on primidone metabolism in patients with epilepsy. *J Neurol* (1975) **209**, 115.
4 Reynolds E H, Fenton G, Fenwick P, Johnson A L and Laundy M. Interaction of phenytoin and primidone. *Br Med J* (1975) **2**, 594.

Phenytoin or phenobarbitone + pyridoxine

Summary

Large doses of pyridoxine can cause a marked reduction in serum phenytoin levels in some patients. Phenobarbitone levels are also reduced.

Interaction

A study in epileptic patients under treatment with phenytoin and phenobarbitone showed that concurrent treatment with pyridoxine (200 mg daily) over a 4-week period reduced the serum phenytoin levels of 7 patients by up to 50%. Reductions in serum phenobarbitone levels were also seen. Not all the patients were affected.

Mechanism

Uncertain. It is suggested that the pyridoxine increases the activity of the liver enzymes concerned with the metabolism of these anticonvulsants.

Importance and management
The documentation is very limited, but the available evidence indicates that a watch should be kept on the serum anticonvulsant levels during the concurrent treatment to ensure that no loss of seizure control occurs. To what extent small doses are likely to cause this interaction is not known. The incidence is uncertain, but apparently not all patients develop this interaction.

Reference
1 Hansson O and Sillanpaa M. Pyridoxine and serum concentrations of phenytoin and phenobarbitone. *Lancet* (1976) **i**, 256.

Phenytoin + salicylates

Summary
There appears as yet to be no confirmation of the assertion that aspirin enhances the actions of phenytoin.

Interaction, mechanism, importance and management
It has been stated that if a 'patient has been taking large quantities of aspirin for headache, . . . the dilantin (phenytoin) is potentiated'.[1] There appears to be no well-controlled clinical evidence for this claim, although salicylates are known to be able to displace phenytoin from plasma protein binding sites.[2,3,4] It is very doubtful if a clinically important interaction normally occurs.

References
1 Toakley J G. Dilantin overdosage. *Med J Aust* (1968) **2**, 639.
2 Ehrnebo M and Odar-Cederlof I. Distribution of phenobarbital and diphenylhydantoin between plasma and cells in blood: effect of salicylic acid, temperature and total drug concentration. *Eur J clin Pharmacol* (1977) **11**, 37.
3 Fraser D G, Ludden T M, Evens R P and Sutherland E W. Displacement of phenytoin from plasma binding sites by salicylate. *Clin Pharmacol Ther* (1980) **27**, 165.
4 Paxton J W. Effects of aspirin on salivary and serum phenytoin kinetics in healthy subjects. *Clin Pharmacol Ther* (1980) **27**, 170.

Phenytoin + sodium valproate

Summary
Conflicting reports state that the serum levels of phenytoin are either raised, or lowered, by sodium valproate. Phenytoin toxicity or an increased seizure frequency may be the result.

Interaction
There seems to be no consistency at all about the reports of the effects of sodium valproate on phenytoin: in some cases the phenytoin serum levels have been seen to rise, and then fall to normal or less than normal levels. In other cases they are reported to have fallen initially, and later risen.

In one study the phenytoin serum concentration of five children taking 6–10 mg/kg a day were seen to have risen by a factor of 2–3 when sodium valproate (dosage not stated) was given at the same time. The phenytoin dosage was accordingly reduced. After 1–3 months' use, the sodium valproate ceased to have any effect on the phenytoin serum levels of 4 of the children. Virtually the same phenytoin dosage was reinstated.[1]

A study, undertaken with 15 patients taking phenytoin and sodium valproate, showed the following: of 11 who stayed on the same dosage of phenytoin, the phenytoin serum concentrations of 7 of them fell, in 3 it stayed the same, and in 1 it rose. Of the other 4 whose phenytoin dosages were altered, 3 of them showed evidence that sodium valproate lowered phenytoin serum levels.[2]

In another study, it was found that during the

first 14 days of combined phenytoin (200–600 mg daily) and sodium valproate (0·6–6·8 g daily) therapy, the phenytoin serum levels of 15 patients fell by an average of 5 μg/ml, and then gradually rose over the next 16–27 days from an average of 16 to 28 μg/ml.[3]

A long-term study, extending over a year, on 8 patients taking sodium valproate and phenytoin, showed that by the end of 10 weeks the serum phenytoin levels of 6 of them had fallen by as much as 50%, but had returned to their original levels by the end of the year.[12]

There are also other cases on record indicating that sodium valproate can cause either a rise or a fall in serum phenytoin levels.[4–8,10–15]

Mechanism

Not understood. Sodium valproate is more highly protein-bound than phenytoin so that a displacement interaction may take place. It has also been observed that the excretion of hydroxylated phenytoin is increased by the presence of the valproate,[9] but how these might relate to one another or account for the interactions seen remains obscure.

Importance and management

Because of the uncertainty of the outcome of concurrent administration, the effects of administering these two drugs should be closely monitored. Much more study is required before a clear picture of this interaction can be presented.

References

1 Windorfer A, Sauer W and Gadeke R. Elevation of diphenylhydantoin and primidone serum concentration by addition of dipropylacetate, a new anticonvulsant drug. *Acta Paediatr Scand* (1975) **64**, 771.

2 Wilder B J, Willmore L J Bruni and Villarreal H J. Valproic acid: interaction with other anticonvulsant drugs. *Neurology* (1978) **28**, 892.

3 Vajda F J E and Morris P M. Pattern of changes in plasma levels of valproate and phenytoin in patients on multiple anticonvulsant therapy. *Clin Exp Pharmacol Physiol* (1978) 7, 288.

4 Haigh D and Forsythe W I. The treatment of childhood epilepsy with sodium valproate. *Develop Med Child Neurol* (1975) **17**, 743.

5 Jeavons P M and Clark J E. Sodium valproate in treatment of epilepsy. *Br Med J* (1974) **2**, 584.

6 Bardy A, Hari R, Lehtovaara R, Majuri H. Valproate may lower serum phenytoin. *Lancet* (1976) **i**, 1297.

7 Bardy A, Hari R, Lehtovaara R and Majuri H. Valproate may lower serum-phenytoin. *Lancet* (1977) **ii**, 1256.

8 Schmidt D, Meinardi H, van der Kleïjn, E. In *Clinical Pharmacology of Antiepileptic Drugs*, pp. 239–40. (Ed) Schneider H, Janz D, Gardner-Thorpe C, Meinardi H and Sherwin A L (1975). Springer-Verlag, New York, Heidelberg, Berlin.

9 Mattson R H, Cramer J A and Williamson P D. Valproic acid in epilepsy: Clinical and pharmacological effects. *Ann Neurol* (1978) **3**, 20.

10 Silberstein P. Sodium valproate for the treatment of childhood epilepsies. *Med J Aust* (1977) **1**, 95.

11 Windorfer A and Sauer W. Drug interactions during anticonvulsant therapy in childhood: diphenylhydantoin, primidone, phenobarbitone, clonazepam, nitrazepam, carbamazepine and dipropylacetate. *Neuropaediatrie* (1977) **8**, 29.

12 Vakil S D, Critchley E M R , Philips J C, Haydock C, Cocks A and Dyer T. The effect of sodium valproate (Epilim) on phenytoin and phenobarbitone blood levels. In *Clinical and Pharmacological Aspects of Sodium Valproate (Epilim) in the Treatment of Epilepsy*, p. 75. Proceedings of a Symposium held at Nottingham University, September 1975.

13 Richens A, Scoular I T, Ahmad S and Jordan B J. Pharmacokinetics and efficacy of Epilim in patients receiving long-term therapy with other antiepileptic drugs. In *Clinical and Pharmacological Aspects of Sodium Valproate (Epilim) in the Treatment of Epilepsy*, p. 78. Proceedings of a Symposium held at Nottingham University, September 1975.

14 Frigo G M, Lecchini S, Gatti G, Perucca E and Crema A. Modification of phenytoin clearance by valproic acid in normal subjects. *Br J clin Pharmac* (1979) **8**, 553.

15 Bruni J, Wilder B J, Willmore I J and Barbour B. Valproic acid and plasma levels of phenytoin. *Neurology* (1979) **29**, 904.

Phenytoin + sulphonamides

Summary

Phenytoin serum levels can be raised, in some cases to toxic concentrations, by the concurrent use of sulphamethizole, sulphamethoxazole, co-trimoxazole and sulphaphenazole. Information about other sulphonamides is lacking, apart from sulphadimethoxine, sulphamethoxypyridazine sulphamethoxydiazine and sulphafurazole (sulfisoxazole) which are reported not to interact.

Interaction

Phenytoin + sulphamethizole, sulphadiazine or sulphaphenazole

A study on 8 patients showed that, after 1 week's treatment with sulphamethizole (1 g four times a day by mouth), the mean half-life of phenytoin taken concurrently was increased from 11·8 to 19·6 h. Three out of 4 patients showed rises in serum phenytoin levels from 22 to 33, from 19 to 23 and from 4 to 7 μg/ml, respectively. The serum phenytoin levels of the fourth patient remained unaltered.[1]

Similar results are described briefly in another study following the observation of phenytoin intoxication in a patient taking both drugs.[2] Sulphaphenazole, sulphadiazine and sulphamethizole are reported in another study to have increased the phenytoin half-life by 237%, 80% and 66%, and the mean metabolic clearance rate by 67%, 45% and 36% respectively.[5]

Phenytoin + co-trimoxazole

A study on 6 patients on phenytoin showed that the concurrent use of co-trimoxazole increased the phenytoin half-life from 13 to 19 h, and decreased the metabolic clearance rate from 41 to 31 ml/min.[3]

In another study sulphamethoxazole + trimethoprim and trimethoprim alone are reported to have increased the phenytoin half-life by 39% and 51% respectively, and the mean metabolic clearance rate by 27% and 30%.[5]

Phenytoin + other sulphonamides

Other reports state that sulphamethoxypyridazine, sulphadimethoxine, sulphafurazole (sulphasoxizole) and sulphamethoxydiazine do not affect the metabolism of phenytoin.[2,4,5]

Mechanism

The sulphonamides which interact would appear to do so by inhibiting the metabolism of phenytoin by the liver, resulting in its accumulation in the body.[5]

Importance and management

The documentation is relatively limited, but it indicates that sulphamethizole, sulphamethoxazole, cotrimoxazole and sulphaphenazole can increase serum phenytoin levels which, in some cases, may lead to phenytoin intoxication. The incidence is uncertain, but some increase probably occurs in most patients. Sulphadimethoxine, sulphamethoxypyridazine, sulphamethoxydiazine and sulphafurazole (sulfisoxazole) are reported not to interact while information about other sulphonamides seems not to be available. A reduction in the dosage of phenytoin where necessary or the use of a non-interacting sulphonamide will accommodate this interaction. The effects of concurrent use with any sulphonamide should be monitored.

References

1 Lumholtz B, Siersbaek-Nielsen K, Skovsted L, Kampmann J and Hansen J M. Sulfamethizole-induced inhibition of diphenylhydantoin, tolbutamide and warfarin metabolism. *Clin Pharmacol Ther* (1975) 17, 731.

2 Siersbaek-Nielsen K, Hansen M, Skovsted L, Lumholtz B and Kampmann J. Sulphamethizole-induced inhibition of diphenylhydantoin and tolbutamide metabolism in man. *Clin Pharmacol Ther* (1973) 14, 148.

3 Hansen J M, Siersbaek-Nielsen K, Skovsted L, Kampmann J P and Lumholtz B. Potentiation of warfarin by co-trimoxazole. *Br Med J* (1975) 1, 684.

4 Hansen J M, Kristensen M, Skovsted L and Christensen L K. Dicoumarol-induced diphenylhydantoin intoxication. *Lancet* (1966) ii, 265.

5 Hansen J M, Kampmann J P, Siersbaek-Nielsen K, Lumholtz I B, Arrøe M, Abildgaard U and Skorsted L. The effect of different sulfonamides on phenytoin metabolism in man. *Acta Med Scand* (1979) Suppl. 624, 106.

Phenytoin + sulthiame

Summary

Phenytoin serum levels can be approximately doubled by the concurrent use of sulthiame which may lead to phenytoin intoxication.

Interaction

A study on 7 epileptic patients under treatment with phenytoin showed that when they were additionally given 400 mg sulthiame daily, the serum levels of 6 of them approximately doubled over a period of 5–25 days, in some cases reaching toxic concentrations. The levels fell once again when the sulthiame was withdrawn. All the patients experienced an increase in side effects, and definite phenytoin intoxication occurred in 2 of them.[1]

A number of other reports confirm this interaction, some of which describe the development of phenytoin intoxication.[2–8]

Mechanism

There is some dispute about the precise mechanism of this interaction, but the available evidence suggests that the sulthiame interferes in some way with the metabolism of the phenytoin by the liver, leading to its accumulation in the body. In one study the phenytoin half-life was found to be approximately doubled (from 28 to 52 h) during treatment with sulthiame.[2,3]

Importance and management

A well-documented and important interaction. The incidence appears to be high. If sulthiame is added to established treatment with phenytoin, increases in the serum levels of phenytoin of up to 75% should be expected.[3,7] Appropriate dosage adjustments of the phenytoin will be necessary to prevent the development of intoxication in most instances.

References

1 Olesen O V and Jensen O N. Drug-interaction between sulthiame (Ospolot®) and phenytoin in the treatment of epilepsy. *Dan Med Bull* (1969) **16**, 154.

2 Houghton G W and Richens A. Inhibition of phenytoin metabolism by sulthiame. *Br J Pharmac* (1973) **49**, 157. P.

3 Houghton G W and Richens A. Inhibition of phenytoin metabolism by sulthiame in epileptic patients. *Br J clin Pharmac* (1974) **1**, 59.

4 Richens A and Houghton G W. Phenytoin intoxication caused by sulthiame. *Lancet* (1973) **ii**, 1442.

5 Houghton G W and Richens A. Inhibition of phenytoin metabolism by other drugs during epilepsy. *Int J Clin Pharmacol* (1975) **12**, 210.

6 Frantzen E., Hansen J M, Hansen O E and Kristensen M. Phenytoin (*Dilantin*) intoxication. *Acta Neurol Scandinav* (1967) **43**, 440.

7 Houghton G W and Richens A. Phenytoin intoxication induced by sulthiame in epileptic patients. *J Neurol Neurosurg Psychiatr* (1974) **37**, 275.

8 Hansen J M, Kristensen L and Skovsted L. Sulthiame (*Ospolot*) as inhibitor of diphenylhydantoin metabolism. *Epilepsia* (1968) **9**, 17.

Phenytoin + theophylline

Summary

Phenytoin serum levels can be reduced by concurrent treatment with theophylline.

Interaction

A study on 14 subjects of a possible interaction between phenytoin and theophylline showed that, after two weeks concurrent use, withdrawal of the theophylline resulted in a 40% rise in the mean serum phenytoin levels of 5 subjects. The mean serum phenytoin level of all the subjects during concurrent use was a little over 9 μg/ml compared with almost 12 μg/ml on phenytoin alone.[1]

Mechanism

The available evidence suggests that the theophylline induces the liver microsomal enzymes resulting in an increase in the metabolism of the phenytoin, and hastening its removal from the body.

Importance and management

It would clearly be prudent to check that seizure control is not made worse if theophylline is given to patients already taking phenytoin, and also that phenytoin intoxication does not develop when the theophylline is withdrawn. Information seems to be limited to this single report, but if it can be taken as a guide the incidence of this interaction may be about 1 in 3. This requires confirmation.

Reference

1 Taylor J W, Hendeles L, Weinberger M, Lyon L W, Wyatt R and Riegelman S. The interaction of phenytoin and theophylline. *Drug Intell Clin Pharm* (1980) **14**, 638.

Phenytoin + tricyclic antidepressants

Summary

Some very limited evidence indicates that imipramine can raise serum phenytoin levels, possibly to toxic concentrations, but nortriptyline and amitriptyline appear not to interact. The potential convulsive activity of the tricyclic antidepressants should be borne in mind if concurrent treatment is considered.

Interaction

During concurrent treatment with phenytoin and imipramine, 75 mg daily, over a 3-month period, the serum phenytoin levels of 2 patients rose. One of them showed an increase from 30 to 60 μmol/l and developed mild signs of intoxication. These signs vanished and the phenytoin levels of both patients fell once the imipramine was withdrawn. One of the patients was also taking nitrazepam and clonazepam, and the other sodium valproate and carbamazepine.[1]

In two other studies it was shown that nortriptyline, 75 mg daily, had a small but insignificant effect on the serum phenytoin levels of 5 patients,[2] and that amitriptyline had no effect on the elimination of phenytoin in 3 subjects.[3]

Mechanism

The evidence suggests that imipramine can inhibit the metabolism of phenytoin which results in its accumulation in the body, but this is not certain.[2] To what extent the other drugs had some part to play is not known.

Importance and management

The evidence is very limited indeed but it indicates that a close watch should be kept on phenytoin blood levels if imipramine is given concurrently. There is not enough data to be certain that nortriptyline and amitryptyline are absolutely safe alternatives, but they would appear to be preferable. Data about other tricyclic antidepressants is lacking. The tricyclic antidepressants as a group have potential convulsive activity,[4] which raises the question of the advisability of giving them to epileptic patients. It has been suggested that the dose of the anticonvulsant should be raised accordingly, but whether this is effective is uncertain.

References

1 Perucca E and Richens A. Interaction between phenytoin and imipramine. *Br J clin Pharmac* (1977) **4**, 485.
2 Houghton G W and Richens A. Inhibition of phenytoin metabolism by other drugs used in epilepsy. *Int J clin Pharmacol* (1975) **12**, 210.
3 Pond S M. Graham G G, Birkett D J, and Wade D N. Effects of tricyclic antidepressants on drug metabolism. *Clin Pharmacol Ther* (1975) **18**, 191.
4 Dallos V and Heathfield K. Iatrogenic epilepsy due to antidepressant drugs. *Br Med J* (1969) **4**, 80.

Phenytoin + viloxazine

Summary

Viloxazine is reported to raise serum phenytoin levels.

Interaction, mechanism, importance and management

The manufacturers of viloxazine warn that phenytoin serum levels may be raised during concurrent use, and that phenytoin intoxication may occur. No further details are given.[1]

Reference

1 *Vivalan* (ICI) 1979–80 Data Sheet Compendium, p. 435. Pharmind Publications Ltd London (1979).

Phenytoin + vitamin D

Summary

Serum phenytoin concentrations are not adversely affected by concurrent treatment with vitamin D.

Interaction, mechanism, importance and management

A controlled trial on 151 epileptic patients, taking phenytoin and calcium showed that the additional administration of 2000 IU/day vitamin D2 over a 3-month period had no significant effect on the serum phenytoin concentrations, although both the experimental and control groups demonstrated a small rise.[1] No special precautions are required.

Reference
1 Christiansen C and Rødbro P. Effect of vitamin D2 on serum phenytoin. A controlled therapeutic trial. *Acta Neurol Scand* (1974) **50**, 661.

Primidone + carbamazepine

Summary
Serum primidone levels may be reduced by the use of carbamazepine.

Interaction, mechanism, importance and management

An extremely brief report on 155 epileptic children indicates that the serum levels of primidone may be reduced by the concurrent use of carbamazepine.[1] No details are given.

Reference
1 Windorfer A and Sauer W. Drug interactions during anticonvulsant therapy in childhood: diphenylhydantoin, primidone, phenobarbitone, clonazepam, nitrazepam, carbamazepin and dipropylacetate. *Neuropädiatrie* (1977) **8**, 29.

Primidone + clonazepam

Summary
Serum primidone levels are reported to be raised to toxic levels by the concurrent use of clonazepam.

Interaction, mechanism, importance and management

The concurrent use of primidone and clonazepam in children between 3 and 15 has been reported to lead to a considerable rise in the concentration of primidone, and to the development of toxic reactions.[1]

Reference
1 Windorfer A and Sauer W. Drug interactions during anticonvulsant therapy in childhood: diphenylhydantoin, primidone, phenobarbitone, clonazepam, nitrazepam, carbamazepine and dipropylacetate. *Neuropädiatrie* (1977) **8**, 29.

Primidone + corticosteroids

Summary
It seems probable that primidone will increase the metabolism of the corticosteroids and invalidate the results of the dexamethasone adrenal suppression tests, but this awaits direct confirmation.

Interaction, mechanism, importance and management

Direct evidence of an interaction seems to be limited to a letter[1] describing a reduction in the effects of dexamethasone in a woman with congenital adrenal hyperplasia who was also undergoing treatment with primidone for petit mal. However, since primidone is metabolized to phenobarbitone, which is known to interact with the corticosteroids, (see p. 435) it seems reasonable to expect a primidone/corticosteroid interaction to take place. The dexamethasone adrenal suppression test results should also be viewed with suspicion in patients taking primidone.

Reference
1 Hancock K W and Levell A. Primidone/dexamethasone interaction. *Lancet* (1978) **ii**, 97.

Primidone + isoniazid

Summary
A single case report describes a rise in serum primidone levels, and a reduction in serum phenobarbitone levels, during concurrent treatment with primidone and isoniazid.

Interaction, mechanism, importance and management
A patient, under treatment with primidone and isoniazid, showed elevated primidone serum levels and reduced serum phenobarbitone levels due, it was demonstrated, to inhibition by the isoniazid of primidone metabolism.[1] The incidence and importance of this interaction is not known, but prescribers should be aware of this reaction if concurrent treatment is undertaken.

Reference
1 Sutton G and Kupferberg H J. Isoniazid as an inhibitor of primidone metabolism. *Neurology* (1975) **25**, 1179.

Sodium valproate + clonazepam

Summary
Limited evidence suggests that enhanced sedation can occur if clonazepam is given to patients taking sodium valproate.

Interaction, mechanism, importance and management
A study on the treatment of epilepsy in children and adolescents with sodium valproate showed that the addition of clonazepam resulted in unwanted effects (drowsiness, absence status) in 9 out of 12 patients. The authors of the report suggested that this combination should be avoided.[1] Enhanced sedation has been briefly described during the concurrent use of sodium valproate and unnamed benzodiazepines in another report.[2]

References
1 Jeavons P M, Clark J E and Mahashwari M C. Treatment of generalized epilepsies of childhood and adolescence with sodium valproate ('Epilim'). *Develop Med Child Neurol* (1977) **19**, 9.
2 Völzke E and Doose H. Dipropylacetate (Dépakine, Ergenyl) in the treatment of epilepsy. *Epilepsia* (1973) **14**, 185.

Sodium valproate + primidone

Summary
Serum levels of primidone can be increased by the concurrent use of sodium valproate leading to sedation. After the continued use of both drugs the interaction may cease to have any effect.

Interaction
The serum primidone concentrations of 7 children taking 10–18 mg/kg daily were seen in one study to have risen by a factor of 2–3 when sodium valproate (dosage not stated) was given at the same time. After 1–3 months, the effect of the valproate had almost disappeared in 3 of the patients, but persisted in 1. The effects on the other 3 are not recorded.[1]

This interaction is described in other reports. Ataxia, drowsiness and marked sedation are reported to have developed during concurrent use.[2-5]

Mechanism
Uncertain. One suggestion is that the sodium valproate initially slows, or blocks, the primidone metabolism, but later the effect is lost,[1] Thus, the serum levels rise because of accumulation, but later return to normal.

Importance and management
An adequately established interaction. A reduction in the dosage of the primidone may be necessary to accommodate this interaction, followed later by an upwards readjustment of the dosage when the effects of the interaction begin to wane.

References
1 Windorfer A. Sauer W and Gadeke R. Elevation of diphenylhydantoin and primidone serum concentrations by addition of dipropylacetate, a new anticonvulsant drug. *Acta Paediatr Scand* (1975) **64**, 771.
2 Wilder B J. Willmore L J, Bruni J and Villarreal H J. Valproic acid: Interaction with other anticonvulsant drugs. *Neurology* (1978) **28**, 892.
3 Haigh D and Forsythe W I. The treatment of childhood epilepsy with sodium valproate. *Develop Med Child Neurol* (1975) **17**, 743.
4 Richens A and Ahmad S. Controlled trial of sodium valproate in severe epilepsy. *Br Med J* (1975) **3**, 255.
5 Volzke E and Doose H. Dipropylacetate (Depakine, Ergenyl) in the treatment of epilepsy. *Epilepsia* (Amst) (1973) **14**, 185.

CHAPTER 8. ANTIHYPERTENSIVE DRUG INTERACTIONS

A drastic, and now abandoned method of reducing hypertension was to sever the nerves of the sympathetic nervous system which innervate the blood vessels. In this way the muscle within the arteries and arterioles was caused to relax, resulting in an expansion in their diameter accompanied by a fall in blood pressure. Surgical sympathectomy of this kind has now been replaced by the use of drugs which cause a reversible relaxation of the blood vessel musculature.

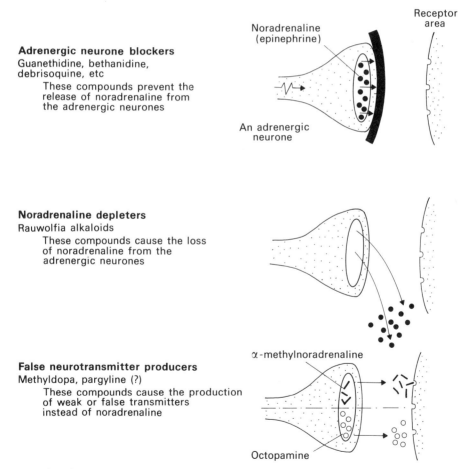

Adrenergic neurone blockers
Guanethidine, bethanidine, debrisoquine, etc
> These compounds prevent the release of noradrenaline from the adrenergic neurones

Noradrenaline depleters
Rauwolfia alkaloids
> These compounds cause the loss of noradrenaline from the adrenergic neurones

False neurotransmitter producers
Methyldopa, pargyline (?)
> These compounds cause the production of weak or false transmitters instead of noradrenaline

Noradrenaline (epinephrine)

Receptor area

An adrenergic neurone

α-methylnoradrenaline

Octopamine

Fig. 8.1. Modes of action of antihypertensives at sympathetic adrenergic neurones. All these drugs prevent noradrenaline (epinephrine) from stimulating the receptors so that normal vasoconstriction of the blood vessels does not occur. A somewhat more detailed and illustrated discussion of the mode of action of adrenergic neurones is to be found on page 12.

Mode of action of the antihypertensive drugs

Some of the antihypertensive drugs affect the sympathetic nervous system at source by interfering with and reducing the output of nervous impulses from the vasomotor centre in the brain. These drugs include the veratrum alkaloids, clonidine, and various sedatives and tranquilizers.

The ganglion blockers interfere with the transmission of the impulses from the brain at the sympathetic ganglia, but since they also affect parasympathetic ganglia as well, their side effects are typically 'anticholinergic'. This group includes mecamylamine, hexamethonium, pempidine and pentolinium. They have now been virtually superseded by drugs which act in other ways.

The most commonly used drugs are those which impair the transmission of the nervous impulses by interfering in some way with the activity of the chemical transmitter, noradrenaline (norepinephrine) at sympathetic nerve endings. The adrenergic neurone blockers (guanethidine, bethanidine, debrisoquine etc.) are taken up into the nerve-endings and prevent the release of noradrenaline (Fig. 8.1.) so that the final transmission link is broken. Methyldopa and pargyline cause the production by the adrenergic neurones of weak or 'false' transmitters which replace the noradrenaline, but have little or no stimulant effects on the receptors within the blood vessels (Fig. 8.1.). Reserpine and the other rauwolfia alkaloids on the other hand

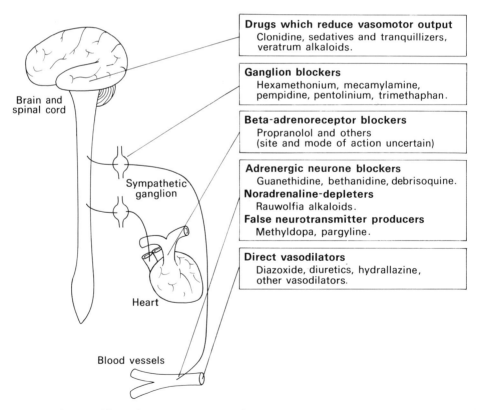

Fig. 8.2. Sites of action of the antihypertensive agents. Only one major site has been illustrated although most drugs affect more than one site.

deplete the adrenergic neurones of noradrenaline (Fig. 8.1.) so that no transmitter is available for release when a nerve impulse arrives.

The antihypertensive actions of the beta-blocking drugs are not fully understood but it has been suggested that they reduce the sympathetic nervous 'drive' to the heart, thereby reducing the force of its output.

A number of other drugs appear to have direct vasodilatory actions on the blood vessels (diazoxide, hydrallazine, diuretics etc.).

The total pharmacology of these drugs is complex and their antihypertensive effects are almost certainly mediated in a number of different ways, but they have been broadly classified in Table 8.1 and their major sites of activity are illustrated in a very

Table 8.1. Antihypertensive drugs

Non-proprietary names	Proprietary names
Adrenergic neurone blockers	
Bethanidine	*Bethanid, Esbatal, Esbaloid*
Bretylium	*Bretylate, Darenthin*
Debrisoquine	*Declinax*
Guanacline	
Guanethidine	*Ismelin*
Guanoclor	*Vatensol*
Guanoxan	*Envacar*
Beta-adrenoreceptor blockers	
See list on page 258.	
False transmitter producers	
Methyldopa	*Aldomet, Dopamet, Hydromet, Aldoril, Medomet, Aldo-*
Methyldopate	*metil, Presinol, Hyperpax, Methoplain, Sembrina*
Pargyline	*Eutonyl*
Noradrenaline depleters (rauwolfia alkaloids)	
Deserpidine	*Harmonyl*
Methoserpidine	*Decaserpyl*
Rauwolfia serpentina	*Hypercal, Hypertane, Hypertensan, Miopressin,*
	Raudixin, Rautrax, Austawolf, Rautensin,
	Rawlina, Lesten, Raufanol, Rautabs, Raupina,
	Raupinetten, Rivadescin, Rauval, Sarpagan,
	Serpetin
Rescinnamine	*Anaprel, Cartic, Moderil*
Reserpine	*Abicol, Seominal, Serpasil, Tensanyl, Alserin,*
	Ebserpine, Neoserp Resercrine, Reserpanca, Serpax
	Serpone, Sertina, Eskaserp, Raurine, Raused, Reserpoid,
	Sandril, Serpate, Serfin, Vioserpine, Reserdrex,
	Ryser, Serpiloid, Tenserp, Sedaraupin
Syrosingopine	*Singoserp*
Ganglion blockers	
Hexamethonium	*Vegolysen*
Mecamylamine	*Inversine, Mevasine*
Pempidine	*Perolysen*
Pentolinium	*Ansolysen*
Trimet(h)aphan	*Arfonad*
Miscellaneous	
Clonidine	*Catapres*
Diazoxide	*Eudemine, Hyperstat, Proglicem*
Diuretics	
Hydrallazine	*Apresoline, Aprelazine, Hyperazin, Lopress*
Veratrum alkaloids	*Puroverine*

simple way in the figures. However for full and detailed information your attention is directed to the standard pharmacology textbooks and reviews.

See Table 8.1 for a list of antihypertensive drug proprietary names.

Interactions

In addition to the interactions discussed in this chapter, there are others involving antihypertensive drugs to be found elsewhere in this book. The index should be consulted for a full list.

Antihypertensive agents + carbenoxolone

Summary
The hypertensive and fluid-retaining effects of carbenoxolone which are seen in some patients may be expected to oppose the effects of antihypertensive agents used concurrently.

Interaction
Although there appear to be few direct reports of adverse interactions between carbenoxolone and the antihypertensive drugs, since carbenoxolone on its own is associated with fluid retention and a rise in blood pressure, antagonism of the antihypertensive response may be expected to occur in some individuals.

> Five out of a total of 10 patients taking 300 mg carbenoxolone daily for the treatment of gastric ulceration, and 2 out of 10 taking 150 mg daily, were observed in one study to have shown a rise in diastolic pressure of 20 mmHg or more.[2]

Numerous other reports describe a rise in blood pressure and fluid retention during carbenoxolone treatment.[1,3-8]

Mechanism
The fluid retention, hypertension and other side-effects associated with carbenoxolone therapy are almost certainly due to its mineralocorticoid-like properties. The evidence for this is, firstly, that these side-effects are not seen with some of the analogues of carbenoxolone such as deglycyrrhizinated liquorice[8] or lauroyl glycyrrhetinic acid[9] which lack mineralcorticoid activity, and secondly, the aldosterone antagonist spironolactone antagonizes the side-effects of carbenoxolone.[4]

Importance and management
The incidence of an increase in blood pressure

during carbenoxolone treatment has been variously reported as being as high as 50%[8] and as low as 4%,[10] whereas fluid retention was found in one study to be absent[1] but in another to affect 46% of the patients.[8] For these reasons patients being treated with carbenoxolone should undergo regular checks on their weight and blood pressure. An increase in the dosage of the antihypertensive agent may be necessary.[1] The manufacturers of carbenoxolone recommend[11] the use of a thiazide diuretic to control oedema and hypertension but not spironolactone which antagonizes the actions of carbenoxolone.

References
1 Bank S and Marks I N. Maintenance carbenoxolone sodium in the prevention of gastric ulcer recurrence. In *Carbenoxolone Sodium*, p. 103. Baron A and Sullivan S (eds) (1970) Butterworths, London.
2 Turpie A G G and Thomson T J. Carbenoxolone sodium in the treatment of gastric ulcer with special reference to side-effects. *Gut* (1965) **6**, 591.
3 Doll R, Langman M J S and Shawdon H H. Effect of different doses of carbenoxolone and different diuretics. In *A Symposium on Carbenoxolone Sodium*, p. 51. Robson A and Sullivan S (eds) (1968). Butterworths, London.
4 Doll R, Langman M J S and Shawdon H H. Treatment of gastric ulcer with carbenoxolone; antagonistic effect of spironolactone. *Gut* (1968) **9**, 42.
5 Montgomery R D and Cookson J B. Comparative trial of carbenoxolone and deglycyrrhizinated liquorice preparation (Caved-S). *Clin Trials J* (1972) **9**, 33.
6 Langman M J S, Knapp D R and Wakley E J. Treatment of chronic gastric ulcer with carbenoxolone and gefarnate: a comparative trial. *Br Med J* (1973) **3**, 84.
7 Horwich L and Galloway R. Treatment of gastric ulcer with carbenoxolone sodium. Clinical and radiological evaluation. *Br Med J* (1965) **2**, 1272.

8 Fraser P M, Doll R, Langman M J S, Misiewicz J J and Shawdon H H. Clinical trial of a new carbenoxolone analogue BX-24, zinc sulphate, and vitamin A in the treatment of gastric ulcer. *Gut* (1972) **13**, 459.
9 Brogden R N, Speight T M and Avery G S. Deglycyrrhizined liquorice: A report of its pharmacological properties and therapeutic efficacy in peptic ulcer. *Drugs* (1974) **8**, 330.
10 Montgomery R D. Side-effects of carbenoxolone sodium: a study of ambulant therapy of gastric ulcer. *Gut* (1967) **8**, 148.
11 ABPI Data Sheet Compendium 1979–80, p. 1148. Pharmind Publications, London (1979).

Antihypertensive agents + fenfluramine

Summary

A small and relatively unimportant enhancement of the blood pressure lowering effects may occur if fenfluramine is used with antihypertensive agents.

Interaction, mechanism, importance and management

Fenfluramine has some hypotensive activity so that if it is given with conventional antihypertensive agents some small adjustment of the dosage may be required. However, in a number of trials involving considerable numbers of obese hypertensive patients who were given 60 mg fenfluramine a day, the changes in blood pressure seen during concurrent treatment with guanethidine, bethanidine, debrisoquine, methyldopa, reserpine, beta-blockers or diuretics were small and, in the context of adverse interactions between drugs, of little or no clinical importance.[1,2,3]

References

1 Waal-Manning J and Simpson F O. Fenfluramine in obese patients on various antihypertensive drugs. Double-blind controlled trial. *Lancet* (1969) **ii**, 1392.
2 Simpson F O and Waal-Manning J. Use of fenfluramine in obese patients on antihypertensive therapy. *S Afr med J* (1971) **45** (*Suppl*), 47.
3 General Practitioner Clinical Trials. Hypotensive effect of fenfluramine in the treatment of obesity. *Practitioner* (1971) **207**, 101.

Antihypertensives + mianserin

Summary

Mianserin hydrochloride does not affect the control of blood pressure with propranolol, propranolol with hydrallazine, guanethidine, bethanidine, or (possibly but not certainly) clonidine.

Interaction

An open study on 3 hypertensive patients being treated with propranolol or propranolol with hydrallazine showed that when they were given 20 mg mianserin three times a day over a period of 3–4 days their mean blood pressures, lying or standing, remained unaffected.[1]

A double-blind study was carried out on 3 hypertensive patients, 1 on bethanidine and 2 on guanethidine, who were given mianserin, 20 mg three times a day, or desipramine 25 mg three times a day. The blood pressure of one of the patients on guanethidine fell but none of them showed evidence that mianserin antagonized the effects of these adrenergic neurone blocking agents. The desipramine raised the blood pressure of one of the patients on guanethidine.[1]

Six hypertensive patients being treated with bethanidine and either mianserin or a placebo in a randomized cross-over study over a 2-week period showed no alteration in the control of their blood pressures.[2]

Mechanism

None.

Importance and management

No special precautions appear to be necessary if mianserin is given to hypertensive patients being treated with propranolol or propranolol with hydrallazine, and this is probably equally true with the other beta-blocking drugs.

No interaction occurs with adrenergic blocking agents such as guanethidine or bethanidine; nor, on the basis of the pharmacology of mianserin, would this be expected since, unlike the tricyclic antidepressants, it does not block their entry into adrenergic neurones.[2] For these reasons no interaction would be expected with debrisoquine or related compounds.

Despite evidence from animal experiments that mianserin may antagonize the effects of clonidine,[3] preliminary studies in volunteers suggest that no interaction takes place in man.[4]

References
1 Burgess C D, Turner P and Wadsworth J. Cardiovascular responses to mianserin hydrochloride: a comparison with tricyclic antidepressant drugs. *Br J clin Pharmac* (1978) **5**, 215.
2 Coppen A, Ghose K, Swade C and Wood K. Effect of mianserin hydrochloride on peripheral uptake mechanisms for noradrenaline and 5-hydroxytryptamine in man. *Br J clin Pharmac* (1978) **5**, 135.
3 Robson R D, Antonaccio M J, Saelens J K and Liebman J. Antagonism by mianserin and classical α-adrenoceptor blocking drugs of some cardiovascular and behavioural effects of clonidine. *Europ J Pharmacol* (1978) **47**, 431.
4 Robson R D. Unpublished data.

Antihypertensives + phenothiazines

Summary
With the exception of the guanethidine-like drugs, the reduction in blood pressure induced by the antihypertensive agents may be exaggerated by the concurrent use of some phenothiazines.

Interaction, mechanism, importance and management
Among the side-effects of chlorpromazine and other phenothiazines is orthostatic hypotension. This is particularly marked with methotrimeprazine. Concurrent use of some antihypertensive agents (excluding the guanethidine-like drugs) may therefore be expected to result in an exaggerated hypotensive response, the extent of which may prove to be unacceptable. For this reason the reaction of patients to the use of both drugs should be monitored, particularly during the first period of treatment. In contrast, the antihypertensive effects of the guanethidine-like drugs can be blocked by the phenothiazines (see p. 232).

A paradoxical increase in blood pressure has been described in one patient with systemic lupus erythematosus and renal disease during concurrent treatment with methyldopa and trifluoperazine. This was due, it has been suggested, to the blocking effect of the phenothiazine on the uptake of the weak 'false transmitter' (see the introduction to this chapter) produced during therapy with methyldopa.[1]

Reference
1 Westervelt F B and Atuk N O. Methyldopa-induced hypertension. *J Amer Med Ass* (1974) **227**, 557.

Antihypertensive agents + phenylbutazone or kebuzone

Summary
The antihypertensive effects of guanethidine and chlorothiazide can be antagonized by phenylbutazone and kebuzone. It seems possible that this will also occur with other antihypertensive agents.

Interaction

Fifteen subjects under treatment with 75 mg guanethidine daily and with a mean blood pressure of 123 mmHg (diastolic + one-third pulse pressure) showed an increase in pressure to 136 mmHg when concurrently treated with 750 mg phenylbutazone or kebuzone daily. A similar rise was seen in 20 other subjects taking chlorothiazide, 50 mg daily, who were also given phenylbutazone. The blood pressure rise represented an approximately two-thirds antagonism of the antihypertensive effects of both guanethidine and chlorothiazide.[1]

Mechanism

Not established. It is probably due to salt and water retention by these pyrazolone compounds.

Importance and management

Data on this interaction are surprisingly limited to this single report and so far seems to be unconfirmed. Antagonism of the antihypertensive effects of these drugs is clearly important. Patients under treatment with guanethidine or thiazides should be checked for a reduction in the antihypertensive response if phenylbutazone, kebuzone or oxyphenbutazone is added. Whether this also occurs with other guanethidine-like drugs or antihypertensive agents is not certain, but if the antagonism is indeed due to salt and water retention, it would seem possible that it will occur with any antihypertensive. This requires confirmation.

Reference

1 Polak F. Die hemmende Wirkung von Phenylbutazon auf die durch einige Antihypertonika hervogerufene Blutdrucksenkung bei Hypertoniker. *Zschr inn Med* (1976) **22**, 375.

Antihypertensive agents or cardiac glycosides + pork

Summary

Hypertension and other reactions have been reported in negro patients after eating very large amounts of pork. This is particularly undesirable in those receiving treatment for hypertension or cardiac failure.

Interaction

Two reports have been published describing acute hypertension and other reactions in negroes who eat large amounts of pork.

A study on 100 negroes in the southern USA who eat extremely large amounts of pork, showed that 35% experienced unpleasant symptoms (dizziness, nausea, eructation, vomiting, headache, blurred vision and gastrointestinal upset including diarrhoea, fainting, scotoma, lacrimation and general malaize) sufficiently often to suggest a direct association between the food and the symptoms.[1]

After eating pork chops on a number of successive days a 42-year-old negro woman experienced severe headache, blurred vision, giddiness, tinnitus, a pounding heart, a blood pressure rise to 240/140 mmHg and a feeling of being seriously ill. These symptoms persisted for several hours but subsided completely when she abstained completely from eating pork.[2]

After eating a considerable amount of fresh pork, the brother of the woman already described suddenly developed hypertension (270/170 mmHg) with haematemesis, haematuria, bloody stools, palpitations, hyperhydrosis and impaired vision, with the syndrome of hypertensive encephalopathy and coma, and then died.[2]

Mechanism

Not known. The author claims that some people are so sensitive to the presence of pork that mere traces of bacon grease or pork seasoning are sufficient to elevate the blood pressure to dangerous levels, but he dismisses the idea that this might be an allergic hypersensitivity reaction.[1]

Importance and control

Strictly speaking this is not an interaction but a direct adverse reaction to food, but it is clearly highly undesirable in those receiving treatment for hypertension or cardiac failure. Salt pork would represent an additional problem. There would seem to be justification for limiting the amount of pork eaten (or pork products such as bacon and sausages) not only because of the reactions described but as a good dietary rule. There is too little information to be able to say whether this adverse reaction is confined to negroes.

References

1. Burch G E, Phillips J H and Wood W. The high-pork diet of the Negro of the Southern United States (Editorial). *Arch Int Med* (1957) **100**, 859.
2 Burch G E. Pork and hypertension *Am Heart J* (1973) **86**, 713.

Beta-blockers, frusemide, bumetanide or thiazides + indomethacin

Summary

The blood-pressure lowering effects of the beta-blockers, thiazides, or frusemide may be reduced by the concurrent use of indomethacin; the therapeutic effectiveness of indomethacin may be reduced by frusemide, and the diuretic effects of bumetanide reduced by indomethacin.

Interactions

(a) Beta-blockers, thiazides or frusemide + indomethacin

A study carried out on 7 hypertensive patients treated with beta-blockers (pindolol, 15 mg daily or propranolol, 80–160 mg daily) showed that when they were given indomethacin, 100 mg daily, over a 10-day period their diastolic pressures rose from 82 to 96 mmHg. Changes in systolic pressures were not statistically significant.[1] These results confirmed previous studies in rabbits.[2]

A study on 4 normal subjects and 6 patients with essential hypertension showed that while frusemide alone (240 mg daily) reduced the mean blood pressure by 13 mmHg, when given with indomethacin as well (200 mg daily) the blood pressure returned to virtually pretreatment levels. Moreover, the normal urinary sodium blood loss induced by frusemide was significantly reduced.[4]

A similar diminution in the antihypertensive effects of propranolol and the thiazide diuretics has been described in another report.[7] Another study has shown that indomethacin can reduce the diuretic effects of bumetanide.[8]

(b) Indomethacin + frusemide

Eight patients with rheumatoid arthritis taking 50 mg indomethacin were found to have significantly reduced serum indomethacin concentrations when they were given 40 mg frusemide at the same time. The effectiveness of the indomethacin in relieving joint tenderness and pain was not statistically altered by the use of frusemide, but the authors of the report say that both tenderness and pain were rated higher with frusemide than without, which on the face of it sounds a somewhat contradictory claim.[5]

Mechanisms

(a) Indomethacin on its own can raise blood pressure. A study on 13 patients with essential hypertension showed that after 3 days' treatment with 150 mg indomethacin a day, their mean systolic blood pressures had risen from 118 ± 9 to 131 ± 8 mmHg.[3] One possible reason is that indomethacin, a known inhibitor of prostaglandin synthesis, may inhibit the production and release by the kidney medulla of pgA and pgE, two prostaglandins which have a powerful dilating effect on peripheral arterioles throughout the body. In their absence the blood pressure may rise.[6] Whether the interaction described is a simple antagonism of the blood-pressure lowering effects of the beta-blockers and frusemide by indomethacin[4,3] or whether a much more complicated interaction in which the antihypertensive effects of these agents is mediated by some involvement with prostaglandin synthesis[1,2,4] is still under investigation.

(b) Not known, but the suggestions put forward include some interference with absorption of the indomethacin by the gut, or possibly a displacement interaction in the plasma.[5]

Importance and management

The documentary evidence is limited but the interaction appears to be adequately established. Some loss of blood-pressure control may be expected if indomethacin is given to patients taking propranolol, pindolol, frusemide, bumetanide or thiazide diuretics. Whether it occurs with other antihypertensives as well is uncertain, but it seems possible. It would clearly be wise to monitor the effects of indomethacin on the blood pressure of any patient using any form of antihypertensive treatment. Similarly the antagonistic effect of indomethacin on the frusemide-induced sodium excretion may be clinically important.

It is difficult to assess how important the presence of frusemide may be on the therapeutic effectiveness of indomethacin, but the authors of the report cited state that in their opinion the two drugs should not be used together.[5]

References

1 Durao V, Prata M M and Goncalves L M P. Modification of antihypertensive effects of β-adrenoceptor-blocking agents by inhibition of endogenous prostaglandin synthesis. *Lancet* (1977) ii, 1005.
2 Durao V and Rico J M G T. Modification by indomethacin of the blood pressure lowering effect of pindolol and propranolol in conscious rabbits. *Europ J Pharmac* (1977) 43, 377.

3 Barrientos A, Alcazar V, Ruilope L, Jarillo D and Rodicio J L. Indomethacin and β-blockers in hypertension. *Lancet* (1978) i, 277.
4 Patak R V, Mookerjee B K, Bentzel C J, Hysert P E, Babej M and Lee J B. Antagonism of the effects of furosemide by indomethacin in normal and hypertensive man. *Prostaglandins* (1975) 10, 649.
5 Brooks P M, Bell P, Lee P, Rooney P J and Dick W C. The effect of frusemide on indomethacin plasma levels. *Br J clin Pharmac* (1974) 1, 485.
6 Lee J B, Patak R V, Moorkerjee B K. Renal prostaglandins and the regulation of blood pressure and sodium and water homeostasis. *Am J med* (1976) 60, 798.
7 Watkins J, Abbott E C, Hensby C N, Webster J and Dollery C T. Attenuation of hypotensive effects of propranolol and thiazide diuretics by indomethacin. *Br med J* (1980) 281, 702.
8 Aggernaes K H. Indometacinehaemning af bumetaniddiurese. *Ugeskr Laeg* (1980) 142, 691.

Clonidine + beta-blockers

Summary

The combined use of clonidine and beta-blockers can have therapeutic benefits, but an isolated report describes antagonism of the hypotensive effects. The rebound hypertension which can follow sudden withdrawal of the clonidine may be worsened by the presence of a beta-blocker.

Interaction

There are two possible problems with the use of these two drugs: (a) during their concurrent use, and (b) following sudden withdrawal of the clonidine.

(a) Concurrent treatment

Clonidine can normally be given with beta-adrenergic blocking drugs with safety and advantage,[4] the total response being greater than with either alone, but an isolated and unexplained report describes what appears to be an antagonistic response.

> When sotalol in daily doses of 160 mg was given to 10 hypertensive patients taking 0·45 mg clonidine daily, the antihypertensive response to clonidine is described as having been abolished in 6 of the patients. Of the 4 patients unaffected, the blood pressures of 2 were lower on combined treatment than with either alone, and the other 2 patients remained unresponsive to treatment.[1]

(b) Beta-blockade following withdrawal of clonidine

Sudden withdrawal of clonidine can result in a severe rebound rise in blood pressure.[2,3,5] This can be greatly exaggerated in the presence of a beta-blocker.

> A woman with a blood pressure of 180/140 mmHg was treated with clonidine to which was added timolol. When the clonidine was discontinued in error, the patient developed a violent throbbing headache, and became progressively confused, ataxic and semicomatose during which she also had a grand mal convulsion. Her blood pressure was found to be 300+/185 mmHg.[2]

A similar response has been described in other reports.[7,8]

Mechanism

The normal additive hypotensive effects seen when clonidine is used with a beta-blocker would seem to result from the two drugs acting in concert at different but complementary sites in the cardiovascular system. The antagonistic effects described[1] are unexplained.

The hypertension which follows clonidine withdrawal is believed to be due to an increase in the levels of circulating catecholamines. Since beta-blockers cause an increase in peripheral resistance (by blocking the normal vasodilator response to noradrenaline) this hypertension would be aggravated.

Importance and management

Although the author of the report[1] describing antagonism between the hypotensive effects of clonidine and sotalol advises that this combination should be avoided until it has been thoroughly investigated, there is very good evidence to show that most patients demonstrate an additive and advantageous hypotensive response.[4,6] Nevertheless an isolated case report of this kind cannot be ignored so that the possibility of this interaction should be borne in mind during combined therapy although its probability is unknown.

The rebound hypertension which can follow the sudden withdrawal of clonidine is a serious reaction. It has been suggested that where patients are taking both drugs the beta-blocker should be withdrawn first of all.[8] However, it should be said that in a study on 5 patients who had previously demonstrated this hypertensive rebound phenomenon it was shown that the reaction could be successfully alleviated by the use of intravenous phentolamine (an alpha-blocker) *and* intravenous propranolol.[3]

References

1 Saarimaa H. Combination of clonidine and sotalol in hypertension. *Br Med J* (1976) **1**, 810.
2 Bailey R R and Neale T J. Rapid clonidine withdrawal with blood pressure overshoot exaggerated by betablockade. *Br med J* (1976) **1**, 942.
3 Hunyor S N, Hansson L, Harrison T S and Hoobler S W. Effects of clonidine withdrawal: Possible mechanisms and suggestions for management. *Br med J* (1973) **2**, 209.
4 Raftos J, Bauer G E, Lewis R G, Stokes G S, Mitchell A S, Young A A and Maclachlan I. Clonidine in the treatment of severe hypertension. *Med J Aust* (1973) **1**, 786.
5 Goldberg A D, Wilkinson P R and Raftery E B. The overshoot phenomenon on withdrawal of clonidine therapy. *Postgrad Med J* (1976) **52** (Suppl 7), 128.
6 Pitkäjärvi T, Ala-Laurila P, Ruosteenoja R, Torsti P and Masar S E. Treatment of hypertension successfully with a diuretic, clonidine or a beta-blocking agent and hydralazine. *Europ J clin Pharmacol* (1977) **12**, 161.
7 Cairns S A and Marshall A J. Clonidine withdrawal. *Lancet* (1976) **i**, 368.
8 Harris A L. Clonidine withdrawal and beta-blockade. *Lancet* (1976) **i**, 596.
9 Reid J L, Dargie H J, Davies D S, Wing L M H, Hamilton C A and Dollery C T. Clonidine withdrawal in hypertension. Changes in blood pressure and plasma and urinary nor-adrenaline. *Lancet* (1977) **i**, 1171.
10 Reza M J. Clonidine-withdrawal syndrome. *Lancet* (1977) **ii**, 89.

Clonidine + tricyclic antidepressants

Summary

The antihypertensive effects of clonidine can be antagonized by the concurrent use of tricyclic antidepressants.

Interaction

In a double-blind trial on 5 hypertensive patients controlled on 600–1800 μg clonidine daily with either chlorthalidone or hydrochlorothiazide, some loss of blood pressure control occurred in 4 of the 5 when given 75 mg desipramine daily. The average blood pressure rise when lying was 22/15 mmHg, and 12/11 mmHg when standing.[2]

Two other cases of this interaction have been described in patients taking 25 and 75 mg imipramine daily.[1,3]

Mechanism

Not understood because the mode of action of clonidine is still under investigation. One theory, based on the results of animal experiments,[4,5] is that clonidine exerts its blood-pressure lowering effects primarily by stimulating alpha-receptors in the rhombencephalon within the brain where the vasomotor centre is located. Stimulation of these receptors activates inhibitory neurones so that the stream of nerve impulses passing out of the brain to the cardiovascular system is reduced.

Experiments with anaesthetized cats[6] have shown that when tricyclic anti-depressants and clonidine are injected into the vertebral artery, which leads directly to the rhombencephalon, the hypotensive effects of clonidine are reduced or abolished. This clearly indicates an interaction in the brain, but just how the two drugs interfere with one another is not clear. An interaction involving peripheral adrenergic neurones as well cannot be excluded.[6]

Importance and management

The documentation is limited but the interaction seems to be established. Only desipramine and imipramine have so far been implicated, but it has been described in animals with amitriptyline, nortriptyline and protriptyline.[7] It would be reasonable to expect this interaction to occur to a greater or lesser degree with the other tricyclic antidepressants until proved otherwise.

This interaction can be accommodated by adjusting the dosage of the clonidine. This was apparently satisfactorily achieved in 10 out of 11 hypertensive patients already taking either ami-triptyline or imipramine who were then administered the clonidine.[8]

References

1 Conolly M E, Paterson J W and Dollery C T. In *Catapres in Hypertension*, p. 167. Conolly M E (ed) (1969) Butterworths, London.

2 Briant R H, Reid J L and Dollery C T. Interaction between clonidine and disipramine in man. *Br med J* (1973) **1**, 522.
3 Coffler D E. Antipsychotic drug interaction. *Drug Intell Clin Pharm* (1976) **10**, 114.
4 van Zwieten P A. The central action of antihyptensive drugs mediated via central α-receptors. *J Pharm Pharmacol* (1973) **25**, 89.
5 Schmitt H, Schmitt H and Fénard S. Evidence for an α-sympathomimetic component in the effects of Catapresan on vasomotor centers: antagonism by piperoxane. *Europ J Pharmacol* (1971) **14**, 98.

6 van Spanning H W and van Zwieten P A. The interference of tricyclic antidepressants with the central hypotensive effect of clonidine. *Europ J Pharmacol* (1973) **24**, 402.
7 van Zwieten P A. Interaction between centrally acting hypotensive drugs and tricyclic antidepressants. *Arch int Pharmacodynam Therap* (1975) **214**, 12.
8 Raftos J. Clonidine in the treatment of severe hypertension. *Med J Aust* (1973) **1**, 786.

Diazoxide + chlorpromazine

Summary

A single case report describes severe hyperglycaemia following the administration of chlorpromazine to a child taking diazoxide and bendroflumethiazide.

Interaction, mechanism, importance and management

A child on long-term treatment for hypoglycaemia with diazoxide, 8 mg/kg, and bendroflumethiazide, 1·25 mg daily, developed a diabetic precoma and severe hyperglycaemia after being given a single 30 mg dose of chlorpromazine.[1] The reason for this response is not understood. Information on this interaction is limited to this one report. Until more is known, phenothiazines such as chlorpromazine should be given with great caution to patients on diazoxide.

Reference

1 Aynsley-Green A and Illig R. Enhancement by chlorpromazine of hyperglycaemic action of diazoxide. *Lancet* (1975) **ii**, 658.

Diazoxide + hydrallazine

Summary

Severe hypotension, in some instances with a fatal outcome, has followed the administration of diazoxide before or after the use of hydrallazine.

Interaction

The blood pressure of a man fell from 220/150 mmHg to 170/120 mmHg after intravenous administration of 3 mg/kg diazoxide. An hour later intravenous administration of 20 mg hydrallazine resulted in a fall to 90/60 with noticeable signs of dizziness and hypotension.[1]

A previously normotensive 25-year-old woman admitted in the 34th week of pregnancy had a blood pressure of 250/150 mmHg which failed to respond to the intravenous administration of magnesium sulphate. It fell transiently to 170/120 mmHg when 15 mg hydrallazine was given. One hour later intravenous administration of 5 mg/kg diazoxide resulted in a blood pressure fall to 60/0 mmHg. Despite the use of large doses of noradrenaline, the hypotension persisted and the patient died.[1]

Two other cases of severe hypotension following the use of hydrallazine and diazoxide are described in this report, and other cases are described in other studies and reports.[3,4] Two of the patients had also received methyldopa.

Mechanism

Not fully understood. Diazoxide reduces blood pressure by its direct relaxant on the smooth muscle of arterioles. The decrease in peripheral resistance which follows is accompanied by a reflex increase in heart rate and the cardiac output rises. The major action of hydrallazine is to lower blood pressure by a not dissimilar relaxation of vascular smooth muscle. It is possible that, in the presence of both vasodilators, the limit of the normal compensatory responses of the cardiovascular system to maintain an adequate blood pressure had been reached.

Importance and management

Hypotension is not an unknown complication of the use of diazoxide but it is unusual.[2,5,6] The advice of the authors of the report cited[1] is that '... diazoxide should be administered with caution to patients being concurrently treated with other potential vasodilatory or catechol-amine depleting agents ...'[1] The results of a study on 10 hypertensive patients given diazoxide (300 mg in 10 s) and propranolol (0·2 mg/kg intravenously following 14 days of 240–340 mg daily) showed that the blood-pressure lowering effects were only slightly increased.[7]

References

1 Henrich W L, Cronin R, Miller P D and Anderson R J. Hypotensive sequelae of diazoxide and hydralazine therapy. *J Am Med Ass* (1977) **237**, 264–5.
2 Miller W E, Gifford R W, Humphrey D C and Vidt D G. Management of severe hypertension with intravenous injections of diazoxide. *Am J Cardiol* (1969) **24**, 870–75.
3 Kumar G K, Pastoor F C, Robayo J R and Razzaque M A. Side effects of diazoxide. *J Am Med Ass* (1976) **235**, 275–6.
4 Tansey W A, Williams E G, Landerman R H and Shwartz M J. Diazoxide. *J Am Med Ass* (1973) **225**, 749.
5 Saker B M, Mathew T H, Eremin J and Kincaid-Smith P. Diazoxide in the treatment of the acute hypertensive emergency. *Med J Aust* (1968) **1**, 592–3.
6 Finnerty F A. Hypertensive encephalopathy. *Am J med* (1972) **52**, 672–8.
7 Mroczek W J, Lee W R, Davidov M E, and Finnerty F A. Vasodilator administration in the presence of beta-adrenergic blockade. *Circulation* (1976) **53**, 985–8.

Diazoxide + hypotensive agents or hypoglycaemic agents

Diazoxide has two main effects and two main therapeutic uses. It lowers blood pressure and is used to control severe hypertension. It also raises blood sugar levels and is used for intractable hypoglycaemia. Each of these two responses is therefore an unwanted side-effect when the other therapeutic use is being exploited. For this reason if other drugs are used concurrently which can either enhance or antagonize either of these two effects (hypoglycaemic agents, antihypertensives, diuretics) the sum of the responses will require careful monitoring and control to ensure that an overall balance is maintained, bearing in mind that some of these other drugs also have dual activity. The thiazide diuretics, for example, can raise blood sugar levels, and the beta blockers can also affect blood sugar levels. See also the previous synopsis.

Debrisoquine + tyramine-rich foods

Summary

Although one study indicated that an interaction between debrisoquine and tyramine-rich food was unlikely, a single case report describes a serious hypertensive reaction in a patient who ate 50 g Gruyère cheese.

Interaction

There are two conflicting reports. One describes a hypertensive reaction while the other indicates that such a response is unlikely:

A study carried out on 4 hypertensive patients taking 40–60 mg debrisoquine daily and who were tested with oral doses of tyramine in water, indicated that only a moderate and unimportant increase in sensitivity to tyramine occurred during treatment with debrisoquine. The authors concluded that hypertensive reactions after eating tyramine-rich foods were unlikely.[1]

A test was carried out on a hypertensive woman treated for a week with doses of debrisoquine progressively increased up to 70 mg a day, who was then given 50 g Gruyère cheese to eat. Within 5 min her blood pressure had risen from 135/85 to 170/90 mmHg, and by the end of an hour had climbed to 195/165 mmHg. After 2 mg phentolamine had been given her blood pressure dropped to 160/95 mmHg but rose again to 200/110 mmHg during the next hour.[2]

Mechanism
Debrisoquine is similar to guanethidine but it also possesses some monoamine oxidase inhibitory characteristics. Unlike the much more potent antidepressant MAO-inhibitors which cause a general inhibition of MAO throughout the body, debrisoquine is much more selective in normal antihypertensive doses and appears not to affect the MAO within the wall of the gut.[1,3] For this reason any tyramine from food is metabolized during absorption and never reaches the general circulation so that no hypertensive interaction would be expected (see p. 370 for a detailed account of the MAOI/tyramine interaction). What then is the explanation of the serious hypertensive reaction described?[2]

One possible answer, based on experimental evidence,[4] is that the particular sample of Gruyère cheese used probably contained extremely large amounts of tyramine. Some of it could have been absorbed through the mucosal lining of the mouth while being chewed, in which case it would by-pass the MAO in the gut. Certainly the rapidity of the response would support this idea. If this is what happened, the tyramine passed around the circulation and released the noradrenaline from the sympathetic neurones associated with the blood vessels causing stimulation of the receptors and a rise in blood pressure.

Importance and management
There is too little data to be able to assess the frequency of this interaction but it can clearly reach serious proportions if it occurs. A list of foods reported to contain significant amounts of tyramine is to be found on page 371.

References
1 Pettinger W A, Korn A, Spiegel H, Solomon H M, Pocelinko R and Abrams W B. Debrisoquin, a selective inhibitor of intraneuronal monoamine oxidase in man. *Clin Pharmacol Ther* (1969) **10**, 667.
2 Amery A and Deloof W. Cheese reaction during debrisoquine treatment. *Lancet* (1970) **ii**, 613.
3 Pettinger W A and Horst W D. Quantifying metabolic effects of antihypertensive and other drugs at the sympathetic neuron level: Clinical and basic correlations. *Ann NY Acad Sci* (1971) **179**, 310.
4 Price K and Smith S E. Cheese reaction and tyramine. *Lancet* (1971) **i**, 130.

Guanethidine and related drugs + alcohol

Summary
Orthostatic hypotension due to guanethidine and related antihypertensives can be exaggerated by the ingestion of alcohol.

Interaction, mechanism, importance and management
Among the commonest side-effects of guanethidine, particularly during early treatment, are dizziness and syncope associated with orthostatic and exertional hypotension. Alcohol causes vasodilation and in some individuals (noted in patients with various types of heart disease[1,2]) lowers the output of the heart. Although reports describing an adverse interaction with guanethidine and alcohol have not been documented, patients may be expected to experience an exaggeration of the hypotensive effects of guanethidine with alcohol, particularly if they stand up quickly, or after exercise. They should be warned to sit or lie down if they feel dizzy, faint or begin to 'black-out', and to limit themselves to moderate amounts of alcohol.

References
1 Gould L, Zahir M, DeMartino A and Gombrecht R F. Cardiac effects of a cocktail. *J Amer Med Ass* (1971) **218**, 1799.
2 Conway N. Haemodynamic effects of ethyl alcohol in patients with coronary heart disease. *Brit Heart J* (1968) **30**, 638.

Guanethidine and
related drugs + diethylpropion

Summary
Limited evidence indicates that no interaction occurs

Interaction, mechanism, importance and management

Although studies[1] in animals indicated that diethylpropion inhibits the effects of guanethidine on blood pressure, a report[2] describing the use of diethylpropion in hypertensive patients who were under treatment with guanethidine, bethanidine or methyldopa suggested that no such antagonism occurs in man.

References
1 Day M D and Rand M J. Antagonism of guanethidine and bretylium by various agents. *Lancet* (1962) ii, 1282.
2 Seedat Y K and Reddy J. Diethylpropion hydrochloride (*Tenuate Dospin*) in the treatment of obese hypertensive patients. *S Afr med J* (1974) **48**, 569.

Guanethidine and related drugs + haloperidol or thiothixene

Summary
The antihypertensive effects of guanethidine can be antagonized by the concurrent administration of haloperidol or thiothixene.

Interaction

A study carried out on 3 hypertensive patients controlled on guanethidine (60–150 mg daily) showed that the addition of haloperidol (6–9 mg daily) raised both their systolic and diastolic blood pressures; in the first patient from 132/95 to 149/99 mmHg; in the second from 125/84 to 148/100 mmHg; and in the third from 138/91 to 154/100 mmHg. One of these patients was subsequently tested with 60 mg thiothixene daily and showed a blood pressure rise from 126/87 to 156/110 mmHg.[1]

These results have been described elsewhere.[2,3]

Mechanism

This interaction occurs because haloperidol and thiothixene antagonize the uptake of the antihypertensive into the adrenergic neurones thereby preventing the guanethidine from continuing to exert its hypotensive actions. This is confirmed by animal experiments.[3] The mechanism of interaction is the same as that seen with guanethidine and the tricyclic antidepressants (see p. 235) or chlorpromazine (see p. 232).

Importance and management

Direct evidence of this interaction appears to be confined to the single report cited, nevertheless it is supported by the well-documented pharmacology of these drugs. It would appear to be an interaction of importance. It patients are treated with both drugs their blood pressure should be closely monitored and appropriate measures taken.

There is no direct evidence of an interaction with other butyrophenones or thioxanthenes and guanethidine (or the other drugs such as bethanidine and debrisoquine which fall into the same group), but it would be prudent to adopt the same precautions. Confirmation of this interaction is needed.

References
1 Janowsky D S, El-Yousef M K, Davis J M, Fann W E and Oates J A. Guanethidine antagonism by antipsychotic drugs. *J. Tenn. State med Assoc* (1972) **65**, 620.
2 Davis J M. Psychopharmacology in the aged. Use of psychotropic drugs in geriatric patients. *J Geriatric Psychiatry* (1974) **7**, 145.
3 Janowsky D S, El-Yousef M K, Davis J M and Fann W E. Antagonism of guanthidine by chlorpromazine. *Am J Psychiatry* (1973) **130**, 808.

Guanethidine and related drugs
+levodopa

Summary
A patient has been described who showed a marked reduction in his guanethidine requirements during concurrent treatment with levodopa.

Interaction
A brief report describes a patient under treatment with guanethidine and a diuretic who, when additionally given levodopa (dose not stated but said to be within the ordinary therapeutic range), required a reduction in his daily dosage of guanethidine from 60 to 20 mg daily. Another patient similarly treated was able to discontinue the diuretic.[1]

Mechanism
Hypotension is one of the recognized side-effects of levodopa so that it seems reasonable to assume that the hypotensive effects of the two drugs are additive.

Importance and management
There appear to be no other reports of the effects of concurrent treatment, but since hypotension is one of the recognized side-effects of levodopa it would clearly be a wise precaution to check that excessive hypotension does not occur if levodopa is added to established treatment with guanethidine.

Reference
1 Hunter K R, Stern G M and Laurence D R. Use of levodopa with other drugs. *Lancet* (1970) ii, 1283.

Guanethidine and related drugs
+mazindol

Summary
The antihypertensive effects of bethanidine and debrisoquine are antagonized by the concurrent use of mazindol. It seems probable that this interaction will also occur with guanethidine.

Interaction
A volunteer subject with mild hypertension and some degree of obesity was given doses of bethanidine (30 mg, three times a day) until his blood pressure, measured after a controlled amount of exercise, was reduced from an average of about 120 mm (diastolic + one-third pulse pressure) to about 80 mm. It was found that a single 2 mg tablet of mazindol was enough to antagonize the antihypertensive effects of bethanidine completely.[1]

It has also been shown in another volunteer that mazindol can also completely antagonize the antihypertensive effects of debrisoquine.[4]

Mechanism
Mazindol is an aryl-substituted tricyclic compound not dissimilar to the tricyclic antidepressants. It seems highly probable that mazindol shares the characteristic of these antidepressants of being able to block the activity of the noradrenaline pump at adrenergic neurones of the sympathetic nervous system.[2,3] This prevents antihypertensives such as debrisoquine and bethanidine from gaining entry to these neurones and of reaching their site of action. As a result their antihypertensive effects are blocked and blood pressure climbs once again.

Importance and management
Although there appear to be only 2 cases of this interaction on record, the known pharmacology of mazindol would lead one to expect this interaction to be of general importance. A similar interaction would be expected with guanethidine and related compounds. The manufacturers advise that these antihypertensives should not be taken until 1 month after withdrawal of the

mazindol, although this is perhaps a little over-cautious since in the case cited[1] a reversal of effects occurred within a few days. It would also be prudent to check for this interaction with clonidine since it is known to be affected by the tricyclic antidepressants. Methyldopa appears not to be affected by mazindol.[4]

References
1 Boakes A J. Antagonism of bethanidine by mazindol. *Br J clin Pharmacol* (1977) **4**, 486.
2 Smith A J and Bant W P. Interactions between post-ganglionic sympathetic blocking drugs and antidepressants. *J Int Med Res* (1975) **3** (Suppl 2), 55.
3 Orme M L'E. Iatrogenic disease. *Medicine* (1972) **4**, 302.
4 Parker J. Wander Pharmaceuticals, England. Private Communication (1976).

Guanethidine and related drugs + monoamine oxidase inhibitors

Summary

The antihypertensive effects of guanethidine can be antagonized by nialamide.

Interaction

Five hypertensive patients whose blood pressure had been controlled with guanethidine (25–35 mg daily) were given a single 50 mg dose of nialamide. Measurement of blood pressure taken 6 h later showed that the antihypertensive effects of the guanethidine in 4 of the 5 had been antagonized to some extent. The mean blood pressure rise was from about 140/85 mmHg to 165/100 mmHg.[1]

Mechanism

Not fully understood.

Importance and management

Information about this interaction seems to be limited to this one report[1] which was a 'single-dose' study. Whether long-term antagonism occurs is uncertain but it would be prudent to monitor the blood pressure response closely during concurrent treatment with guanethidine and any MAOI. Whether other guanethidine-like antihypertensives (debrisoquine, bethanidine etc.) interact similarly is not certain.

One of the initial pharmacological actions of guanethidine is to cause the release of noradrenaline from nerve endings. During MAOI treatment greater than usual amounts are present so that the addition of guanethidine might result in excessive sympathetic stimulation. Whether this happens in practice is uncertain but prescribers should be alert to the possibility.

Reference

1 Gulati O D, Dave B T, Gokhale S D and Shah K M. Antagonism of adrenergic neuron blockade in hypertensive subjects. *Clin Pharmacol Ther* (1966) **7**, 510.

Guanethidine and related drugs + phenothiazines

Summary

Chlorpromazine antagonizes the antihypertensive effects of guanethidine.

Interaction

After controlling the blood pressures of 2 severely hypertensive patients with 80 mg guanethidine, both were additionally administered daily doses of 200–300 mg chlorpromazine. The standing diastolic blood pressure of one rose over a period of 10 days from 94 to 112 mmHg and continued to climb to 116 mmHg even when the chlorpromazine was withdrawn, before falling to 106 mmHg. The other patient reacted similarly: his diastolic pressure rose firstly from 105 to 127 mmHg and then on to 150 mmHg even when the chlorpromazine was withdrawn.[1]

A study[2] was carried out on 4 hypertensive patients who were firstly controlled on guanethidine (60–150 mg daily) and then given 100–400 mg daily doses of chlorpromazine as well. Two of the patients were tested twice with different dose regimens. Highly significant increases in diastolic pressures were seen in every case. For example, one of the patients controlled with 60 mg guanethidine daily showed a blood pressure rise from 121/97 to 179/118 mgHg following concurrent treatment with 400 mg chlorpromazine. Some of the patients exhibited a 'rebound' rise in pressure when the chlorpromazine was withdrawn.

The authors of these two reports also describe the same or similar work elsewhere.[3,4]

Mechanism
Before guanethidine can exert its hypotensive actions it must first of all be taken up into the adrenergic nerve endings by the noradrenaline (norepinephrine) 'pump' which normally transports noradrenaline. Chlorpromazine prevents the entry of guanethidine into these nerve endings, as a result of which the guanethidine fails to exert its actions and the blood pressure begins to climb once again to its former levels. This is essentially the same mechanism of interaction as that seen with the tricyclic antidepressants to which chlorpromazine is closely related[5] and has been confirmed by experiments in animals.[3]

Importance and management
Direct documentary evidence of this interaction is very limited[1,2,3,4] but the well-understood pharmacology of both drugs and the close relationship of chlorpromazine to the tricyclic antidepressants which interact similarly would suggest that this is likely to be a common reaction, although there may be considerable differences in the extent to which individual patients will react.[2,5] It is clinically important because the therapeutic benefits of the guanethidine can be partially or totally abolished leaving the patient unprotected against the damaging effects of hypertension.

The smallest dose of chlorpromazine used in the documented studies of this interaction was 100 mg daily with 90 mg guanethidine. This raised the blood pressure from 113/82 to 153/105 mmHg. It seems reasonable to expect that smaller doses will induce this interaction to a lesser extent, but possibly still of clinical significance.

There is almost no direct evidence about whether other phenothiazines interact similarly. One study[6] indicated that no interaction takes place with prochlorperazine, but very short-term single-dose studies like this one are by no means reliable predictors of what may happen during chronic therapy and indeed this study showed that single doses of amitriptyline had no significant effect on the action of guanethidine! It would therefore be prudent to monitor the antihypertensive response of any patient on guanethidine very closely who is treated with any phenothiazine.

Haloperidol and thiothixene interact like chlorpromazine but to a lesser extent (see p. 230)[2] so that neither the butyrophenones nor the thioxanthenes would seem to be safe alternatives. On the other hand molindone has been found not to interact with guanethidine.[7]

It is not certain whether other antihypertensives, bethanidine and debrisoquine, interact with chlorpromazine, but on the basis of their known pharmacology it would be expected.

References
1 Fann W E, Janowsky D S, Davis J M and Oates J A. Chlorpromazine reversal of the antihypertensive action of guanethidine. *Lancet* (1971) **ii**, 436.
2 Janowsky D S, El-Yousef M K, Davis J M, Fann W E and Oates J A. Guanethidine antagonism by antipsychotic drugs. *J Tenn State Med Assoc* (1972) **65**, 620.
3 Janowsky D S, El-Yousef M K, Davis J M and Fann W E. Antagonism of guanethidine by chlorpromazine. *Am J Psychiatry* (1973) **130**, 808.
4 Davis J M. Psychopharmacology in the aged. Use of psychotropic drugs in geriatric patients. *J Geriatric Psychiatry* (1974) **7**, 145.
5 Tuck D, Hamberger B and Sjoqvist F. Drug interactions: effect of chlorpromazine on the uptake of monoamines into adrenergic neurons in man. *Lancet* (1972) **ii**, 492.
6 Ober K F and Wang R I H. Drug interactions with guanethidine. *Clin Pharmacol Ther* (1973) **14**, 190.
7 Simpson L L. Combined use of molindone and guanethidine in patients with schizophrenia and hypertension. *Am J Psychiatry* (1979) **136**, 1410.

Guanethidine and related drugs + pizotifen

Summary
An isolated case report describes antagonism of the antihypertensive effects of debrisoquine by pizotifen.

Interaction

A man with severe focal glomerulonephritis and severe hypertension which was satisfactorily controlled with debrisoquine, 30 mg daily, timolol 10 mg and frusemide 40 mg 8-hourly, was additionally given treatment with pizotifen (*Sandomigran*) as a prophylactic for migraine. Over the next few weeks his blood pressure climbed from 130/90 mmHg to 195/145 mmHg. It was found impossible to lower the pressure with either diazoxide or prazosin, but within 48 h of withdrawing the pizotifen the pressure has fallen to 105/82, and later stabilized at 140/90 mmHg.[1]

Mechanism

Not known. A suggestion put forward by Sandoz, the manufacturers of pizotifen, is that since this antimigraine preparation is structurally similar to the tricyclic antidepressants, it may possibly antagonize the actions of debrisoquine in a similar way by blocking the uptake of the antihypertensive into adrenergic neurones (see p. 235).

Importance and management

Although information is limited to this single report, it would be wise to check for the development of this interaction in any patient on debrisoquine or any other guanethidine-like antihypertensive to whom pizotifen is additionally given.

Reference

1 Bailey R R. Antagonism of debrisoquine sulphate by pizotifen (*Sandomigran*). NZ Med J (1976) 1, 449.

Guanethidine and related drugs + sympathomimetic amines with indirect actions

Summary

The antihypertensive effects of guanethidine and related drugs can be antagonized by the concurrent use of drugs with indirect sympathomimetic activity (e.g. amphetamines, ephedrine, pseudoephedrine, phenylpropanolamine, methylphenidate, etc.).

Interaction

Guanethidine + amphetamines, ephedrine or methylphenidate

When 16 hypertensive patients controlled on 25–35 mg guanethidine daily were additionally treated with dextroamphetamine (10 mg orally), methylphenidate (20 mg orally), ephedrine (90 mg orally) or methamphetamine (30 mg intramuscularly), the antihypertensive response was completely abolished and the pressures in some instances rose higher than before treatment with guanethidine.[1]

Bethanidine + phenylpropanolamine

The blood pressure of a hypertensive woman, which had been effectively reduced by treatment with 20 mg bethanidine a day, returned to pretreatment levels (220/140 mmHg) when, over a period of 36 h, she was given three spansules of *Ornade* (phenylpropanolamine 50 mg, chlorpheniramine 8 mg, isopropamide 2·5 mg).[2]

Bretylium + amphetamine

An investigation prompted by the observation that 4 patients on amphetamines failed to show a fall in blood pressure in response to bretylium, showed that when 7 patients, satisfactorily controlled on bretylium, were given 25 mg amphetamine early in the morning and another 25 mg dose at lunchtime, their blood pressures rapidly rose to pretreatment levels. Two-and-a-half hours after the last dose of amphetamine the blood pressures of most of them were beginning to fall once again.[3]

Other reports describe similar interactions between guanethidine and dextroamphetamine,[6] guanethidine and methamphetamine[5] and an unnamed adrenergic neurone blocker and ephedrine.[4]

Mechanism

Before adrenergic neurone blocking drugs such as guanethidine can exert their hypotensive actions they must be taken up into the adrenergic neurones of the sympathetic nervous system using the noradrenaline (norepinephrine) 'pump'. Once inside they prevent the normal release of noradrenaline which maintains the tone of the blood vessel muscles, so that the blood pressure falls.

Indirectly acting sympathomimetic amines such as the amphetamines also act on the same neurones. They not only prevent guanethidine being taken up into the neurones, but they can also displace quanethidine already there,[10] so that the blood-pressure lowering effects of guanethidine are abolished. These amines raise blood pressure by causing the release of noradrenaline from the neurones, and they may also have a direct vasoconstrictor action as well which raises blood pressure. Thus the actions of guanethidine are not only antagonized, but the pressure may be raised even higher than before treatment.[7-12]

Importance and management

An established and important interaction. The therapeutic benefits of the antihypertensive therapy can be abolished by the concurrent use of these sympathomimetics. Not every combination of antihypertensive and sympathomimetic has been investigated in man, but on the basis of their well-understood pharmacology there is good reason to expect them all to behave similarly. Patients taking these antihypertensives should be particularly warned against taking proprietary over-the-counter preparations for the relief of coughs, colds (or the nasal stuffiness which is a common side-effect) if they contain sympathomimetic amines of this kind.

References

1 Gulati O D, Dave B T, Gokhale S D and Shah K M. Antagonism of adrenergic neuron blockade in hypertensive subjects. *Clin Pharmacol Ther* (1966) **7**, 510.

2 Misage J R and McDonald R H. Antagonism of hypotensive action of bethanidine by 'common cold' remedy. *Br Med J* (1970) **2**, 347.

3 Wilson R and Long C. Action of bretylium antagonized by amphetamine. *Lancet* (1960) **ii**, 262.

4 Starr K J and Petrie J C. Drug interactions in patients on long-term oral anticoagulant and antihypertensive adrenergic neuron-blocking drugs. *Br Med J* (1972) **2**, 133.

5 Laurence D R and Rosenheim M L. Ciba Foundation Symposium on adrenergic mechanisms, p. 201. London (1960).

6 Ober K F and Wang R I H. Drug interactions with guanethidine. *Clin Pharmacol Ther* (1973) **14**, 190.

7 Day M D and Rand M J. Antagonism of guanethidine and bretylium by various agents. *Lancet* (1962) **ii**, 1282.

8 Day M D and Rand M J. Evidence for a competitive antagonism of guanethidine by dexamphetamine. *Brit J Pharmacol* (1963) **20**, 17.

9 Day M D. Effect of sympathomimetic amines on the blocking action of guanethidine, bretylium and xylocholine. *Brit J Pharmacol* (1962) **18**, 421.

10 Feagin O T, Morgan D H, Oates J A and Shand D G. The mechanism of the reversal of the effect of guanethidine by amphetamines in cat and man. *Brit J Pharmacol* (1970) **39**, 253.

11 Starke K. Interactions of guanethidine and indirect-acting sympathomimetic amines. *Arch Int Pharmacodyn Therap* (1972) **195**, 309.

12 Boura A L A and Green A F. Comparison of bretylium and guanethidine: tolerance and effects on adrenergic nerve function and responses to sympathomimetic amines. *Brit J Pharmacol* (1962) **19**, 31.

Guanethidine and related drugs + tricyclic antidepressants

Summary

The antihypertensive effects of guanethidine, bethanidine and debrisoquine are antagonized by the concurrent administration of tricyclic antidepressants such as desipramine, imipramine, amitriptyline and others. Doxepin taken in doses of 200 mg or more a day interacts similarly, but in smaller doses appears not to do so.

Interaction

The antihypertensive effects of guanethidine, bethanidine and debrisoquine can be rapidly and completely antagonized by the concurrent administration of the older type of tricyclic antidepressant (amitriptyline, desipramine, imipramine, nortriptyline, protriptyline etc) and to a lesser extent by some of the more recent ones (maprotiline, doxepin, iprindole). Two examples from many:

A study on 5 hypertensive patients, controlled on 50–150 mg guanethidine daily, showed that when they were also given 50–75 mg desipramine or 20 mg protriptyline daily over a period of 1–9 days, their average blood pressure (diastolic pressure + one-third pulse pressure) rose by 27 mmHg. When the antidepressant was withdrawn, the full antihypertensive effect of guanethidine was not re-established for an average of 5 days.[1]

A report on 2 hypertensive patients, treated with 60 and 240 mg debrisoquine daily respectively, stated that when they were also given 75 mg desipramine daily for between 1 and 6 days, their blood pressures (diastolic + one-third pulse pressure) rose from 88 to 127 mmHg and from 80 to 107 mmHg.[3]

Other reports have been published of the antagonism of guanethidine by desipramine,[2,3] imipramine,[4,5] amitriptyline,[6-8] protriptyline,[3] and nortriptyline;[17] of bethanidine by desipramine,[1-3,9] imipramine,[8,10] amitryptyline,[10] and nortriptyline;[10] and of debrisoquine by amitriptyline.[8,10]

In some instances the interaction develops

rapidly and fully within a very few hours and may continue for many days. For example, only two 25 mg doses of desipramine (less than a day's dosage) completely antagonized the effects of bethanidine in a patient for an entire week[2] whereas the interaction with guanethidine may take several days to develop fully. It may also take many days after withdrawal of the tricyclic antidepressant for its effects on these antihypertensives to disappear.

Mechanism

Before these guanidine antihypertensives can exert their hypotensive actions they must first of all be taken up into the adrenergic nerve endings associated with the blood vessels by the 'pump' which normally transports noradrenaline (norepinephrine). The tricyclic antidepressants not only enter these neurones by the same means but they can also successfully compete with the antihypertensives for the 'pump' so that the latter fail to reach their site of action.[19,20] As a result of this competition, the antihypertensives are prevented from exerting their actions and consequently the blood pressure climbs once again to its former levels. The tricyclic antidepressants, though similar to one another, are not identical in their behaviour. This is also true of the guanidine antihypertensives so that the rate of development, the duration and the extent of the interactions between them are not absolutely identical but reflect their individual pharmacological characteristics as well as the individual differences between patients.

Importance and management

An extremely well-documented and well-established interaction. The benefits of the antihypertensive therapy can be completely abolished leaving the patient unprotected against the damaging effects of hypertension. Many of the possible combinations of antihypertensive and tricyclic antidepressant have been shown to interact and it seems reasonable to expect that the others (with the possible exception of doxepin, maprotiline and iprindole) will behave in a similar fashion.

This interaction can be accommodated by raising the dose of antihypertensive to balance the effects of the antidepressant, but this runs the real risk of severe hypotension if the antidepressant is withdrawn.[6,8] More satisfactory ways are to choose a different antidepressant or to change to another antihypertensive agent.

(a) Choosing a different antidepressant

Maprotiline appears to interact in only a few patients[8,11] but there seems to be no way of predicting who will be affected. The antagonism by doxepin does not take place until doses of about 200 mg daily are reached. Progressively higher doses partially inhibit the antihypertensive effects, until at 300 mg or more per day doxepin interacts to the same extent as the other tricyclics.[9,12–16] If the daily dose is kept below these interacting levels it may be used, although it would clearly be prudent to monitor the effects closely. Iprindole acts largely on adrenergic neurones in the CNS and not on peripheral neurones so that on theoretical grounds it would seem possible that it may not interact, but there is as yet no direct evidence which confirms this.

An alternative would be to select an antidepressant from another group such as mianserin hydrochloride which does not interact with the guanidine antihypertensives (see p. 221).

(b) Choosing a different antihypertensive

Clonidine not only interacts with the tricyclics in a similar way to the interaction described here (see p. 226) but there is also the risk of central depression and sedation which could aggravate existing depression. Depression is also associated with methyldopa and the rauwolfia derivatives, and there is some evidence that very occasionally the former can interact adversely with the tricyclic antidepressants (see p. 238).

One recommendation which has been made is to use diuretics, beta-blockers and vasodilators instead[18] which do not interact with the tricyclic antidepressants and do not have inherent depressive activity.

References

1 Mitchell J R, Arias L and Oates J A. Antagonism of the antihypertensive action of guanethidine sulfate by desipramine hydrochloride. *J Am Med Ass* (1967) **202**, 973.

2 Oates J A, Mitchell J R, Feagin O T, Kaufmann J S and Shand D G. Distribution of guanidium antihypertensives—mechanism of their selective action. *Ann NY Acad Sci* (1971) **197**, 302.

3 Mitchell J R, Cavanaugh J H, Arias L. and Oates J A. Guanethidine and related agents. III. Antagonism by drugs which inhibit the norepinephrine pump in man. *J Clin Invest* (1970) **49**, 1596.

4 Leishmann A W D, Matthews H L and Smith A J. Antagonism of guanethidine by imipramine. *Lancet* (1963) **i**, 112.

5 Boston Collaborative Drug Surveillance Program. Adverse reactions to the tricyclic antidepressant drugs. *Lancet* (1972) **i**, 529.

6 Meyer J F, McAllister C K and Goldberg L I. Insidious and prolonged antagonism of guanethidine by amitriptyline. *J Am Med Ass* (1970) **213**, 1487.

7 Ober K F and Wang R I H. Drug interactions with guanethidine. *Clin Pharmacol Ther* (1973) **14**, 190.

8 Smith A J and Bant W P. Interactions between post-ganglionic sympathetic blocking drugs and antidepressants. *J Int Med Res* (1975) **3**, (Suppl 2), 55.

9 Oates J A, Fann W E and Cavanaugh J H. Effect of doxepin on the norepinephrine pump. A preliminary report. *Psychosomatics* (1969) **10** (*Suppl*), 12.
10 Skinner C, Coull D C and Johnston A W. Antagonism of the hypotensive action of bethanidine and debrisoquine by tricyclic antidepressants. *Lancet* (1969) **ii**, 564.
11 Briant R H and George C F. The assessment of potential drug interaction with a new tricyclic antidepressant drug. *Br J clin Pharmac* (1974) **1**, 113.
12 Fann W E, Cavanaugh J H, Kaufmann J S, Griffith J D, Davis J M, Janowsky D S and Oates J A. Doxepin: Effects on transport of biogenic amines in man. *Psychopharmacologica* (1971) **22**, 111.
13 Gerson I M, Friedman R and Unterberger H. Non-antagonism of anti-adrenergic agents by a dibenzoxepine (preliminary report). *Dis Nerv Syst* (1970) **31**, 780.
14 Ayd F I. Long-term administration of doxepin (*Sinequan*). *Dis Nerv Syst* (1971) **32**, 617.
15 Ayd F J. Doxepin with other drugs. *Southern med J* (1973) **66**, 465.
16 Ayd F J. Maintenance doxepin (*Sinequan*) therapy for depressive illness. *Dis Nerv Syst* (1975) **36**, 109.
17 McQueen E G. New Zealand Committee on Adverse Reactions: Ninth Annual Report 1974. *NZ Med J* (1974) **2**, 305.
18 Cocco G and Agué C. Interactions between cardioactive drugs and antidepressants. *Europ J Clin Pharmacol* (1977) **11**, 389.
19 Cairncross K D. On the peripheral pharmacology of amitriptyline. *Arch Int Pharmacodyn* (1965) **154**, 438.
20 Atkinson R, Watkinson B and Weetman D F. The interaction between desmethylimipramine and guanethidine on the rabbit ileum. The importance of the noradrenaline uptake process in the reversal of guanethidine-induced adrenergic neurone blockade. *Arch Int Pharmacodyn Therap* (1972) **198**, 385.

Methyldopa + barbiturates

Summary

The effects of methyldopa are not altered by the concurrent use of phenobarbitone.

Interaction

Conflicting data, some of it indicating that the effects of methyldopa may be reduced by phenobarbitone, but other more direct evidence showing that no interaction occurs.

A controlled study on 6 subjects who were treated with 2 g methyldopa and 330 mg phenobarbitone daily showed that their serum catecholamine levels were lower than those of a control group who were not treated with phenobarbitone.[1]

Other studies, in hypertensive subjects under long-term treatment with 750–1500 mg methyldopa daily, showed that the concurrent treatment with 100 mg phenobarbitone daily had no effects on plasma concentrations of methyldopa or on the ratio of methyldopa to its metabolite, methyldopa-O-sulphate.[2,3]

Mechanism

None.

Importance and management

The second of the two studies cited[2,3] is by far the more direct since the actual amounts of methyldopa were measured, so that it would seem that no interaction takes place. The original suggestion[1] that phenobarbitone might increase the rate of metabolism of methyldopa by enzyme induction, thereby reducing the serum levels and its effects, is not established.

References

1 Kaldor A., Juvancz P, Demeczky M, Sebestynen K and Palotas J. Enhancement of methyldopa metabolism with barbiturate. *Br med J* (1971) **3**, 518.
2 Kristensen M, Jørgensen M and Hansen T. Plasma concentration of alfamethyldopa and its main metabolite, methyldopa-O-sulphate during long-term treatment with alfamethyldopa with special reference to possible interaction with other drugs given simultaneously. *Clin Pharmacol Ther* (1973) **14**, 139.
3 Kristensen M, Jørgensen M and Hansen J. Barbiturates and methyldopa metabolism. *Br med J* (1973) **1**, 49.

Methyldopa + haloperidol

Summary

Three cases have been reported of dementia occurring when haloperidol was added to an established methyldopa regimen, but uneventful concurrent use has also been described.

Interaction

Two patients who had been taking methyldopa for an extended period without problems developed a dementia syndrome (USA terminology) within a week of the addition of haloperidol. One of the patients who had been taking 1 g methyldopa daily for 3 years developed psychic retardation, inability to do calculations, recent memory impairment and ideas of reference with accompanying inappropriate suspicion within 3 days of starting to take 8 mg haloperidol daily. The other patient who had been taking 1·5 g methyldopa for 18 months showed a slowing of mental and motor performance, transient disorientation, inability to concentrate and intermittent inability to recognize his own writing within 3 days of starting to take 6 mg haloperidol daily. These mental symptoms cleared completely within 72 h of withdrawing the haloperidol.[1]

A case of severe irritability and aggressive behaviour has been described in another patient treated with these drugs.[3]

Mechanism

Not understood. Among the side-effects of methyldopa relevant to this interaction are sedation, depression and dementia; and of haloperidol, drowsiness, dizziness and depression.

Importance and management

These reports must be viewed alongside another report[2] of a trial extending over 4 weeks with 10 schizophrenic patients on 500 mg methyldopa and 10 mg haloperidol daily. Among the important side effects were somnolence (8 patients) and dizziness (6 patients) but no serious interaction of the kind described above. It would clearly be prudent to be on the alert for the possible development of this interaction if these drugs are given together, but concurrent use need not be avoided.

References

1 Thornton W E. Dementia induced by methyldopa with haloperidol. *New Eng J med* (1976) **243**, 1222.
2 Chouinard G, Pinard G, Serrano M and Tetreault L. Potentiation of haloperidol by α-methyldopa in the treatment of schizophrenic patients. *Curr. Ther Res.* (1973) **15**, 473.
3 Nadel I and Wallach M. Drug interaction between haloperidol and methyldopa. *Brit J Psychiat* (1979) **135**, 484.

Methyldopa + salbutamol

Summary

Severe hypotension attributed to the use of salbutamol infusion in the presence of methyldopa has been observed.

Interaction

Three cases of acute hypotension have been reported following the use of salbutamol infusion to postpone delivery in premature labour in women already receiving 2–2·5 g methyldopa daily for the hypertension of pregnancy.[1]

Mechanism

It has been suggested that this reaction is due to peripheral vasodilation due to stimulation of the beta-receptors.

Importance and management

This report[1] was issued on 16 February 1979 by the manufacturers of salbutamol infusion as a general warning about the concurrent use of salbutamol infusion with either methyldopa or any other drug with an acute hypotensive effect. There is as yet nothing to suggest that salbutamol given orally will interact similarly.

Reference

1 Allen and Hanbury Ltd. Letter. 16 February 1979.

Methyldopa + tricyclic antidepressants

Summary

Although an isolated case report describes antagonism of methyldopa by amitriptyline, other very limited evidence indicates that an interaction is normally unlikely. Depression can accompany the use of methyldopa.

Interaction

The antihypertensive effects of methyldopa are antagonized by the tricyclic antidepressants *in animals*, but only a single isolated case report describes this antagonism in man. Another report states that no interaction occurs.

> A hypertensive man whose blood pressure was controlled with methyldopa (700 mg daily) and a thiazide diuretic, demonstrated tremor, agitation, a pulse rate of 148 and a blood pressure rise from 120–150/80–90 mmHg to 170/110 mmHg within 10 days of starting concurrent treatment with amitryptyline, 75 mg daily. A week after withdrawing the amitriptyline, his pulse rate was 100 and his blood pressure 160/90 mmHg.[1]
>
> A study on three hypertensive patients who had been taking methyldopa in doses of 2·5–3·0 g for 15–28 days demonstrated no antagonism of the antihypertensive effects when concurrently treated with 75 mg desipramine daily for 5–6 days. In fact the blood pressure (diastolic + one-third pulse pressure) fell by an average of about 5 mmHg.[2]

Mechanism

The mechanism of the response seen in man is not understood. No interaction would be expected because methyldopa, unlike guanethidine, does not use the noradrenaline pump to gain entry to the neurones. In animals the antagonism seems to occur within the brain, possibly within the rhombencephalon.[3,4]

Importance and management

The data are very sparse indeed. It is difficult to draw any firm general conclusions on only two reports but the controlled study (on 3 patients) suggests that normally no interaction takes place. Nevertheless it would still be prudent to check for signs of antagonism if amitriptyline or any other tricyclic antidepressant is given to patients on methyldopa.

Methyldopa can induce depression so that it may not be appropriate for depressed patients requiring antihypertensive treatment.

References

1 White A G. Methyldopa and amitriptyline. *Lancet* (1965) **ii**, 441.
2 Mitchell J R, Cavanaugh J H, Arias L and Oates J A. Guanethidine and related agents. III. Antagonism by drugs which inhibit the norepinphrine pump in man. *J Clin Invest* (1970) **49**, 1596.
3 Van Spanning H W and van Zwieten P A. The interaction between alpha-methyl-dopa and tricyclic antidepressants. *Int J Clin Pharmacol* (1975) **11**, 65.
4 Van Zwieten P A. Interaction between centrally acting hypotensive drugs and tricyclic antidepressants. *Arch int Pharmacodyn Therap* (1975) **214**, 12.

Mecamylamine + urinary alkalinisers or acidifiers

Summary

The excretion of mecamylamine is decreased in alkaline urine and increased in acid urine.

Interaction, mechanism, importance and management

Mecamylamine is a basic substance, the excretion of which is affected by the pH of the urine. Retention of the mecamylamine occurs if the urine is made alkaline (with for example sodium bicarbonate or acetazolamide), whereas its excretion is increased in acid urine. A more detailed account of this interaction mechanism is outlined on page 9.

Rauwolfia alkaloids + tricyclic antidepressants

Summary

The rauwolfia alkaloids cause depression and are usually regarded as contraindicated in patients requiring treatment for depression, but there are a few reports of their successful use with the tricyclic antidepressants in the treatment of some resistant forms of depression.

Interaction
Although the rauwolfia alkaloids cause depression and are not therefore usually given to patients already with depression, a few reports describe their successful use when combined with tricyclic antidepressants:

Rauwolfia-induced depression

Out of a total of 270 patients who were under treatment with various extracts of rauwolfia for hypertension, 63 patients (23%) developed depressive episodes within about 7 months of starting treatment. Of these patients 51 were taking 750 μg or more daily.[1]

Depression and sedation resulting from treatment with the rauwolfia alkaloids is very well recognized[2] and animals treated with reserpine have been used by pharmacologists as experimental models of depression for testing the activity of compounds with potential antidepressant activity.[3,4]

Rauwolfia alkaloids + tricyclic antidepressants

Fourteen out of 15 patients with endogenous depression resistant to imipramine responded well to treatment with doses of up to 300 mg imipramine and 7·5–10 mg reserpine a day after an initial manic response. Among the side-effects were diarrhoea and flushing of the skin.[5]

There are other reports describing the concurrent use of reserpine with desipramine[6] and imipramine[7] but the latter report seriously questions the advantages claimed by other workers.

Mechanism
The rauwolfia alkaloids such as reserpine cause adrenergic (noradrenaline-releasing) and serotoninergic (5-hydroxytryptamine-releasing) neurones to become depleted of their normal stores of neurotransmitter, the result being that very reduced amounts are available for release by nerve impulses. Because of these effects at adrenergic sympathetic nerve endings associated with blood vessels the rauwolfia alkaloids can be used as hypotensive agents. The brain possesses both types of neurones and failure in nervous transmission at this level is believed to be responsible for the sedation and severe depression which can occur.

The antidepressant actions of the tricyclics, on the other hand, are believed to be due to their ability to inhibit the normal return of noradrenaline into adrenergic neurones in the CNS, so that the transmitter accumulates in the receptor area and enhances transmission. The rauwolfia alkaloids and the tricyclic antidepressants would appear therefore to have actions which are mutually opposed. Perhaps the transient hyperexcitability and mania which follows their concurrent use represents a manifestation of the large amounts of neurotransmitter in the receptor areas in the brain derived from the nerve endings as they lose their transmitter in response to the reserpine, associated with the inability of the nerve endings to remove the transmitter from the receptor area due to the actions of the antidepressant. There is no obvious reason why reserpine with a tricyclic antidepressant should be more effective than the tricyclic alone.

Importance and management
As a general principle the rauwolfia alkaloids should be avoided in patients being treated with a tricyclic antidepressant or who have a history of depression. Only in carefully controlled situations and with patients unresponsive to other forms of antidepressant treatment should this drug combination be used. The development of mania is a possibility.

References
1 Bolte E, Marc-Aurele J, Brouillet J, Beauregard P, Verdy M and Genest J. Mental depressive episodes during rauwolfia therapy for arterial hypertension with special reference to dosage. *Can med Ass J* (1959) **80**, 291.
2 Quetsch R, Achor R W P, Litin E M and Faucett R L. Depressive reactions in hypertensive patients: A comparison of those receiving no specific antihypertensive treatment. *Circulation* (1959) **19**, 366.
3 Kinnard W J, Barry H, Watzmann N and Buckley J P. In *Antidepressant Drugs*. Proceedings of the 1st International Symposium, Milan 1966. International Congress Series, no. 122, p. 89. Excerpta Medica Foundation.
4 Garratini S and Jori A. Interactions between imipramine-like drugs and reserpine on body temperature. In *Antidepressant Drugs*. Proceeding of the 1st International Symposium, Milan 1966. International Congress Series No 122, p. 179. Excerpta Medica Foundation.
5 Haskovec L and Rysanek K. The action of reserpine in imipramine-resistant depressive patients. A clinical and biochemical study. *Psychopharmacologia* (1967) **11**, 18.
6 Poldinger W. Combined administration of desipramine and reserpine or tetrabenazine in depressed patients. *Psychopharmacologia* (1963) **4**, 308.
7 Carney M W P, Thakurdas H and Sebastian J. Effects of imipramine and reserpine in depression. *Psychopharmacologia* (1969) **14**, 349.

CHAPTER 9. ANTIPARKINSONIAN DRUG INTERACTIONS

These drugs have been classified together because their major therapeutic application is in the treatment of Parkinson's disease, although some of them have uses for other conditions. 'Parkinson's disease' is named after Dr James Parkinson who, a century-and-a-half ago in his 'Essay on the shaking palsy', described the four main signs of the disease—muscle rigidity, tremor, muscular weakness and hypokinesia—which are displayed in varying degrees by patients with this condition, and which may also appear in other disorders. Similar symptoms may also be displayed as unwanted side-effects of therapy with certain drugs.

The basic cause of Parkinson's disease remains unsolved, but the seat of the disease is known to lie in the basal ganglia of the brain, particularly the corpus striatum and in the substantia nigra. It is believed that the normal extrapyramidal control of skeletal muscle activity depends upon a balance being maintained between the activity of the nerve fibres in this area which use acetycholine as a transmitter substance (cholinergic fibres) and those which use dopamine (dopaminergic fibres). In Parkinson's disease this balance is drastically upset by a loss in the ability to produce dopamine (due to a degeneration of some of the dopaminergic fibres) so that the cholinergic system comes to be in dominant control (see the illustration in Fig. 9.1). Much of the treatment of Parkinson's disease is based on an attempt to redress this balance either by limiting the activity of the cholinergic system with anticholinergic drugs, and/or by 'topping up' the dopaminergic system with dopamine administered in the form of levodopa, or with other agents such as amantadine and bromocriptidine which increase dopaminergic activity in the brain.

Anticholinergic agents

The belladonna alkaloids (hyoscine, atropine etc.) were used originally but these have largely been superseded by some of the more selective drugs such as benztropine, benzhexol (trihexiphenidyl,) and others listed in Table 9.1. Among the peripheral side-effects of these drugs are urinary retention, paralytic ileus, blurred vision, precipitation of glaucoma and inhibition of thermoregulatory sweating. Central side-effects include depression, confusion and delerium.

Amantadine

Originally an antiviral compound, but found to have antiparkinsonian effects due, it is thought, to some augmentation of dopaminergic activity in the brain.

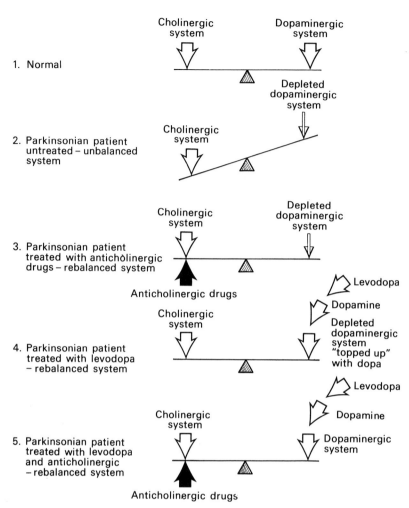

Fig. 9.1. A series of diagrams to illustrate (1) the normal balance between the cholinergic and dopaminergic systems in the basal ganglia of the brain; (2) the imbalance in Parkinson's disease which can be rebalanced by the use of anticholinergic drugs (3) or levodopa (4), or even both (5).

Bromocriptidine

Bromocriptidine is also a stimulant of dopaminergic receptors. By this means it also inhibits the release of prolactin. Among its side-effects are nausea, constipation, postural hypotension, dizziness and headache.

Levodopa

Dopamine itself cannot penetrate the blood–brain barrier so that its precursor, dopa, is used instead and this is then converted within the brain to dopamine by the enzymic activity of dopa-decarboxylase. The original DL–racemic mixture proved to have more serious side-effects than L-Dopa (levodopa) so this isomer is now used exclusively. More recently it has become common to include with the levodopa enzyme-inhibitory compounds such as carbidopa (in *Sinemet*) or benserazide (in *Madopar*). These

Table 9.1. Antiparkinsonian drugs

Non-proprietary names	Proprietary Names
Anticholinergics	
Benapryzine	*Brizin*
Benzhexol (trihexiphenidyl)	*Antispas, Antitrem, Aparkane, Artane, Novohexidyl, Peragit, Pargitane, Pipanol, Tremin, Trihexy, Trinol, Trixyl*
Benztropine	*Congentin, Congentinol*
Biperiden	*Akineton, Akinophyl*
Caramiphen	
Chlorphenoxamine	*Clorevan, Phenoxene, Systral*
Cycrimine	*Pagitane*
Dexetimide	*Tremblex*
Diethazine	*Diparcol*
Ethopropazine (profenamine)	*Lysivane, Parsidol, Parkin*
Methixene	*Methyloxan, Tremaril, Tremarit, Tremoquil, Tremonil, Trest*
Orphenadrine (mephenamine)	*Disipal, Mephenamin, Norflex, Orpadrex*
Procyclidine	*Kemadrin, Osnervan*
Tigloidine	*Tiglyssin*
Amantadine	*Contenton, Mantadix, Symmetrel, Virofral*
Bromocriptidine	*Parlodel*
Levodopa (L-Dopa)	*Bendopar, Berkdopa, Brocadopa, Dopar, Dopastral Emeldopa, Helfo-Dopa, Larodopa, Ledopa, Levopa, Sobidop A, Speciadopa, Syndopa, Veldopa*
Levodopa + benserazide	*Madopar*
Levodopa + carbidopa	*Sinemet*
Piribedil	*Trivastal*

compounds prevent the 'wasteful' enzymic metabolism of the levodopa, which goes on outside the brain, in the mucosa of the gut, the liver and the kidneys and allow higher plasma levels of the levodopa to be achieved with lower oral doses and fewer side-effects.

In addition to the interactions with levodopa and other antiparkinson drugs discussed in this chapter, there are others dealt with elsewhere in this book. The index should be consulted for a full list.

Amantadine + amphetamine, CNS stimulants or anticonvulsants

Summary
The manufacturers of amantadine state that concurrent use with these drugs is not recommended.

Interaction, mechanism, importance and management
The manufacturers of amantadine (Geigy) recommend that it should not be given with amphetamines or other CNS stimulants, nor to those who are subject to convulsions. Similar precautions

are recommended elsewhere.[1] The extent of the data on which these recommendations are made is not stated.

Reference
1 Anon. Symmetrel. *New Ethicals* (1969) 10, 41.

Amantadine + anticholinergics

Summary
The effects of anticholinergic drugs may be enhanced by amantadine, possibly leading to anticholinergic toxicity.

Interaction, mechanism, importance and management
Martindale's Extra Pharmacopœia, 27th edn, states that amantadine can enhance the effects of benzhexol, benztropine and orphenadrine and that their dosage should be reduced during concurrent use. It has also been pointed out elsewhere[1] that hallucinations (central anticholinergic toxicity) can occur, but the documentation for this is very sparse.

Reference
1 Dallos V., Heathfield K, Stone P and Allen F A D. Use of amantadine in Parkinson's disease. Results of a double-blind trial. *Br Med J* (1970) 4, 24.

Anticholinergic agents and drugs with anticholinergic side-effects + butyrophenones, phenothiazines, thioxanthenes and tricyclic antidepressants

Summary
These drugs are frequently administered together with advantage and without hazard, but serious and even life-threatening interactions can occur. These include heat-stroke in hot and humid conditions, severe constipation and adynamic ileus, and atropine-like psychoses. The antiparkinsonian anticholinergics used to counteract the extrapyramidal effects of neuroleptics (chlorpromazine, haloperidol etc.) may also reduce or abolish their therapeutic effects.

For the sake of clarity these interactions have been subdivided into four: (a) heat stroke, (b) constipation and adynamic ileus, (c) atropine-like psychoses and (d) antagonism of neuroleptic effects.

Interaction (a): heat stroke in hot and humid conditions
Three patients were admitted to hospital in Philadelphia for drug-induced hyperpyrexia during a hot and humid period. In each case their skin and mucous membranes were dry and the pulse fast (120/min). The first was taking daily doses of chlorpromazine, 500 mg, chlorprothixene 200 mg, and benztropine, 6 mg. The second was taking chlorpromazine 600 mg, trifluoperazine 12 mg and benztropine 2 mg daily. And the third was on haloperidol 8 mg and benztropine 2 mg daily. There was no evidence of infection.[1]

Three patients died of heat-stroke during a humid heat-wave in the mid-western states of the USA in 1969. All had rectal temperatures of 108°F and showed hot, dry skin and no sweating. The first was taking chlorpromazine 500 mg and trifluoperazine 15 mg daily; the second, fluphenazine enanthate 37·5 mg intramuscularly every fortnight, with benztropine 2 mg and benzhexol 4 mg daily; the third was taking promazine 450 mg and benztropine 2 mg daily.[2]

There are other reports similarly describing heat-stroke in patients taking chlorpromazine and benztropine or other phenothiazines and atropine-like drugs,[4] or chlorpromazine with amitriptyline and benztropine.[5] The danger of heat-stroke in patients taking atropine and atropine-like compounds was recognized more than half-a-century ago, and the warning has been repeated many times.[13,14]

Mechanism

Anticholinergic drugs inhibit the parasympathetic nervous system by which the sweat glands are innervated. When, therefore, the ambient temperature rises, the major heat-losing mechanism (the evaporation of sweat) is partially or wholly inactivated. Phenothiazines, thioxanthenes and butyrophenones may also have anticholinergic activity, but in addition they also impair to a greater or lesser extent the ability of the body to maintain a constant temperature, when exposed to either heat or cold, by their actions upon the thermoregulatory mechanisms in the hypothalamus. So, when the ambient temperature rises, the body temperature rises as well. The tricyclic antidepressants also have anticholinergic activity and can disrupt the central hypothalamic temperature control. Thus, when these drugs are taken together in particularly hot and humid conditions and when the need to reduce the temperature is great, patients become '. . . little more able to control their internal responses to heat than are reptiles . . .',[5] but unlike poikilothermic animals they are unable to sustain life once the temperature exceeds a certain point.

Interaction (b): constipation and adynamic ileus

Eight cases of adynamic ileus with faecal impaction have been reported in patients under treatment with phenothiazines (chlorpromazine, levopromazine, thioridazine, perphenazine), imipramine and benztropine or trihexiphenidyl, or a combination of two or more of these drugs for schizophrenia or depression. Five were successfully treated but recognition of the condition was too late in some of the cases and 3 patients died.[6]

Other cases have been reported involving chlorpromazine with amitriptyline,[9] nortriptyline[9] or benztropine and trifluoperazine.[7] In the last case the patient died from peritonitis following the adynamic ileus.

Mechanism

Anticholinergic drugs reduce intestinal motility which, in the extreme, results in total gut stasis.

Additive effects can occur if two or more drugs with anticholinergic effects are taken together.

Interaction (c): atropine-like psychosis

Three elderly patients taking imipramine or desipramine demonstrated excitement, confusion and hallucination when concurrently treated with 6 mg benzhexol daily.[11]

Three patients taking part in a double-blind study to investigate this interaction, and who were taking a phenothiazine as well as benztropine mesylate for the parkinsonian side-effects, developed an intermittent toxic confusional state (marked disturbance of short-term memory, impaired attention, disorientation, anxiety, visual and auditory hallucinations) with peripheral anticholinergic signs.[12]

Mechanism

These responses closely resemble the central effects of atropine or belladonna poisoning, and appear to result from the additive effects of these drugs. In the second study cited[12] the toxicity was rapidly and dramatically reversed by the injection of physostigmine salicylate. This compound possesses anticholinesterase activity which raises the levels of acetylcholine in the receptor area where the blockage exists and allows the transmitter to stimulate the receptors normally.

Interaction (d): antagonism of the neuroleptic effects

Anticholinergic drugs used routinely to prevent or counteract the extra-pyramidal effects of neuroleptic agents may also reduce or abolish the therapeutic effects:

Studies in psychiatric patients taking chlorpromazine, 300–600 mg daily, showed that when benzhexol, 8 mg daily, was added the plasma chlorpromazine levels fell from a range of 140–300 ng/ml to less than 30 ng/ml. This, it was demonstrated, is too low for patients to develop clinical improvement. When the benzhexol was withdrawn, the plasma chlorpromazine levels rose again and clinical improvement was seen.[18,21]

A double-blind investigation[15,16] carried out on 10 acute schizophrenic on haloperidol ($1 \cdot 5$–60 mg daily) indicated that when they were additionally given 6 mg benztropine, some of the actions of the haloperidol on social avoidance behaviour were reversed, but cognitive integrative function was unaffected.

Other studies have confirmed that benzhexol reduces plasma levels of chlorpromazine[17,22] and that orphenadrine reduces the plasma levels and the effects of chlorpromazine.[10]

Mechanism

Not fully understood. Animal studies[21] indicate

that it may occur because the anticholinergic reduces peristaltic movement and mixing which is necessary for maximal absorption of the neuroleptic. But this probably not the whole story.

Importance and management

These are established interactions. While these drugs have been very widely used together with apparent advantage and without complication, it is important that prescribers should be aware of the potential hazards and disadvantages, particularly when high doses are used.

Patients should be suitably warned to minimize outdoor exposure and/or exercise in hot and humid climates, particularly if they are receiving high doses of antipsychotic/anticholinergic medications. A close watch should be instituted for severe constipation and for the rapid development of complete stasis of the gut which can have a fatal outcome if overlooked. A central anticholinergic psychosis can develop, the diagnosis of which may be difficult because of the overlap which occurs between the basic psychotic symptoms of the patient and those induced by the medication. Withdrawal of one or more of the drugs concerned, or reduction of the dosage and/or appropriate symptomatic treatment should be used to control these interactions.

It has been estimated[19] that somewhere between a third and a half of the patients taking neuroleptics are also given anticholinergic drugs to counteract or prevent the troublesome extrapyramidal reactions which can occur. This figure is high compared with the 7% who were found in one study actually to need this additional medication.[20] Although there are, as yet, only a few reports which show that these antiparkinson drugs can cancel or reduce the effects of some neuroleptics, there are now good arguments for not giving these two types of drugs together as a matter of course unless there are clear clinical indications for doing so.

References

1 Westlake R J and Rastegar A. Hyperpyrexia from drug combinations. *J Amer Med Ass* (1973) **225**, 1250.
2 Kollias J and Bullard R W. The influence of chlorpromazine on the physical and chemical mechanism of temperature regulation in the rat. *J Pharmacol Exp Ther* (1964) **145**, 373.
3 Zelman S and Guillan R. Heat stroke in phenothiazine-treated patients: a report of three fatalities. *Am J Psychiat* (1970) **126**, 1787.
4 Sarnquist F and Larson C P. Drug induced heat stroke. *Anesthesiology* (1973) **39**, 348.
5 Reimer D R, Mohan J and Nagaswami S. Heat dyscontrol syndrome in patients receiving antipsychotic, antidepressant and anti-parkinson drug therapy. *J Florida Med Ass* (1974) **61**, 573.
6 Warnes H, Lehmann and H E and Ban T A. Adynamic ileus during psychoactive meditation. A report of three fatal and five severe cases. *Canad Med Ass J* (1967) **96**, 1112.
7 Giorano J, Huang A and Canter J W. Fatal paralytic ileus complicating phenothiazine therapy. *S Med J* (1975) **68**, 351.
8 Burkitt E A and Sutcliffe C K. Paralytic ileus after amitriptyline (*Tryptizol*) *Br Med J* (1961) **2**, 1648.
9 Milner G and Hills N F. Adynamic ileus and nortriptyline. *Br Med J* (1966) **1**, 841.
10 Loga S, Curry S and Lader M. Interactions of orphenadrine and phenobarbitone with chlorpromazine: plasma concentrations and effects in man. *Br J clin Pharmac* (1975) **2**, 197.
11 Rogers S C. Imipramine and benzhexol. *Br Med J* (1967) **1**, 500.
12 Davis J M. Psychopharmacology in the aged. Use of psychotropic drugs in geriatric patients. *J Geriatric Psychiatry* (1974) **7**, 145.
13 Wilcox W H. The nature, prevention and treatment of heat hyperpyrexia. *Br Med J* (1920) **1**, 392.
14 Litman R E. Heat sensitivity due to autonomic drugs. *J Amer Med Ass* (1952) **149**, 635.
15 Singh M M and Smith J M. Reversal of some therapeutic effects of an antipsychotic agent by an antiparkinsonian drug. *J Nerv Ment Dis* (1973) **157**, 50.
16 Singh M and Smith J M. Reversal of some therapeutic effects of haloperidol in schizophrenia by antiparkinson drugs. *Pharmacologist* (1971) **13**, 207.
17 Chan T, Sakalis G and Gershon S. Some aspects of chlorpromazine metabolism in humans. *Clin Pharmacol Ther* (1973) **14**, 133.
18 Rivera-Calimlim L, Castenada L and Lasagna L. Significance of plasma levels of chlorpromazine. *Clin Pharmacol Ther* (1973) **14**, 144.
19 Prient R F. Unpublished surveys from the NIMH collaborative project on drug therapy in chronic schizophrenics and the VA collaborative project on interim drug therapy in chronic schizophrenics. Quoted in *Int Drug Therap Newsletter* (1974) **9**, 29.
20 Klett C J and Caffey E M. Evaluating the long-term need for antiparkinson drugs by chronic schizophrenics. *Arch Gen Psychiat* (1972) **26**, 374.
21 Rivera-Calimlim L, Castenada L and Lasagna L. Chlorpromazine and trihexiphenidyl interaction in psychiatric patients. *Pharmacologist* (1973) **15**, 212.
22 Rivera-Calimlim L, Nasrallah H, Strauss J and Lasagna L. Clinical response and plasma levels: effect of dosage schedules and drug interactions on plasma chlorpromazine levels. *Am J Psychiat* (1976) **133**, 647.

Bromocriptidine + alcohol

Summary

Some very limited evidence suggests that the adverse effects of bromocriptidine may be enhanced by those who take alcohol.

Interaction, mechanism, importance and management

Intolerance to alcohol has been briefly mentioned in one report in patients taking bromocriptidine for acromegaly.[1] In another[2] 2 patients with high prolactin levels are described as having developed the side-effects of bromocriptidine even in low doses while continuing to drink. When they abstained, they experienced a marked reduction in the frequency and severity of side-effects, even with higher doses of bromocriptidine. This, it is suggested, may be due to some alcohol-induced increase in the sensitivity of dopamine receptors.[1] Although the evidence is extremely limited, it would seem sensible for patients on bromocriptidine to avoid alcohol, particularly if side-effects develop.

References

1 Wass J A H, Thorner M O, Morris D V, Rees L H, Mason A S, Jones A E and Besser E M. Long-term treatment of acromegaly with bromocriptidine. *Br Med J* (1977) **1**, 875.
2 Ayres J and Maisey M N. Alcohol increases bromocriptidine side-effects. *New Eng J Med* (1980) **302**, 806.

Bromocriptidine + griseofulvin

Summary

A single case report describes antagonism of the effects of bromocriptidine by griseofulvin when used in the treatment of acromegaly.

Interaction, mechanism, importance and management

An isolated case has been reported of a patient who, while under treatment for acromegaly with bromocriptidine, was given griseofulvin for a mycotic infection. The effects of the bromocriptidine were blocked until the griseofulvin was withdrawn. The mechanism of this interaction and its general importance are not known, but prescribers should be aware of it if considering their concurrent use in patients under treatment for parkinsonism.

Reference

1 Schwinn G, Dirks H, McIntosh C and Kobberling J. Metabolic and clinical studies in patients with acromegaly treated with bromocriptidine over 22 months. *Europ J clin Invest* (1977) **7**, 101.

Levodopa + antacids

Summary

The concurrent use of some antacids may increase the absorption of levodopa, but the effects are probably of limited importance.

Interaction

A study in man of the effects of a magnesium–aluminium hydroxide antacid on the absorption of C^{14}-levodopa showed that it caused the peak serum levels to be elevated and to occur sooner.[1]

Another study[2] using an unnamed antacid reported similar results, while yet another was unable to confirm this interaction when using *Magaldrate* (monalium hydrate).[3]

Mechanism

The most probable explanation is that alkalinization of the gastric contents by the antacids accelerates the rate of passage of the levodopa through the stomach and away from the gastric mucosa where it is inactivated. Thus more is available (and sooner) for absorption in the small intestine.[1]

Importance and management

The extent to which the absorption of levodopa is likely to be affected is uncertain because of patient variability and the differences in the ability of antacids to alter the rate of gastric emptying. Prescribers should, however, be aware of this interaction, but it is doubtful if it is normally likely to be of great importance.

References

1 Rivera-Calimlim L, Dujovne C A, Morgan J O, Lasagna L and Bianchine J R. Absorption and metabolism of L-dopa by the human stomach. *Europ J clin Invest* (1971) 1, 313.
2 Pocelinko G B T and Solomon H M. The effect of an antacid on the absorption and metabolism of levodopa. *Clin Pharmacol Ther* (1972) 13, 149.
3 Leon A S and Spiegel H E. The effect of antacid administration on the absorption and metabolism of levodopa. *J Clin Pharmacol* (1972) 12, 263.

Levodopa + anticholinergics

Summary

Although anticholinergic drugs are very widely used with levodopa, there is evidence that they can reduce the absorption of levodopa and diminish its therapeutic effects.

Interaction

The effects of levodopa can be reduced by the concurrent use of anticholinergics.

A study on 6 normal volunteers and 6 patients with Parkinson's disease showed that the administration of benzhexol (trihexyphenidyl) lowered the peak serum levels and reduced the absorption of levodopa in about half the subjects by an average of about 16–20%.[1]

A patient who required 7 g levodopa daily while taking homatropine developed levodopa toxicity when the homatropine was withdrawn and he was subsequently restabilized on 4 g levodopa daily.[2]

This interaction has been described in another report.[3]

Mechanism

The most probable explanation of this interaction is that the anticholinergics delay gastric emptying and this gives the gastric mucosa more time to metabolize the levodopa wastefully,[4] so that much less is available by the time the small intestine is reached where levodopa is primarily absorbed. If this theory is correct, drugs such as metoclopramide which stimulate gastric mobility should increase levodopa absorption and this has been shown to be the case.[5]

Importance and management

Although anticholinergic drugs are almost certainly the most commonly co-administered drugs during levodopa therapy, good evidence indicates that its effects can be diminished. One of the studies cited[1] indicates that the incidence may be as high as 50%. Prescribers should be on the alert for a reduced levodopa response if anticholinergics are added to established levodopa treatment, or for levodopa toxicity following their withdrawal.

References

1 Algeri S, Cerletti C, Curcio M, Morselli P L, Bonollo L, Buniva M, Minazzi M and Minoli G. Effect of anticholinergic drugs on gastrointestinal absorption of L-Dopa in rats and man. *Europ J Pharmacol* (1976) 35, 293.
2 Fermaglich J and O'Doherty D S. Effect of gastric motility on levodopa. *Dis Nerv Syst* (1972) 33, 624.
3 Birket-Smith E. Abnormal involuntary movements in relation to anticholinergics and levodopa therapy. *Acta Neurol Scand* (1975) 52, 158.
4 Rivera-Calimlim L, Morgan J P, Dujovne C A, Bianchine J R and Lasagna L. L-Dopa absorption and metabolism by the human stomach. *J Clin Invest* (1970) 49, 79.
5 Mearrick P T, Wade D N, Birkett D J and Morris J. Metoclopramide, gastric emptying and l-dopa absorption. *Aust NZ J med* (1974) 4, 144.

Levodopa + benzodiazepines

Summary
The therapeutic effects of levodopa can be antagonized in some patients by chlordiazepoxide, diazepam, or nitrazepam. It is uncertain whether it also occurs with other benzodiazepines.

Interaction
The antiparkinsonian effects of levodopa are antagonized in some patients by the concurrent use of a benzodiazepine.

> A report of a double-blind study on 8 patients treated with levodopa and various benzodiazepines (mostly in unstated doses but described as being within the normal therapeutic range) stated that no adverse interaction occurred in 3 patients on chlordiazepoxide or in 1 patients on oxazepam. A dramatic deterioration in the control of parkinsonism was seen in a patient given 5 mg diazepam twice a day from which he spontaneously recovered. Two out of 3 other patients given nitrazepam also showed marked deterioration but failed to react in the same way when rechallenged with nitrazepam in three further tests.[1]

There are other reports of this interaction occurring with chlordiazepoxide (9 patients)[2,3,5] and diazepam (3 patients).[6]

Mechanism
Not known.

Importance and management
An established interaction, but there is too little data available to assess its incidence. It is clear that it can adversely affect the control of parkinsonism in some, but not all, patients. For this reason there is no general contraindication to their concurrent use but, if any of them are used, patients should be closely monitored for signs of deterioration in the control of parkinsonism. Only chloriazepoxide, diazepam and nitrazepam have been implicated, but it would seem reasonable to be on the alert for other benzodiazepines to behave similarly until there is good evidence to the contrary.

References
1 Hunter K R, Stern G M and Laurence D R. Use of levodopa with other drugs. *Lancet* (1970) ii, 1283.
2 Mackie L. Drug antagonism. *Br med J* (1971) ii, 651.
3 Schwartz G A and Fahn S. Newer medical treatments in parkinsonism. *Med Clin N Amer* (1970) 54, 773.
4 Brogden R N, Speight T M and Avery G S. Levodopa: A review of its pharmacological properties and therapeutic use with particular reference to Parkinsonism. *Drugs* (1971) 2, 262.
5 Wodak J, Gilligan B S, Veale J L, and Dowty B J. Review of 12 months' treatment with L-dopa in Parkinson's disease, with remarks on unusual side effects. *Med J Aust* (1972) 2, 1277.

Levodopa + beta-blockers

Summary
Concurrent treatment normally appears to be favourable but the long-term effects of the elevated growth hormone levels are uncertain.

Interaction, mechanism, importance and management
There seems little reason to avoid the concurrent use of levodopa and the beta-blockers because the effects are reported either to be favourable or not usually undesirable.

Dopamine, derived from levodopa, stimulates beta-receptors in the heart and can cause cardiac arrhythmias which may be reduced or blocked by the use of propranolol.[1] An enhancement of the levodopa effects and a reduction in tremor in some[2] but not all patients[3,5] have been described. There is, however, evidence[4] that growth hormone levels are substantially elevated, but to what extent this might prove during long-term treatment to be adverse appears not to have been assessed.

References
1 Goldberg L I and Whitsett T L. Cardiovascular effects of levodopa. *Clin Pharmacol Ther* (1971) **12**, 376.
2 Kissel P, Tridon P and André J M. Levodopa–propranolol therapy in parkinsonian tremor. *Lancet* (1974) **ii**, 403.
3 Sandler M, Fellows L E, Calne D B and Findley L J. Oxprenolol and levodopa in parkinsonian patients. *Lancet* (1975) **i**, 168.

4 Camanni F and Massara F. Enhancement of levodopa-induced growth hormone stimulation by propranolol. *Lancet* (1974) **i**, 942.
5 Marsden C D, Parkes J D and Rees J E. Propranolol in Parkinson's disease. *Lancet* (1974) **ii**, 410.

Levodopa + clonidine

Summary

Antagonism of the effects of levodopa by clonidine has been observed in two patients.

Interaction, mechanism, importance and management

Two patients taking levodopa with carbidopa who were concurrently treated with clonidine showed a worsening of their parkinsonism due, it was suggested, to stimulation by the clonidine of alpha-adrenergic receptors within the CNS which antagonized the antiparkinson effects of the levodopa. The data are much too limited to comment constructively on the general importance of this interaction, but it would be prudent to be on the alert for the development of this interaction during concurrent use.[1]

Reference
1 Shoulson I and Chase T N. Clonidine and the anti-parkinsonian response to L-dopa or piribedil. *Neuropharmacology* (1976) **15**, 25.

Levodopa + methionine

Summary

The effects of levodopa can be antagonized by methionine.

Interaction

The therapeutic benefits of levodopa therapy can be reversed by methionine:

> Fourteen patients with Parkinson's disease under treatment with levodopa were given a low-methionine diet for a period of 8 days. Three out of the seven patients who were then given a placebo showed some subjective improvement, whereas 5 out of the other 7 who were treated with 4·5 g methionine daily showed a definite worsening of their symptoms (gait, tremor, rigidity etc.). The deterioration ceased once the methionine was withdrawn.[1]

This report confirms the results of a previous study.[2]

Mechanism
Unknown.

Importance and management
The data are very limited but it indicates that large doses of methionine should not be given to patients under treatment with levodopa. Some of the multivitamin preparations contain methionine, but whether in normal dosages they are likely to have a significant effect on the response to levodopa is uncertain.

References
1 Pearce L A and Waterbury L D. L-methionine: a possible levodopa antagonist. *Neurology (Minneap)* (1974) **24**, 640.
2 Pearce L A and Waterbury L D. L-methionine: a possible L-dopa antagonist. *Neurology (Minneap)* (1971) **21**, 410.

Levodopa + methyldopa

Summary
Although methyldopa occasionally induces parkinsonian-like symptoms, it can enhance the actions of levodopa and permit a reduction in the dosage in some patients. The side-effects of the levodopa are however sometimes made worse. A small enhancement of the effects of methyldopa can also occur.

Interaction
Levodopa and methyldopa when taken together can each enhance the effects of the other.

(a) Enhancement of the effects of levodopa
A double-blind crossover trial on 10 patients with Parkinson's disease who had previously been treated with levodopa alone for periods of 12–40 months showed that the optimum daily dosage of levodopa (5·5 g) fell by 78% when using the highest doses of methyldopa studied (1920 mg daily), and by 50% when the dosage of methyldopa was 800 mg daily.[1]

A one-third[2] and a two-thirds[3] reduction in levodopa requirements during concurrent methyldopa treatment have been described in other reports.

(b) Enhancement of the hypotensive effects of methyldopa
An investigation carried out on 18 patients with Parkinson's disease showed that levodopa and methyldopa when taken together lowered the blood pressure in doses which, when given singly, did not alter the pressure. Fifteen of them were given daily doses of 1–2 g levodopa with 500 mg methyldopa, and the other 3 received 1·75–2·5 g levodopa with 500 mg methyldopa. The mean fall in pressure was about 12/6 mmHg. No change in the control of the Parkinson's disease was seen but the investigation only extended over a few days.[4]

Mechanism
Not known. One theory to account for the enhancement of the effects of levodopa is that the methyldopa prevents the enzymic decarboxylation of the levodopa outside the CNS so that more is available to exert its therapeutic effects.[1,6] Some support for this idea comes from the fact that occasionally methyldopa on its own induces parkinsonian-like symptoms which might be attributed to a reduction in the amounts of dopamine in the CNS caused (possibly?) by inhibition of dopa-decarboxylase.

As far as the increased hypotension is concerned, this might simply result from the additive combined effects of the two drugs, but just how levodopa mediates its blood-pressure lowering effect is not clear.

Importance and management
These interactions are established. Although there have been some reports that methyldopa on its own can cause a reversible parkinsonian-like syndrome[6,7,8] there appears not only to be no contraindication to its use with levodopa, but evidence to show that it can often enhance its actions. A reduction in the dosage of levodopa is possible. The reports cited above[1,2,3] quote figures of between 30 and 78%. These figures should not be interpreted as a recommendation to use the two drugs together, but only to indicate that there are usually no serious problems associated with concurrent therapy. However, the possibility of an adverse response should not be dismissed.

The enhancement of the hypotensive effects of methyldopa by levodopa is small. It has been recommended[4] that methyldopa should only be given to patients on levodopa in a hospital where the blood pressure can be monitored and the dosages controlled.

References
1 Fermaglich J and Chase T N. Methyldopa or methyldopahydrazine as Levodopa synergists. *Lancet* (1973) **1**, 1261.
2 Mones K J. Evaluation of alpha methyl dopa and alpha methyldopa hydrazine with L-dopa therapy. *NY State J med* (1974) **74**, 47.
3 Fermaglich J and O'Doherty D S. Second generation of L-dopa therapy. *Neurology* (1971) **21**, 408.
4 Gibberd F B and Small E. Interaction between levodopa and methyldopa. *Br med J* (1973) **2**, 90.
5 Smith S E. The pharmacological actions of 3,4-dihydroxyphenyl-α-methylalanine (α-methyldopa), an inhibitor of 5-hydroxytryptophan decarboxylase. *Brit J Pharmacol* (1960) **15**, 319.
6 Groden B M. Parkinsonism occurring with methyldopa treatment. *Br Med J* (1963) **1**, 1001.
7 Peaston M J T. Parkinsonism associated with alpha methyldopa therapy. *Br Med J* (1964) **2**, 168.
8 Strang R R. Parkinsonism occurring during methyldopa therapy. *Can med Ass J* (1966) **95**, 928.

Levodopa or whole broad beans + monoamine oxidase inhibitors

Summary

Patients under treatment with MAOI for hypertension or depression should not be given levodopa, nor should they eat whole broad beans which contain dopa, because a serious hypertensive reaction can occur. An interaction with compound levodopa preparations containing carbidopa or benserazide (*Sinemet, Madopar*) is unlikely but the manufacturers still list the MAOI among their contraindications.

Interaction

A sharp and serious rise in blood pressure was seen in a patient who had been treated with phenelzine daily for 10 days and who was given 50 mg levodopa by mouth. Within an hour his blood pressure had risen from 135/90 mmHg to about 190/130 mmHg, and even after the intravenous injection of 5 mg phentolamine (an alpha-adrenoreceptor blocker) it climbed over the next 10 min to 200/135 mmHg, before falling in response to a further 4 mg injection of phentolamine. Next day the experiment was repeated with 25 mg levodopa but no changes in blood pressure were seen, and 3 weeks after withdrawal of the phenelzine even 500 mg levodopa had no effect on the blood pressure.[1]

Similar cases of severe hypertension, accompanied in many instances by flushing, throbbing and pounding in the head, neck and chest, and lightheadedness, have been described in numerous other case reports and studies involving pargyline,[2] nialamide,[3,4] tranylcypromine,[4,5,7] phenelzine[6] and isocarboxazid.

A serious hypertensive reaction has similarly been decribed in patients on monoamine oxidase inhibitors who have eaten *whole* cooked broad beans (*Vicia faba*, L.) which normally contain dopa. The reports involve pargyline,[8] phenelzine[9] and an unnamed MAOI.[10]

Mechanism

Not fully understood. Levodopa is enzymatically converted in the body, firstly to dopamine and then to noradrenaline (norepinephrine):

$$\text{Dopa} \xrightarrow{\text{dopa-decarboxylase}} \text{Dopamine} \rightarrow$$
$$\text{Noradrenaline (norepinephrine)}$$

Both dopamine and noradrenaline are normally under enzymic attack by monoamine oxidase, but in the presence of an MAO-inhibitor this attack is suppressed, which means that the total levels of dopamine and noradrenaline are increased. Precisely how this then leads to a sharp rise in blood pressure is not clear, but either dopamine or noradrenaline, or both, directly or indirectly, stimulate the alpha-receptors of the cardiovascular system.

Importance and management

An important, serious and well-documented interaction. During treatment with any monoamine oxidase inhibitor, whether for depression or hypertension, and for a period of 2–4 weeks after withdrawal, patients should not be given levodopa. The same precautions apply to the eating of whole cooked broad beans, the dopa being contained in the pods but not in the beans.[8,9] If accidental ingestion takes place, the hypertensive reaction can be controlled by the intravenous injection of an alpha-adrenoreceptor blocker such as phentolamine.

This interaction has been shown to be inhibited in man by the presence of dopa decarboxylase inhibitors[5] such as carbidopa (in *Sinemet*) and beserazide (in *Madopar*) so that a serious interaction is very much less likely to occur with these preparations. Even so the manufacturers of both list the MAOI among their contraindications although *Madopar* has been used successfully with an MAOI in the treatment of parkinsonism.[11]

References

1 Hunter K R, Boakes A J, Laurence D R and Stern G M. Monoamine oxidase inhibitors and L-dopa. *Br Med J* (1970) 3, 388.
2 Hodge J V. Use of monoamine oxidase inhibitors. *Lancet* (1965) i, 764.
3 Friend D G, Bell W R and Kline N S. The action of L-dihydroxyphenylalanine in patients receiving malamide. *Clin Pharmacol Ther* (1965) 6, 362.
4 Horwitz D, Goldberg L I, and Sjoerdsma A. Increased blood pressure responses to dopamine and norepinephrine produced by monoamine oxidase inhibitors in man. *J Lab Clin med* (1960) 56, 747.
5 Teychenne P F, Calne D B, Lewis P J and Findley L J. Interactions of levodopa with inhibitors of monoamine oxidase and L-aromatic amino acid decarboxylase. *Clin Pharmacol Ther* (1975) 18, 273.
6 Schildkraut J J, Klerman G, Friend I and Greenblatt M. Biochemical and pressor effects of oral D,L-dihydroxy-

phenyalanine in patients pretreated with antidepressant drugs. *Ann NY Acad Sci* (1963) **107**, 1005.

7 Sharpe J, Marquez-Julio A and Ashby P. Idiopathic orthostatic hypotension treated with levodopa and MAO inhibitor: A preliminary report. *Can Med Ass J* (1972) **107**, 296.

8 Hodge J V, Nye E R and Emerson G W. Monoamine oxidase inhibitors, broad beans and hypertension. *Lancet* (1964) **i**, 1108.

9 Bromley D J. Monoamine-oxidase inhibitors. *Lancet* (1964) **i**, 1181.

10 McQueen E G. Interactions with monoamine oxidase inhibitors. *Br Med J* (1975) **3**, 101.

11 Birkmayer W, Riederer P, Ambrozi L and Youdim M B H. Implications of combined treatment with 'Madopar' and L-deprenil in Parkinson's disease. *Lancet* (1977) **i**, 439.

12 McGilchrist J M. Interactions with monoamine oxidase inhibitors. *Br Med J* (1975) **2**, 591.

Levodopa + papaverine

Summary

The therapeutic effects of levodopa in the treatment of Parkinson's disease are antagonized by the concurrent use of papaverine.

Interaction

A woman with long-standing parkinsonism, well controlled on levodopa and later on levodopa with carbidopa, began to show a steady worsening of her parkinsonism within a week of beginning to take, in addition, 100 mg papaverine hydrochloride daily. The deterioration continued until the papaverine was withdrawn, when the normal response returned within a week. Four other patients showed a similar response.[1]

Two other almost identical cases have been described in another report.[2]

Mechanism

Not understood. One suggestion is that the papaverine might act by blocking the dopamine receptors in the striatum of the brain, thereby inhibiting the effects of the levodopa.[1,3] Another is that the papaverine may have a reserpine-like action on the vesicles of adrenergic neurones.[1,4]

Importance and management

The evidence is limited (a total of 7 patients) but strong enough to indicate clearly that papaverine should not be given to patients with parkinsonism, whether or not they are being treated with levodopa.

References

1 Duvoisin R C. Antagonism of levodopa by papaverine. *J Amer Med Ass* (1975) **231**, 845.

2 Posner D M. Antagonism of levodopa by papaverine. *J Amer Med Ass* (1975) **233**, 768.

3 Gonzalez-Vegas J A. Antagonism of dopamine-mediated inhibition in the nigro-striatal pathway: A mode of action of some catatonia-inducing drugs. *Brain Res* (1974) **80**, 219.

4 Cebeddu L X and Weiner N. Relationship between a granular effect and exocytic release of norepinephrine by nerve stimulation. *Pharmacologist* (1974) **16**, 190.

Levodopa + piperidine

Summary

The beneficial effects of levodopa and the associated dyskinesia are both antagonized by piperidine hydrochloride. An experimental study.

Interaction, mechanism, importance and management

A study on 11 patients with Parkinson's disease and levodopa-induced dyskinesia showed that piperidine hydrochloride, in daily doses of 700–6300 mg over periods of 10–33 days, diminished the dyskinesia but also antagonized the effects of levodopa and allowed the re-emergence of the parkinsonian symptoms. This is probably because piperidine has cholinergic properties which would upset the cholinergic/dopaminergic balance (see the introduction to this chapter) for which the levodopa had originally been given. This was essentially an experimental study undertaken in the hope that piperidine might be used to block the dyskinesia but not the beneficial effects of levodopa. There would seem, therefore, to be no therapeutic value in the concurrent use of these two drugs.

Reference
1 Tolosa E S, Cotzias G C, Papavasilou P S and Lazarus C B. Antagonism by piperidine of levodopa effects in Parkinson's disease. *Neurology* (1977) **27**, 875.

Levodopa + phenothiazines or butyrophenones

Summary
Phenothiazines and butyrophenones can antagonize the effects of levodopa. The antipsychotic effects and extrapyramidal side-effects of the phenothiazines can be antagonized by levodopa.

Interaction, mechanism, importance and management
Phenothiazines (chlorpromazine etc.) and butyrophenones (haloperidol, droperidol) block dopamine receptors in the brain and can therefore upset the balance between cholinergic and dopaminergic components within the corpus striatum and substantia nigra (see the introduction to this chapter on p. 241). As a consequence, they can not only induce the development of extrapyramidal (parkinson-like) symptoms, but they can aggravate parkinsonism and antagonize the effects of levodopa used in its treatment.[1,2] For this reason they are generally regarded as contraindicated in patients under treatment for Parkinson's disease, or only to be used with great caution in carefully controlled conditions. Non-phenothiazine antiemetics which do not antagonize the effects of levodopa include cyclizine (*Marzine*) and diphenidol (*Vontrol*).

The extrapyramidal symptoms which frequently occur with the phenothiazines have been treated with varying degrees of success with levodopa, but the levodopa may also antagonize the antipsychotic effects of the phenothiazines.[3]

References
1 Duvoisin R C. Diphenidol for levodopa-induced nausea and vomiting. *J Amer med Ass* (1972) **221**, 1408.
2 Campbell J B. Long-term treatment of Parkinson's disease with levodopa. *Neurology* (1970) **20**, 18.
3 Yaryura-Tobias J A. Action of L-dopa in drug-induced extrapyramidalism. *Dis Nerv Syst* (1970) **31**, 60.

Levodopa + phenylbutazone

Summary
A single case report describes antagonism of the effects of levodopa by phenylbutazone.

Interaction, mechanism, importance and management
A single case has been reported[1] in which the abnormal involuntary movements caused by levodopa and its therapeutic effects were lessened by the concurrent use of phenylbutazone. The reason for this is not known. Prescribers should be aware of this isolated case but there is far too little information available to make any useful statement about its general importance or management.

Reference
1 Wodak J, Gilligan B S, Veale J L and Dowty B J. Review of 12 months' treatment with L-dopa in Parkinson's disease, with remarks on unusual side-effects. *Med J Aust* (1972) **2**, 1277.

Levodopa + phenytoin

Summary

The effects of levodopa can be antagonized by the concurrent use of phenytoin.

Interaction

In a report on 5 patients undergoing treatment with levodopa for Parkinson's disease and experiencing levodopa-induced side effects, the concurrent use of phenytoin was found not only to relieve the dyskinesias, but also to antagonize its beneficial effects.[1]

Mechanism

Unknown.

Importance and management

This seems to be the only report of this interaction and the data are too limited to assess its general importance, but it would indicate that concurrent use of phenytoin and levodopa should probably be avoided. More study is needed.

Reference

1 Mendez J S, Cotzias G C, Mena I and Papavasilou P S. Diphenylhydantoin blocking of levodopa effects. *Arch Neurol* (1975) **32**, 44.

Levodopa + pyridoxine (vitamin B6)

Summary

The effects of levodopa can be antagonized by the concurrent use of pyridoxine in daily doses of 5 mg or more. No interaction occurs with levodopa–carbidopa preparations.

Interaction

(a) Levodopa + pyridoxine

An investigation on 25 patients being treated with levodopa showed that if they were also given high doses of pyridoxine (750–1000 mg daily) the effects of the levodopa were completely antagonized within 3 to 4 days, and some antagonism was evident within 24 h. 50–100 mg a day reduced or abolished the effects of the levodopa, and an increase in the signs and symptoms of parkinsonism occurred in 8 of 10 patients taking only 5–10 mg pyridoxine a day.[1]

The antagonism of the effects of levodopa by pyridoxine has been described in numerous other reports.[2-11]

(b) Levodopa + carbidopa + pyridoxine

A study carried out on 6 chronic levodopa-treated patients with Parkinson's disease showed that when they were given 250 mg levodopa with 50 mg pyridoxine their mean plasma levels of levodopa fell by 70% (from 356 to 109 ng/ml). With levodopa and carbidopa the mean plasma levels rose almost three-fold (to 845 ng/ml), and with 50 mg pyridoxine as well a further slight increase occurred (to 891 ng/ml), although the plasma-integrated area fell 22% from that obtained with levodopa/carbidopa.[11]

Mechanism

The enzymatic conversion of levodopa to dopamine requires pyridoxal-5-phosphate (derived from pyridoxine) as a co-factor, so it seems probable that when the dietary amounts of pyridoxine are increased the general metabolism of the levodopa throughout the body is accelerated, and even less is available to reach the CNS.[11] This would explain the reduction in the control of the disease although it has also been suggested that the pyridoxine might also alter the metabolism of the levodopa by Schiff-base formation.

Carbidopa (also called MK-486, or alpha-methyl-dopa-hydrazine) is an inhibitor of dopa-decarboxylase which prevents the peripheral ('wasteful') metabolism of levodopa and so allows much larger amounts of levodopa to reach the CNS, even if quite low oral doses are given. So even in the presence of large amounts of pyridoxine the peripheral metabolism remains unaffected, and the serum levels of levodopa remain virtually unaltered.

Importance and management

An important, well-documented and well-established interaction. Doses of pyridoxine as low as 5 mg a day have been shown to cause partial antagonism of the effects of levodopa[1] so that vitamin supplements and other preparations containing significant amounts of pyridoxine should be avoided. Martindale's Extra Pharmacopoeia, 27th edn, lists numerous over-the-counter preparations containing varying amounts of pyridoxine (ranging from 0·1 to 25 mg pyridoxine in each tablet or capsule), many of which could undoubtedly interact to a significant degree with levodopa. It is difficult to justify the use of pyridoxine to reduce the side effects of levodopa when the same result can be achieved by lowering the dose.

Some breakfast cereals are fortified with pyridoxine and other vitamins, but since, for example, a normal serving of fortified *Kellogg's Corn Flakes* or *Rice Krispies* (UK preparations) contains only about 0·6 mg pyridoxine (a whole 500 g (1·1 lb) packet contains a total of only 9·0 mg) there seems little reason to exclude them from the diet. Nor is there any good clinical evidence to suggest that a low-pyridoxine diet is desirable. Indeed it may be harmful since the normal dietary requirements are about 2 mg a day.

The problem can be totally solved by using a levodopa/carbidopa preparation with which pyridoxine does not interact. This is the answer for those patients with any condition where a pyridoxine supplement is necessary.

References
1 Duvoisin R C, Yahr M D and Coté L D. Pyridoxine reversal of L-dopa effects in parkinsonism. *Trans Amer Neurol Ass* (1969) **94**, 81.
2 O'Reilly S. Pyridoxine reversal of L-dopa effects in parkinsonism. *Trans Amer Neural Ass* (1969) **94, 81.**
3 Markham C H. Pyridoxine reversal of L-dopa effects in parkinsonism. *Trans Amer Neurol Ass* (1969) **94, 81.**
4 Schwab R S. Pyridoxine reversal of L-dopa effects in parkinsonism. *Trans Amer Neural Ass* (1969) **94, 81.**
5 Celesia G G and Barr A N. Psychosis and other psychiatric manifestations of levodopa therapy. *Arch Neurol* (1970) **23**, 193.
6 Carter A B. Pyridoxine and parkinsonism. *Br Med J* (1973) **4**, 236.
7 Cotzias G C and Papavasiliou P S. Blocking the negative effects of pyridoxine on patients receiving levodopa. *J Amer med Ass* (1971) **215**, 1504.
8 Leon A S, Spiegel H E, Thomas G and Abrams W B. Pyridoxine antagonism of levodopa in parkinsonism. *J Amer Med Ass* (1971) **218**, 1924.
9 Hildick-Smith M. Pyridoxine in parkinsonism. *Lancet* (1973) **ii**, 1029.
10 Yahr M D and Duvoisin R C. Pyridoxine and levodopa in the treatment of parkinsonism. *J Amer Med Ass* (1972) **220**, 861.
11 Mars H. Metabolic interactions of pyridoxine, levodopa and carbidopa in Parkinson's disease. *Arch Neurol* (1974) **30**, 444.

Levodopa + rauwolfia alkaloids

Summary
The therapeutic effects of levodopa in the treatment of parkinsonism can be antagonized by the concurrent use of rauwolfia alkaloids

Interaction, mechanism, importance and management
Neuroleptic agents such as reserpine deplete the brain of monamines, including dopamine, or block their activity and thereby diminish or prevent the effects of dopamine.[1] This reserpine-induced loss directly opposes the effects of administered levodopa. There are sound pharmacological reasons for believing that this is an interaction of clinical importance. A reduction in the antiparkinson activity of levodopa by reserpine has been observed.[2] The rauwolfia alkaloids should be avoided in patients under treatment for parkinsonism, whether or not they are taking levodopa.

References
1 Bianchine J R and Sunyapridakul L. Interactions between levodopa and other drugs: significance in the treatment of Parkinson's disease. *Drugs* (1973) **6** 364
2 Yahr M D. Personal communication (1977).

Levodopa + tricyclic antidepressants

Summary

The effects of levodopa may be reduced by the concurrent use of tricyclic antidepressants, but the reduction is probably normally too small to be of much importance. An isolated case of hypertensive crisis has been reported in a patient given metoclopramide as well.

Interactions

(a) A study in man showed that the concurrent use of imipramine, 100 mg daily, for 3 days, caused a reduction in the absorption of levodopa from the gastrointestinal tract.[1]

(b) A woman with Parkinson's disease being treated with digoxin, cyclopenthiazide and amitriptyline (20 mg at night) was also administered *Sinemet* (levodopa 100 mg + carbidopa 10 mg) half a tablet, and metoclopramide, 10 mg, each given three times a day. Over the next 36 h her blood pressure climbed from 190/110 mmHg to 270/140 mmHg, and remained elevated until the amitriptyline, metoclopramide and *Sinemet* were withdrawn.[2]

Mechanism

A probable explanation of (a) is that the tricyclic antidepressants have anticholinergic activity, which slows the gastric emptying, and this allows more time for the gastric mucosa to metabolize the levodopa wastefully, thereby reducing the amount available for absorption[5] (see also page 248).

The hypertensive reaction in (b) is not understood. Theoretically amitryptyline might potentiate the pressor effects of noradrenaline derived from the levodopa, but in practice this normally does not occur. Whether the metoclopramide had some part to play is not clear.

Importance and management

Information about these two interactions is extremely limited. The tricyclic antidepressants have been used successfully and apparently uneventfully in treating depression in patients with Parkinson's disease.[3,4,6] Concurrent use of levodopa and the tricyclics need not be avoided, but it should be confirmed that the effects of the levodopa are not diminished. Prescribers should also be aware of the isolated hypertensive crisis cited when metoclopramide was used as well, but there is insufficient evidence to comment on its general importance.

References

1 Morgan J P, Rivera-Calimlim L, Messiha F, Sandaresan P R and Trabert N. Imipramine-mediated interference with levodopa absorption from the gastrointestinal tract in man. *Neurology* (1975) **25**, 1029.
2 Rampton D S. Hypertensive crisis on a patient given *Sinemet*, metoclopramide, and amitriptyline. *Br Med J* (1977) **3**, 607.
3 Yahr M D. The treatment of parkinsonism—Current concepts. *Med Clin N Amer* (1972) **56**, 1377.
4 Calne D B and Reid J L. Antiparkinsonian drugs: Pharmacological and therapeutic aspects. *Drugs* (1972) **4**, 49.
5 Messcha F S and Morgan J P. Imipramine-mediated effects on levodopa metabolism in man. *Biochem Pharmac* (1974) **23**, 1503.
6 van Wiegeren A and Wright J. Observations on patients with Parkinson's disease treated with L-dopa. I. Trial and evaluation of L-dopa therapy. *SA Med J* (1972) **46**, 1262.

Piribedil + clonidine

Summary

The antiparkinsonian effects of piribedil can be antagonized by clonidine.

Interaction, mechanism, importance and management

Five patients taking piribedil who were concurrently treated with clonidine showed a worsening of their parkinsonism due, it was suggested, to stimulation by the clonidine of alpha-adrenergic receptors within the CNS which antagonized the antiparkinson effects of the levodopa. The data are much too limited to comment constructively on the general importance of this interaction, but it would be prudent to be on the alert for the development of this interaction during concurrent use.

Reference

1 Shoulson I and Chase T N. Clonidine and the anti-parkinsonian response to L-dopa or piribedil. *Neuropharmacology* (1976) **15**, 25.

CHAPTER 10. BETA-ADRENORECEPTOR BLOCKER DRUG INTERACTIONS

The adrenoreceptors of the sympathetic nervous system are of two types, namely alpha (α) and beta (β). The beta-adrenoreceptor blocking drugs (more briefly and commonly known as the beta-blockers) are sufficiently selective to block only the beta-receptors and this property is therapeutically exploited to reduce the normal sympathetic stimulation of the heart. The activity of the heart in response to stress and exercise is reduced, its consumption of oxygen is diminished, and in this way the angina of effort can be treated. The beta-blockers can also be used in the treatment of cardiac arrhythmias and hypertension, and this too is believed to be due to their beta-blocking activity.

Some of the beta-blocking drugs are sufficiently selective to demonstrate that all beta-receptors are not identical, but can be further subdivided into two groups, β_1 and

Table 10.1. Beta-blocking drugs

Non-proprietary names	Proprietary names
Cardioselective (block β_1 receptors only)	
Acebutalol	*Sectral*
Atenolol	*Tenormin*
Bunitrolol	
Metoprolol	*Betaloc, Lopressor, Seloken*
Practolol	*Eraldin, Dalzic*
Tolamolol	
Non-selective (block β_1 and β_2 receptors)	
Alprenolol	*Aptin, Betacard, Guernal, Tenorectic*
Bufetolol	*Adobiol*
Bufuralol	
Bunitrolol	
Bunolol	
Bupranolol	*Betadran, Betadrenol, Looser*
Inpea	
Nadolol	*Corgard*
Oxprenolol	*Trasicor*
Penbutolol	
Pindolol	*Visken, Viskaldix*
Propranolol	*Avlocardyl, Dociton, Herzul, Inderal, Kemi, Berkolol, Sumial*
Sotalol	*Sotazide, Betacardone, Sotacor*
Timolol	*Blockadren, Betim, Prestim*
Toliprolol	*Doberol*

In addition labetalol (*Trandate*) blocks β_1, β_2 and α-receptors.

β_2. The former are found in the heart and the latter in the bronchi. Since one of the unwanted side-effects of generalized beta-blockade is the loss of the normal noradrenaline-stimulated bronchodilation (leading to bronchospasm), there was some considerable therapeutic advantage in the development of these 'cardioselective' β_1 blocking drugs (such as practolol, metoprolol etc.) which leave the β_2-receptors virtually unaffected. These cardioselective beta-blockers are therefore particularly valuable in patients such as asthmatics where bronchospasm is clearly unacceptable, although it should be pointed out that their selectivity is by no means absolute (see page 265). Table 10.1 lists most of the cardioselective and non-selective beta-blocking drugs which have been produced commercially.

In addition to the interactions with the beta-blockers detailed in this chapter, there are others discussed elsewhere. A full list is to be found in the Index.

Beta-blockers + anaesthetics (general)

Summary

Although the cardiac rate and output can fall markedly during anaesthesia in patients taking beta-blockers, concurrent use is not contraindicated provided appropriate precautions are taken, such as the use of atropine to prevent excessive vagal tone and the avoidance of certain anaesthetic agents (ether, chloroform, cyclopropane, trichloroethylene, methoxyflurane).

Interaction

The cardiac rate and output can fall during anaesthesia in patients on beta-blocking drugs.

A study on patients receiving general anaesthesia with nitrous oxide, oxygen and 1% halothane showed that the presence of oxprenolol (2 mg), alprenolol (5 mg) or practolol (15 mg) given intravenously caused marked reductions in cardiac output (mean reduction 25% but individually as high as 40%), a fall in heart rate (means 12%) and a sustained rise in central venous pressure.[1]

Similar responses have been described elsewhere in patients under halothane anaesthesia treated with propranolol or alprenolol,[2] and there are numerous other studies of this interaction. One method of accommodating this reaction has been to withdraw the beta-blocker before the operation and in two detailed reports this was achieved successfully and relatively uneventfully.[3,4]

Mechanism

In the presence of drugs which block the beta-adrenoreceptors of the heart, one of the normal responses of the body to stress is severely impaired. This exaggerates the hazards of hypotension and bradycardia.

Importance and management

Concurrent use is not contraindicated provided precautions are taken. The intravenous injection of atropine (1–2 mg) will protect against the bradycardia due to the unrestrained vagal dominance.[5] It is also advised that ether, chloroform, cyclopropane and trichloroethylene are avoided.[5] Animal and clinical data suggest that methoxyflurane should also be included because of its myocardial depressant effects.[6,7]

Temporary withdrawal of the beta-blocker has been advocated but it appears to be neither necessary nor advisable because the sudden interruption of treatment can expose patients to the development of severe angina or dysrhythmias.[5,8]

It has been suggested[3] that hypotension during concurrent use should be controlled by decreasing the depth of anaesthesia, increasing IV fluid administration, altering surgical manipulation and position of the patients, and administering vasopressors such as ephedrine. Additional further treatment can be undertaken with an isoprenaline (isoproteronol) drip, although larger doses than usual will be needed to compete for the beta-receptors; 5–20 μg/min has been used. Glucagon as a 5–10 mg IV bolus followed by a 1 mg/min IV drip has proved effective; 250–1000 mg $CaCl_2$ given slowly intravenously will also bypass beta-adrenoreceptor blockade.[3]

References

1 Stephen G W, Davie I T and Scott D B. Haemodynamic effects of beta-receptor blocking drugs during nitrous oxide/halothane anesthesia. *Brit J Anaesth* (1971) **43**, 320.
2 Jorfeldt L, Löfström B, Möller J and Rosén A. Cardiovascular effects of beta-receptor blocking drugs during halothane anaesthesia in man. *Acta anaesthes Scandinav* (1970) **14**, 35.
3 Kaplan J A and Dunbar R W. Propranolol and surgical anesthesia. *Anesth Analg* (1976) **55**, 1.
4 Kaplan J A, Dunbar R W and Bland J W. Propranolol and cardiac surgery; a problem for the anesthesiologist? *Anesth Analg* (1975) **54**, 571.
5 Inderal Tablets and Infection. *Data Sheet Compendium 1979–80*, p. 422. Pharmind Publications, London (1979).
6 Viljoen J F, Estafanous F C and Kellner G A. Propranolol and cardiac surgery. *J Thorac Cardiovasc Surg* (1972) **64**, 826.
7 Saner C A, Foëx P, Roberts J G and Bennett M J. Methoxyflurane and practolol: a dangerous combination. *Brit J Anaesth* (1975) **47**, 1025.
8 Shand D G. Propranolol withdrawal. *New Eng J Med* (1975) **293**, 449.

Beta-blockers + antacids

Summary

Some preliminary evidence indicates that aluminium hydroxide may cause a marked reduction in the absorption of propranolol from the gut. Evidence about other antacids and beta-blockers is lacking.

Interaction

A study on 5 subjects who were treated concurrently with single doses of propranolol, 80 mg, and aluminium hydroxide, 30 ml, showed that the maximum plasma concentration of propranolol and the area under the plasma concentration time curve were both reduced by almost 60%.[1]

Mechanism

Uncertain. The reduction in absorption could possibly be related to a delay in gastric emptying induced by the antacid.

Importance and management

Information appears to be limited to this one report, moreover, it is a single-dose study and not therefore necessarily a reliable predictor of what may happen in patients on chronic treatment with propranolol. Until more data are available, and considering the extent of the reduction (60%) it would seem wise to separate the dosages of the antacid and propranolol by as long a time interval as possible. Information about other antacids and beta-blockers is not available. More study is required.

Reference

1 Dobbs J H, Skoutakis V A, Acchardio S R and Dobbs B R. Effects of aluminium hydroxide on the absorption of propranolol. *Curr Ther Res* (1977) **21**, 887.

Beta-blocking agents + barbiturates

Summary

The serum levels of alprenolol and metoprolol are reduced by the concurrent use of pentobarbitone, but the effect of this on the clinical response has not been determined.

Interaction

The serum levels of some of the beta-blocking drugs may be reduced by the concurrent use of barbiturates.

(a) Alprenolol + pentobarbitone

A study on 5 normal subjects showed that the area under the plasma concentration/time curve after a 200 mg oral dose of alprenolol was reduced by about 80% (from 706 to 154 μg/ml) following the administration of 100 mg pentobarbitone for 10–14 days.[1]

(b) Metoprolol + pentobarbitone

A study on eight normal subjects showed that the area under the plasma concentration time curve after a 100 mg dose of metoprolol was reduced by an average of 32% after treatment with 100 mg pentobarbitone at bedtime for 10 days.

Mechanism

Barbiturates, such as pentobarbitone, are potent liver enzyme inducing agents and can enhance the metabolism and clearance of drugs from the body. Since the oral but not intravenous dose of alprenolol[1] was affected in the study cited,[1] it is thought that the reduced plasma concentrations were due to an increase in the metabolism of the beta-blocker during its passage through the liver on its way into the general circulation (a so-called 'first pass' effect).

Importance and management

Information is limited but, on the basis of the studies described, a reduction in the effects of alprenolol and metoprolol by pentobarbitone may be expected. The extent to which this affects the treatment of angina or hypertension has not been studied but particularly in the case of alprenolol where the reduction in serum concentration was found to be 80%, a clinically important reduction in response seems highly likely. It is not known whether this interaction takes place with other beta-blockers, but it would be prudent to watch for a reduction in the clinical response if barbiturates are used with beta-blockers which are extensively metabolised. All the barbiturates are potent enzyme-inducing agents so that interaction may be expected to take place with barbiturates other than pentobarbitone, but no interaction apart from those cited has yet been documented.

References

1 Alván G, Piafsky K, Lind M and von Bahr C. Effect of pentobarbital on the disposition of alprenolol. *Clin Pharmacol Ther* (1977) **22**, 316.
2 Haglund K, Seideman P, Collste P, Borg K-O and von Bahr C. Influence of pentobarbital on metoprolol plasma levels. *Clin Pharmacol Ther* (1979) **26**, 326.

Beta-blockers + cimetidine

Summary

Elevated serum propranolol levels and reduced resting pulse rates have been described in patients concurrently taking cimetidine. Profound bradycardia has been seen with atenolol. Labetalol also appears to be affected.

Interaction

The observation that a patient taking cimetidine developed profound sinus bradycardia (36 beats/minute) when atenolol was added for the treatment of angina, prompted further study of this possible interaction in another patient. It was found that after taking 200 mg cimetidine three times a day and 400 mg at night for a period of two weeks, the serum levels of propranolol over the 12 h following a single 80 mg dose were markedly raised. The area under the concentration/time curve was increased by 340% and the serum levels increased between 3 and 6 times.[1]

This interaction has been confirmed in another study.[3]

Another brief report on 3 normal subjects stated that the bioavailability of labetalol was increased about 80% by the use of cimetidine, 400 mg four times a day for 3 days.[2]

Mechanism

Uncertain. The suggestion is that the cimetidine inhibits the metabolism of the propranolol by the liver, thereby allowing it to accumulate[1,3] and reduces the liver blood flow.[3]

Importance and management

Information seems to be limited to these reports, but they serve to alert prescribers to the possibility of an enhancement of the effects of these beta-blockers, in the presence of cimetidine. More study is needed. There seems as yet to be no information about other beta-blockers.

References

1 Donovan M A, Heagerty A M, Patel L, Castleden M and Pohl J E F. Cimetidine and bioavailability of propranolol. *Lancet* (1981) **i**, 164.
2 Daneshmend T K and Roberts C J C. Cimetidine and bioavailability of labetalol. *Lancet* (1981) **i**, 565.
3 Feeley J., Wilkinson G R. and Wood A J J. Reduction of liver blood flow and propranolol metabolism by cimetidine. *New Eng J Med* (1981) **304**, 692.

Beta-blockers + ergotamine

Summary

The concurrent use of propranolol and ergotamine (in *Cafergot*) for the treatment of migraine is usually safe and effective, but two adverse reactions have been described.

Interaction

A man whose recurrent migraine headaches had been reasonably well controlled over a 6-year period with two daily suppositories of *Cafergot* (ergotamine tartrate 2 mg, caffeine 100 mg, butalbital 100 mg, belladonna leaf alkaloids 250 μg) developed progressively painful and purple feet a short while after additionally beginning to take 30 mg propranolol daily. When he eventually resumed taking *Cafergot* alone there was no further evidence of peripheral vasoconstriction.[1]

A man with a history of migraine, easily relieved by *Cafergot*, was given propranolol for the treatment of angina and cardiac arrhythmias. The migraine attacks were exacerbated, becoming more frequent and severe, and proved refractory to the ergot until the propranolol was withdrawn.[2]

These two reports contrast with another stating that concurrent use in 50 patients was effective and uneventful.[3]

Mechanism

Uncertain. One suggestion[1] to explain the severe vasoconstruction is that since the ergot alkaloids induce vasoconstriction, and propranolol blocks the vasodilatory effects of the adrenaline, the two effects would enhance one another. Another report suggests that the patient might have been taking an overdose.[3] There is no explanation for the second case described.

Importance and management

There are only two reports of adverse interactions and good evidence that concurrent use is usually safe and effective, but it would clearly be prudent to be on the alert for any signs of an adverse response.

References

1 Baumrucker J F. Drug interaction—propranolol and cafergot. *New Eng J med* (1973) **288**, 916.
2 Blank N K and Rieder M J. Paradoxical response to propranolol in migraine. *Lancet* (1973), **ii**, 1336.
3 Diamond S. Propranolol and ergontaine tartrate (cont.) *New Eng J Med* (1973) **289**, 159.

Beta-blockers + dextromoramide

Summary

Two cases of bradycardia and severe hypotension have been observed in patients during the pre-surgical period following the use of propranolol and dextromoramide.

Interaction, mechanism, importance and management

Two women about to undergo partial thyroidectomy were given 30 mg propranolol and dextromoramide (1·25 and 4 mg respectively) by injection during the preoperative period following the induction of anaesthesia. Each developed marked bradycardia and severe hypotension which responded rapidly to the intravenous injection of atropine.[1] The reasons for this response are not understood.

Reference

1 Cabanne F, Wilkening M, Caillard B, Foissac J C and Aupecle P. Interférences médicamenteuses induites par l'association propranolol–dextromoramide. *Anesth Anal Réan* (1973) **30**, 369.

Beta-blockers + glucagon

Summary
The hyperglycaemic effects of glucagon may be reduced by propranolol.

Interaction, mechanism, importance and management

A study on 5 normal subjects showed that the hyperglycaemic activity of glucagon was reduced to some extent in the presence of propranolol. The mechanism of this is uncertain. A similar response would be expected in patients under treatment with propranolol. Whether this is also true of the other beta-blockers is not confirmed.

Reference
1 Messerli F H, Kuchel O and Tolis G. Effects of beta-adrenergic blockade on plasma cyclic AMP and blood sugar responses to glucagon and isoproteronol in man. *Int J Clin Pharmacol* (1976) **14**, 189.

Beta-blockers + halofenate

Summary
Halfenate can cause a marked reduction in the serum levels and therapeutic effects of propranolol. This may possibly prove to be hazardous in those under treatment for angina where sudden withdrawal is known to exacerbate coronary insufficiency.

Interaction

A crossover study in 4 healthy subjects who were given either 80 or 160 mg propranolol or a placebo for 2 days, after taking halofenate, 1 g daily, for 21 days, showed that the steady-state plasma levels of the propranolol were reduced by 74 and 81% respectively. The cardiac response to isoprenaline correlated with the reduction in beta-blockade in 3 of the 4 subjects.[1]

Mechanism

Uncertain. One postulate is that the halofenate increased the metabolism and clearance of the propranolol from the body.[1]

Importance and management

Information is very limited but the study cited was well controlled. Because the reduction in the serum levels is so large and because the morbidity of those with coronary insufficiency is increased by the sudden withdrawal of propranolol,[2] it is clearly most important that patients on therapy with both drugs should be carefully checked for a reduction in the response to propranolol. Information about the effect of halofenate on other beta-blockers appears to be lacking.

References
1 Huffman D H, Azarnoff D L, Shoeman D W and Dujorne C A. The interaction between halofenate and propranolol. *Clin Pharmacol Therap* (1976) **19**, 807.
2 Miller R R, Olson H G, Amsterdam E A and Mason D T. Propranolol withdrawal rebound phenomenon: Exacerbation of coronary events after abrupt cessation of anti-anginal therapy. *New Eng J Med* (1975) **293**, 416.

Beta-blockers + nifedipine

Summary
Two cases of heart failure and another of excessive hypotension have been described in patients on beta-blockers when additionally given nifedipine

Interaction, mechanism, importance and management

Two patients with angina under treatment with beta-blockers (alprenolol, propranolol) developed heart failure when nifedipine, 10 mg three times a day, was additionally given. The signs of heart failure disappeared when the nifedipine was withdrawn.[1] In another report[2] one out of 15 patients with hypertension and exertional angina developed hypotension when nifedipine (10 mg twice daily) was added to their treatment with atenolol (50–100 mg daily), prazocin (9 mg daily) and diuretics. The situation was controlled by withdrawal of the nifedipine.

Concurrent use is not contraindicated, but these reports emphasize the need for particular care if combined treatment is undertaken.

References
1 Anastassiades C J. Nifedipine and beta-blocker drugs. *Brit Med J* (1980) **281**, 1251.
2 Opie L H and White D A. Adverse interaction between nifedipine and beta-blockade. *Brit Med J* (1980) **281**, 1462.

Beta-blockers + phenothiazines

Summary

The serum levels of propranolol can be raised by the concurrent use of chlorpromazine. Serum chlorpromazine levels can be raised by the use of propranolol.

Interaction

A study on 4 normal subjects and 1 hypertensive patient, all of whom were taking propranolol, 80 mg 8-hourly, showed that the concurrent administration of chlorpromazine, 50 mg 8-hourly, raised the mean steady-state propranolol serum levels by 70% (from 41·5 to 70·2 ng/ml). The increase was considerable in some of the subjects but barely detectable in others. Another subject on propranolol not included in this study climbed out of bed 2 h after his first dose of chlorpromazine and promptly fainted. He was found to have a pulse-rate of 35–40 and a blood pressure of 70/0 mmHg. He was given 3 mg atropine within a few minutes of the collapse, when his pulse rate rose to 85 and blood pressure to 120/70 mmHg.[1]

Another case of hypotension during the concurrent use of chlorpromazine and sotalol has also been reported.[2] It has also been shown that chlorpromazine serum levels can be markedly raised by the concurrent use of propranolol.[4]

Mechanism

Pharmacokinetic evidence[1] suggests that chlorprorazine inhibits the metabolism of propranolol resulting in its accumulation. This is confirmed by in-vitro experiments with rat tissue.[3]

The severe hypotension described in one patient,[1] mild postural hypotension in another[1] and hypotension in a third[2] may have resulted from the additive hypotensive effects of both chlorpromazine and propranolol, but this is not certain.

Importance and management

The data are very limited but indicate that additive hypotensive effects may occur during concurrent treatment. If the dosage of propranolol is established in the presence of the chlorpromazine, it should be borne in mind that subsequent withdrawal of the phenothiazine might result in inadequate therapeutic concentrations of the propranolol. This has not yet been confirmed.

Information about other beta-blockers and phenothiazines is not available.

References
1 Vestal R E, Kornhauser D M, Hollifield J W and Shand D G. Inhibition of propranolol metabolism by chlorpromazine. *Clin Pharmacol Ther* (1979) **25**, 19.
2 Baker L, Barcai A, Kaye R and Haque N. Beta-adrenergic blockade and juvenile diabetes: acute studies and long-term therapeutic trial. *J Pediat* (1969) **75**, 19.
3 Shand D G and Oates J A. The metabolism of propranolol by rat liver microsomes and its inhibition by phenothiazine and tricyclic antidepressants. *Biochem Pharmacol* (1971) **20**, 1720.
4 Peet M, Middlemiss D N and Yates R A. Pharmacokinetic interaction between propranolol and chlorpromazine in schizophrenic patients. *Lancet* (1980) **ii**, 978.

Beta-blockers + salicylates

Summary
There is evidence that no interaction occurs between alprenolol and sodium salicylate.

Interaction, mechanism, importance and management

Sodium salicylate has no significant effect on the pharmacological response to alprenolol in man despite a theory that some interference with metabolism migh occur. Information about other salicylates and beta-blockers is lacking.[1]

Reference
1 Johnsson G, Regardh C G and Sölvell L. Lack of biological interaction of alprenolol and salicylate in man. *Europ J clin Pharmacol* (1973) **6**, 9.

Beta-blockers + sympathomimetics (bronchodilators)

Summary
Non-selective beta-blockers (e.g. propranolol) are contraindicated in asthmatics. The safety of cardioselective beta-blockers (eg metoprolol) in asthmatic patients is by no means absolutely certain, but no adverse interaction would be expected during the concurrent use of sympathomimetic bronchodilators (eg isoprenaline).

Interaction
(a) Non-selective beta-blockers (see Table 10.1 on page 258)

These drugs are contraindicated in asthmatic subjects because they prevent normal bronchodilation and exacerbate asthma.[1,2]

(b) Cardioselective beta-blockers (see Table 10.1 on page 258) + *sympathomimetic bronchodilators*.

Although in theory these drugs do not affect the beta-receptors in the bronchi, there are cases on record of severe broncho-spasm following their use, and their so-called cardioselectivity is by no means an absolute guarantee that some patients will not react adversely. There is however evidence that no adverse interaction occurs with sympathomimetic bronchodilators.

A study in 29 patients with chronic bronchial asthma under treatment with practolol, 200 mg daily, showed that the effects of terbutaline, 5 mg three times a day, were unaltered and no subjective or objective worsening of the asthmatic symptoms was seen.[3]

Similar results have been described in other studies with metoprolol[1,2] or practolol[1] and isoprenaline.

Mechanism
Non-selective beta-blockers block the beta-receptors in the bronchi as well as the heart so that the normal bronchodilation which is under the control of the sympathetic nervous system does not take place. Thus the bronchoconstriction of asthma is exacerbated. Selective beta-blockers on the other hand preferentially block beta-1 receptors in the heart, leaving the beta-2 receptors in the bronchi largely unaffected so that the beta-2 stimulating bronchodilators have their normal activity.

Importance and management
It is clearly important to avoid the use of non-selective beta-blockers in asthmatic subjects. Even the use of eyedrops containing the non-selective beta-blocker, timolol, has been reported to precipitate an asthmatic attack.[4] The cardioselective beta-blockers are by no means necessarily safe substitutes for the non-selective beta-blockers in patients with chronic obstructive airway disease who require bronchodilators, although the evi-

dence suggests that an adverse interaction with the sympathomimetics (isoprenaline, terbutaline, salbutamol) is unlikely. It might be safer to consider alternative drugs for hypertension or angina in patients who also need treatment for broncho-spasm.

References

1 Thiringer G and Svedmyr N. Interaction of orally adminis-tered metoprolol, practolol and propranolol with isoprenaline in asthmatics. *Europ J Clin Pharmacol* (1976) **10**, 163.

2 Johnsson G, Svedmyr N and Thiringer G. Effects of intra-venous propranolol and metoprolol and their interaction with isoprenaline on pulmonary function, heart rate and blood pressure in asthmatics. *Europ J Clin Pharmacol* (1975) **8**, 175.

3 Formgren H and Eriksson N E. Effects of practolol in combination with terbutaline in the treatment of hyperten-sion and arrhythmias in asthmatic patients. *Scand J Resp Dis* (1975) **56**, 217.

4 Charan N B and Lakshminarayan S. Pulmonary effects of topical timolol. *Arch Int Med* (1980) **120**, 843.

CHAPTER 11. ORAL CONTRACEPTIVE DRUG INTERACTIONS

The oral contraceptives are of three main types: the 'combined' oestrogen–progestogen preparations; the sequential type which also contains both steroids, but the doses of each are varied throughout the cycle; and the progestogen-only preparations. There are now a very large number of oral contraceptive preparations marketed worldwide, some of which are listed in Table 11.1. The oestrogens used are either ethinyloestradiol, in doses of 20–50 μg, or mestranol, in doses of 50–100 μg. The progestogens are either those derived from 19-nortestosterone (e.g. norethynodrel, ethynodiol acetate, norgestrel, norethisterone, lynoestrenol) or more rarely from 17α-hydroxyprogesterone (e.g. megestrol) in doses ranging from about 0·25–5·0 mg.

Combined contraceptives

Most of these are taken for 20–21 days, followed by a period of 7 days during which withdrawal bleeding occurs. Some of them (e.g. *Minovlar Ed* and *Norinyl 1/28*) also include 6 or 7 tablets of lactose which can be taken during this period so that the daily habit of taking a tablet is not broken. These combined contraceptives act in several ways. The oestrogenic component suppresses ovulation, and the progestogen acts to change the endometrial structure so that even if conception were to occur, implantation would be unlikely. In addition the cervical mucus becomes unusually viscous which inhibits the free movement of the spermatozoa.

Sequential contraceptives

These preparations follow the normal menstrual cycle hormonal changes, but inhibit ovulation. The progestogen component ensures that the menstrual cycle flow is more moderate than would occur with the oestrogen only.

Progestogen-only contraceptives ('mini pill')

The so-called 'minipills' (because the dosages of the progestogen are low) are taken continuously. They do not inhibit ovulation, but they probably act by increasing the viscosity of the cervical mucus so that movement of the sperm is retarded, and by causing changes in the endometrium which inhibit successful implantation.

In addition to the interactions of the oral contraceptives discussed in this chapter, there are others dealt with elsewhere. A full list is to be found in the Index.

Table 11.1. Various formulations of combination progestogen–oestrogen oral contraceptive preparations, containing 19-nortestosterone derivatives as progestogens

Progestogen (dose in mg)	Oestrogen (dose in μg)				
	Ethinyl-oestradiol 50	Mestranol			
		50	75	80	100
Ethynodiol diacetate					
0·5	1	—	—	—	14
1·0	2	—	—	—	15
Lynoestrenol					
1·0	—	—	—	—	16
2·5	3	—	11	—	—
Norethisterone (Norethindrone)					
0·5	—	—	—	—	17
1·0	—	10	—	13	—
2·0	—	—	—	—	18
Norethisterone acetate					
1·0	4	—	—	—	—
2·5	5	—	—	—	—
3·0	6	—	—	—	—
4·0	7	—	—	—	—
Norethynodrel					
2·5	—	—	—	—	19
5·0	—	—	12	—	—
Norgestrel					
(d) 0·25	8	—	—	—	—
(dl) 0·5	9	—	—	—	—

1 *Demulen 50*
  Ovulen 0·5/50
2 *Edulen*
  Ovulen 1/50
3 *Minilyn*
4 *Minovlar*
  Norlestrin 1 mg
  Orlest
  Zotane 1/50
5 *Norlestrin 2·5 mg*
6 *Controlvar*
  Gynovlar
7 *Anovlar*

8 *Neogynon*
  Ovran
  Nordiol
9 *Eugynon**
  Ovral
10 *Norinyl-1 (or 1 + 50)*
  Ortho-Novin† 1/50
11 *Anacyclin*
  Lyndiol
12 *Conovid*
  Enovid 5 mg
13 *Ortho-Novin† 1/80*
  Norinyl 1 + 80

14 *Edulen*
  Demulen
  Ovulen 0·5 mg
15 *Ovulen 1·0 mg*
16 *Microcyclin*
  Ovostat
17 *Ortho-Novin† 0·5 mg*
18 *Norinyl-2*
  Ortho-Novin† 2 mg
19 *Conovid E*
  Enovid E
  Novol
  Oralyn

* Eugynon 30 contains 30 μg instead of 50 μg of ethinyloestradiol.
† Also spelt 'Ortho-Novum'.

Reproduced with permission from *Textbook of Pharmacology*, Bowman and Rand (eds) (1980) Blackwell Scientific Publications.

Oral contraceptives + antacids

Summary
Some in-vitro evidence suggests that there is the possibility that magnesium trisilicate might reduce the reliability of the oral contraceptives.

Interaction, mechanism, importance and management

An in-vitro study showed that some steroids commonly found in oral contraceptives were adsorbed by a suspension of magnesium trisilicate in water (see Table 11.2).

Elution experiments with dilute hydrochloric acid showed that not more than 35% of the steroids was eluted from the antacid within 3 hours, and a dissolution test with *Anovlar 21* demonstrated that the presence of 0·5 mg% magnesium trisilicate almost completely adsorbed the norethisterone after 3 h.[1]

These experiments suggest that the concurrent use of magnesium tricilicate, and possibly other antacids and adsorbents, might reduce the bioavailabiltiy of the contraceptives to such an extent that a normal menstrual cycle with ovulation could recommence. Contraceptive failure attributed to the use of antacids appears not to have been described, but the possibility of such an interaction ought not to be dismissed.

Reference

1 Khalil S A H. The in-vitro uptake of some oral contraceptive steroids by magnesium trisilicate. *J Pharm Pharmac* (1976) **28**, (*Suppl*), 47P.

Table 11.2. Percentage adsorption by a 1% suspension of magnesium trisilicate in water

Steroid, and its initial concentration	0·5 mg%	1·0 mg%
Ethisterone	87·6	93·1
Mestranol	81·0	—
Norethisterone	49·2	49·8
Ethinyloestradiol	5·5	6·3

After S A H Khalil.[1]

Oral contraceptives + anti-asthmatic preparations

Summary

No recorded interactions, but asthma is included by some manufacturers of oral contraceptives among their 'special precautions' because the asthmatic condition may be affected (not necessarily adversely).

Interaction, mechanism, importance and management

There have been some instances in which women have developed allergic conditions such as allergic rhinitis, atopic eczema, urticaria or asthma while taking oral contraceptives.[1-3] In contrast there are instances where the pre-existing asthma and other allergic conditions have improved.[2] For this reason it has been claimed that '. . . it is always worth giving an oral contraceptive a trial for the patients with any of these complaints [eczema, asthma, vasomotor rhinitis, migraine] as there is an even chance that she will be improved; if the condition is aggravated, it will return to its previous state as soon as the medication is stopped.[1]

References

1 Mears E. Oral contraceptives. *Lancet* (1964) **i**, 980.
2 Falliers C J. Oral contraceptives and allergy. *Lancet* (1974) **ii**, 515.
3 Horan J D and Lederman J J. Possible asthmogenic effect of oral contraceptives. *Canad Med Ass J* (1968) **99**, 130.

Oral contraceptives + antibiotics and anti-infective agents

Summary

Cases of oral contraceptive failure attributed to the concurrent use of chloramphenicol, dapsone, erythromycin, cephalexin with clindamycin, nitrofurantoin, co-trimoxazole or sulphamethoxypyridazine have been reported.

Interaction

Two women have been very briefly reported who became pregnant while taking an oral contraceptive. One had also been treated with chloramphenicol, and the other with sulphamethoxypyridazine. Break-through bleeding was observed in both women following the use of these two drugs.[1,2] Other single cases of contraceptive failure have been attributed to the concurrent use of chloramphenicol, dapsone, erythromycin, cephalexin with clindamycin, nitrofurantoin, and co-trimoxazole.[3]

Mechanism

Not understood. Suppression of intestinal bacteria, as suggested with the tetracyclines (see p. 275) is a possible explanation.

Importance and management

There appear to be only isolated cases of interactions with these drugs on record, but prescribers should be aware of these reports. Whether alternative forms of contraception should be advised routinely is uncertain. The comments relating to the management of the contraceptive/penicillin interaction would seem to be applicable to these drugs as well (see p. 272).

References

1 Hempel E, Böhm W, Carol W and Klinger G. Medikamentose Enzyminduktion und hormonal Kontrazeption. Zbl Gynäk (1973) 95, 1451.
2 Hempel E. Personal communication (1975).
3 Back D J, Breckenridge A M, Crawford F E, MacIver M, Orme L E and Rowe P H. Interindividual variation and drug interactions with hormonal steroid contraceptives. Drugs (1981) 21, 46.

Oral contraceptives + anticonvulsants

Summary

The oestrogen/progestogen oral contraceptives are not reliable during concurrent treatment with phenytoin, primidone, barbiturates, or possibly carbamazepine. Intermediate break-through bleeding and spotting may take place and pregnancies have occurred. Epileptic seizure control may also be disturbed.

Interaction

Concurrent use can result in (a) failure of the contraceptive to prevent pregnancy and (b) a disturbance of seizure control.

(a) Contraceptive failure

The first report was published in 1972 of an epileptic woman, taking 200 mg phenytoin and 50 mg sulthiame daily, with ferrous gluconate and folic acid, who became pregnant despite the regular use of an oral contraceptive containing ethinyloestradiol 0·05 mg and norethisterone acetate, 3 mg.[1]

Since this report appeared, at least another 25 pregnancies have been reported in epileptic women taking a variety of oestrogen/progestogen contraceptives and anticonvulsant drugs, in various combinations, but including either phenytoin, a barbiturate or primidone.[2–6,11] There is also some evidence implicating carbamazepine as well.[13] The Committee on the Safety of Medicines in the UK has also received another 23 reports[12] making a total of 49 known cases in the 1972–80 period.

(b) Disturbance of seizure control

Epilepsy is included by most manufacturers of oral

contraceptives among the 'special precautions' because seizure control may sometimes be made worse, but it is also true that it may remain unaltered or even improve:

> An epileptic woman under treatment with phenobarbitone and phenytoin became much worse while taking *Lyndiol* but improved when *Gynovlar* and later *Ovulen* were substituted.[7]

Other reports describe 20 epileptics taking a variety of anticonvulsants whose condition was unaltered when administered *Norinyl-1* as well.[8] A woman on phenytoin and phenobarbitone was completely free of fits until she discontinued the unnamed oral contraceptive she had been taking.[9]

Mechanism
The available evidence strongly suggests that oral contraceptive failure occurs because phenytoin, the barbiturates and primidone act as potent liver enzyme inducing agents which increase the rate of metabolism of the components of the oral contraceptive. This may also be true of carbamazepine. These anticonvulsants can also lower the concentration of free and active molecules of the progestogen by increasing their binding to sex-hormone binding globulin. The biological activity of the steroids is thereby reduced allowing the normal menstrual cycle and ovulation to recommence.[2]

Changes in seizure control have been attributed to changes in fluid retention which can influence seizure frequency.[7,8]

Importance and management
Failure of the contraceptive in the presence of anticonvulsants is well-established but its incidence it not known. One of the signs of developing failure is intermediate break-through bleeding and spotting. Two courses of action have been suggested to accommodate this interaction: one is to use contraceptives containing 50 μg ethinyloestradiol;[11,12] if break-through bleeding still occurs, give in addition a preparation containing 30 μg ethinyloestradiol.[12] The alternative is to use a mechanical form of contraception. It is also important to be on the alert for changes in seizure control.

References
1 Kenyon I E. Unplanned pregnancy in an epileptic. *Br Med J* (1972) **1**, 686.
2 Hempel von E, Bohm W, Carol W and Klinger G. Medikamentöse Enzyminduktion und hormonale Kontrazepcion. *Zbl Gynäk* (1973) **95**, 1451.
3 Janz D and Schmidt D. Anti-epileptic drugs and failure of oral contraceptives. *Lancet* (1974) **i**, 1113.
4 Janz D and Schmidt D. Anti-epileptic drugs and the safety of oral contraceptives. Paper delivered to the German Section of the International League against Epilepsy, Berlin, 1 September 1974.
5 Belaisch J, Driguez P and Janaud A. Influence de certains médicaments sur l'action des pilules contraceptives. *Nouv Presse Méd* (1976) **5**, 1645.
6 Gagnaire J C, Tchertchian J, Revol A and Rochet Y. Grossesses sous contraceptifs oraux chez les patientes recevant des barbituriques. *Nouv Presse Méd* (1975) **4**, 3008.
7 McArthur J. Notes and comments. Oral contraceptives and epilepsy. *Br Med J* (1967) **3**, 162.
8 Espir M, Wallace M E and Lawson J P. Epilepsy and oral contraception. *Br Med J* (1969) **1**, 294.
9 Copeman H. Oral contraceptives. *Med J Aust* (1963) **2**, 969.
10 Back D J and Orme M L'E. Drug interactions with oral contraceptive steroids. *Prescriber's Journal* (1977) **17**, 137.
11 Coulam C B and Annegers J F. Do anticonvulsants reduce the efficacy of oral contraceptives? *Epilepsia* (1979) **20**, 519.
12 Editorial. Drug interaction with oral contraceptive steroids. *Br Med J* (1980) **3**, 93.
13 Hempel E and Klinger W. Drug stimulated biotransformation of hormonal steroid contraceptives. Clinical implications. *Drugs* (1976) **12**, 442.

Oral contraceptives + antihypertensive agents

Summary
Oral contraceptive-induced hypertension is frequently inadequately controlled by antihypertensive therapy

Interaction, mechanism, importance and management
Virtually all women who take oestrogen-containing oral contraceptives demonstrate some rise in blood pressure. One study[1] on 83 women showed that the average rise was 9·2/5·0 mmHg, and it is about twice as likely to occur as in those not taking an oral contraceptive. There are many reports confirming this response but, despite extensive work, the reasons for the blood pressure rise are by no means fully understood although much of the work has centred around the increases seen in the activity of the renin–angiotensin system. Once the contraceptive is withdrawn,

the blood pressure usually returns to its former levels.[2]

Attempts to control gross rises in pressure using guanethidine, methyldopa and other antihypertensive agents have been less than satisfactory, probably because these agents act on the sympathetic nervous system and would therefore be unlikely to have a major influence on renin–angiotensin-induced vasoconstriction. Clezy in one report stated that '. . . concurrent medication with guanethidine and oral contraceptives made satisfactory control of hypertension difficult or impossible'.[3] Other reports similarly describe a poor or ineffective response to methyldopa or guanethidine in many patients.[4,5]

The hypertension associated with, or exacerbated by, the use of oral contraceptives may therefore not respond adequately to conventional antihypertensive treatment.

References
1 Weir R J, Briggs E, Mack A, Naismith L, Taylor L and Wilson E. Blood pressure in women taking oral contraceptives. *Br Med J* (1974) **1**, 533.
2 Anon. Editorial. Hypertension and oral contraceptives. *Br Med J* (1978) **1**, 1570.
3 Clezy T M. Oral contraceptives and hypertension: the effect of guanethidine. *Med J Aust* (1970) **1**, 638.
4 Wallace M R. Oral contraceptives and severe hypertension. *Aust NZ J Med* (1971) **1**, 49.
5 Woods J W. Oral contraceptives and hypertension. *Lancet* (1967) **iii**, 653.

Oral contraceptives + penicillins

Summary
Contraceptive failure and pregnancies attributed to the concurrent use of penicillins, and ampicillin in particular, have been reported on a number of occasions.

Interaction
The first report of oral contraceptive failures attributed to the use of a penicillin antibiotic was published in 1976:

> A woman had two unwanted pregnancies while on *Minovlar* (ethinyloestradiol 0·05 mg + norethisterone 1 mg). She had also been treated for tonsillitis with wide-spectrum antibiotics, particularly ampicillin. There was no history of diarrhoea or vomiting. Another woman who had been using *Minovlar* for 5 years, with no history of break-through bleeding, lost a quantity of blood similar to a normal period loss within a day of starting to take *Penbritin* (ampicillin), 1 capsule four times a day. There was no evidence of diarrhoea or vomiting. Details of a third case are not available.[1,2]

The British Committee on the Safety of Medicines now have in their records 15 further cases of contraceptive failure in women on penicillin antibiotics: 3 on ampicillin, 3 on ampicillin with either fusidic acid, tetracycline or flucloxacillin, 2 on amoxycillin, 1 on talampicillin, 2 on phenoxymethyl-penicillin (one also taking oxytetracycline), and 4 on 'penicillin'.[8] In another experimental study with ampicillin and penicillin sporadic bleeding disturbances were observed.

In contrast, a controlled study failed to demonstrate this interaction in most of the subjects:-

> A study in 11 volunteers given *Demulen* (50 μg ethinyloestradiol + 1 mg ethynodiol diacetate) showed that when concurrently treated with 250 mg ampicillin, four times a day, over days 1–16 of two menstrual cycle periods, no significant changes in serum levels of follicle-stimulating hormone, luteinizing hormone, oestradiol, progesterone or testosterone binding globulin capacity were seen, although two individuals noted break-through bleeding. One also reported spotting during the use of a placebo.[6]

Mechanism
Not understood. It has been observed that ampicillin given to women in the latter weeks of pregnancy decreases the urinary oestriol levels by nearly 70%[3,4] and phenoxymethylpenicillin behaves in a similar way,[5] but whether these antibiotics interfere with exogenous hormones of the type contained in oral contraceptive preparation, and how this might make them less effective, is not clear. The mechanism suggested for the interaction involving tetracycline (see p. 275) might possibly be applicable to the penicillin antibiotics.

Importance and management
Penicillins have been widely prescribed for many years and must have been given to women taking oral contraceptives on a very large number of occasions, but this interaction has only been

suspected relatively recently. Evidence from reports where drugs have been taken in uncontrolled situations is difficult to evaluate, but the number of cases now on record is sufficiently large for this interaction to be taken seriously. Preliminary data[8] and common experience would seem to suggest that the majority of women may not be at risk, but as yet there seems to be no way of predicting who is likely to be affected.

Some prescribers may consider it prudent to warn patients taking both drugs that spotting and break-through bleeding are signs of diminished contraceptive effectiveness, and additional alternative forms of contraception should be used. The more cautious might suggest using an alternative contraceptive method routinely during concurrent use.

References

1 Dossetor E J. Drug interactions with oral contraceptives. *Br Med J* (1975) **4**, 467.
2 Dossetor E J. Personal communication (1976).
3 Willman K and Pulkkinen M O. Reduced maternal plasma and urinary oestriol during ampicillin treatment. *Am J Obstet Gyn* (1971) **109**, 893.
4 Tikkanen M J, Aldercreutz H and Pulkinnen M O. Effect of antibiotics on oestrogen metabolism. *Br Med J* (1973) 1, 369.
5 Pulkkinen M O and Willman K. Maternal oestrogen levels during penicillin treatment. *Br med J* (1971) **4**, 48.
6 Friedman C I, Huneke A L, Kim M H and Powell J. The effect of ampicillin on oral contraceptive effectiveness. *Obst Gynec* (1980) **55**, 33.
7 Hempel E. Personal communication (1978).
8 Back D J, Breckenridge A M, Crawford F E, MacIver M, Orme L E and Rowe P H. Interindividual variation and drug interactions with hormonal steroid contraceptives. *Drugs* (1981) **21**, 46.

Oral contraceptives + rifampicin

Summary

The ovulation-inhibitor (oestrogen–progestogen) oral contraceptives may not prevent conception and pregnancy in those taking rifampicin. *See also the following synopsis.*

Interaction

Break-through bleeding and pregnancy can occur if rifampicin is used concurrently:

> In the first report of this interaction, a marked increase was described in the frequency of intermediate break-through bleeding in 51 women being treated with rifampicin and ovulation inhibitor oral contraceptives.[1]
>
> In a later report, 62 out of 88 women (i.e. 70%) taking combined oral contraceptives, and who were treated with rifampicin, are described as having developed menstrual cycle disorders of various kinds. Five pregnancies in women taking both types of drug are also mentioned.[2,3]

Other reports have described pregnancies or a disturbance in the menstrual cycles of a large percentage of women using oral contraceptives and rifampicin.[4–8] At least 15 pregnancies have been reported.

Mechanism

Rifampicin is a potent inducer of the drug metabolizing enzymes in the liver. In-vitro experiments[9,10] with liver microsomes taken from patients pretreated with 600 mg rifampicin daily for 6 days have shown that the normal rate of aromatic hydroxylation of ethinyloestradiol (the major pathway for its metabolism and inactiva-

tion in human beings) was increased four-fold, and it can reasonably be assumed that this occurs in vivo as well. There is also good evidence that rifampicin causes a significant reduction in the serum levels of norethisterone which is the progestogen component of many of the combined contraceptives.[12] The reduced levels of these steroids which result would appear to be insufficient to prevent the re-establishment of a normal menstrual cycle and this would explain the break-through bleedings and the pregnancies which have occurred. Mestranol, which is used as an alternative to ethinyloestradiol in a large number of combined and sequential contraceptives, is the 3-methyl ether derivative of ethinyloestradiol and must be demethylated[11] in the body to the parent compound to have effective oestrogenic activity, so it seems highly probable that it will also be affected by the enzyme-inductive effects of rifampicin.

Importance and management

A well-documented and well-established interaction. There is no detailed information about the failure rate, but all women undergoing treatment with rifampicin should use an alternative form of contraception if pregnancy is to be avoided with certainty. The low-dose oestrogen contraceptives would seem likely to be particularly vulnerable.

Evidence against other anti-tubercular drugs is very limited. In one study[2] where rifampicin was substituted by streptomycin, only 1 out of 26 showed a menstrual cycle disorder, but a case of contraceptive failure attributed to the concurrent use of rifampicin with streptomycin and isoniazid has been reported.[13] There is also another case involving isoniazid alone.[13]

References

1 Reimers D and Jezek A. Rifampicin und andere Antituberkulotika bei gleichzeitiger ovaler Kontrazeption. *Prax Pneumol* (1971) **25**, 255.
2 Reimers D, Nocke-Finck L and Breuer H. Rifampicin causes a lowering in efficacy of oral contraceptives by influencing oestrogen excretion. Reports on Rifampicin: XII International Tuberculosis Conference, Tokyo, September 1974.
3 Reimers D, Nocke-Finck L and Breuer H. Rifampicin, 'pill' do not go well together. *J Amer Med Ass* (1974) **227**, 608.
4 Kropp R. Rifampicin und Ovulationshemmer. *Prax Pneumol* (1974) **28**, 270.
5 Bessot J-C, Vandevenne A, Petitjean R and Burghard G. Effets opposés de la rifampicine et de l'isoniazide sur le métabolisme des contraceptifs oraux? *Nouv Presse méd* (1977) **6**, 1568.
6 Hirsch A. Pilules endormies. *Nouv Presse méd* (1973) **2**, 2957.
7 Piguet B, Muglioni J F and Chaline G. Contraception orale et rifampicine. *Nouv Pressé Med* (1975) **4**, 115.
8 Skolnick J L, Stoler B S, Katz D B and Anderson W H. Rifampicin, oral contraceptives and pregnancy. *J Amer Med Ass* (1976) **236**, 1382.
9 Bolt H M, Kappus H and Bolt M. Rifampicin and oral contraception. *Lancet* (1974) **i**, 1280.
10 Bolt H M, Kappus H and Bolt M. Effect of rifampicin treatment on the metabolism of oestradiol and 17 alpha-ethinyloestradiol by Human Liver Microsomes. *Europ J Clin Pharmacol* (1975) **8**, 301.
11 Bolt H M and Bolt W H. Pharmacokinetics of mestranol in man in relation to its oestrogenic activity. *Europ J Clin Pharmacol* (1974) **7**, 295.
12 Back D J, Breckenridge A M, Crawford F, MacIver M, Orme M L'E, Park B K, Rowe P H and Smith E. The effect of rifampicin on norethisterone pharmacokinetics. *Europ J clin Pharmacol* (1979) **15**, 193.
13 Back D J, Breckenridge A M, Crawford F E, MacIver M, Orme L E and Rowe P H. Interindividual variation and drug interactions with hormonal steroid contraceptives. *Drugs* (1981) **21**, 46.

Oral contraceptives + rifampicin

Summary

The serum levels of norethisterone (the active ingredient of some of the progestogen-only oral contraceptives) can be markedly reduced by the concurrent use of rifampicin. The reliability of this type of contraceptive in the presence of rifampicin is now in some doubt. *See also the previous synopsis.*

Interaction

A study on 9 women who were given an oral contraceptive (*Minovlar*—ethinyloestradiol 0·05 mg + norethisterone 1·0 mg) showed that the rate of clearance of the norethisterone was markedly increased by the use of rifampicin, 450–600 mg daily. The serum norethisterone half-life and the area under the curve (AUC) after a single 1 mg dose of norethisterone were reduced about 50%. In one of the women who was on long-term oral contraceptive therapy the 12 h plasma norethisterone concentration was reduced by the rifampicin by more than 80% (from 12·3 to 2·3 ng/ml).[1]

Mechanism

Rifampicin is a known enzyme-inducing agent which increases the rate of metabolism and loss of a number of drugs in man. The study cited[1] included measurements of various indices of enzyme induction and it seems most probable that the results described were due to an increase in the metabolism—and therefore a loss in the biological activity of—norethisterone by rifampicin, due to its enzyme inductive effects.

Importance and management

At least two of the progestogen-only contraceptives (*Micronor*—Ortho, *Noriday*—Syntex) contain only norethisterone, 0·35 mg. If, as has been demonstrated, the serum levels of norethisterone can be reduced by rifampicin to below 20% of the usual levels, there would seem to be the distinct risk that a normal menstrual cycle could recommence. Although at the moment there are no reports of contraceptive failures due to this interaction, until there is good evidence confirming that it is quite safe for women to use this type of contraceptive, it would seem prudent to use an alternative contraceptive method during rifampicin treatment.

Reference

1 Back D J, Breckenridge A M, Crawford F, MacIver M, M L'E Orme, Park B K, Rowe P H and Smith E. The effect of rifampicin on norethisterone pharmacokinetics. *Europ J clin Pharmacol* (1979) **15**, 193.

Oral contraceptives + tetracyclines

Summary
Cases of pregnancy and of break-through bleeding while taking oral contraceptives have been attributed to the concurrent use of tetracycline or oxytetracycline.

Interaction

A woman who had been taking *Microgynon 30* (ethinyloestradiol 30 μg and D-norgestrel 150 μg) for 2 years was treated for sinusitis with tetracycline, 500 mg 6-hourly for 3 days and then 250 mg 6-hourly for 2 days. Three months later she was found to be pregnant. The clinical evidence indicated that she must have ovulated while taking the tetracycline or in the week afterwards. There was no evidence of nausea or vomiting, or of failure to take the contraceptive, which might have accounted for the pregnancy.[1]

A case of break-through bleeding and another of pregnancy have been observed during the concurrent use of an oral contraceptive and tetracycline.[1,2] The British Committee on the Safety of Medicines have reports of two cases of contraceptive failure with tetracycline, and four cases with oxytetracycline.[3]

Mechanism

Not understood, but one suggestion has been made. Normally the contraceptive steroids take part in the enterohepatic circulation, that is to say they are repeatedly absorbed by the gut and re-secreted in the bile in the form of steroid conjugates which are then hydrolysed by bacteria in the gut before further re-absorption. If these bacteria are decimated by the use of an antibiotic, these steroid conjugates fail to undergo bacterial hydrolysis and would therefore not be reabsorbed, resulting in lower-than-normal concentrations of circulating steroids and, presumably, in an inadequate suppression of the normal menstrual cycle.[1] This explanation, however, fails to answer the question of why tetracycline-induced oral contraceptive failure is, apparently, such a rare event.

Importance and management

There appear to be only these few cases on record. Until more information becomes available it would seem prudent for women taking oral contraceptives, particularly the low-dose variety, to take additional precautions during treatment with tetracycline or oxytetracycline if they wish to be sure of preventing pregnancy. Whether an interaction is likely with other tetracyclines is not known.

Reference

1 Bacon J F and Shenfield G M. Pregnancy attributable to interaction between tetracyline and oral contraceptives. *Br Med J* (1980) 1, 293.
2 Lesqueux A. Grossesse sous contraceptif oral après prise de tétracycline. *Louvain Med* (1980) 99, 413.
3 Back D J, Breckenridge A M, Crawford F E, MacIver M, Orme L' E and Rowe P H. Interindividual variation and drug interactions with hormonal steroids. *Drugs* (1981) 21, 46

Oral contraceptives + tobacco

Summary
The risk of coronary heart disease in women in the 40–41 age group on oral contraceptives may possibly be increased if they also smoke.

Interaction, mechanism, importance and management

Although strictly speaking not a 'drug' interaction in the narrowest sense of the term, the possible long-term effects of smoking in women taking oral contraceptives are important. A survey in a population of Leiden in Holland showed that women in the 40–41 age group taking the pill who also smoked, had a lower level of high-density lipoprotein in their serum than women who neither smoked nor took the pill. The significance of this finding is that low levels of high-density lipoprotein are a major risk factor in the development of coronary heart disease.[1]

Reference
1 Arntzenius A C, van Gent C M, van der Voort H, Stegerhoek C I and Styblo K. Reduced high-density lipoprotein in women aged 40–41 using oral contraceptives. *Lancet* (1978) i, 1221.

Contraceptives + triacetyloleandomycin

Summary

Severe pruritis and jaundice have been observed in women taking oral contraceptives who were administered triacetyloleandomycin.

Interaction

A report describes 10 cases of cholestatic jaundice and pruritis in women taking oral contraceptives and triacetyloleandomycin. All had been using the contraceptive for 7–48 months, and were given the antibiotic in 250 or 500 mg doses four times a day. The pruritis was intense, lasting 2–24 days, and preceded the jaundice which, in 8 of the patients, persisted for over a month.[1]

There are other reports of this reaction,[2–5] one of which describes 24 cases.[5]

Mechanism

Uncertain. Hepatotoxicity has been associated with the use of both types of drugs. The reaction suggests that their damaging effects on the liver may be additive.

Importance and management

An established interaction, and important. The incidence is uncertain. Caution should be exercised if these two potentially hepatotoxic agents are used together. It would seem preferable to use an alternative antibiotic. It is curious that so far all the reports are French.

References
1 Miguet J P, Monange C, Vuitton D, Allemand H, Hirsch J P, Carayon P and Gisselbrecht H. Ictère cholestatique survenu après administration de triacétyloléandomycine: interférence avec les contraceptifs oraux? Dix observations. *Nouv Presse Méd* (1978) 7, 4304.
2 Perol R, Hincky J and Desnos M. Hépatites cholestatiques lors de la prise de troléandomycine chez deux femmes prenant des estrogènes. *Nouv Presse méd* (1978) 7, 4302.
3 Goldfain D and Chauveinc L. Ictère cholestatique chez des femmes prenant simultanément de la triacétyloléandomycine et des contraceptifs oraux. *Nouv Presse méd* (1979) 8, 1099.
4 Rollux R, Plottin F, Mingat J and Bessard G. Ictère après association estroprogestatif-troléandomycine. Trois observations. *Nouv Presse méd* (1979) 8, 1694.
5 Miguet J P, Vuitton D, Pessayre D, Allemand H, Metreau J M, Poupon R, Capron J P and Blanc F. Jaundice from troleandomycin and oral contraceptives. *Ann Intern Med* (1980) 92, 434.

Contraceptives + vitamins

Summary

The oral contraceptives have been reported to raise serum levels of vitamin A, and lower levels of pyridoxine, folic acid, cyanocobalamin and ascorbic acid.

Interaction, mechanism. importance and management

There is evidence that the use of oral contraceptives can result in a biochemical deficiency of a number of vitamins, although clinical deficiency does not necessarily manifest itself. Serum concentrations of cyanocobalamin can be lowered[1] and folate deficiency with anaemia attributed to the use of oral contraceptives has been described. [2,3] Reduced levels of ascorbic acid[4,5] and pyridoxine,[6,7] and raised levels of vitamin A[8] have been reported. These changes in vitamin requirements induced by the oral contraceptives are reviewed in detail elsewhere.[9] Treatment of pyridoxine deficiency has been shown to cause an improvement in the mood of depressed women on oral contraceptives.[11]

Routine prophylactic treatment with vitamins for women on oral contraceptives has been advised by some authors,[10] but questioned by others[12,13] because an increased intake of some vitamins in some circumstances may be harmful. For example, in areas of the world where protein malnutrition is rife, a pyridoxine supplement might lead to an undesirable increase in amino-acid catabolism in patients on a low daily intake of protein.[12] One author's 'comment' on the indiscriminate supplementation of the diet with vitamins is that '... the use of multivitamin preparations by women on oral contraceptives can hardly be justified'.[13]

References

1 Wertalik L F, Metz E N, LoBuglio A F, and Balcerzak S P. Decreased serum B12 levels with oral contraceptive use. *J Amer Med Ass* (1972) **221**, 1371.
2 Streiff R R. Folate deficiency and oral contraceptives. *J Amer med Ass* (1970) **214**, 214.
3 Meguid M M and Loebl W Y. Megaloblastic anaemia associated with the oral contraceptive pill. *Postgrad Med J* (1974) **60**, 470.
4 Harris A B, Pillay M and Hussein S. Vitamins and oral contraceptives. *Lancet* (1975) **ii**, 82.
5 Briggs M and Briggs M. Vitamin C requirements and oral contraceptives. *Nature* (1972) **238**, 277.
6 Bennick H J T C and Schreurs W H P. Disturbance of tryptophan metabolism and its correction during hormonal contraception. *Contraception* (1974) **9**, 347.
7 Doberenz A R, van Miller J P, Green J R and Beaton J R. Vitamin B6 depletion in women using oral contraceptives as determined by erythrocyte glutamic–pyruvic transaminase activities. *Proc Soc Exp Biol Med* (1971) **137**, 1100.
8 Wild J, Schorah C J and Smithells R W. Vitamin A, pregnancy and oral contraceptives. *Brit Med J* (1974) **1**, 57.
9 Larsson-Cohn U. Oral contraceptives and vitamins: A review. *Amer J Obstet Gynec* (1975) **121**, 84.
10 Briggs M and Briggs M. Oral contraceptives and vitamin requirements. *Med J Aust* (1975) **1**, 407.
11 Adams P W, Wynn V, Seed M and Folkhard J. Vitamin B6, depression and oral contraception. *Lancet* (1974) **ii**, 515.
12 Adams P W, Wynn V, Rose D P, Folkhard J, Seed M and Strong R. Effect of pyridoxine hydrochloride (vitamin B6) upon depression associated with oral contraception. *Lancet* (1973) **i**, 897.
13 Wynn V. Vitamins and oral contraceptive use. *Lancet* (1975) **i**, 561.

CHAPTER 12. CYTOTOXIC
DRUG INTERACTIONS

The cytotoxic agents (antineoplastics) are used in the treatment of malignant disease in conjunction with radiotherapy, surgery and immunosuppressants such as the corticosteroids and lymphocytic antisera. They also find application in the treatment of skin conditions such as psoriasis.

They are, generally speaking, highly toxic substances with a low therapeutic index so that a quite small increase in their activity can lead to the development of serious and life-threatening toxicity. A list of the agents which are discussed appears in Table 12.1.

Unlike most of the other interaction synopses in this book, much of the information is derived from animal experiments and still requires confirmation in man. The reason for including these theoretical data is that drugs in this group generally do not lend themselves readily to the kind of clinical studies which can be undertaken with other drugs, and there would seem to be justification in this instance for including indirect evidence from animal experiments. The aim is not to make definite predictions, but to warn prescribers of the interaction possibilities.

Table 12.1. Cytotoxic agents

Non-proprietary names	Proprietary names
Actinomycin (dactinomycin)	Cosmegen, Lyovac
Azathioprine	Imuran, Imurek, Imurel
Bleomycin	Blenoxane
Carmustine (BCNU)	
Cis-platinum (CPDD)	
Colaspase (asparaginase)	Crasnitin, Kidrolase, Laspar
Cyclophosphamide	Cytoxan, Endoxan (A), Enduxan, Genoxal, Procytox, Sendoxan
Cytarabine (cytosine arabinoside)	Cytosar, Alexan, Aracytine
Doxorubicin (adriamycin)	Adriblastina, Farmiblastina, Adriacin
Fluorouracil (5-Fu)	Efudix, Fluoroplex
Hydroxyurea	Hydrea Litalir
Lomustine (CCNU)	
Mercaptopurine	Purinethol
Methotrexate (amethopterin)	Ledertrex
Meturedepa	Turloc
Mithramycin	Mithracin
Procarbazine	Natulan, Matulane, Natulanar
Streptozocin	
Thiotepa	Tifosyl
Vincristine	Oncovin

278

In addition to the interactions with the cytotoxic agents discussed in this chapter, there are others dealt with elsewhere in this book. A full list is to be found in the Index.

Actinomycin-D + doxorubicin + mithramycin

Summary

A case of fatal cardiomyopathy attributed to the concurrent use of actinomycin-D with doxorubicin (adriamycin) and mithramycin has been described.

Interaction, mechanism, importance and management

A single report describes cardiomyopathy, apparently due to the use of actinomycin-D, doxorubicin and mithramycin which had a fatal outcome. The general importance of this is uncertain, but it would seem prudent to be on the alert for evidence of changes in cardiac function in patients treated with these drugs.[1]

Reference
1 Kushner J P, Hansen V L and Hammar S P. Cardiomyopathy after widely separated courses of adriamycin exacerbated by actinomycin-D and mithramycin. *Cancer* (1975) **36**, 1577.

Azathioprine or mercaptopurine + allopurinol

Summary

The effects of mercaptopurine and azathioprine are markedly enhanced by the concurrent use of allopurinol. The dosage of the cytotoxic agent should be reduced to a third or a quarter if toxicity is to be avoided.

Interaction

(a) Mercaptopurine + allopurinol

A study in 7 patients with chronic granulocytic leukaemia, treated with 50 mg mercaptopurine daily, showed that when additionally given 400 mg allopurinol daily their granulocyte level fell by an amount equivalent to that expected with four to five times the dose of mercaptopurine.[1]

In another study, profound pancytopenia rapidly developed in 3 children with acute leukaemia in remission with mercaptopurine, 2·5 mg/kg/day, and allopurinol, 10 mg/kg/day. When the dose of mercaptopurine was halved, no untoward side-effects were noted.[2]

Other reports and studies in man[5] and animals confirm[4] these findings.

(b) Azathioprine + allopurinol

A patient treated with 300 mg allopurinol a day developed pancytopenia following the additional administration of 150 mg azathioprine daily.[3]

Mechanism

Azathioprine is chemically related to 6-mercaptopurine and represents an alternative form of the same drug because it is firstly metabolized in the body to active 6-mercaptopurine. This compound, whether derived from azathioprine or directly administered, is enzymatically oxidized to an inactive compound (6-thiouric acid) by the enzyme xanthine oxidase and excreted. Allopurinol inhibits the activity of this enzyme so that in its presence the mercaptopurine accumulates and, if the dosage of the cytotoxic drug remains unaltered, the toxic potentialities (leucopenia, thrombocytopenia etc.) are realized. In effect the patient suffers gross overdosage.

Importance and management

A well-documented and well-established interaction. During concurrent treatment with allopurinol the dosages of azathioprine or mercaptopurine should be reduced to about a third or a quarter to prevent the development of toxicity.

References
1 Rundles R W, Wyngaarden J B, Hitchings G H, Elion G B and Silberman H R. Effects of a xanthine oxidase inhibitor on thiopurine metabolism, hyperuricaemia and gout. *Trans Assoc Am Phys* (1963) **76**, 126.
2 Levine A S, Sharpt H L, Mitchell J, Krivit W and Nesbit M. Combination therapy with 6-mercaptopurine (NSC-755) and allopurinol (NSC-1390) during induction and maintenance of remission of acute leukaemia in children. *Cancer Chemotherap Reports* (1969) **53**, 53.
3 Glogner P and Heni N. Panzytopenie nach kombinationsbehandlung mit allopurinol und azathioprin. *Med Welt* (1976) **27**, 1545.
4 Ragab A H, Gilkerson E and Myers M. The effect of 6-mercaptopurine and allopurinol on granulopoiesis. *Cancer Res* (1974) **34**, 2246.
5 Vogler W R, Bain J A, Huguley C M, Palmer H G and Lowrey M E. Metabolic and therapeutic effects of allopurinol in patients with leukaemia and gout. *Amer J Med* (1966) **40**, 548.

Bleomycin + oxygen

Summary
The use of normal concentrations of oxygen during anaesthesia may enhance the pulmonary toxicity of bleomycin.

Interaction, mechanism, importance and management
A study of 17 patients under treatment with bleomycin showed that the incidence of pulmonary toxicity, in some instances with a fatal outcome, was enhanced in those who during and immediately following anaesthesia had received normal concentrations of oxygen. The authors of the study suggest that reduced oxygen levels may prevent the full development of these toxic effects.[1]

Reference
1 Goldiner P L, Carlon C G, Cvitkovic E, Schweizer O and Howland W S. Factors influencing postoperative morbidity and mortality in patients treated with bleomycin. *Br Med J* (1978) **1**, 1664.

Carmustine (BCNU) + cimetidine

Summary
Clinical evidence shows that cimetidine can increase the bone marrow depressant effects of carmustine.

Interaction
Six out of 8 patients treated with carmustine, 80 mg/m^2/day for 3 days, cimetidine, 300 mg 6-hourly, and steroids demonstrated marked leucopenia and thrombocytopenia (less than 500 white cells and 8000 platelets) after the first administration. Biopsy confirmed the marked decrease in granulocytic elements. In comparison only 6 out of 40 patients who were similarly treated, but without cimetidine, showed comparable white cell and platelet depression.[1]

Mechanism
Not understood, but both drugs are recognized bone marrow depressants which would appear to be additive during concurrent treatment.[1,2]

Importance and management
The data are limited to this one report, but the reaction would seem to be established. Prescribers should be aware of the bone-marrow depressant potentialities of these two drugs and take appropriate precautions.

References
1 Selker R G, Moore P and LoDolce D. Bone-marrow depression with cimetidine plus carmustine. *New Eng J Med* (1978) **299**, 834.
2 Klotz S and Kay B. Cimetidine and agranulocytosis. *Ann Intern Med* (1978) **88**, 579.

Cis-platinum + gentamicin and cephalothin

Summary
Acute renal failure has been attributed to the use of gentamicin and cephalothin following treatment with cis-platinum.

Interaction, mechanism, importance and management
Four patients treated with cis-dichlorodiammineplatinum (II) (CPDD) in dosages ranging from low to very high (8 doses of 0·5 mg/kg; 5 mg/kg) who were subsequently given gentamicin/cephalothin therapy developed severe acute renal failure which persisted until death. Autopsy revealed extensive renal tubular necrosis. It would appear that renal tubular damage caused by the CPDD can be grossly enhanced by these antibiotics which are recognized to have nephrotoxic potentialities. These antibiotics, it is recommended, should be given with great caution, and probably not at all, to patients under treatment with CPDD.[1]

References
1 Gonsalez-Vitale J C, Hayes D M, Cvitkovic E and Sternberg S S. Acute renal failure after cis-Dichlorodiammineplatinum (II) and gentamicin–cephalothin therapies. *Cancer Tret. Rep* (1978) **62**, 693.

Cyclophosphamide + allopurinol

Summary
The incidence of serious bone marrow depression induced by cyclophosphamide is markedly increased by the concurrent use of allopurinol.

Interaction
A retrospective epidemiological survey[1] of patients who had been treated with cyclophosphamide showed that the incidence of serious bone marrow depression was 57·7% in 26 patients who had also received allopurinol, and 18·8% in 32 patients who had not: a three-fold increase.

Mechanism
Not understood. One suggestion[1] is that apart from its effects as an inhibitor of xanthine oxidase, allopurinol also inhibits pyrimidine synthesis[2,3] and is converted to an allopurinol nucleotide. If this metabolite were to inhibit enzymes normally regulated by purine and pyrimidine ribonucleotides, then inhibition of normal biosynthesis might enhanced the effects of various antimetabolites which can depress the activity of the bone marrow. This requires experimental confirmation.

Importance and management
The report described[1] covered a 4-year period, and the increase in bone marrow depression was evident in all four hospitals from which the data were obtained. It would appear to be an established interaction, but there are no other confirmatory reports. The authors of the report conclude that 'conceivably, addition of allopurinol to the treatment regimen may render chemotherapy more effective at the expense of bone marrow depression . . . ., there seem to be good grounds for re-evaluating the routine practice of administering allopurinol prophylactically'. This interaction requires further study, but it would seem that the routine administration of allopurinol to all patients given cyclophosphamide to avoid hyperuricaemia is not a practice to be recommended.

References
1 Boston Collaborative Drug Surveillance Programme. Allopurinol and cytotoxic drugs. Interaction in relation to bone marrow depression. *J Amer Med Ass* (1974) **227**, 1036.
2 Fox R M. Royse-Smith D, O'Sullivan W J. Orotidinuria induced by allopurinol. *Science* (1970) **168**, 861–2.
3 Kelley W N and Beardmore T D. Allopurinol: alteration in pyrimidine metabolism in man. *Science* (1970) **169**, 388–90.

Cyclophosphamide + barbiturates

Summary

Despite some animal data, the evidence from studies in man suggests that neither the toxicity nor the therapeutic effects of cyclophosphamide are significantly affected by the barbiturates.

Interaction, mechanism, importance and management

There is evidence from a number of animal studies that the barbiturates and other potent liver enzyme-inducing agents may affect the activity of cyclophosphamide,[1,2] but the studies undertaken in man indicate that although some changes in the pharmacokinetics of cyclophosphamide occur, neither the toxicity nor the therapeutic effects of cyclophosphamide are significantly altered.[3,4]

References

1 Donelli M G, Colombo T and Garattini S. Effect of cyclophosphamide on the activity and distribution of pentobarbital in rats. *Biochem Pharmacol* (1973) **22**, 2609.
2 Alberts D S and Van Daalen Wetters T. The effect of phenobarbital on cyclophosphamide antitumour activity. *Cancer Res* (1976) **36**, 2785.
3 Bagley C M, Bostick F W and De Vita V T. Clinical pharmacology of cyclophosphamide. *Cancer Res* (1973) **33**, 226.
4 Jao J Y, Jusko W J and Cohen J L. Phenobarbital effects on cyclophosphamide pharmacokinetics in man. *Cancer Res* (1972) **32**, 2761.

Cyclophosphamide + chloramphenicol

Summary

Some limited evidence indicates that chloramphenicol may inhibit the production of the therapeutically active metabolites of cyclophosphamide, thereby reducing its activity.

Interaction and mechanism

Cyclophosphamide itself is inactive, but after administration it is metabolized within the body to active alkylating metabolites. Animal studies[1] have shown that pretreatment with chloramphenicol reduces the activity (lethality) of cyclophosphamide because, it is believed, the antibiotic inhibits its metabolic conversion to these active metabolites. Studies in 5 patients have shown that this can also occur in man.[2] The administration of 2 g chloramphenicol daily was found to prolong the mean half-life of the cyclophosphamide from 7·5 to 11·5 h.

Importance and management

The documentation is very limited. More study is required. A reduction in the activity of cyclophosphamide may occur if chloramphenicol is used concurrently. The extent to which this will affect treatment with cyclophosphamide is uncertain.

References

1 Dixon R L. Effect of chloramphenicol on the metabolism and lethality of cyclophosphamide in rats. *Proc Soc Exp Biol Med* (1968) **127**, 1151.
2 Faber O K, Mouridsen H T and Skovsted L. The effect of chloramphenicol and sulphaphenazole on the biotransformation of cyclophosphamide in man. *Br J clin Pharmac* (1975) **2**, 281.

Cyclophosphamide + corticosteroids

Summary

Single doses of prednisone can reduce the activity of cyclophosphamide, but longer-term treatment increases its activity.

Interaction and mechanicm

Cyclophosphamide itself is inactive, but after administration it is metabolized within the body to active alkylating metabolites. Single doses of prednisone have been shown to inhibit the activation of cyclophosphamide in man[1] and animals,[2] probably due to competition for the drug-metabolizing enzymes in the liver. Longer-term treatment on the other hand (50 mg/day for 1–2 weeks) has been shown in man to have the opposite effect and increases the rate of activation of the cyclophosphamide, probably due to the induction of the liver enzymes.

Importance and management

The documentation is extremely limited. More study is required. Changes in the activity of cyclophosphamide, possibly with the development of toxicity, should be watched for if corticosteroids are used, but whether other corticosteroids behave in the same way as prednisone is uncertain.

References
1 Faber O K and Mouridsen H T. Cyclophosphamide activation and corticosteroids. *New Eng J Med* (1974) **291**, 211.
2 Sladek N E. Therapeutic efficacy of cyclophosphamide as a function of inhibition of its metabolism. *Cancer Res* (1972) **32**, 1848.

Cyclophosphamide + dapsone

Summary
Some extremely limited evidence suggests that dapsone might be responsible for a reduction in the activity of cyclophosphamide.

Interaction, mechanism, importance and management

An unexplained and undetailed report[1] has described patients with leprosy on dapsone and cyclophosphamide who demonstrated inhibition of the leucopenia normally associated with cyclophosphamide treatment. Whether this indicates a reduction in the effects of cyclophosphamide is uncertain, but it would seem prudent to be on the alert for a depressed therapeutic response to cyclophosphamide during concurrent treatment with dapsone. More data are required.

Reference
1 Quoted by Warren R D and Bender R A. Drug interactions with antineoplastic agents. *Cancer Treatment Reports* (1977) **61**, 1231.

Cyclophosphamide + sulphonamides

Summary
Some very limited evidence suggests that sulphaphenazole may increase or decrease the activity of cyclophosphamide.

Interaction, mechanism, importance and management

A study in 7 subjects on a 50 g dose of cyclophosphamide who were given 2 g sulphaphenazole for 9–14 days, showed that the half-life of cyclophosphamide was unchanged in 3, longer in 2 and shorter in the remaining 2. The reasons are not known. Whether this has any practical importance or not is, as yet, uncertain, but it would seem prudent to be on the watch for changes in the response to cyclophosphamide if sulphaphenazole is given concurrently.

Reference
1 Faber O K, Mouridsen H T and Skovsted L. The effect of chloramphenicol and sulphaphenazole on the biotransformation of cyclophosphamide in man. *Br J clin Pharmac* (1975) **2**, 281.

Cytarabine (cytosine arabinoside) + methotrexate

Summary

Animal experiments suggest that the outcome of combined use may not necessarily be therapeutically advantageous.

Interaction, mechanism, importance and management

Although synergism has been observed, there is some limited evidence from animal experiments that antagonism may also occur between these drugs. This suggests that the clinical outcome of concurrent use is by no means certain.

Reference

1 Tattersall M N H, Connors T A and Harrap K R. Interaction of methotrexate and cytosine arabinoside. *Lancet* (1972) **ii**, 1378.

Cytotoxic agents + vaccines

Summary

Generalized infection can occur in patients on cytotoxics because the immune response of the body is suppressed.

Interaction, mechanism, importance and management

Since the cytotoxic agents are immunosuppressants, the response of the body to infection is reduced and immunization with live vaccines may result in a generalized and potentially life-threatening infection. For example, a woman who was under treatment with methotrexate, 15 mg daily, for psoriasis and who was vaccinated against smallpox, developed a generalized vaccinial infection. For this reason extreme care should be exercised in patients receiving cytotoxic agents.

Reference

1 Allison J. Methotrexate and smallpox vaccination. *Lancet* (1968) **ii**, 1250.

Doxorubicin + barbiturates

Summary

Animal studies indicate that the effects of doxorubicin (adriamycin) may be reduced by the concurrent use of barbiturates. This requires confirmation in man.

Interaction, mechanism, importance and management

Studies with mice have shown that the serum levels of doxorubicin are depressed and the clearance rate increased by the concurrent use of phenobarbitone. It is possible that this is due to the enzyme-inductive properties of the phenobarbitone. Whether a similar interaction occurs in man is uncertain, but the possibility should be borne in mind during concurrent treatment with phenobarbitone or any other barbiturate.[1]

Reference

1 Reich S D and Bachur N R. Alterations in adriamycin efficacy by phenobarbital. *Cancer* (1976) **36**, 3803.

Doxorubicin + beta-blockers

Summary
Animal data suggest that additive cardiotoxicity may occur with doxorubicin (adriamycin) and propranolol. This awaits clinical confirmation.

Interaction, mechanism, importance and management
Experiments with mice[1] have shown that when doxorubicin (adriamycin) in doses of 18 and 23 mg/kg, and propranolol in doses of 1 and 10 mg/kg were given concurrently, the mortality was significantly increased compared with the mortality seen with either drug alone. This may be because both drugs inhibit the activity of two cardiac CoQ_{10} enzymes (succinoxidase, NADH oxidase) which are essential for mitochondrial respiration so that cardiotoxicity is increased. There is no clinical confirmation of this interaction in man but the authors of the report warn that the administration of both drugs may be contraindicated. Doxorubicin has been associated with the development of ventricular quadrigeminy in a patient who was given an infusion of 60 mg over 1 min. Later, when the patient died from leukaemia, a postmortem revealed pathological changes in the heart muscle.[2]

References
1 Choe J Y. Combs A B and Folkers K. Potentiation of the toxicity of adriamycin by propranolol. *Res Comm Chem Pathol Pharmacol* (1978) **21**, 577.
2 Cosgriff T M. Doxorubicin and ventricular arrhythmia. *Ann Int Med* (1980) **92**, 435.

5-Fluorouracil + allopurinol

Summary, interaction, mechanism, importance and management
It has been suggested that allopurinol may inhibit the anti-tumour response to 5-fluorouracil in man, but this awaits confirmation.[1]

Reference
1 Tisman G and Wu S J G. Allopurinol modulation of high-dose fluorouracil toxicity. *Lancet* (1979) **i**, 1353.

5-Fluorouracil + aminoglycosides

Summary
Neomycin can delay the gastrointestinal absorption of 5-fluorouracil but the clinical importance of this is uncertain.

Interaction, mechanism, importance and management
Some preliminary information from a study in a number of patients under treatment with 5-fluorouracil showed that although the neomycin caused some delay in the absorption of the 5-fluorouracil, the effects were generally too small to reduce the therapeutic response, except possibly in one instance. Although not confirmed it would seem probable that this interaction occurs because the neomycin can induce a gastrointestinal malabsorption syndrome. If neomycin, paromomycin or kanamycin are used in patients on 5-fluorouracil, the possibility of this interaction should be borne in mind.[1]

Reference
1 Bruckner H W and Creasey W A. The administration of 5-fluorouracil by mouth. *Cancer* (1974) **33**, 14.

Hydroxyurea + CNS depressants

Summary
Enhanced CNS depression may occur.

Interaction, mechanism, importance and management
Hydroxyurea has CNS-depressant effects and causes drowsiness. These effects may be expected to be additive with other drugs possessing these characteristics (e.g. alcohol, antiemetics, phenothiazines, antihistamines, barbiturates, hypnosedatives, cough suppressants, narcotics, tricyclic antidepressants etc.)

Lomustine (CCNU) + theophylline

Summary
A single case has been reported of bleeding and thrombocytopenia attributed to the use of theophylline with lomustine.

Interaction
An asthmatic woman taking theophylline, and under treatment for medulloblastoma with vincristine, lomustine and prednisone, developed severe epistaxis and thrombocytopenia 3 weeks after the third cycle of chemotherapy. This was attributed to the concurrent use of theophylline with lomustine.[1]

Mechanism
Unknown. It is suggested that the theophylline inhibited the activity of phosphodiesterase within the blood platelets, thereby increasing cyclic AMP levels and disrupting their normal function.[1] This theory would seem to be supported by an experimental study.[2]

Importance and management
The data are far too limited to act as more than a warning of the possibility of increased thrombopathia and myelotoxicity during the concurrent use of theophylline and lomustine.

References
1 Zeltzer P M and Feig S A. Theophylline-induced lomustine toxicity. *Lancet* (1979) **ii**, 960.
2 DeWys W D and Bathina S. Synergistic anti-tumour effect of cyclic AMP elevation (induced by theophylline) and cytotoxic drug treatment. *Proc Am Assoc Cancer Res* (1978) **19**, 104.

Mercaptopurine + doxorubicin

Summary
The hepatotoxicity of mercaptopurine can be increased by doxorubicin (adriamycin).

Interaction, mechanism, importance and management
A study carried out on 11 patients under treatment with mercaptopurine showed that liver damage induced by the mercaptopurine was enhanced by the concurrent use of doxorubicin. Since azathioprine is converted to mercaptopurine within the body, it would seem probable that enhanced hepatotoxicity may also be seen with this drug and doxorubicin.

Reference
1 Minow R A, Stern M H and Casey J H. Clinico-pathological correlation of liver damage in patients treated with 6-mercaptopurine. *Cancer* (1976) **38**, 1524.

Methotrexate + alcohol

Summary

There is some inconclusive evidence indicating that alcohol may enhance the risk of methotrexate-induced hepatic cirrhosis and fibrosis.

Interaction, mechanism, importance and management

It has been claimed that alcohol can enhance the hepatotoxicity of methotrexate.[2] This is supported by a study in which 3 out of 5 patients with cirrhosis caused by methotrexate were reported to have taken alcohol concurrently,[1] but the evidence is by no means conclusive and no direct causal relationship has been established. The manufacturers of methotrexate (Lederle) advise the avoidance of drugs, including alcohol, which have hepatotoxic potentialities.

References

1 Tobias H and Auerbach R. Hepatotoxicity of long-term methotrexate therapy. *Arch Int Med* (1973) **132**, 391.
2 Pai S II, Werthamer S and Zak F G. Severe liver damage caused by treatment of psoriasis with methotrexate. *NY State J Med* (1973) **73**, 2585.

Methotrexate + aminoglycoside antibiotics

Summary

There is evidence that the gastrointestinal absorption of methotrexate can be markedly reduced by the concurrent use of paromomycin. Whether some of the other aminoglycosides interact similarly is uncertain.

Interaction

A study in 10 patients under treatment for small cell bronchogenic carcinoma with methotrexate showed that concurrent treatment with a range of oral antibiotics (paromomycin, vancomycin, polymyxin B, nystatin) reduced the gastrointestinal absorption of the methotrexate by over one third.[1]

Mechanism

Uncertain. Paromomycin (in common with some other aminoglycosides) is associated with a malabsorption syndrome[2] which may have been responsible for this interaction, but the extent to which the other antibiotics may have had a part to play is not known.

Importance and management

The documentation is very limited. The extent of the reduction in methotrexate absorption (one third) is so large that it would seem to be clinically important. If methotrexate is given with paromomycin (or neomycin, kanamycin) a close watch should be kept for a reduction in the therapeutic response.

References

1 Cohen M H, Creaven P J, Fossieck B E, Johnston A V and Williams C L. Effect of oral prophylactic broad spectrum nonabsorbable antibiotics on the gastrointestinal absorption of nutrients and methotrexate in small cell bronchogenic carcinoma patients. *Cancer* (1976) **38**, 1556.
2 Keusch G T, Troneale F J and Buchanan R D. Malabsorption due to paromomycin. *Arch int Med* (1970) **125**, 273.

Methotrexate + barbiturates

Summary

Animal studies suggest that phenobarbitone may enhance the alopecia caused by methotrexate.

A study in rats showed that severe alopecia could be induced by the concurrent administration of methotrexate and phenobarbitone in dosages which when given alone failed to cause any hair

loss. Whether this similarly occurs in man awaits confirmation.[1]

Reference
1 Basu T K, Williams D C and Raven R W. Methotrexate and alopecia. *Lancet* (1973) ii, 331.

Methotrexate + chloramphenicol, phenytoin, PAS, sodium salicylate, sulphamethoxypyridazine, tetracycline or tolbutamide

Summary
Animal experiments suggest that the toxicity of methotrexate may be enhanced by the concurrent use of these drugs, but this has yet to be confirmed in man.

Interaction
Male mice treated for 5 days with each of four doses of methotrexate, (1·53–12·25 mg/kg) administered intravenously, were each treated with non-toxic doses of the drugs listed above by intraperitoneal injection immediately afterwards. These drugs '... appeared to be capable of decreasing the lethal dose and/or decreasing the median survival time of methotrexate-treated mice.[1] That is to say, the toxicity of the methotrexate was increased.

Mechanism
Not understood. Displacement of the methotrexate from plasma-protein binding sites could result in a rise in the levels of unbound and active methotrexate, and in the case of the salicylates to a decrease in the renal clearance (see p. 291).

Importance and management
One cannot use the results of animal experiments and apply them uncritically to man. However, it would be prudent to be on the alert for the possibility of increased methotrexate toxicity if any of the drugs listed are used with methotrexate. There is already evidence that this occurs in man with the salicylates (p. 291).

Reference
1 Dixon R L. The interaction between various drugs and methotrexate. *Toxicol Appl Pharmacol* (1968) 12, 308.

Methotrexate + corticosteroids

Summary
Some very inconclusive evidence suggests that the corticosteroids may possibly enhance the toxicity of methotrexate in some instances. The efficacy of methotrexate may also possibly be reduced by hydrocortisone with cephalothin.

Interaction, mechanism, importance and management
Although methotrexate and the corticosteroids have been used together successfully (for example in the treatment of psoriatic arthritis where a 50% reduction in the corticosteroid dosage was poss-

ible,[2]) a number of fatalities have also been reported.

Two patients under treatment with psoriasis with methotrexate, 5 mg daily for 5–7 days, and who were on long-term corticosteroid therapy, died apparently from severe bone marrow depression. One was also on chloramphenicol.[1] Another patient taking 30 mg prednisone daily for psoriasis and who was given 50 mg, 100 mg and 150 mg methotrexate by injection at 10-day intervals, developed severe leucopenia and thrombocytopenia.[2] Yet another patient, debilitated from arthritis and prolonged corticosteroid therapy, died of a generalized systemic moniliasis infection after two doses of methotrexate. She had no haematological abnormalities.[4]

In-vitro experiments with blast cells from 7 patients with acute myelogenous leukaemia indicate that the intracellular uptake of methotrexate was reduced by the presence of cephalothin (21 μg/ml) and hydrocortisone (20 μg/ml) which are normal achievable clinical serum concentrations.[5]

All of this information suggests that particular care should be exercised during concurrent use to confirm that the clinical outcome is, as intended, advantageous.

References
1 Haim S and Alray G. Methotrexate in psoriasis. *Lancet* (1967) **i**, 1165.
2 Black R L, O'Brien W M, Van Scott E J, Auerbach R, Eisen A Z and Bunim J J. Methotrexate therapy in psoriatic arthritis. *JAMA* (1964) **189**, 743.
3 Schewach-Millet M and Ziprkowski L. Methotrexate in psoriasis. *Br J Derm* (1968) **80**, 534.
4 Roenigk H H, Fowler-Bergfeld W and Curtis G H. Methotrexate for psoriasis in weekly oral doses. *Arch Derm* (1969) **99**, 86.
5 Bender A R, Bleyer W A, Frisby S A and Oliverio V J. Alterations in methotrexate uptake in human leukaemia cells by other agents. *Cancer Res.* (1975) **35**, 1305.

Methotrexate + 5-fluorouracil

Summary
In-vitro and animal data indicate that the cytotoxic effects of methotrexate and 5-fluorouracil may possibly be reduced by concurrent use. This has yet to be confirmed in man.

Interaction
Although there are as yet no human data on this possible interaction, in-vitro and animal data suggest that the cytotoxic effects of methotrexate and 5-fluorouacil (5-FU) can be diminished by concurrent use. Some of the data are conflicting.

> Tests on tumour cells grown in culture indicate that methotrexate interferes with and reduces the activity of 5-fluorodeoxyuridine (FldUrd) given at the same time. Since this compound is believed to act in the same way as 5-FU, the question was initially raised whether methotrexate similarly interacts with 5-FU.[1]
>
> In-vitro studies carried out in the L1210 cell system, in the Friend leukaemia system, and in human bone marrow, confirmed that in the presence of methotrexate the activity of 5-FU (as measured by the suppression of de novo DNA synthesis) is considerably reduced.[2]

Other reports relating to this interaction have also been published.[3-6]

Mechanism
Both 5-FU and a similar compound, FldURD, are metabolized in the body to a third compound, FldUrd monophosphate, which is the active cyto-toxic agent. This monophosphate inhibits the activity of an enzyme (thymidilate synthetase) which takes part in the biosynthesis of DNA. Thus these two drugs indirectly inhibit the synthesis of DNA and thereby impair the growth of tumour cells.

FldUrd can inhibit the enzymic activity of thymidilate synthetase by becoming strongly and irreversibly bound to it, but only in the presence of a co-factor (5,10,methylenetetrahydrofolic acid). It seems, however, that methotrexate inhibits the synthesis of this co-factor and thereby weakens the activity of FldUrd and, by implication, 5-FU as well. Thus any antagonistic effects of methotrexate on the activity of 5-FU can be explained.

Importance and management
One cannot uncritically extrapolate the results of tissue culture or animal experiments to man. Moreover, there is already considerable debate about the time-scheduling of administration,[3] and discussion about whether combinations of methotrexate and 5-FU are antagonistic or even additive.[6] The available evidence (if it does nothing else) indicates that these two drugs ought not to

be given together without a full awareness that they may possibly be less effective than each drug given singly.

References

1 Maugh T H. Cancer chemotherapy: an unexpected drug interaction. *Science* (1976) **194**, 310.
2 Waxman S and Bruckner H. Antitumour drug interactions: additional data. *Science* (1976) **194**, 672.
3 Bertino J, Sawicki W L, Lindquist C A and Gupta V S. Schedule-dependent antitumour effects of methotrexate and 5-fluorouracil. *Cancer Res* (1977) **37**, 327.
4 Tattersall M N H, Jackson R C, Connors T A and Harrap K R. Combination chemotherapy: the interaction of methotrexate and 5-fluorouracil. *Eur J Cancer* (1973) **9**, 733.
5 Waxman S, Rubinoff M, Greenspan E and Bruckner H. Interaction of methotrexate (MTX) and 5-fluorouracil (5FU); effect on de novo DNA synthesis. *Proc Am Assoc Cancer Res* (1976) **17**, 157.
6 Brown I and Ward H W C. Therapeutic consequences of antitumour drug interactions: methotrexate and 5-fluorouracil in the chemotherapy of C3H mice with transplanted mammary adenocarcinoma. *Cancer Letters* (1978) **5**, 291.

Methotrexate + phenylbutazone

Summary

Two cases have been reported of severe methotrexate toxicity (one of the patients died) following the concurrent use of phenylbutazone.

Interaction

A man treated for unstable psoriasis with intermittent low oral doses of methotrexate (an average of 15 mg weekly over 24 h) which had been well tolerated for some considerable time, developed widespread superficial skin erosion and pyrexia after taking 200 mg phenylbutazone daily for 2 days before his weekly dose of methotrexate. The high fever persisted for 10 days.[1]

A woman with chronic plaque-type psoriasis developed buccal and widespread cutaneous ulceration estimated at one third of her body surface, within 6 days of beginning treatment with 2·5 mg methotrexate and 600 mg phenylbutazone daily. She died 5 days later from septicaemia following bone marrow depression.[1] She had had both drugs on previous occasions without adverse effects.

Mechanism

Not known. The clinical features, certainly in the second case, are those of methotrexate toxicity and overdosage. The authors of the report postulate that the phenylbutazone (a highly bound drug) displaced the methotrexate (another highly bound drug) from its binding sites on plasma proteins, thereby increasing the concentrations of free, and biologically active, methotrexate.

Importance and management

The evidence for this interaction appears to be limited to these two cases; nevertheless, because the reaction is potentially so serious it would be prudent to give these drugs together with great caution. The same precautions would also seem to be appropriate with oxyphenbutazone.

Reference

1 Adams J D and Hunter G A. Drug interaction in psoriasis. *Aust J Derm* (1976) **17**, 39.

Methotrexate + probenecid

Summary

The serum levels of methotrexate are markedly increased by the concurrent use of probenecid which may call for a considerable reduction in methotrexate dosage if excessive toxicity is to be avoided.

Interaction

A study in man of the effects of using probenecid and methotrexate injection together showed that the serum levels of methotrexate at 24 h were four times higher than in those who had not received probenecid.[1, 4] (0·40 mg/L compared with 0·09 mg/L.)

Mechanism

Studies in rats have shown that probenecid inhibits the excretion of methotrexate by the renal and biliary routes, and a similar inhibitory effect on renal excretion has been seen in monkeys.[2,3] This is probably the mechanism of this interaction in man. A reduction in elimination will lead to an accumulation of the methotrexate and a rise in serum levels.

Importance and control

In the case of rats[3] the toxicity of methotrexate has been clearly shown to be substantially increased by the use of probenecid and it would seem reasonable to expect that this could equally well occur in man. A reduction in the dosage of methotrexate may well be necessary if these two drugs are used together. This has been recommended.[4] Further study is required.

References

1 Aherne G W, Piall E, Marks V, Mould G and White W F. Prolongation and enhancement of serum methotrexate concentrations by probenecid. *Br Med J* (1978) 1, 1097.
2 Bourke R S, Chhada G, Bremer A, Watnable O and Tower D B. Inhibition of renal tubular transport of methotrexate by probenecid. *Cancer* (1975) 35, 110.
3 Kates R E, Tozer T N and Sorby D L. Increased methotrexate toxicity due to concurrent probenecid administration. *Biochem Pharmacol* (1976) 25, 1485.
4 Aherne G W, Marks V, Mould G P, Piall E and White W F. The interaction between methotrexate and probenecid in man. *Brit J Pharmacol* (1978) 6, 369P.

Methotrexate + salicylates

Summary

Severe and even fatal methotrexate toxicity can result from the concurrent use of methotrexate and aspirin.

Interaction

The development of lethal pancytopenia in 2 patients treated with methotrexate and aspirin lead to a retrospective review of the records of 176 patients who had been treated with intra-arterial infusions of methotrexate for epidermoid carcinoma of the oral cavity. This showed that concurrent use of aspirin increased the incidence of haemopoietic complications and death. A rapid fall in absolute and relative white cell counts was seen after salicylates, even after a single dose. Six out of 7 patients who developed a rapid and serious pancytopenia had had salicylates. Similar results were observed in experiments carried out on mice.[4]

Methotrexate toxicity and hepatotoxicity have been described in 3 patients taking methotrexate for psoriasis and who were concurrently receiving aspirin.[3,5]

Mechanism

Not fully understood, but clinical and experimental evidence suggests that two different mechanisms acting in concert may be involved. Methotrexate is a highly plasma-protein bound compound which can be displaced by salicylates. The levels of bound methotrexate fall by about 30% and levels of unbound, and biologically active, methotrexate rise accordingly.[1,2] It has also been shown in patients with disseminated malignancies that sodium salicylate competes with and reduces the renal excretion of methotrexate by about 35%. Both of these mechanisms acting together would result in increased amounts of active circulating methotrexate, and, since the therapeutic dosages closely approach toxic levels, a quite small increase could account for the toxicity described.

Importance and management

A serious interaction, adequately but not extensively documented. Although both drugs have been used together without the development of toxicity,[6] it would be prudent to avoid concurrent use whenever possible. The interaction has been described with aspirin, and it seems possible that it will also occur with other salicylates. This requires confirmation.

References

1 Liegler D G, Henderson E S, Halin M A and Oliverio V T. The effect of organic acids on renal clearance of methotrexate in man. *Clin Pharmacol Therap* (1969) 10, 849.
2 Dixon R L, Henderson E S and Rall D P. Plasma protein binding of methotrexate and its displacement by various drugs. *Fed Proc* (1965) 24, 454.
3 Baker H. Intermittent high dose oral methotrexate therapy in psoriasis. *Br J Dermatol* (1976) 82, 65.
4 Zuik M and Mandel M A. Methotrexate–salicylate interaction: a clinical and experimental study. *Surgical Forum* (1975) 26, 567.
5 Dubin H V and Harrell E R. Liver disease associated with methotrexate treatment of psoriatic patients. *Arch Dermatol* (1970) 102, 498.
6 Black R L, O'Brien W M, Van Scott E J, Auerbach R, Eisen A Z and Bunin J J. Methotrexate therapy in psoriatic arthritis. *J Amer Med Ass* (1964) 189, 743.

Procarbazine + CNS depressants
or antihypertensive agents

Summary
The effects of drugs which can cause CNS depression or lower blood pressure may possibly be enhanced in the presence of procarbazine.

Interaction, mechanism, importance
and management
Procarbazine can cause CNS depression ranging from mild drowsiness to profound stupor. The incidence is variously reported as being 31%, 14% and 8%.[1-3] Additive CNS depression may therefore be expected if other drugs possessing CNS-depressant activity are given concurrently.

Orthostatic hypotension has been described in 4 out of 48 patients on procarbazine.[3] Elsewhere a patient with hypertension and Hodgkin's disease has been reported whose blood pressure returned to normal when treated with procarbazine.[4] Additive hypotensive effects may therefore be seen with the concurrent use of antihypertensive drugs.

References
1 Brunner K W and Young C W. A methylhydrazine derivative in Hodgkin's disease and other malignant neoplasms: therapeutic and toxic effects studied in 51 patients. Ann Int med (1965) 63, 69.
2 Stolinsky D C, Solomon J, Pugh R P, Stevens A R, Jacobs E M, Irwin L E, Wood D A, Steinfeld J L and Bateman J R. Clinical experience with procarbazine in Hodgkin's disease, reticulum cell sarcoma, and lymphosarcoma. Cancer (1970) 26, 984.
3 Samuels M L, Leary W B, Alexanian R, Howe C D and Frei E. Clinical trials with N-isopropyl-α-(2-methylhydrazino)-p-toluamide hydrochloride in malignant lymphoma and other disseminated neoplasia. Cancer (1967) 20, 1187.
4 Frei E. Quoted as a personal communication by De Vita V T, Hahn M A and Oliverio V T in Monoamine oxidase inhibition by a new carcinostatic agent, N-isopropyl-α-(2-methylhydrazino)-p-toluamide (MIH). Proc Soc exp Biol Med (1965) 120, 561.

Procarbazine + tyramine-containing foods
and sympathomimetic amines

Summary
Whether the monoamine-oxidase inhibitory properties of procarbazine can cause an adverse interaction with certain sympathomimetic amines is uncertain. An itching skin reaction attributed to an interaction with cheese has been reported in one patient.

Interaction
The manufacturers of procarbazine state that 'Natulan is a weak MAO inhibitor and therefore interaction with certain foodstuffs and drugs, although very rare, must be borne in mind.' This is apparently based on the results of animal experiments which have shown that procarbazine possesses monoamine oxidase inhibitory properties which are weaker than pheniprazine.[1] Whether in fact procarbazine can interact with indirectly acting sympathomimetic amines (e.g. phenylpropanolamine, amphetamines etc.) or the tyramine in certain foodstuffs (e.g. cheese) to cause a hypertensive crisis is uncertain. Direct reports of such an interaction appear to be lacking, although an itching skin eruption observed after the ingestion of cheese which was attributed to the MAO-inhibitory properties of procarbazine has been described.[2]

References
1 De Vita V T, Hahn M A and Oliverio V T. Monoamine oxidase inhibition by a new carciostatic agent, N-isopropyl-α-(2-methylhydrazino)-p-toluamide (MIH). Proc Soc exp Biol Med (NY) (1965) 120, 561.
2 Cooper I A, Madigan R C, Motteran R, Maritz J S and Turner C N. Combination chemotherapy (MOPP) in the management of advanced Hodgkin's disease. A progress report on 55 patients. Med J Aust (1972) 1, 41.

Stretozotocin + phenytoin

Summary

A single case report indicates that phenytoin can antagonize the cytotoxic effects of stretozotocin.

Interaction, mechanism, importance and management

A patient with an organic hypoglycaemic syndrome, due to a metastatic apud cell carcinoma of the pancreas, who was treated with 2 g stretozotocin every 4 days together with 400 mg phenytoin daily, failed to show the expected response to stretozotocin until the phenytoin was withdrawn. It would seem that the phenytoin protects the beta cells of the pancreas from the cytotoxic effects of the stretozotocin by some mechanism as yet not understood. Although this is an isolated case report its authors recommend that concurrent use of these two drugs should be avoided.

Reference
1 Koranyi L and Gero L. Influence of diphenylhydantoin on the effect of stretozotocin. *Br Med J* (1979) **1**, 127.

Vincristine + colaspase, isoniazid and pyridoxine

Summary

Vincristine neurotoxicity may possibly be considerably enhanced by the concurrent use of these drugs.

Interaction, mechanism, importance and management

Severe neurotoxicity has been described in 3 patients who were under treatment with vincristine. One of them was also taking colaspase, and the other two were concurrently receiving isoniazid and pyridoxine. A definite relationship between the development of this serious toxicity and the use of these drugs has not been established, but the evidence suggests that particular care should be exercised if they are given to patients on vincristine.[1]

Reference
1 Hildebrand J and Kenis Y. Vincristine and neurotoxicity. *New Eng J Med* (1972) **287**, 517.

CHAPTER 13. DIGITALIS GLYCOSIDE INTERACTIONS

Plant extracts containing cardiac glycosides have been in use for thousands of years. The ancient Egyptians were familiar with squill, as were the Romans who used it as a heart tonic and diuretic. The foxglove was mentioned in the writings of Welsh physicians in the thirteenth century and features in *An account of the Foxglove and some of its Medical Uses*, published by William Witterning in 1785, in which he described its application in the treatment of 'dropsy' or the oedema which results from heart failure.

The most commonly used cardiac glycosides today are those obtained from members of the foxglove family, *Digitalis purpurea* and *D. lanata*. The leaves of these two plants are the source of a number of purified glycosides (e.g. digitoxin, digoxin, gitoxin, lanatoside C, and others), of gitalin (an amorphous mixture largely composed of digitoxon and digoxin), and of powdered whole leaf digitalis. Occasionally ouabain or strophanthin (also of plant origin) are used for particular situations, while for a number of years the Russians have exploited convallatoxin, an extract of lily of the valley. All of these cardiac glycosides have similar actions, but they differ in their potency and in their rates of elimination, and this determines how much is given and how often. Table 13.1 lists many of the cardiac glycosides in use.

Table 13.1. Cardiac glycosides

Non-proprietary names	Proprietary names
Acetyldigitoxin	*Aclanid(e)*
Acetyldigoxin	*Acygloxine, Dioxanin (α-isomer), Lanadigin Novodigal (β-isomer), Sandolanid*
Acetyl strophanthidin	
Delanoside	*Cedilanid-D*
Digitalis leaf	*Digiforitis, Digiglusin, Digitora, Digialysat, Pil-Digis*
Digitoxin	*Crystodigin, Digilong, Digimed, Digimerck, Ditaven, Digitox, Digitrin, Purodigin*
Digoxin	*Cardiox, Coragoxine, Dialoxin, Digolan, Davoxin, Digacin, Fibroxin, Lanicor, Lanoxin, Lanatoxin, Lanacrist, Natigoxine Nativelle, Rougoxin, Winoxin,*
Gitalin	*Cristaloxin, Gitalgin*
Lanatoside-A	*Adilgan*
Lanatoside-C	*Cedilanid, Celadigal, Cetosanol, Lanimerck, Lanocide*
Ouabain (strophanthin-G)	*Purostrophan, Stodival, Strophoperm*
Strophanthin-K	*Kombetin, Strophantine, Strophosid*

Digitalization

The cardiac glycosides have two main actions and two main applications: for the treatment of congestive heart failure, and for cardiac arrythmias and fibrillation. Because the most commonly used glycosides are derived from digitalis, the achievement of the desired therapeutic serum concentration of any cardiac glycoside is usually referred to as 'digitalization'.

It is usual to begin treatment by administering a large loading dose so that the therapeutic concentrations are achieved reasonably quickly, but once this has been reached the amount is reduced to a maintenance dose which is intended to keep a nice balance between the drug intake and drug clearance. This has to be done carefully because the therapeutic ratio of the cardiac glycosides is low, that is to say there is a fairly narrow gap between serum concentrations which are therapeutic and those which are toxic. Normal therapeutic levels are about one third of those which are fatal, and serious toxic cardiac arrhythmias begin at about two thirds of the fatal levels. If a patient is over-digitalized he will begin to show signs of digitalis intoxication. He may first lose his appetite, then begin to be nauseated, and vomit. Visual disturbances may also be experienced, headache, drowsiness, occasionally diarrhoea, and the pulse rate can fall as low as 40 beats/min. Death can take place from cardiac arrhythmias which are associated with total AV block. Patients under treatment for cardiac arrhythmias can therefore demonstrate arrhythmias when they are both under- as well as over-digitalized, which complicates the decision to increase or reduce the dosage.

Interactions of the cardiac glycosides

The pharmacological actions of these glycosides are the same, but their rates and degree of absorption, metabolism and clearance are different and this determines the dosages used. For example the half life of digoxin is 30–40 h. This compares with 4–6 days for digitoxin, and is reflected in their daily maintenance doses of 0·125–0·5 mg and 0·15 mg respectively. It is therefore most important not to extrapolate an interaction seen with one glycoside and apply it uncritically to any other.

Because the therapeutic ratio of the cardiac glycosides is low, a quite small change in serum levels may lead to inadequate digitalization or to toxicity. For this reason interactions which have a relatively modest effect on serum levels may sometimes have serious consequences.

Digitalis glycosides + aminoglycoside antibiotics

Summary
The serum levels of digoxin can be reduced by the concurrent use of neomycin. Whether kanamycin and other digitalis glycosides interact similarly is uncertain.

Interaction

A study in normal subjects showed that the oral administration of neomycin depressed and delayed the gastrointestinal absorption of digoxin. Separating the administration of the two drugs by several hours still resulted in depressed absorption.[1,2]

Mechanism

Neomycin can induce a reversible gastrointestinal malabsorption syndrome which can reduce the absorption of several drugs. The failure to prevent the interaction by separating the administration would lend support to this mechanism, rather than to the idea that a chemical interaction takes place which makes the digoxin less soluble.

Importance and management

The documentation is limited, but the interaction seems to be established and potentially important. A fall in the serum levels of digoxin and in its therapeutic effects should be expected if neomycin is given. A larger oral dose will probably be required, because separating the administration of the two drugs is not effective. Whether other digitalis glycosides interact similarly appears not to have been documented. Kanamycin can also induce a malabsorption state but to a lesser extent. Whether it also interacts is not certain.

References

1 Lindenbaum J, Maulitz R M, Saha J R, Shea N and Butler V P. Impairment of digoxin absorption by neomycin. *Clin Res* (1972) **20**, 410

2 Lindenbaum J, Maulitz R M, and Butler V. Inhibition of digoxin absorption by neomycin. *Gastroenterology* (1976) **71**, 399.

Digitalis glycosides + amiodarone

Summary

One report claims that serum digoxin levels can be markedly increased and toxicity may develop if amiodarone is given concurrently. Another states that no interaction occurs.

Interaction

The observation that several patients on digoxin developed signs of digitalis toxicity and unexpectedly high serum levels when amiodarone was added, prompted further study of this interaction:

Seven patients who had been on constant daily doses of digoxin for at least a fortnight showed a mean rise in serum digoxin levels of 69% (from 1·17 to 1·98 μg/l) over a 7-day period when they were concurrently treated with amiodarone, 200 mg three times a day. Two other patients showed similar rises when treated with 600 mg amiodarone daily.[1]

In another report the concurrent use of amiodarone in similar doses is said to have had virtually no effect on serum digoxin levels.[2]

Mechanism

Not understood. One idea is that the highly tissue-bound amiodarone may displace digoxin from its tissue-binding sites, thereby raising the plasma concentrations. Another is that it may interfere with the excretion of the digoxin.[1]

Importance and management

The evidence is limited and seems to be confined to these reports. The interaction is not established. The authors point out that the digitalis toxicity which can develop may be incorrectly interpreted as being a direct effect of the amiodarone '. . . leading to inappropriate modification of treatment'. Their present practice is to allow for the interaction by halving the maintenance dose of digoxin when amiodarone is added.[1] More study is needed.

Reference

1 Moysey J O, Jaggarao N S V, Grundy E N and Chamberlain D A. Amiodarone increases plasma digoxin concentations. *Brit Med J* (1981) **282**, 272.

2 Achilli A. and Serra N Amiodarone increases plasma digoxin concentrations. *Brit Med J* (1981) **282**, 1630.

Digitalis glycosides +
antacids or kaolin-pectin

Summary

Despite evidence that the absorption from the gut of digoxin can be reduced by the concurrent administration of aluminium hydroxide, magnesium carbonate, magnesium hydroxide, bismuth carbonate, kaolin-pectin, and magnesium trisilicate, a clinical study indicates that the interaction with aluminium hydroxide and magnesium trisilicate may not be clinically important. Digitoxin possibly interacts similarly, but not lanatoside C. β-acetyldigoxin appears not to interact with aluminium-magnesium hydroxide. The administration of these drugs should be separated as much as possible.

Interaction

A study on 10 normal subjects who were given 0·75 mg digoxin (*Lanoxin*) with 60 ml of either 4% aluminium hydroxide gel, kaolin-pectin, 8% magnesium hyroxide gel, or magnesium trisilicate showed that the culmulative 6-day urinary digoxin excretion expressed as a percentage of the original dose was as follows: Control 40%; alumium hydroxide 31%; magenesium hydroxide 27%; kaolin-pectin 23%[1]

These results are consistent with two other reports, one of which describes a 62% reduction in the absorption of digoxin with kaolin-pectin.[2] The other describes an 11% reduction with aluminium hydroxide, 15% with bismuth carbonate and light magnesium carbonate, and 99·5% with magnesium trisilicate.[3] In-vitro studies with digitoxin suggest that it may possibly interact similarly[4] but lanatoside C probably does not.[5] The bioavailability of β-acetyldigoxin has been shown to be unaffected by the concurrent use of *Alucol* (aluminium and magnesium hydroxide).[7]

In contrast, no interaction was observed in a clinical study:

Four patients on chronic medication with 250–500 μg digoxin were concurrently treated with either 10 ml aluminium hydroxide mixture BPC, three times a day or 10 ml magnesium trisilicate mixture, BPC, three times a day. Neither antacid reduced the bioavailability of the digoxin and none of the patients showed any reduction in the control of their symptoms.[6]

Mechanism

Not fully understood. One suggestion[1,4] is that the digoxin may be adsorbed by the antacids and kaolin-pectin, particularly by the magnesium trisilicate, but to a less extent by the magnesium and aluminium hydroxides. However, it seems probably that some other, as yet unidentified, mechanism also has some part to play. The notion that alterations in the motility of the gut might be involved is seriously doubted by one group of workers.[1]

Importance and management

Despite the reports cited, the clinical importance of the interactions between digoxin and these drugs is not established. It would be prudent to be on the alert for signs of underdigitalization, and sensible to follow the normal recommendation of giving the antacid drug between meals, and the digoxin as a single daily dose before or with food.[6] More study is needed.

References

1 Brown D D and Juhl R P, Lewis K, Schrott M and Bartels B. Decreased bioavailability of digoxin due to antacids and kaolin-pectin. *New Eng J Med* (1976) **295**, 1034
2 Albert KS, Ayres J W, Disanto A R, Weidler D J, Sakmar E, Hallmark M R, Stoll R G, Desante K A and Wagner J G. Influence of kaolin-pectin suspension on digoxin bioavailability. *J Pharm Sci* (1978) **67**, 1582.
3 McElnay J C, Harron D W G, D'Arcy P F and Eagle M R G. Interaction of digoxin with antacid constituents. *Br Med J* (1978) **i**, 1554.
4 Khalil S A H. The uptake of digoxin and digitoxin by some antacids. *J Pharm Pharmac* (1974) **26**, 961.
5 Aldous S and Thomas R Absorption and metabolism of lanatoside C. *Clin Pharmacol Ther.* (1977) **21**, 647.
6 Cooke J and Smith J A. Absence of interaction of digoxin with antacids under clinical conditions. *Brit Med J* (1978) **2**, 1166.
7 Bonelli J, Hruby K, Magometschigg D, Hitzenberger G and Kaik G. The bioavailability of β-acetyldigoxin alone and combined with aluminium hydroxide and magnesium hydroxide. *Int J Clin Pharmacol* (1977) **15**, 337.

Digitalis glycosides + barbiturates

Summary

On the basis of experiments in man a reduction in the response to digitoxin may be expected if phenobarbitone is given concurrently, but as yet there are no direct reports of an adverse interaction.

Interaction

The metabolism of digitoxin can be increased by the concurrent use of phenobarbitone resulting in reduced serum digitoxin levels. Some studies have failed to demonstrate this interaction:

> A study on 3 patients taking digitoxin, 2 of whom were also phenobaribitone, showed that treatment with phenobarbitone markedly increased the metabolism of digitoxin to digoxin. While taking 96 mg phenobarbitone daily for 13 days the rate of conversion in one patient rose from 4 to 27%.[1]
>
> A study on patients taking 0·1 mg digitoxin daily and who were also given 180 mg phenobarbitone daily for 12 weeks showed that the steady-state serum digitoxin levels fell by 50%. In associated studies it was also found that the half-life of digitoxin decreased from about 8 to 5 days during phenobarbitone treatment.[2,3]
>
> A short-term study on three groups of 10 normal subjects who were given either 0·8 mg acetyldigitoxin, 0·4 mg digitoxin or 1 mg digoxin daily failed to show any effect on the serum concentrations of these cardiac glycosides when 100 mg phenobarbitone daily was being taken concurrently for 7–9 days.[4]

Mechanism

The most plausible explanation of this interaction is that the hepatic metabolism of the digitoxin to digoxin and other metabolites is increased by the phenobarbitone. This would account for the fall in serum digitoxin levels[2] and a rise in the excretion of digoxin[1] which is a major metabolic product of digitoxin. Although digoxin is also an active cardiac glycoside, its duration of action (half-life about $1\frac{1}{2}$ days) is considerably shorter than digitoxin and a much larger dose is required to achieve the same degree of digitalization. Thus an increased conversion of digitoxin to digoxin means a marked reduction in the total activity of the two glycosides.

It is not immediately obvious why the last study cited[4] failed to demonstrate this interaction, except to point out that it was, relatively speaking, only short term (7–9 days) whereas one of the other studies[2] lasted 12 weeks and used virtually double the dose of phenobarbitone.

Importance and management

Although there is good experimental evidence from studies in man that long-term treatment with phenobarbitone can reduce the serum levels of digitoxin by a considerable degree (as much as 50% in one of the studies) there is, surprisingly, no evidence that this interaction has proved to be a serious problem in practice. Nevertheless, patients taking both drugs should be monitored for under-digitalization and, where necessary, the dose of digitoxin should be increased. The other barbiturates are also potent enzyme-inducers so that the same precautions similarly apply to them although there is as yet no direct clinical evidence that they interact.

Any interaction (by no means a certainty) which may take place between digoxin and phenobarbitone is less likely to be as marked because digoxin is cleared rapidly from the body and any effects of enzyme induction are likely to be smaller.

References

1 Jelliffe R W. and Blankenhorn D H. Effect of phenobarbital on digitoxin metabolism. *Clin Res* (1966) **14**, 160.
2 Solomon H M, Reich S, Gaut Z, Pocelinko R and Abrams W B. Induction of the metabolism of digitoxin in man by phenobarbital. *Clin Res* (1971) **19**, 356.
3 Soloman H M and Abrams W B. Interactions between digitoxin and other drugs in man. *Amer Heart* (1972) **83**, 277.
4 Káldor A, Somogyi G Y, Debreczeni L A and Gachalyi B. Interaction of heart glycosides and phenobarbital. *Int J Clin Pharmacol* (1975) **12**, 403.

Digitalis glycosides + beta-blockers

Summary
Concurrent use is common but controversial. Excessive and potentially fatal bradycardia can occur if beta-blockers are used to control digitalis-induced arrhythmias unless appropriate precautions are taken.

Interaction, mechanism, importance and management

Digitalis glycosides and beta-blockers are commonly used together, although there is some controvery about whether concurrent use is beneficial.[1,2] Cardiac arrhythmias and cardiac flutter, which can occur in digitalis intoxication, can be controlled with propranolol, but under these circumstances patients appear to be particularly sensitive to the actions of propranolol and show marked bradycardia.[3] There have been fatalities. It has been suggested[4] that, if propranolol is used in this situation, it would be wise to give the patient a test dose of 5 mg or less before giving a full dose, or to combine the full dose with a protective dose of atropine. Atropine can be used in this way because it blocks the normal parasympathetic (heart slowing) activity which, if not adequately balanced by sympathetic (heart accelerating) activity results in further bradycardia.

References
1 O'Reilly M, Goldberg E and Chaithiraphan S. Propranolol and digitalis. *Lancet* (1974) **i**, 138.
2 Crawford M H, LeWinter M, Karliner J S and O'Rourke R A. Propranolol and digitalis. *Lancet* (1974) **i**, 458.
3 Turner J R B. Propranolol in the treatment of digitalis-induced and digitalis-resistant tachycardias. *Amer J Cardiol* (1966) **18**, 450.
4 Watt D A L. Sensitivity to propranolol after digoxin intoxication. *Br Med J* (1968) **3**, 413.

Digitalis glycosides + calcium preparations

Summary
The intravenous administration of calcium preparations should be undertaken with great caution in patients on digitalis because of the danger of causing life-threatening digitalis-induced heart arrhythmias.

Interaction
The activity of digitalis is enhanced by an increase in serum calcium levels and reduced by a reduction in serum calcium levels.

Increased serum Ca^{2+}
Two patients who were given digitalis intramuscularly and calcium chloride or gluconate intravenously died following the development of heart arrhythmias. No absolutely certain causative relationship was established.[1]

Reduced serum Ca^{2+}
A patient with congestive heart failure and atrial fibrillation was resistant to the actions of digoxin in the usual therapeutic range ($1 \cdot 5$–$3 \cdot 0$ ng/ml) until his serum calcium levels had been raised from $6 \cdot 7$ to about $8 \cdot 5$ mg% by the administration of high calcium levels and oral vitamin D therapy.[2]

Disodium edetate which lowers ionic calcium levels in the serum has been used successfully in the treatment of digitalis intoxication.[3,4,5] So too have sodium and potassium citrate.[6]

Mechanism
The total picture of the way the digitalis glycosides act on the heart is not even now fully understood, but there is good evidence to show that the glycosides increase the uptake of calcium into cardiac muscle cells by acting on cell membranes, and the activity of digitalis in increased by raised calcium levels. Conversely it is reduced when calcium levels are lowered by compounds which remove calcium such as EDTA.[3,4,5] If the activity of digitalis is enhanced it can lead to digitalis intoxication and heart arrhythmias which can be lifethreatening.

Importance and managment

The report cited[1] seems to be the only direct clinical evidence in the literature that intravenous administration of calcium to patients on digitalis can have a serious outcome, although there is plenty of less direct evidence which would lead one to expect that it might be so. It has been suggested that calcium be given slowly or in small amounts to patients who are digitalized in order to avoid transient calcium levels greater than 15 mEq/l, which can occur if large or rapid doses of calcium are given intravenously.[7]

References

1 Bower J O and Mengle H A K. The additive effects of calcium and digitalis. A warning with a report of two deaths. *J Amer Med Ass* (1936) **106**, 1151.

2 Chopra D, Janson P and Sawin C T. Insensitivity to digoxin associated with hypocalcaemia. *New Eng J Med* (1977) **296**, 917.

3 Jick S and Karsh R. The effect of calcium chelation on cardiac arrhythmias and conduction disturbances. *Amer. J Cardiol* (1959) **43**, 287.

4 Szekely P and Wynne N A. Effects of calcium chelation on digitalis induced cardiac arrhythmias. *Br Heart J* (1963) **25**, 589.

5 Rosenbaum J L, Mason D and Seven M. The effect of disodium EDTA on digitalis intoxication. *Amer. J Med Sci* (1960) **240**, 77.

6 Barbieri F F, Gold H, Lang T W, Bernstein H and Corday E. Sodium and potassium citrate salts for the treatment of digitalis toxicity. *Amer J Cardiol* (1964) **14**, 650.

7 Nola G T, Pope S and Harrison D C. Assessment of the synergistic relationship between serum calcium and digitalis. *Amer Heart J* (1970) **79**, 499.

Digitalis glycosides + carbamazepine

Summary

An enhancement of digitalis-induced bradycardia has been attributed to the use of carbamazepine.

Interaction, mechanism, importance and management

An observation made in 1968 that carbamazepine might have been responsible for the enhancement of bradycardia due to digitalis is as yet unconfirmed.[1]

References

1 Killian J M and Fromm G H. Carbamazepine in the treatment of neuralgia. Use and side effects. *Arch Neurol* (1968) **19**, 129.

Digitalis glycosides + carbenoxolone

Summary

Carbenoxolone is generally regarded as contraindicated in patients requiring digitalis treatment because it can raise the blood pressure, cause fluid retention and reduce serum potassium levels.

Interaction, mechanism, importance and management

The side-effects of carbenoxolone therapy include an increase in blood pressure (both systolic and diastolic), fluid retention and a reduced serum potassium. The incidence of these side-effects is said in some reports to be as high as 50%, and although others quote lower figures, it is clear that they are not an uncommon occurrence. Hypertension and fluid retention occur early in carbenoxolone treatment, whereas a reduced serum potassium develops later and may take place in the absence of the other two.[1-4] The hypokalaemia may also be exacerbated if thiazide diuretics are used to control fluid retention without the use of suitable potassium supplements. For example, severe hypokalaemia has been described in a patient treated with chlorthalidone and carbenoxolone without potassium supplementation.[5]

For all these reasons carbenoxolone should not be used in patients with congestive heart failure who are taking digitalis glycosides unless stringent precautions are taken. It is debatable whether this could be justified now that cimetidine is available.

References

1 Geismar P, Mosebech J and Myren J. A double-blind study of the effect of carbenoxolone sodium in the treatment of gastric ulcer. *Scand J Gastroenterol* (1973) **8**, 251.

2 Turpie A G G and Thomson T J. Carbenoxolone sodium in the treatment of gastric ulcer with special reference to side effects. *Gut* (1965) **6**, 591.

3 Langman M J S, Knapp D R and Wakley E. Treatment of chronic gastric ulcer with carbenoxolone and gefarnate: a comparative trial. *Br Med J* (1973) **3**, 84.

4 Davis G J, Rhodes J and Caleraft B J. Complications of carbenoxolone therapy. *Br Med J* (1974) **3**, 400.

5 Descamps C. Rhabdomyocosis and acute tubular necrosis associated with carbenoxolone and diuretic treatment. *Br Med J* (1977) **1**, 272.

Digitalis glycosides + cholestyramine

Summary

Although cholestyramine can reduce the gastrointestinal absorption of digoxin and digitoxin, and thereby reduce the serum cardiac glycoside levels attained, the clinical importance of these interactions has not been adequately assessed. It can be avoided by giving the cholestyramine $1\frac{1}{2}$ h after the cardiac glycoside.

Interaction

A study carried out with 12 volunteers who were given 0·75 mg digoxin showed that the cumulative 6-day recovery of digoxin from the urine was reduced from 40·5 to 33·1% when 4 g cholestyramine was given concurrently.[1]

Other reports describe a fall in serum digoxin levels during concurrent treatment with cholestyramine[2] and an increase in the loss of digoxin and its metabolites in the faeces during concurrent long-term use.[3] A reduction in the half-life of digitoxin from 10 to $6\frac{1}{2}$ days has also been reported,[4] and the same workers have described similar results in another report.[5] The mean half-life of digitoxin is reported elsewhere to have been reduced from 142 to 84 hours by cholestyramine.[8]

Mechanism

By no means fully understood. Although it is well recognized that cholestyramine can bind with drugs within the gut, thereby reducing their bioavailability, it is doubtful if this interaction can be accounted for quite as simply. It is probable that some interference with the enterohepatic cycle takes place, but as one study showed[3] the effects of concurrent use are varied and inconsistent. More work is needed to elucidate the total picture.

Importance and management

A reduction in the absorption of both digoxin and digitoxin by cholestyramine has been clearly demonstrated, but the practical importance of these interactions and the extent to which the treatment of patients with these glycosides is impaired by this interaction appears not to have been determined. Nevertheless it would be prudent to be on the alert for signs of under-digitalization. Long-term studies have shown that the interaction can be avoided if the cholestyramine is taken $1\frac{1}{2}$ h after either of these glycosides.[6] An alternative may be to use β-methyldigoxin, which other studies suggest may be minimally affected by the presence of cholestyramine.[7]

References

1 Brown D D, Juhl R P and Warner S L. Decreased bioavailability of digoxin produced by dietary fibre and cholestyramine. *Amer J Cardiol* (1977) **39**, 297.

2 Smith T W. New approaches to the management of digitalis intoxication. In *Symposium on digitalis*, Glydendal Norsk Forlag, Oslo (1973) 312.

3 Hall W H, Shappell S D and Doherty J E. Effect of cholestyramine on digoxin absorption and excretion in man. *Amer J Cardiol* (1977) **39**, 213.

4 Caldwell J H and Greenberger N J. Cholestyramine enhances digitalis excretion and protects against lethal intoxication. *J Clin Invest* (1970) **49**, 16a.

5 Caldwell J H, Bush C A and Greenberger N J. Interruption of the enterohepatic circulation of digitoxin by cholestyramine. *J Clin Invest* (1971) **50**, 2638.

6 Bazzano G and Bazzano G S. Effect of digitalis binding resins on cardiac glycoside plasma levels. *Clin Res* (1972) **20**, 24.

7 Hahn K-J and Weber E. Effect of cholestyramine on absorption of drugs. In *Frontiers of Internal Medicine* (1975), p. 409. 12th Int Cong Internal Med, Tel Aviv, 1974. Karger, Basel.

8 Carruthers S G and Dujovne C A. Cholestyramine and spironolactone and their combination in digitoxin elimination. *Clin Pharmacol Ther* (1980) **27**, 184.

Digitalis + colestipol

Summary

There is evidence indicating that the activity of the digitalis glycosides may be reduced by the concurrent use of colestipol.

Interaction

Colestipol is an ion-exchange resin similar to cholestyramine which can bind with the digitalis glycosides. A study in which colestipol was used to treat digitalis intoxication in 5 patients (4 on digitoxin and 1 on digoxin), showed that the administration of 10 g colestipol, followed by 5 g every 6–8 h, shortened the period of intoxication compared with some other patients not given colestipol. The digitoxin plasma half-life was shortened from 9·3 to 2·75 days, and the digoxin half-life of the 1 patient was shortened to 16 h from 1·8–2·0 days in the control patients.[1]

Mechanism

In-vitro studies confirm that colestipol binds with the digitalis glycosides.[1] Since these glycosides take part in the enterohepatic cycle (i.e. they are excreted in the bile and later reabsorbed), the presence of colestipol would reduce the amount available for reabsorption and hasten the removal of digitalis from the body.

Importance and management

The documentation is limited, but it indicates that a reduction in the activity of the digitalis glycosides would be expected if colestipol were used concurrently. If the colestipol is given $1\frac{1}{2}$ h after the glycosides no interaction occurs.[2]

References

1 Bazzano G and Bazzano G S. Digitalis intoxication. Treatment with a new steroid-binding resin. *J Amer Med Ass* (1972) **220**, 828.

2 Bazzano G and Bazzano G S. Effect of digitalis-binding resins on cardiac glycoside plasma levels. *Clin Res* (1972) **20**, 24.

Digitalis glycosides + potassium-depleting diuretics (chlorthalidone, ethacrynic acid, frusemide, thiazides)

Summary

The potassium loss caused by these diuretics can increase the activity and the toxicity of the digitalis glycosides. It is common practice to given potassium supplements.

Interaction

An extensive study on a large number of patients treated with digoxin showed that almost 1 in 5 had some toxic reactions attributable to the use of the glycoside. Of these, 16% had demonstrable hypokalaemia (less that 3·5 mEq/l) which was associated with the concurrent use of potassium-depleting diuretics, notably hydrochlorothiazide and frusemide.[1]

Numerous other studies and reports similarly describe the increase in digitalis toxicity which occurs with potassium depletion[2-5] although there is at least one discordant report.[6]

Mechanism

Not fully understood. The cardiac glycosides inhibit the activity of the enzyme sodium-potassium adenosine triphosphatase which is concerned with the transport of sodium and potassium across the membrane of the myocardial cells, and this (it is postulated) is associated with an increase in the availability of calcium ions concerned with the contraction of the cells. Potassium loss caused by these diuretics exacerbates the potassium loss from the myocardial cells, thereby increasing the activity, and the toxicity of the digitalis. Some loss of magnesium may also have a part to play. The mechanism of this interaction is still being debated.

Importance and management

An extremely well-established and well-known interaction of practical importance. Only a few selected references have been listed. It is only a short step from effective therapy with digitalis to a state of intoxication, for which reason potassium and magnesium levels should be monitored and, wherever necessary, potassium supplements should be given to offset the potassium loss caused by these diuretics. Many, but not all, patients require additional potassium. There is the risk of inducing hyperkalaemia if the supplement is given 'blind' without monitoring.

References

1 Shapiro S, Slone D, Lewis G P and Jick H. The epidemiology of digoxin. A study in three Boston hospitals. *J Chron Dis* (1969) 22, 361.
2 Steiness E and Olesen K H. Cardiac arrhythmias induced by hypokalaemia and potassium loss during maintenance digoxin therapy. *Br Heart J* (1976) 38, 167.
3 Binnion P E. Hypolalaemia and digoxin-induced arrhythmias. *Lancet* (1975) i, 343.
4 Poole-Wilson P A, Hall R and Cameron I R. Hypokalaemia, digitalis, and arrhythmias. *Lancet* (1975) i, 575.
5 Shapiro W and Tuabert K. Hypolalaemia and digoxin-induced arrhythmias. *Lancet* (1975) ii, 604.
6 Ogilvie R I and Ruedy J. An educational program in digitalis therapy. *J Amer Med Ass* (1972) 222, 50.

Digitalis + edrophonium

Summary

Excessive bradycardia and AV block may occur in patients on digitalis given edrophonium.

Interaction, mechanism, importance and management

The rapid intravenous injection of 10 mg edrophonium has proved to be a useful vagotonic drug in the differentiation of cardiac arrhythmias, but it has been recommended that it should not be given to patients with auricular flutter or tachycardia taking digitalis because of the risk of producing atrioventricular block due to the additive heart-slowing effects.[1] This recommendation is reinforced by a case in which bradycardia, atrioventricular block and asystole developed as a result of concurrent use.[2]

Reference

1 Reddy R C V, Gould L and Gomprecht R F. Use of edrophonium (Tensilon) in the evaluation of cardiac arrhythmias. *Amer Heart J* (1971) 82, 742.
2 Gould L, Zahir M and Gomprecht R F. Cardiac arrest during edrophonium administration. *Amer Heart J* (1971) 81, 437.

Digitalis glycosides + dietary fibre

Summary

The absorption of digoxin from the gut can be reduced by the presence of large amounts of crude fibre in the diet if the two are taken together.

Interaction

A study carried out with 12 normal adult volunteers who were given 0·75 mg digoxin showed that the cumulative 6-day recovery of digoxin from the urine was reduced from 40·5% to 33·0% when ingested with a meal containing 5 g crude fibre. An identical reduction was seen when concurrently taken with 4 g cholestyramine instead, whereas a normal amount of dietary fibre (0·75 g) had no effect.[1]

Mechanism

Not fully established, but it seems very probable that the digoxin binds to the fibre within the gut so that less is available for absorption.

Importance and management

Information is limited, but the interaction seems to be established. A long-term study would give absolute confirmation. The authors of the paper cited suggest that taking the digoxin with meals of high or unknown fibre content should be avoided since the absorption can be considerably reduced. This could lead to under-digitalization. Meals containing a normal amount of crude fibre do not affect absorption. Since it seems that taking digoxin $1\frac{1}{2}$ hours before cholestyramine can prevent the cholestyramine/digoxin interaction[2], it seems possible that a similar precaution might be effective for patients on a high fibre diet. An average 40 g ($1\frac{1}{3}$ oz) serving of Kellogg's *All-Bran* contains about 10 g dietary fibre.

References

1 Brown D D, Juhl R P and Warner S L. Decreased bioavailability of digoxin produced by dietary fibre and cholestyramine. *Amer J Cardiol* (1977) **39**, 297.
2 Bazzano G and Bazzano G S. Effect of digitalis-binding resins on cardiac glycoside plasma levels. *Clin Res* (1972) **20**, 24.

Digitalis glycosides + indomethacin

Summary

Indomethacin is reported to have induced digitalis toxicity in 3 premature infants.

Interaction, mechanism, importance and management

Three premature infants treated for 3 days with digoxin (loading dose 40 μg/kg; maintenance 10 μg/kg/day) showed evidence of digitalis toxicity when they were concurrently given 0·2 mg/kg indomethacin. Each of the three developed prolonged periods of bradycardia and ST segment elevation. Studies subsequently carried out in rabbits suggested that indomethacin may possibly raise serum digoxin levels and lower the volume of distribution.[1]

The general importance of this possible interaction in adults is not known, but it would seem prudent to be on the alert for signs of digitalis toxicity in patients stabilized on digoxin who are given indomethacin. More study is required.

References

1 Mayes L C and Boerth R C. Digoxin–indomethacin interaction. *Pediatric Res* (1980) **14**, 469.

Digitalis glycosides + metoclopramide

Summary

Serum digoxin levels may be lowered by about a third if metoclopramide and slowly dissolving solid forms of digoxin are given concurrently. No interaction is likely with digoxin in liquid form or in fast-dissolving preparations which fulfil current BP or USP requirements.

Interaction

A study on 11 patients taking a slow-dissolving formulation of digoxin showed that concurrent treatment with metoclopramide (10 mg three times a day for 10 days) reduced the serum digoxin levels by about 36% (from 0·72 to 0·46 ng/ml).[1]

Mechanism

The most likely reason for this reduction in digoxin absorption is that the metoclopramide increases the motility of the gut to such an extent that full dissolution and absorption of digoxin is unfinished by the time it is lost in the faeces.

Importance and management

Metoclopramide is unlikely to affect the absorption of solid-form, fast-dissolving digoxin preparations (those fulfilling the BP and USP requirements) or digoxin in liquid form, but it may affect those preparations which are slow-dissolving. A reduction in serum digoxin levels of a third could result in underdigitalization. There is no information about digitoxin but an interaction would not be expected because it is more completely absorbed than digoxin. Direct information about the digitalis/metoclopramide interaction seems to be limited to the one paper quoted.[1]

References
1 Manninen V, Apajalahti A, Melin J and Kavesoja M. Altered absorption of digoxin in patients given propantheline and metoclopramide. *Lancet* (1973) i, 398.

Digitalis glycosides + neuromuscular blockers

Summary

Serious cardiac arrhythmias may develop in patients receiving digitalis who are given suxamethonium. In contrast, tubocurarine has been used to treat cardiac arrhythmias.

Interaction

In a study on 17 digitalized patients, initially anaesthetized with sodium thiamylal and then maintained with nitrous oxide and oxygen, it was found that serious ventricular arrhythmias occurred in 8 patients following the intravenous injection of 40–100 mg suxamethonium. Three of the others had immediate and definite ST/T wave changes, and the remaining 6 showed frequent multifocal premature ventricular contractions. Similar findings were seen in animal experiments.[1]

There are other reports of this interaction.[2,3] In contrast, five out of eight patients with ventricular arrhythimias returned to normality when given 15–30 mg tubocurarine, and another returned to a regular nodal rhythm from ventricular tachycardia.[1]

Mechanism

Not understood. One possibility is that the suxamethonium may cause the rapid removal of potassium from the myocardial cells which could precipitate arrhythmias due to digitalis toxicity.

Importance and management

Information is limited but the interaction appears to be established. Suxamethonium should be avoided, or used with great caution, in patients receiving digitalis glycosides.

References
1 Dowdy E G and Fabian L W. Ventricular arrhythmias induced by succinylcholine in digitalized patients. A preliminary report. *Anaesth Analg* (1963) 42, 501.
2 Perez H R. Cardiac arrythmia after succinylcholine. *Anesth Analg* (1970) 49, 33.
3 Smith R B and Petrusack J. Succinylcholine, digitalis, and hypercalcaemia: a case report. *Anesth Analg* (1972) 51, 202.

Digitalis glycosides + phenylbutazone

Summary

A single case report describes a marked reduction in serum digitoxin levels caused by the concurrent use of phenylbutazone.

Interaction

A study on a patient with normal renal and hepatic function taking 0·1 mg digitoxin daily, showed that on each of two occasions when he was concurrently treated with 300 mg phenylbutazone daily the serum digitoxin levels were approximately halved.[1]

Mechanism

Not understood. The suggestion is that the phenylbutazone acts as an enzyme-inducing agent which increases the rate of metabolism and loss from the body of the digitoxin.[1]

Importance and management

Information seems to be limited to this single report. It would seem wise to watch for under-digitalization if phenylbutazone is added to established treatment with digitoxin, but much more study is required to establish the general importance of this interaction

Reference

1 Solomon H M, Reich S, Spirt N and Abrams W B. Interactions between digitoxin and other drugs *in vitro* and *in vivo*. *Ann NY Acad Sci* (1971) 179, 362.

Digitalis glycosides + phenytoin

Summary

Phenytoin has proven value in the treatment of digitalis-induced heart arrhythmias. Whether excessive bradycardia is a potential hazard is uncertain. A marked reduction in serum-digitoxin levels during chronic concurrent treatment with phenytoin has been described in 1 patient.

Interaction

(a) Treatment of digitalis toxicity

In a report on a number of patients requiring treatment for digitalis-induced heart arrhythmias, 20 out of a total of 24 patients with ventricular arrhythmias are described who returned to sinus rhythm after the intravenous administration of phenytoin (5 mg/kg).[1]

There are a number of other reports describing the successful use of phenytoin in the treatment of digitalis toxicity.[2,3,4]

(b) Long-term concurrent treatment with digitoxin and phenytoin

The serum digitoxin levels of a man taking digitoxin were observed to fall on each of three occasions when he was concurrently treated with phenytoin. On the third occasion, while taking 0·2 mg digitoxin daily, the addition of 900 mg phenytoin a day caused a fall in serum digitoxin levels over a period of 7–10 days from about 25 to 10 μg/ml.[5]

Mechanism

Phenytoin probably prevents arrhythmias by reducing the uptake of calcium into heart muscle cells. This has a stabilizing action on the responsiveness of these cells to stimulation and at the same time it increases the AV and intraventricular conduction. The overall result is that the toxic threshold dosage at which arrhythmias occur is raised. However, the cardiac-slowing effect of digitalis is not opposed by phenytoin (at least in dogs)[7] and the lethal dose is unaltered, so the combined bradycardia may result in sudden cardiac arrest.

Phenytoin is a known enzyme-inducing agent so that the fall in serum digitoxin levels in the single case cited[5] may have been due to a phenytoin-induced increase in the metabolism and clearance of the digitoxin.

Importance and management

The value of phenytoin in the treatment of digitalis-induced arrhythmias is established,[1-4] although the authors of the last of these reports warn that phenytoin should not be used in patients with a high degree of heart block or marked bradycardia. This is borne out by experiments in dogs which showed that sudden cardiac arrest could occur.[7] The dosage of phenytoin used in the treatment of digitalis-induced arrhythmias in one of the reports cited was 5 mg/kg.[1] Another recommends 100 mg administered intravenously every 5 min, and after control has been achieved the drug can be given orally in doses of 400–600 mg/day until the serum digitalis levels are back to the normal range.[8] An unexplained report describes a mongol patient given phenytoin, 200 mg daily, for grand mal seizures and digoxin, 0·25 mg daily, for mitral insufficiency who developed marked bradycardia (34 beats/min) and complete heart block.[6] But in what way this reaction is related to the cardiopathy seen in mongols and what its general relevance may be to non-mongol patients is not clear.

Information about the effects on serum digitoxin levels seems to be confined to the one report cited,[5] so that its general applicability is as yet not known, but until more work is published on this interaction it would be prudent to check that patients on digitoxin who are subsequently given phenytoin as well do not become underdigitalized.

There appears to be nothing documented about an interaction between any of the other cardiac glycosides with phenytoin in man.

References

1 Helfant R H, Seuffert G W, Patton R D, Stein E and Damato A N. The clinical use of diphenylhydantoin (Dilantin) in the treatment and prevention of cardiac arrhythmias. *Am Heart J* (1969) **77**, 315.
2 Lang T W, Bernstein H, Barbieri F, Gold H and Corday E. Digitalis toxicity. Treatment with diphenylhydantoin. *Arch Intern Med* (1965) **116**, 573.
3 Karliner J S. Intravenous diphenylhydantoin sodium (dilantin) in cardiac arrhythmias. *Dis Chest* (1967) **51**, 256.
4 Rosen M R, Lisak R, and Rubin I L. Diphenylhydantoin in cardiac arrhythmias. *Am J Cardiol* (1967) **20**, 674.
5 Solomon H M, Reich S, Spirt N and Abrams W B. Interactions between digitoxin and other drugs *in vitro* and *in vivo*. *Ann NY Acad Sci* (1971) **179**, 362.
6 Viukari N M A and Aho K. Digoxin–phenytoin interaction. *Br Med J.* (1970) **2**, 51.
7 Scriabine A, Kostis J, Nigri A, Bellet S, Morgan G and Rival J. Some aspects of interaction between diphenydantoin and digoxin by simultaneous administration in dogs. *Toxicol Appl Pharmacol* (1970) **17**, 708.
8 Bigger J T and Strauss H C. Digitalis toxicity: Drug interactions promoting toxicity and the management of toxicity. *Seminars in Drug Treatment* (1972) **2**, 147.

Digitalis glycosides + propantheline

Summary

Serum digoxin levels may be raised by a third or more if propantheline and slowly dissolving solid forms of digoxin are given concurrently. No interaction is likely with digoxin in liquid form or in a fast-dissolving preparation which fulfils current BP or USP requirement.

Interaction

The absorption by the gut of digoxin from slowly dissolving formulations may be increased by propantheline:

The serum digoxin levels rose in 9 of 13 patients by 30% (from 1·02 to 1·33 ng/ml) while taking propantheline (15 mg for 10 days) with a slowly dissolving formulation of digoxin. In 3 patients the digoxin concentrations remained unaltered and fell slightly in 1. An associated study on 4 normal subjects given digoxin in liquid form, with and without propantheline, showed that serum digoxin levels were higher than those seen when given in tablet form, and they remained unaffected by propantheline.[1]

The same workers in a subsequent study on 8 subjects using two different formulations of digoxin were able to show that propanetheline (10 mg three times a day) increased the digoxin serum levels by 40% (from 0·96 to 1·35 ng/ml) with a slow-dissolving preparation, but only about 4% (from 1·69 to 1·75 ng/ml) with a fast-dissolving formulation.[2]

Mechanism

Propantheline is an anticholinergic agent which reduces the motility of the gut and prolongs the transit time of materials passing through. This allows the slow-dissolving formations of digoxin more time to pass into solution and more is therefore available for absorption. Thus the serum levels are elevated. It has also been suggested that since propantheline inhibits the flow of bile (into which about 10% of the digoxin is secreted) more digoxin is retained and this might also account for some of the increase in serum digoxin levels.[3] No interaction is likely with formulatons in liquid form or which dissolve rapidly.

Importance and management

The interaction is only of importance if brands of digoxin are used which dissolve slowly. Because a 30–40% rise in serum levels may be enough to put concentrations into the toxic range, patients on both drugs should be monitored carefully. Most formulation, such as those which fulfil the BP or USP standards (e.g. *Lanoxin*), are unlikely to interact. Under-digitalization is a possibility if propantheline is withdrawn. There seems to be no evidence of an interaction with other anticholinergic drugs, and no interaction of any importance is likely with formulations which dissolve rapidly or are in liquid form. Digitoxin is also better absorbed from the gut than digoxin so that an interaction with propantheline would not be expected.

References

1 Manninen V, Apajalahti A, Melin J and Kavesoja M. Altered absorption of digoxin in patients given propantheline and metoclopramide. *Lancet* (1973) i, 398.
2 Manninen V. Effect of propantheline and metoclopramide on absorption of digoxin. *Lancet* (1973) i, 1118.
3 Thompson W G. Altered absorption of digoxin in patients given propantheline and metoclopramide. *Lancet* (1973) i, 783.

Digitalis glycosides + quinidine or quinine

Summary

The serum concentrations of digoxin can be more than doubled by the concurrent administration of quinidine which may lead to the development of digitalis intoxication. A smaller rise has been described with quinine.

Interaction

A study[1] on 12 patients showed that when quinidine (600 mg twice a day) was added to an established digoxin regimen, the mean digoxin serum levels rose by almost 90% (from 0·85 to 1·16 ng/ml). Only one of the six whose digoxin levels rose above the normal therapeutic range showed signs of digitalis intoxication.[1]

A retrospective study of 27 patients showed that when quinidine was administered, the serum digoxin levels of 25 of them rose significantly. The levels more than doubled (from 1·3 to 3·2 ng/ml) in 17 who continued to take the same dose of digoxin. Sixteen showed typical signs of digitalis intoxication (nausea, vomiting, anorexia) which resolved in 10 of them when the digoxin was either reduced or withdrawn, and in 5 of them when the quinidine was withdrawn, leaving the digoxin dosages unaltered[2]

This effect of quinidine on digoxin serum levels has been reported in other studies on a considerable number of patients.[3,5,8–14,16] There is some evidence that no quinidine–digitoxin interaction occurs.[15] Quinine in doses of 300 mg four times a day has been shown to raise steady state serum digoxin levels by about 75%.[17]

Mechanisms

Clinical investigations[4,5] into the mechanism of this interaction have shown that quinidine inhibits renal excretion of digoxin. In one study on 4 patients the digoxin/creatinine clearance ratio was 0·74 during quinidine therapy and 1·11 after withdrawal.[4] In another study on 15 patients the digoxin/creatinine ratio was 0·85 compared with 1·22 in 44 other patients not taking quinidine.[5]

Normally digoxin is cleared from the body by glomerular filtration and tubular excretion, but there is evidence of tubular re-absorption as well.[6,7] Just which of these is affected by the quinidine is not known, and indeed whether other non-renal mechanisms such as displacement from tissue binding may also be involved[8] requires further investigation.

Importance and management

An established and important interaction. If the digoxin serum levels are markedly increased, concentrations may be reached which are toxic. For this reason quinidine should only be given to patients on digoxin if the serum levels and clinical effects can be monitored carefully and suitable adjustments to the digoxin dosage made. Similarly, if quinidine is withdrawn, an upward readjustment of the digoxin dosage should be expected. It would seem prudent to apply the same precautions with quinine. See also the digoxin/quinidine/pentobarbitone interaction on page 309.

References

1 Ejvinsson G. Effect of quinidine on plasma concentrations of digoxin. *Br Med J* (1978) 1, 279.
2 Leahey E B, Reiffel J A, Drusin R E, Heisenbuttel R H, Lovejoy W P and Bigger J TH. Interactions between quinidine and digoxin *J Am Med Ass* (1978) **240**, 533.
3 Hooymans P M and Merkus F W H M. Effect of quinidine on plasma concentration of digoxin. *Br Med J* (1978) 2, 1022.
4 Doering W and Konig E. Anstieg der Digoxinkonzentration im Serum unter Chinidinmedikation. *Med Klin* (1978) **73**, 1085.
5 Hooymans P M and Merkus F W H M. The mechanism of the interaction between digoxin and quinidine. *Pharm Weekblad Sci Ed* (1979) i, 36.

6 Steiness E Renal tubular secretion of digoxin. *Circulation* (1974) **50**, 103.
7 Halkin H, Sheiner L B, Peck C C and Melmon K. Determinants of the renal clearance of digoxin. *Clin Pharmacol Therap* (1975) **17**, 385.
8 Hager W D, Fenster P, Mayersohn M, Perrier D, Graves P, Marcus F I and Goldman S. Digoxin–quinidine interaction. Pharmacokinetic evaluation. *New Eng J Med* (1979) **300**, 1238.
9 Chapron D J, Mumford D and Pitegoff G I. Apparent quinidine-induced digoxin toxicity after withdrawal of pentobarbital. A case of sequential drug interactions. *Arch Int Med* (1979) **139**, 363.
10 Holt D W, Hayler A M, Edmonds M E and Ashford R F. Clinically significant interaction between digoxin and quinidine. *Br Med J* (1979) **2**, 1401.
11 Risler T, Peters U, Grabensee B and Seipel L. Quinidine–digoxin interaction. *New Eng J Med* (1980) **302**, 175.
12 Pedersen K E and Hvidt S. Quinidine–digoxin interaction. *New Eng J Med* (1980) **302**, 176.
13 Powell J R, Fenster P E, Hager W D, Graves P, Wandell M W and Conrad K. Quinidine–digoxin interaction. *New Eng J Med* (1980) **302**, 176.
14. Doering W. Quinidine–digoxin interaction Pharmacokinetics, underlying mechanism and clinical implications. *New Eng J Med* (1979) **301**, 400.
15. Keller F and Kreutz G. Keine Chinidin-interaktion mit digitoxin. *Dtsch Med Wschr* (1980) **105**, 701.
16. Reid P K and Meek A G. Digoxin–quinidine interaction. *Johns Hopkins Med J* (1979) **145**, 227
17. Avonson J K. and Carver J G. Interaction of digoxin with quinine. *Lancet* (1981) **i**, 1418.

Digitalis glycosides +
quinidine and pentobarbitone

Summary

A case has been reported in which the digoxin-quinidine interaction (development of digoxin toxicity) only manifested itself when a third drug, pentobarbitone, was withdrawn.

Interaction

The effects of quinidine on the elimination of digoxin can be reduced by the presence of potent enzyme-inducing agents such as pentobarbitone:

A woman in her nineties who had been taking 100 mg pentobarbitone at bedtime for at least a year developed paroxysmal atrial fibrillation and was treated with 0·25 mg digoxin daily and 200 mg quinidine sulphate every 6 h. Because her serum quinidine levels remained consistently below the therapeutic range, the quinidine half-life was measured and found to be unusually short (1·6 h compared with the normal 10). Within about 3 weeks of withdrawing the pentobarbitone, the half-life of the quinidine was found to have lengthened to 6·1 h, the quinidine and digoxin levels were elevated, and the patient showed signs of digoxin toxicity.[1]

Mechanism

It would seem that in the presence of the pentobarbitone (a known and potent liver enzyme-inducing agent) the serum levels of quinidine were kept unusually low and its effects on the elimination of digoxin were comparatively small.

As a result the quinidine/digoxin interaction was contained. Once the enzyme-inducing agent was withdrawn, the serum levels of the quinidine climbed and the quinidine/digoxin interaction (see p. 308), which results in elevated digoxin levels, was able to manifest itself fully.

Importance and management

This interaction, though unusual, is clearly of importance. The precipitation of the quinidine–digoxin interaction by the withdrawal of the pentobarbitone emphasizes the need to be alert to the possible consequences of withdrawing potent enzyme-inducing agents from patients who continue to take other drugs whose metabolism may have been affected by concurrent therapy. This is particularly true of drugs like digoxin where the maintenance of serum levels within a fairly narrow range is important.

Reference

1 Chapron D J, Mumford D and Pitegoff G J. Apparent quinidine-induced digoxin toxicity after withdrawal of pentobarbital. A case of sequential drug interactions. *Arch Int Med* (1979) **139**, 363.

Digitalis glycosides + rauwolfia alkaloids

Summary

Concurrent use of digitalis and the rauwolfia alkaloids is not uncommon but the incidence of arrhythmias appears to be increased, particularly in those with atrial fibrillation. Excessive bradycardia and hypotension have also been described.

Interaction

Concurrent use of these two groups of drugs is by no means uncommon, but (a) there is evidence that the incidence of cardiac arrhythmias may be increased; and (b) excessive bradycardia and syncope have also been described.

(a) Increased cardiac arrhythmias

A report describes 3 patients treated with digoxin and either reserpine or whole root *Rauwolfia serpentina* who subsequently developed various arrhythmias: atrial tachycardia with 4:1 Wenckebach irregular block; ventricular bigeminy and tachycardia; and atrial fibrillation. A large number of other patients had received both drugs with impunity.[1]

A comparative study on a group of patients, all of whom were taking rauwolfia alkaloids, showed that the incidence of premature ventricular systoles was roughly doubled amongst those concurrently taking digitalis: 7 out of 15 taking both drugs showed arrhythmias compared with only 3 out of 15 on rauwolfia alone.[2]

The sensitivity of the myocardium to digitalis was tested on 15 patients with congestive heart failure using acetyl strophanthidin in the presence and absence of reserpine. In 5 of the 9 patients with atrial fibrillation it was found that reserpine reduced the tolerated dose of strophanthidin. Eight out of the 9 exhibited advanced toxic rhythms during acute digitalization compared with only 1 patient who responded in this way in the absence of reserpine.[3]

(b) Excessive bradycardia and syncope

A man on digoxin (0·25 and 0·375 mg on alternative days) and reserpine (0·25 mg daily) developed a very slow heart rate, sinus bradycardia and carotid sinus supersensitivity and was admitted to hospital because of syncope. The problem remitted when reserpine was withdrawn.[4]

Mechanism

Not fully understood. A possible explanation is that the rauwolfia alkaloids deplete the sympathetic nerve supply (i.e., accelerator) to the heart of its neurotransmitter which allows the parasympathetic or vagal supply (i.e., heart slowing) to have full rein. In the presence of digitalis which also causes heart slowing, the total bradycardia could become excessive. In this situation the rate could be so slow that ectopic foci which would normally be swamped by a faster, more normal beat, begin to 'fire', leading to the development of arrhythmias. The syncope described in the single case[4] could be accounted for in a similar way; that is a combination of bradycardia in association with the other hypotensive effects of reserpine elsewhere in the cardiovascular system.

Importance and management

Concurrent treatment with digitalis and the rauwolfia alkaloids is not unusual. One group of authors, despite having described adverse reactions in 3 patients given these two groups of drugs, conclude by saying that 'time has proven the safety of the combination'.[1] However, they continue with the proviso that '... the development of arrhythmias must be anticipated and appropriate steps taken at their appearance ...'. One might also add that there appears to be a particular risk of arrhythmias in patients with atrial fibrillation (8 out of 9 in one of the reports cited[3]), and with digitalized patients who are given reserpine parenterally because of the sudden release of catecholamines which takes place.[4] Excessive bradycardia with syncope has also been described.[4] Some caution is therefore advisable if these drugs are given together.

References

1 Dick H L H, McCawley E L and Fisher W A. Reserpine–digitalis toxicity. *Arch Intern Med* (1962) **109**, 49.
2 Schreader C J and Etzl M M. Premature ventricular contractions due to rauwolfia therapy. *J Amer Med Ass* (1956) **162**, 1256.
3 Lown B, Ehrlich L, Lipschultz B and Blake J. Effect of digitalis in patients receiving reserpine. *Circulation* (1961) **24**, 1185.
4 Bigger J T and Strauss H C. Digitalis toxicity: drug interactions prompting toxicity and the management of toxicity. *Seminars in Drug Treatment* (1972) **2**, 147

Digitalis glycosides + rifampicin

Summary

The serum levels of digitoxin can be halved by the concurrent use of rifampicin. Digoxin is probably little affected, but this requires confirmation

Interaction

A comparative study on tuberculous patients and normal subjects given 0·1 mg digitoxin daily showed that the serum digitoxin levels of the patients taking rifampicin were approximately 50% of those not on rifampicin (18·4 ng/ml compared with 39·1 ng/ml). The half-life of digitoxin was found to be reduced by the presence of the rifampcin from 8·2 to 4·5 days.[1]

Another study in man reported a reduction in digitoxin half-life from 12 to 3 days due to rifampicin,[2] and a case report describes a patient whose serum digitoxin levels were considerably more than halved when rifampicin was given.[3]

Mechanism

It seems probable that rifampicin, a recognized and potent liver enzyme-inducing agent, increases the metabolism and loss of the digitoxin from the body.

Importance and management

This appears to be an established interaction. Patients should be checked for under-digitalization during concurrent therapy with rifampicin and digitoxin. Whether digoxin is similarly affected is uncertain, but it seems unlikely because digoxin is normally not metabolized to any great extent.

References

1 Peters U, Hausmen T-U and Gross-Brockhoff F. Einfluss von Tuberkulostatika auf die Pharmakokinetik des Digitoxins. *Deut Med Wochenschr* (1974) 99, 2381.
2 Zilly W, Breimer D D and Richter E. Pharmacokinetic interactions with rifampicin. *Clin Pharmacokinetics* (1977) 2, 61.
3 Boman G, Eliasson K and Odarcederlöf I. Acute cardiac failure during treatment with digoxin—an interaction with rifampicin. *Br J Clin Pharmacol* (1980) 10, 89.

Digitalis glycosides + spironolactone

Summary

There is evidence that serum digoxin levels may possibly be raised by the use of spironolactone. Serum digitoxin levels may also be altered. The importance of these changes is not known for certain.

Interaction

(a) Digoxin + spironolactone

Eight patients were given single 0·1 mg intravenous doses of tritiated digoxin before and after 15 days' treatment with 150 mg spironolactone daily. The total body clearance of digoxin'. . . remained unaltered . . . ' although the figures quoted were 109 ± 39 ml/min before spironolactone, and 90 ± 40 ml/min afterwards.[1]

Four patients with arteriosclerotic disease and 4 normal subjects were given single 0·75 mg intravenous doses of digoxin before and after 5 days' treatment with 200 mg spironolactone daily. The total clearance of digoxin was reduced by about 25%.[2]

(b) Digitoxin + spironolactone

A study in 6 normal subjects who had received 0·1 or 0·15 mg digitoxin daily for 30 days showed that when they were then treated with 300 mg spironolactone daily the mean half-life of the digitoxin was increased from 141 to 192 h.[5]

Another study showed that the concurrent use of 400 mg spironolactone and digitoxin resulted in a 20% reduction in the volume of distribution of the digitoxin. Changes in the urinary excretion of digitoxin and its metabolites also occurred. The half-life of the tritiated digitoxin used was reduced from 256 to 204 h by the spironolactone.[4]

Spironolactone has been shown to reduce digitoxin poisoning in rats.[6]

Mechanism

Uncertain. Spironolactone can inhibit the renal tubular excretion of digoxin.[3] Digoxin is cleared from the body by the liver and kidneys, elimination by the kidneys being both by glomerular filtration and tubular secretion. With normal doses of digoxin the glomerular filtration is almost at capacity so that the inhibition by spironolactone of the tubular secretion may have an effect on the total clearance. There is also evidence that spironolactone affects both the metabolism and the urinary excretion of digitoxin.[4]

Importance and management

The available evidence does not give a clear picture of the clinical importance of these interactions. More study is needed. However, the effects of concurrent use should be monitored to ensure that serum digitalis levels are not altered undesirably.

References

1 Ohnhaus E E and Masson A. The influence of therapeutic doses of spironolactone on the liver microsomal enzyme system and digoxin elimination in man. *Br J clin Pharmac* (1977) **15**, 639.
2 Waldorff S, Andersen J D, Heeboll–Nielsen N, Nielsen O G, Moltke E and Steiness E. Spironolactone-induced changes in digoxin kinetics. *Clin Pharmacol Ther* (1978) **24**, 162.
3 Steiness E. Renal tubular secretion of digoxin circulation (1974) **50**, 103.
4 Wirth K E, Frölich J C, Hollifield J W, Falkner F C, Sweetman B S, and Oates J A. Metabolism of digitoxin in man and its modification by spironolactone. *Europ J clin Pharmacol* (1976) **9**, 345.
5 Carruthers S G and Dujovne C A. Cholestyramine and spironolactone and their combination in digitoxin elimination. *Clin Pharmacol Ther* (1980) **27**, 184.
6 Solymoss B, Toth S, Varga S and Selye H. Protection by spironolactone and oxandrolone against chronic digitoxin or indomethacin intoxication. *Toxicol Appl Pharmacol* (1971) **18**, 586.

Digitalis glycosides + sodium diatrizoate

Summary

The results of animal studies suggest that patients on digitalis glycosides may have an increased risk of serious reactions to sodium diatrizoate in intravenous urography.

Interaction, mechanism, importance and management

Studies in mice with strophanthin-K and sodium diatrizoate indicate that a synergistic increase in their lethality may occur during concurrent use, possibly related to the diatrizoate ion. The direct relevance of this to man is uncertain and much more study is required, but the authors of the report consider that patients on cardiac glycosides should be considered to have a higher than normal risk of serious reactions to intravenous injections of contrast media.[1]

Reference

1 Fischer H W, Morris T W, King A N and Harnish P P. Deleterious synergism of a cardiac glycoside and sodium diatrizoate. *Invest Radiol* (1978) **13**, 340.

Digitalis glycosides + sulphasalazine

Summary

Serum levels of digoxin can be reduced by up to 50% by the concurrent use of sulphasalazine. Whether digitoxin levels are similarly affected is not known.

Interaction

The observation that a patient under treatment with 8 g sulphasalazine daily had low serum digoxin levels prompted a cross-over study in 10 normal subjects who were given 0·5 mg digoxin alone, and later after 6 days' treatment with sulphasalazine.

Some of the subjects were given only 2 g sulphasalazine daily, whereas others were taking up to 6 g a day. The absorption of the digoxin was found to be reduced, varying between the subjects from 50% to virtually nothing, depending upon the dosage of sulphasalazine used.[1]

Mechanism

Not understood.

Importance and management

The documentation is limited but the interaction appears to be established. It has been suggested that serum digoxin levels should certainly be monitored during concurrent use.[1] In the one patient examined, separating the times of administration was not found to be useful. Whether digitoxin might prove to be less affected is not known.

Reference

1 Juhl R P, Summers R W, Guillory J K, Blaug S M, Cheng F H and Brown D. Effect of sulfasalazine on digoxin biovailability. *Clin Pharmacol Ther* (1976) **20**, 387.

Digitalis glycosides + verapamil

Summary

Serum levels of digoxin can be markedly raised by the concurrent use of verapamil.

Interaction, mechanism, importance and management

A very brief report states that in the course of treating 41 patients over a 5-year period with verapamil, 240 mg daily, it was observed that the serum levels of digoxin were increased in all but two of the patients from 0·96 to 1·63 ng/ml. There was no mention of digitalis intoxication.[1] The mechanism of this interaction is not understood. Information on this interaction seems to be limited to this one report, but it would appear to be important. More study is needed. An isolated case of asystole in a man taking digoxin who was given verapamil intravenously has also been described.[2]

References

1 Klein H O, Lang R, Segni E D and Kaplinsky E. Verapamil-digoxin interaction. *New Eng J Med* (1980) **303**, 160.
2 Kounis N G. Asystole after verapamil and digoxin. *Brit J Clin Prac* (1980) **34**, 57.

CHAPTER 14. HYPOGLYCAEMIC AGENT INTERACTIONS

The hypoglycaemic agents are used to control diabetes mellitus, a disease in which there is partial or total failure of the beta-cells within the pancreas to secrete into the circulation enough of the hormone insulin, in some cases there being evidence to show that the disease results from the presence of factors which oppose the activity of insulin.

With insufficient insulin, the body tissues are unable to take up and utilize the glucose which is in circulation in the blood. Because of this, glucose (derived from the digestion of food and elsewhere) which would normally be removed and stored in the liver and tissues throughout the body, accumulates and boosts the glucose in the blood to such grossly elevated proportions that the kidney is unable to cope with such a load and glucose appears in the urine. Raised blood sugar levels (hyperglycaemia) with glucose and ketone bodies in the urine (glycosuria and ketonuria) are among the manifestations of this serious disturbance in the metabolic chemistry of the body which, if untreated, can lead on to the development of diabetic coma and death.

There are two main types of diabetes: one is the juvenile type which, as its name implies, develops early in life and occurs when the ability of the pancreas suddenly, and often almost totally, fails to produce insulin. This type of diabetes is sometimes referred to as being 'labile' or 'brittle' because it is often quite difficult to achieve and maintain a stable metabolic balance. The other form of diabetes is the maturity-onset type and is most often seen in those over 40. This occurs when the pancreas gradually loses the ability to produce insulin so that the disease develops over a period of months or years. The maturity-onset diabetes is often associated with being over-weight and this type of diabetes can very often be quite satisfactorily controlled without the use of hypoglycaemic agents of any kind by losing weight and adhering to an appropriate diet. In contrast, juvenile diabetes always calls for dietary control and a hypoglycaemic agent.

The mode of action of the hypoglycaemic agents

Insulin

Insulin extracted from the pancreatic tissue of pigs and cattle is so similar to human insulin that it can be used in replacement therapy. It is administered, not by mouth, but by injection in order to bypass the enzymes of the gut which would digest and destroy it like any other protein. Although animal insulins like these are 'foreign' proteins, most diabetics do not produce a significant amount of antibodies against them even after many years of daily use. There are now very many formulations of insulin, some of them designed to delay absorption from the subcutaneous or intramuscular tissue into which the injection is made, so that repeated daily injections can be avoided, but all of them sooner or later release insulin into the circulation where it acts to replace or top-up the insulin from the human pancreas.

Sulphonylurea and biguanide oral hypoglycaemic agents

The sulphonylurea and other sulphonamide-related compounds such as tolbutamide, chlorpropamide and glymidine (an extensive list is shown in Table 14.1) were the first synthetic compounds used in medicine as hypoglycaemic agents and they have the obvious advantage of being taken by mouth. They act by stimulating the remaining functional beta-cells of the pancreas to grow and secret insulin which, with a restricted diet, controls the blood sugar levels and permits a normal metabolism to occur. Clearly they can only be effective in those diabetics whose pancreas still has the

Table 14.1. Oral hypoglycaemic agents

Approved or generic name	Proprietary names
Sulphonylureas	
Acetohexamide	*Dimelor, Dymelor, Ordimel*
Carbutamide	*Invenol, Nadisan*
Chlorpropamide	*Chloromid, Chloronase, Diabetal, Diabetoral, Diabinese, Diabines, Melitase, Novopropamide, Stabinol*
Glibenclamide (glyburide)	*Daonil, Diabeta, Euglucon*
Glibornuride	*Glutril, Gluborid*
Gliclazide	*Diamicron*
Glipentide	—
Glipzide	*Glibenese, Mindiab, Minidiab, Minodiab*
Gliquidone	*Glurenorm*
Glisoxepide	*Pro-diaban*
Glybuzole	*Gludiase*
Glycopyramide	*Deamelin-S*
Glycylamide	*Diaboral(E)*
Glydanile sodium	—
Metahexamide	*Isodiane*
Tolazamide	*Diabewas, Norglycin, Tolanase, Tolinase, Tolisan*
Tolbutamide	*Arcosal, Artosin, Chembutamide, Dolipol, Insalange-D, Ipoglicone, Mellitol, Mobenol, Neo-Dibetic, Novobutamide, Nigloid, Oramide, Oribetic, Orinase, Pramidex, Rastinon, Westcotol*
Sulfonamide-related compounds	
Gliflumide	—
Glymidine (glycodiazine)	*Glyconormal, Gondafon, Lycanol, Redul*
Biguanides	
Buformin	*Silubin, Sindiatal*
Metformin	*Diabex SR, Diabexyl, Diguanil, Glucophage, Hanrymellin, Metiguanide, Obin*
Phenformin	*DBI, DB Retard, Dibein, Dibotin, Dipar, Glucopostin, Insoral (also used for carbutamide) Meltrol*

capacity to produce some insulin, so that they are only of use in maturity-onset diabetes.

The mode of action of the other types of synthetic oral hypoglycaemic agent, the biguanides such as metformin and phenformin, is obscure but they do not stimulate the pancreas like the sulphonylureas to release insulin, but appear to facilitate the uptake and utilization of glucose by the cells. Their use is restricted to maturity-onset diabetes because they are not effective unless insulin, either from the pancreas or by injection, is also available. The biguanides are currently somewhat under a cloud because they appear to be associated with the occurrence of lactic acidosis.

Other oral hypoglycaemic agents

Outside orthodox Western medicine, there are herbal preparations which are used in the treatment of diabetes and which appear to have hypoglycaemic properties when taken orally. Blueberries were used traditionally by the Alpine peasants; bitter gourd or karela (*Momordica charantia*) is an established part of the herbal treatment in the Indian subcontinent and elsewhere; and the Chinese herbals also contain remedies for diabetes. The mode of action of all of these and their efficacy await formal clinical evaluation.

Interactions

The commonest interactions are those which result in a rise or a fall in blood glucose levels, thereby disturbing the control of diabetes. A number of examples are to be found in this chapter. Other interactions where the hypoglycaemic is the affecting agent are described elsewhere. A full listing is to be found in the Index.

Hypoglycaemic agents + alcohol

For the sake of clarity these interactions have been subdivided into two sections, (a) Insulin + Alcohol, and (b) Oral Hypoglycaemic Agents + Alcohol, but to obtain the full picture the comments and data in the 'Summary' and 'Importance and Management' subheadings should be read in conjunction.

(a) INSULIN + ALCOHOL

Summary
Diabetics should either avoid alcohol altogether or only drink with great moderation because alcohol can impair the normal homoeostatic response to hypoglycaemia. Under the influence of alcohol they may become careless with their food and insulin administration, and less able to recognize the signs of hypoglycaemia. Some drinks (beer being one) contain sugar.

Interaction

Alcohol can augment the glucose-lowering actions of insulin, particularly in those with an inadequate diet. A reduced glucose tolerance has also been seen.

> Over a 3-year period 5 insulin-dependent diabetics were hospitalized with severe hypoglycaemia after going on the binge. Two of them died without recovery from the initial coma, and the other 3 suffered permanent damage to the nervous system. A subsequent study on 6 volunteers given standard insulin tolerance tests showed that the extent of the insulin-induced hypoglycaemia was not affected by alcohol but the return to normal was prolonged.[1]

Mechanism

The normal homoeostatic response to hypoglycaemia is the conversion of glycogen within the liver to glucose and its release into the circulation. If the liver glycogen stores are low (this is likely in alcoholics and others who neglect their diet) the liver turns to the formation of new glucose from amino acids (neoglucogenesis). This response is inhibited by the presence of alcohol so that the hypoglycaemia is inadequately compensated, and may progress into a full-scale coma.[1]

Importance and management

Alcohol is not totally contraindicated in diabetic patients but there are very good reasons why they should only drink very moderately.

Patients befuddled with drink may become casual and irresponsible with their diet or may fail to eat properly; careless with the timing and administration of their insulin, giving themselves too much, or too little, and possibly in an unhygienic manner; less able to recognize and respond to the signs of hypoglycaemia. Alcohol also interferes with the homoeostatic response to hypoglycaemia and, in diabetics with an inadequate diet, this makes them particularly vulnerable to the hypoglycaemic actions of alcohol. A drunken stupor can also confuse the recognition and diagnosis of a hypoglycaemic coma if it occurs. In addition beer and some other drinks contain some sugar so that the maintenance of a good dietary balance may be more difficult.

Reference

1 Arky R A, Veverbrandts E and Abramson E A. Irreversible hypoglycaemia. *J Amer med Ass* (1968) **206**, 575.

(b) ORAL HYPOGLYCAEMIC AGENTS + ALCOHOL

Summary

In addition to the points outlined under 'Insulin + Alcohol', disulfiram-like reactions not infrequently occur in patients taking chlorpropamide who drink. This reaction is rare with the other sulphonylureas. The half-life of tolbutamide is reduced in alcoholic subjects. Alcohol may precipitate lactic acidosis in phenformin-treated patients.

Interactions

Sulphonylureas + alcohol

> About one third of those on chlorpropamide who drink alcohol, even in quite small amounts, experience a disulfiram-like reaction within 5–20 min, usually lasting 30–60 min but occasionally for much longer. A warm, tingling, or burning sensation affects the face and sometimes the neck and arms as well. Lightheadedness, headache, palpitations and breathlessness also occur frequently.[1] Vomiting has also been described.[8]

This reaction has been described in numerous other reports involving large numbers of patients on chlorpropamide[3,5-7] but very much more rarely with glipizide,[1] glibenclamide,[1,9] or tolbutamide.[4,6,20] Flushing and a decreased tolerance to alcohol has also been described in one patient on tolazamide.[2]

A comparative study in man showed that the mean half-life of tolbutamide in alcoholic subjects was reduced by about one third (from 384 to 232 min).[10]

Biguanides + alcohol

A well-controlled comparative study on 5 ketosis-resistant maturity-onset diabetics taking 50–100 mg phenformin daily and given either glucose alone, alcohol alone or glucose with alcohol showed that in the presence of the alcohol (equivalent to about 3 oz whisky) their blood lactate and lactate–pyruvate levels were markedly raised. Two of them attained blood lactate levels of more than 50 mg%. One of these two had previously described nausea, weakness and malaise while taking phenformin and alcohol.[13]

The ingestion of alcohol is described in other reports as having preceded the onset of phenformin-induced lactic acidosis[14–16,18] or a rise in blood lactate levels.[17]

> In a study on 33 diabetics treated with 75–150 mg of phenformin daily 10 of them are reported to have lost the desire for alcohol and several of them complained of a metallic taste.[19]

Mechanisms

The disulfiram-like reaction with the sulphony-lureas is not understood. It appears to be genetically determined and is particularly associated with non insulin dependent diabetics,[1] but it is not accompanied by the significant rises in blood acetaldehyde levels which have been described with disulfiram.[5] One suggestion is that it is an exaggeration of the normal response of small blood vessels to ethyl alcohol.[5] Another is that it results from some change in the metabolism of 5-hydroxytryptamine.[21]

The decreased half-life of tolbutamide in alcoholic patients would appear to be due to the inducing effects of alcohol on the liver microsomal enzymes.[10–12]

The raised blood lactate levels seen during the concurrent use of alcohol and phenformin is also not understood. However, the metabolic conversion of alcohol to acetaldehyde, and of lactate to pyruvic acid, both require the reduction of NAD to NADH, so it is tempting to postulate that the presence of alcohol (coupled with its general inhibitory actions on the liver) may depress the lactate→pyruvate reaction and result in the accumulation of lactic acid.[13]

Importance and management

The general principles outlined under this sub-heading in 'Insulin + Alcohol' also apply to the oral hypoglycaemic agents with the following additional points applicable to particular oral hypoglycaemic agents.

Sulphonylureas

The disulfiram-like reaction, first seen in 1956, is extremely well documented and affects a large number of those on chlorpropamide (the incidence is variously stated to be between 13%[7] and 33%[5]). It is relatively rare with other sulphonylureas so that a wide range of non-interacting alternatives is available. Alcoholic patients given tolbutamide (possibly other sulphonylureas as well) may require above-average doses because of the increased rate of clearance of the hypoglycaemic agent.

Biguanides

Although some patients on biguanides continue to drink there is the possibility that it may precipitate lactic acidosis. Heavy drinking should certainly be avoided. A metallic taste and an increased intolerance to alcohol may act as deterrents.

References

1 Leslie R D G and Pyke D A. Chlorpropamide–alcohol flushing: a dominantly inherited trait associated with diabetes. Br Med J (1978) 2, 1519.
2 McKendry J B R and Gfeller K F. Clinical experience with the oral antidiabetic compound, tolazamide. Canad med Ass J (1967) 96, 531.
3 Klink D D, Fritz R D and Franke G H. Disulfiram-like reaction to chlorpropamide (Diabinese). Wisconsin Med J (1969) 68, 134.
4 Dolger H. Experience with the tolbutamide treatment of 500 cases of diabetes on an ambulatory basis. Ann NY Acad Sci (1957) 71, 275.
5 Fitzgerald M G, Gaddie R, Malins J M and O'Sullivan D J. Alcohol sensitivity in diabetics receiving chlorpropamide. Diabetes (1962) 11, 40.
6 Signorelli S. Tolerance for alcohol in patients on chlorpropamide. Ann NY Acad Sci (1959) 74, 900.
7 Daeppen J P, Hofstetter J R, Curchod B and Saudan Y. Traitment oral du diabete par un nouvel hypoglycémiant, le P 607 ou Diabinese. Schweiz med Woch (1959) 89, 817.
8 Canessa I, Valiente S and Mella I. Clinical evaluation of chlorpropamide in diabetes mellitus. Ann NY Acad Sci (1959) 74, 752.
9 Stowers J M. Alcohol and glibenclamide. Br Med J (1971) 3, 533.
10 Carulli N, Manenti F, Gallo M and Salvioli G F. Alcohol–drugs interaction in man: alcohol and tolbutamide. Europ J clin Invest (1971) 1, 421.
11 Kater R M H, Roggin G, Tobon F, Zieve P and Iber F L. Increased rate of clearance of drugs from the circulation of alcoholics. Amer J Med Sci (1969) 258, 35.
12 Kater R M H, Tobon F and Iber F L. Increased rate of tolbutamide metabolism in alcoholic patients. J Amer Med Ass (1969) 207, 363.
13 Johnson H K and Waterhouse C. Relationship of alcohol and hyperlactatemia in diabetic subjects treated with phenformin. Am J Med (1968) 45, 98.
14 Davidson M B, Bozarth W R, Challoner D R and Goodner C J. Phenformin hypoglycemia and lactic acidosis. Report of an attempted suicide. New Eng J med (1966) 275, 886.
15 Gottlieb A, Duberstein J and Geller A. Phenformin acidosis. New Eng J Med (1962) 267, 806.
16 Maclachlan M J and Rodman G P. Effects of food, fast and alcohol on serum uric acid and acute attacks of gout. Am J. Med (1967) 42, 38.
17 Roštlapil J, Zelenka K and Křišťan M. Nebezpečí užití alkoholu při léčení biguanidy. Vnitřní Lékařstiví (1979) 25, 374.
18 Schaffalitzky de Muckadell O B, Køster A and Jensen S L. Fenformin–alkohol-interaktion. Ugeskr Laeg (1973) 135, 925.
19 Lisboa P E, Branco-Castel N and Sá Marques M M. Anorexia for alcohol: a side-effect of phenethylbiguanide. Lancet (1961) i, 678.
20 Büttner H. Athanolunverträglichkeit beim Menschen nach Sulfonylharnstoffen. Dtsch Arch Klin Med (1961) 207, 1.
21 Podgainy H and Bressler R. Biochemical basis of sulphony-lurea-induced antabuse syndrome. Diabetes (1968) 17, 678.

Hypoglycaemic agents + allopurinol

Summary

One study describes an increase in the half-life of chlorpropamide during therapy with allopurinol. An enhanced hypoglycaemic response would seem possible.

Interaction

A brief report describes 7 patients given allopurinol and chlorpropamide concurrently. The half-life of chlorpropamide in 1 patient with gout but normal renal function exceeded 200 h (normal 36 h) after 10 days' treatment with allopurinol. In 2 others, the half-life was extended to 44 and 55 h. The other 3 patients were given allopurinol for only 1 or 2 days and the half-life of chloropamide remained unaltered.[1]

Mechanism

Not understood. It has been suggested that it possibly involves some competition for renal tubular mechanisms.[1]

Importance and management

Information is limited to this single report. The incidence is not known. Prescribers should be alert to the possibility of an increase in the activity of chlorpropamide leading to excessive hypoglycaemia in patients treated with both drugs. Nothing seems to have been documented about allopurinol and other hypoglycaemic agents.

Reference

1 Petitpierre B, Perrin L, Rudhardt M, Herrera A and Fabre J. Behaviour of chlorpropamide in renal insufficiency and under the effects of associated drug therapy. *Int J clin Pharmacol* (1972) **6**, 120.

Hypoglycaemic agents + amiloride

Summary

There is some limited evidence that diabetic patients may possibly be predisposed to the development of amiloride-induced hyperkalaemia.

Interaction, mechanism, importance and management

Two cases of hyperkalaemia (6·5 mEq/l or more) occurred in 4 hypertensive diabetic patients treated with amiloride. One of them died. It is suggested that diabetics may have some electrolyte abnormality which predisposes them to this condition during the use of potassium-retaining diuretics. The manufacturers of *Moduretic* (amiloride with hydrochlorothiazide)—MSD—issued a warning that renal status should be determined before giving amiloride, and that the diuretic should be discontinued before giving glucose tolerance tests. Strictly speaking this is not an interaction but an adverse response to amiloride in patients who need hypoglycaemic agents.

Reference

1 McNay J and Oran E. Possible predisposition of diabetic patients to hyperkalaemia following administration of a potassium-retaining diuretic, Amiloride (MK 870). *Metabolism* (1970) **19**, 58.

Hypoglycaemic agents + anabolic steroids

Summary

Nandrolone, methandienone (methandrostenolone) and testosterone may reduce the dosage requirements of the hypoglycaemic agents in some patients. Whether other anabolic steroids behave similarly is uncertain.

Interaction

Some, but not all, anabolic steroids can reduce blood sugar levels and enhance the blood sugar lowering effects of conventional hypoglycaemic agents in diabetic patients.

> In a study on 54 diabetic patients who were under treatment with nandrolone phenpropionate or decanoate, it was found that there was an average reduction in insulin requirements of 40% (range 10–90%).[1]

Other reports similarly describe this response with insulin and nandrolone,[2,3] tolbutamide with methandienone (methandrostenolone),[4] and insulin with testosterone.[5,6]

Mechanism

Uncertain.

Importance and management

An established interaction, but the overall picture is far from complete because not all the steroids have been thoroughly investigated and it appears that they do not all behave identically. The situation is also complicated by the fact that steroid-induced changes in blood sugar levels may occur in poorly muscled, emaciated patients, but not in well-muscled individuals. In general some reduction in the hypoglycaemic agent dosage requirements should be looked for, but it may not be realized in all cases. Interactions involving methandienon (methandrostenolone), nandrolone and testosterone have been documented, but the response with stanozolol[7] is uncertain.

References

1 Houtsmuller A J. The therapeutic applications of anabolic steroids in ophthalmology biochemical results. *Acta Endocrinol* (1961) **39**, (suppl 63), 154.
2 Dardenne U. The therapeutic applications of anabolic steroids in ophthalmology. *Acta Endocrinol* (1961) **39** (suppl 63), 143.
3 Weissel W. Anabolic steroid in malignant or complicated diabetes mellitus. *Wien Klin Wchnschr* (1962) **74**, 234.
4 Landon J, Wynn V, Samols E and Bilkus D. The effect of anabolic steroids on blood sugar and plasma insulin levels in man. *Metabolism* (1963) **12**, 924.
5 Sirek O V and Best C H. The protein anabolic effect of testosterone. *Endocrinology* (1953) **52**, 390.
6 Talaat M, Habib Y A and Habib M. The effect of testosterone on the carbohydrate metabolism of normal subjects. *Arch Int Pharmacodyn* (1957) **3**, 215.
7 Pergola F. Stanozolol, a new anabolic agent. Study on 200 cases. *Prensa méd argent* (1962) **49**, 274.

Hypoglycaemic agents + anaesthetics

Summary

Halothane and thiopentone–nitrous oxide appear to have relatively unimportant effects on blood sugar and insulin levels. A change from oral antidiabetic therapy to insulin may be advisable if the surgical procedures are very extensive.

Interaction

Table 14.2 (p. 321) summarizes the findings of ten studies carried out on a large number of patients.

Mechanism

Extremely complex and by no means fully understood.

Importance and management

Among the work summarized in the table, halothane[2] or nitrous oxide–thiopentone[1] have been recommended as anaesthetics for diabetics because they neither increase the blood sugar, or growth hormone levels significantly nor do they decrease insulin levels. A change from oral hypoglycaemics to insulin prior to anaesthesia has been a not uncommon practice, but it would seem that there is now an increasing tendency to leave the patient's antidiabetic treatment unchanged[9,10] although one recommendation is that those undergoing extensive and prolonged procedures should be switched to insulin.[11]

References

1 Yoshimura N, Kodama K and Yoshitake J. Carbohydrate metabolism and insulin release during ether and halothane anaesthesia. *Br J Anaesth* (1971) **43**, 1022.
2 Oyama T and Takasawa T. Effect of halothane anaesthesia and surgery on human growth hormone and insulin levels in plasma. *Br J Anaesth* (1971) **43**, 573.
3 Merin R G, Samuelson P N and Schalch D S. Major inhalation anaesthesics and carbohydrate metabolism. *Anaesth Analg* (Curr Res L971) **50**, 625.
4 Allison S P, Tomlin P J and Chamberlain M J. Some effects of anaesthesia and surgery on carbohydrate and fat metabolism. *Br J Anaesth* (1969) **41**, 588.
5 Oyama T, Takiguchi M and Kudo T. Metabolic effects of anaesthesia: effect of thiopentone–nitrous oxide anaesthesia on human growth hormone and insulin levels in plasma. *Can Anaesth Soc J* (1971) **18**, 442.

Table 14.2. The effects of anaesthetics on blood sugar and insulin levels.

Anaesthetic	Patients	Glucose load	Insulin levels (μU/ml)		Glucose levels (mg%)		References
			Before	After	Before	After	
Ether-N$_2$O	10	—	16	25 at 30' 28 at 60'	83	118 at 60'	1
Ether-N$_2$O	19	—	38	30 at 30' 30 at 45'	85	124 at 45'	7
Halothane-N$_2$O	8	—	17	14 at 60'	80	88 at 60'	1
Halothan-N$_2$O	20	—	11	10 at 45'	83	93 at 45'	2
Halothane-N$_2$O	5	—	16	15 at 30'	78	102 at 30'	3
Halothane-N$_2$O	4	—	18	14 at 20'	84	94 at 20'	4
Thiopentone-N$_2$O	20	√	12	12 at 45'	92	135 at 45'	5
Methoxyflurane-N$_2$O	5	—	8	8 at 30'	84	103 at 30'	3
Methoxyflurane-N$_2$O	20	—	23	19 at 45'	99	108 at 45'	8
Droperidol-N$_2$O	25	√	16	24 at 45'	102	169 at 30'	6

After Hagan and Kendall.[9]

6 Oyama T and Takiguchi M. Effects of neuroleptanaesthesia on plasma levels of growth hormone and insulin. *Br J Anaesth* (1970) **42**, 1105.

7 Oyama T and Takasawa T. Effects of diethyl ether anaesthesia and surgery on carbohydrate and fat metabolism in man. *Can Anaesth Soc J* (1971) **18**, 51.

8 Oyama T and Takasawa J. Effect of methoxyflurane anaesthesia and surgery on human growth hormone and insulin levels in plasma. *Can Anaesth Soc J* (1970) **17**, 347.

9 Hagan J J and Kendall C H G. Insulin and oral antidiabetic drugs. *Int Anesthesiol Clinics* (1975) **13**, 127.

10 Fletcher J, Langman M J S and Kelloch T D. Effects of surgery on blood sugar levels in diabetes mellitus. *Lancet* (1965) **ii**, 52.

11 Stehling L. Clinical anaesthesia: Pharmacology of Adjuvant Drugs. *Philadelphia* (1973) vol. 10, p. 239.

Hypoglycaemic agents + anticoagulants

Summary
The hypoglycaemic effects of some sulphonylureas are enhanced by some oral anticoagulants. Acute hypoglycaemic episodes have been described. The effects of one anticoagulant, dicoumarol, are enhanced by a sulphonylurea. Bleeding has been described. Only a few sulphonylurea/anticoagulant pairs are known to interact, and may only do so in a few patients.

Interaction
Enhanced hypoglycaemia and enhanced hypoprothrombinaemia have been described during concurrent use. A summary of the information documented:

(a) Dicoumarol + tolbutamide
Acute hypoglycaemic episodes; tolbutamide half-life prolonged;[1-4,15,16] haemorrhage, prothrombin times prolonged.[7,8,16] Some studies state that the anticoagulant effects are unaltered.[9,10]

(b) Phenindione or warfarin + tolbutamide
Stated to be no interaction.[3,8]

(c) Dicoumarol + chlorpropamide
Acute hypoglycaemic episode, chlorpropamide half-life prolonged.[5]

(d) Nicoumalone (acenocoumarol) + chlorpropamide
Chlorpropamide half-life prolonged.[6]

(e) Phenprocoumon + glibenclamide, glibornuride, tolbutamide or insulin

Anticoagulant effects unaltered by these hypoglycaemic agents.[10,13] Half-life of glibornuride slightly increased[13] but the pharmacokinetics of glibenclamide[14] and the hypoglycaemic effects of tolbutamide stated to be unaltered.[3] A number of these are case reports on one or two individuals, whereas others are studies undertaken to gain more information about the interactions.

Mechanisms

The enhanced hypoglycaemic effects of tolbutamide and chlorpropamide induced by the dicoumarol are probably a result of the inhibition of the liver microsomal enzymes concerned with their metabolism, resulting in the accumulation of these sulphonylureas in the body, but there is also in-vitro evidence that the anticoagulant may also be able to displace them from their plasma protein binding sites[11] so that two interaction mechanisms may be involved.

The increase in the anticoagulant effects of dicoumarol induced by tolbutamide[6,8] may have been due to a plasma-protein binding interaction,[12] but a pharmacokinetic study has shown that in the case of phenprocoumon several different mutually opposing processes may be involved which may cancel each other out and produce a 'silent' interaction.

Importance and management

The total number of reports on these interactions is relatively small, most of them being listed here. Dicoumarol in combination with tolbutamide is the best documented, and the outcome of concurrent use is potentially serious. Potentially serious interactions may also occur with either dicoumarol or nicoumalone (acenocoumarol) with chlorpropamide. The incidence of none of these interactions is known, but there is enough evidence to indicate that these pairs of potentially interacting drugs should be avoided unless the effects can be closely monitored.

Warfarin and phenprocoumon may prove to be non-interacting alternatives to dicoumarol and nicoumalone (acenocoumarol), and there seem to be no interactions on record with the newer sulphonylureas glibenclamide and glibornuride, but it must be emphasized that the evidence is very limited.

Patients on any anticoagulant with a sulphonylurea should be closely watched for possible interactions. A retrospective search[8] through the records of 57 patients on maintenance therapy with tolbutamide who were subsequently also treated with dicoumarol or warfarin, showed no evidence of adverse interactions, probably because they would have been routinely stabilized on the anticoagulant even if an interaction had been taking place. This indicates that concurrent use can be safe and uneventful.

References

1 Spurney O M, Wolf J W, Devins G S. Protracted tolbutamide-induced hypoglycaemia. *Arch Intern Med* (1965) **115**, 53.
2 Solomon H M and Schrogie J J. Effect of phenyramidol and bishydroxycoumarin on the metabolism of tolbutamide in human subjects. *Metabolism* (1967) **16**, 1029.
3 Kristensen M and Hansen J M. Potentiation of the tolbutamide effect by dicoumarol. *Diabetes* (1967) **16**, 211.
4 Jähnchen E, Meinertz T, Gilfrich H-J and Groth U. Pharmacokinetic analysis of the interaction between dicoumarol and tolbutamide in man. *Europ J Clin Pharmacol* (1976) **10**, 349.
5 Kristensen M and Hansen J M. Accumulation of chlorpropamide caused by dicoumarol. *Acta Med Scand* (1968) **183**, 83.
6 Petitpierre B, Perrin L, Rudhardt M, Herrera A and Fabre J. Behaviour of chlorpropamide in renal insufficiency and under the effect of associated drug therapy. *Int J Clin Pharmacol* (1972) **6**, 120.
7 Chaplin H and Cassell M. Studies on the possible relationship of tolbutamide to dicoumarol in anticoagulant therapy. *Amer J Med Sci* (1958) **235**, 706.
8 Poucher R L and Vecchio T J. Absence of tolbutamide effect on anticoagulant therapy. *J Amer Med Ass* (1966) **197**, 121.
9 Jähnchen E, Gilfrich H J, Groth U and Meinertz T. Pharmacokinetic analysis of the dicumarol–tolbutamide interaction. *Naunyn-Schmiedberg's Arch Pharmacol* (1975) **287**, (Suppl) 88.
10 Heine P, Kewitz H and Wiegboldt K-A. The influence of hypoglycaemic sulphonylureas on the elimination and efficacy of phenprocoumon following a single oral dose in diabetic patients. *Europ J Clin Pharmacol* (1976) **10**, 31.
11 Judis J. Displacement of sulfonylureas from human serum proteins by coumarin derivatives and cortical steroids. *J Pharm Sci* (1973) **62**, 232.
12 Welch R M, Harrison Y E, Conney A H and Burns J J. An experimental model in dogs for studying interactions of drugs with bishydroxycoumarin. *Clin Pharmacol Therap* (1969) **10**, 817.
13 Eckhardt W, Rudolph R, Sauer H, Schuber W R and Undeutsch J. Zur pharmakologischen Interferenz von Glibornurid mit Sulfaphenazol, Phenylbutazon und phenprocoumon beim Menschen. *Arzneimittel-Forsch* (1972) **22**, 2212.
14 Schulz E and Schmidt F H. Über den Einfluss von Sulphaphenazol, Phenylbutazon und Phenprocumarol auf die Elimination von Glibenclamid beim Menschen. *Vern Dtsch Ges Inn Med* (1970) **76**, 435.
15 Fontana G, Addavii F and Peta G. Su di uno casa di coma ipoglicemico in corso di terapia con tolbutamide e dicumarolici. *G Clin Med* (1968) **49**, 849.
16 Schwartz J F. Tolbutamide-induced hypoglycaemia in Parkinson's disease. A case report. *J Amer Med Ass* (1961) **176**, 107.

Hypoglycaemic agents + asparaginase

Summary

Asparaginase can induce diabetes mellitus. Changes in hypoglycaemic agent dosage requirements may occur.

Interaction

Three patients with acute lymphocytic leukaemia developed diabetes mellitus after treatment with asparaginase: two of them 2 and 4 days after a single dose of L-asparaginase, and another patient 2 days after a fourth dose. Plasma insulin was undetectable. The normal insulin response returned in 1 patient after 23 days, whereas the other 2 patients showed a suboptimal response 2 weeks and 9 months afterwards.[1]

In another study, 5 out of a total of 39 patients developed hyperglycaemia and glycosuria after treatment with asparaginase.[2]

Mechanism

Not understood. Suggestions include the inhibition of insulin synthesis, and direct damage to the Islets of Langerhans.[1]

Importance and management

Not strictly speaking an interaction, but it is clear that patients already under treatment for diabetes should be closely observed for changes in their hypoglycaemic agent dosage requirements during asparaginase treatment. It seems not unreasonable to expect that they may possibly be more sensitive to the toxic effects of asparaginase on the pancreas than non-diabetics.

References

1 Gailani S, Nussbaum A, Takao O and Freeman A. Diabetes in patients treated with asparaginase. *Clin Pharmacol Ther* (1971) **12**, 487.
2 Ohnuma T, Holland J F, Freeman A and Sinks L. Biochemical and pharmacological studies with asparaginase in man. *Cancer Res* (1970 **30**, 2297.

Hypoglycaemic agents + aspirin

Summary

Although aspirin can lower blood sugar levels, small analgesic doses have not been reported to cause excessive hypoglycaemia. Some modification of the hypoglycaemic agent dosage might be necessary if large doses are used, but reports of adverse interactions due to aspirin in therapeutic doses appear to be lacking.

Interaction

The effects of the hypoglycaemic agents can be enhanced by concurrent treatment with aspirin.

(a) Insulin + aspirin

Twelve juvenile diabetics being treated with insulin were additionally given either 300 mg aspirin (patients under 60 lb) or 600 mg (patients over 60 lb) four times a day for a week. Blood glucose levels measured on the morning following this period of treatment were reduced by an average of about 15% (from 188 to 159 mg%).[1] No significant changes in insulin requirements were necessary.

Eight patients who had been receiving 12–48 units of insulin zinc suspension daily required no insulin when treated for 2–3 weeks with aspirin in doses large enough to give blood concentrations of 350–450 μg/ml. Six other patients were able to reduce their insulin requirements by approximately a half (from 22–112 units to 10–72 units).[6]

(b) Chlorpropamide + aspirin

The glucose tolerance curve of a patient on chlorpropamide (500 mg daily) was considerably reduced by the concurrent administration of aspirin in doses sufficient to achieve salicylate serum levels of 26 mg%. Blood glucose levels were lowered about two thirds.[2]

Mechanism

Aspirin has inherent hypoglycaemic activity in diabetic patients and in relatively large doses has been used successfully on its own in the treatment of diabetes.[3,5] How it does this is not known for certain, but a likely postulate is that it alters the peripheral utilization of glucose.

In addition, a direct interference takes place with chlorpropamide. A study on a single individual showed that calcium aspirin (2 g three times a day) increased the serum chlorpropamide levels (0·5 g a day) from 10 to 13·5 mg%; simultaneously the serum salicylate levels were increased from 5·4 to 11·7 mg%.[2] This may have been due to some interference with renal tubular excretion, but other in-vitro data show that salicylate displaces the sulphonylureas from protein-binding sites in the serum and increases the amount of unbound (i.e. biologically active) sulphonylurea.[4]

There are therefore a number of ways by which this enhanced hypoglycaemic effect could occur, but whether one or all or even other mechanisms are also responsible is not known.

Importance and management
Information on this interaction is surprisingly sparse, although it appears to be established. Aspirin can be expected to enhance the actions of insulin and the oral hypoglycaemic agents to some extent, but from the data available, supported by the common experience of diabetics, it seems that excessive and undesirable hypoglycaemia is an unlikely event with small doses used for analgesia. However, some caution would be appropriate with larger doses. The reports in the literature seem to be confined to aspirin with either insulin or chlorpropamide. The possibility of an interaction should be borne in mind with any other hypoglycaemic agent, although considering the extremely wide usage of aspirin one might have expected that any generally serious interaction would have come to light by now. Much more work is needed to assess the importance of this interaction.

References
1 Kay R, Athreya B H, Kunzman E E and Baker L. Antipyretics in patients with juvenile diabetes mellitus. *Amer J Dis Child* (1966) **112**, 52.
2 Slowers J M, Constable L W and Hunter R B. A clinical and pharmacological comparison of chlorpropamide and other sulfonylureas. *Ann NY Acad Sci* (1959) **74**, 689.
3 Gilgore S G and Rupp J J. The long-term response of diabetes mellitus to salicylate therapy. Report of a case. *J Amer Med Ass* (1962) **180**, 65.
4 Wishinsky H, Glasser E J and Perkal S. Protein interactions of sulfonylurea compounds. *Diabetes* (1962) **11** (*Suppl*) 18.
5 Reid J, Macdougall A I and Andrews M M. Aspirin and diabetes mellitus. *Br Med J* (1957) **2**, 1071.
6 Reid J and Lightbody T D. The insulin equivalence of salicylate. *Br Med J* (1959) **1**, 897.

Hypoglycaemic agents + barbiturates

Summary
The hypoglycaemic effects of glymidine are reported not to be affected by phenobarbitone.

Interaction, mechanism, importance and management
A study in man showed that the hypoglycaemic effects of the oral hypoglycaemic agent glymidine were unaffected by concurrent treatment with phenobarbitone.[1]

Reference
1 Gerhards E, Kolb K H and Schulz P E. Uber 2-Benzolsulfonyla-mino-5(beta-methoxy-äthoxy)-pyrimidin (Glycodiazin). V. In vitro- und in vivo-Versuche zum Einfluss von Phenyl-äthylbarbitursäure (Luminal) auf en Stoffwechsel und die blutzuckersendkende Wirkung des Glycodiazins. *Naunyn-Schmied. Arch Pharmack u exp Path* (1966) **255**, 200.

Hypoglycaemic agents + benzodiazepines

Summary
An isolated case of hyperglycaemia associated with the use of chlordiazepoxide has been reported.

Interaction

A woman with maturity-onset diabetes of 27 years' duration, stably but imperfectly controlled on 45 u isophane insulin suspension daily, showed a rise in her fasting blood sugar levels from 200 to almost 400 mg/100 ml during a 3-week period while taking 40 mg chlordiazepoxide daily. Four other maturity-onset diabetics, two controlled on diet alone and the other two on tolbutamide, showed no changes in blood sugar levels while taking chlordiazepoxide.[1]

This reaction has also been reported in animal studies.[2] No change in the half-life of chlorpropamide in man is said to have occurred in another study when diazepam was given concurrently.[3]

Mechanism

Not understood.

Importance and management

Only one case of this interaction has been reported. Concurrent use need not be avoided but prescribers should be aware of this interaction.

References

1 Zumoff B and Hellman L. Aggravation of diabetic hyperglycemia by chlordiazepoxide, *J Amer Med Ass* (1977) **237**, 1960.

2 Rutishauser M. Beeinflussung des Kohlenhydrat-stoffwechsels des Rattenhirns durch Psychopharmaka mit sedativer Wirkung. *Arch Exp Pathol* (1963) **245**, 396.

3 Petitpierre B, Perrin L, Rudhardt M, Herrera A and Fabre J. Behaviour of chlorpropamide in renal insufficiency and under the effect of associated drug therapy. *Int J Clin Pharmacol* (1972) **6**, 120.

Hypoglycaemic agents + beta-blocking agents

Summary

Propranolol increases the incidence and severity of hypoglycaemic episodes in some diabetic patients, accompanied by an undesirable rise in blood pressure. The hypoglycaemic warning sign of tachycardia may not occur, although sweating may be increased. Other more cardioselective beta-blockers may interact to a lesser extent than propranolol or not at all.

Interactions

Two different but related interactions can occur with some, but possibly not all, beta-blockers: the incidence and severity of hypoglycaemic episodes may be increased, and an undesirable rise in diastolic pressure may occur.

Hypoglycaemia

A woman who had previously shown signs of some hypoglycaemia 2–3 hours after a meal was treated with 80 mg propranolol daily for angina. Over a period of 6 months she was admitted to hospital on three occasions in hypoglycaemic coma. Her blood pressure was observed to be 200/90 mmHg and her pulse rate 52.[1]

A poorly controlled diabetic man treated with insulin was also given 40 mg propranolol daily. He subsequently experienced four episodes of severe hypoglycaemia, two of them with coma, but none once the propranolol was withdrawn. His insulin requirements remained unchanged throughout.[1]

Similar episodes or enhanced hypoglycaemic responses have been described in other diabetic and non-diabetic patients taking propranolol[10–13] and

oxprenolol (with glibenclamide, phenformin and thyroxine)[8].

Hypertension

When 14 normal subjects were treated with insulin alone, their blood sugar levels fell to 30 mg%, all experienced hypoglycaemic symptoms, their heart rates increased and their diastolic pressures were reduced. The hypoglycaemic response was the same when given insulin with propranolol, but the heart-rate already slowed by the propranolol became even slower at the onset of hypoglycaemia and both the systolic and diastolic pressures rose. The diastolic rise was about 20 mmHg but in one instance rose above 120 mmHg.[2]

Changes in the cardiovascular response have been described in other studies[10] in normal subjects.

Mechanism

Not fully understood, but a possible explanation has been put forward. The normal physiological response of the body to reduced blood sugar levels is the mobilization of sugar stored in the liver under the stimulation of adrenaline released from the adrenals. This stimulates the conversion of stored glycogen into glucose, and its release into the circulation.

Unselective beta-blockers such as propranolol block both the beta-2 receptors in the heart, as well as the beta-1 receptors concerned with glycogenolysis. The normal reflex mobilization of sugar which occurs when blood sugar levels fall too low is therefore attenuated so that the recovery from hypoglycaemia is prolonged, and in diabetics prone to hypoglycaemia it may allow a full-scale hypoglycaemic episode to occur.

The adrenaline released as a result of the hypoglycaemia also affects the cardiovascular system. Normally it would increase the heart rate but with the beta-receptors of the heart already blocked this does not occur. The hypertensive response probably comes about because with the beta-receptor stimulant action of adrenaline already blocked, the alpha-receptors (which cause vasoconstriction) are stimulated unopposed. The rise in blood pressure which follows would stimulate the baro-receptor reflexes and could account for some of the bradycardia which has been observed. Thus the blood pressure rises, but the normal tachycardia associated with hypoglycaemia is not seen.

Importance and management

An established interaction, and potentially serious. The incidence is uncertain but probably small. A survey in 1968 in conjunction with the British Diabetic Association identified 152 diabetics on propranolol out of a total of 80,000 diabetics.[5] None had experienced hypoglycaemia attributable to propranolol. There is no clear total contraindication to concurrent use, but very good reasons for caution. The problem of identifying patients particularly at risk remains unsolved, but those already prone to hypoglycaemia would seem to fall into this category. On theoretical

grounds and from indirect evidence (studies in normal subjects and animals) the cardioselective blockers atenolol,[15] acebutalol[4] and tolamolol[7] appear to be less likely to interact, but this requires confirmation in diabetics. Information about metoprolol is equivocal.[4]

All diabetics on any type of beta-blocker should be warned that some of the premonitory signs of hypoglycaemia, in particular tachycardia, may be masked, although sweating may even be increased.[9]

References

1 Kotler M N, Berman L and Rubenstein A H. Hypoglycaemia precipitated by propranolol. *Br Med J* (1966) **11**, 1389.
2 Lloyd-Mostyn R H and Oram S. Modification by propranolol of cardiovascular effects of induced hypoglycaemia. *Lancet* (1975) **1**, 1213.
3 Persson I and Eskar P. Carbohydrate tolerance during beta-adrenergic blockade in hypertension. *Europ J Clin Pharmacol* (1973) **5**, 151.
4 Newman R J. Comparison of propranolol, metoprolol, and acebutolol an insulin-induced hypoglycaemia. *Br Med J* (1976) **2**, 447.
5 Fitzgerald J D. Effects of propranolol on blood sugar, insulin and free fatty acids. *Diabetologia* (1968) **5**, 339.
6 Brown J H and Riggilo D A. Effect of sotalol (MJ 199) and propranolol on insulin-induced hypoglycaemia in the rat (32897). *Proc Soc Exp Biol Med* (1968) **127**, 1258.
7 Baird J R C and Carter A J. Assessment of effects of β-blocking drugs on blood glucose levels and insulin hypoglycaemia in rats. *Europ. J Pharmacol* (1974) **25**, 275.
8 McQueen E G. New Zealand Committee on Adverse Drug Reactions. Ninth Annual Report 1974. *NZ Med J* (1974) **80**, 305.
9 Molnar G W. Propranolol enhancement of hypoglycaemic sweating. *Clin Pharmacol Ther* (1974) **15**, 490.
10 Abramson E A, Arky R A and Woeber K A. Effects of propranolol on the hormonal and metabolic responses to insulin-induced hypoglycaemia. *Lancet* (1966) **ii**, 1386.
11 Simpson T. Propranolol and hypoglycaemia. *Lancet* (1967) **i**, 508.
12 Felley J. Beta-blockers for diabetics. *Lancet* (1977) **i**, 950.
13 Ball K D and Thomson C. Diabetics and beta-blockers. *Pharm J* (1979) **286**, 24.
14 Deacon S P. Beta-blocking drugs in diabetes. *Br Med J* (1978) **1**, 106.
15 Deacon S P and Barnet D. Comparison of atenolol and propranolol during insulin-induced hypoglycaemia. *Br med J* (1976) **11**, 272.
16 Davidson N McD, Corrall R J M, Shaw T R D and French E B. Observations in man of hypoglycaemia during selective and non-selective beta-blockade. *Scot Med J* (1977) **22**, 69.

Hypoglycaemic agents + chloramphenicol

Summary

The hypoglycaemic effects of tolbutamide and chlorpropamide can be enhanced by chloramphenicol. Acute hypoglycaemia has been described. Information about other sulphonylureas is lacking.

Interaction

Chloramphenicol can increase the hypoglycaemic effects of tolbutamide and chlorpropamide

> While taking 2 g chloramphenicol daily a man was additionally started on a course of 2 g tolbutamide daily. Three days later he suffered a typical hypoglycaemic collapse and was found to have serum tolbutamide levels three to four times higher than expected.[1,2]

Another case of hypoglycaemic coma has been described with tolbutamide and chloramphenicol.[6] Studies in diabetic patients have shown that 2 g daily doses of chloramphenicol can approximately double the half-lives of tolbutamide[2] and chlorpropamide[3], and double the serum concentrations of tolbutamide.[3] Other studies using 1 g daily doses of chloramphenicol similarly showed a doubling of the serum concentrations of tolbutamide, and blood sugar level reductions of 25–30%.[4,5]

Mechanism

The evidence available indicates that chloramphenicol inhibits the activity of the liver microsomal enzymes concerned with the metabolism of the hypoglycaemic agents. This results in their accumulation in the body, reflected in prolonged half-lives, increased serum levels, reduced blood sugar levels and occasionally acute hypoglycaemia.[1-6]

Importance and management

An established interaction. The chloramphenicol–tolbutamide interaction is well documented, but less information is available about chlorpropamide. An enhanced hypoglycaemic response to these sulphonylureas should be expected in most patients if concurrent use is undertaken. Appropriate precautions should be taken. Some patients may show a particularly exaggerated response. A simpler and safer solution would be to use an alternative non-interacting antibiotic.

Information about other sulphonylureas appears not to be available although most manufacturers list chloramphenicol as one of the drugs which interact with every sulphonylurea. This is almost certainly a precaution on their part based on the known interactions with tolbutamide and chlorpropamide, but direct information about other sulphonylureas appears to be lacking. More study is needed.

References

1 Hansen J M and Kristensen M. Tolbutamide in the treatment of Parkinson's disease. A double blind trial. *Dan Med Bull* (1965) **12**, 181.

2 Christensen L K and Skovsted L. Inhibition of drug metabolism by chloramphenicol. *Lancet* (1969) **ii**, 1397.

3 Petitpierre B, Perrin L, Rudhardt M, Herrera A and Fabre J. Behaviour of chlorpropamide in renal insufficiency and under associated drug therapy. *Int J Clin Pharmacol* (1972) **6**, 120.

4 Brunová E, Slabachová Z and Platilová H. Influencing the effect of dirastan (tolbutamide). Simultaneous administration of chloramphenicol in patients with diabetes and bacterial urinary tract inflammation. *Čas Lék čes* (1974) **113**, 72.

5 Brunová E, Slabachová Z, Platilová H, Pavlík F, Grafnetterová J and Dvorácek K. Interaction of tolbutamide and chloramphenicol in diabetic patients. *Int J Clin Pharmacol* (1977) **15**, 7.

6 Ziegelasch H-J. Extreme Hypoglykämie unter kombinierter Behandlung mit Tolbutamid, n-1-Butylbiguanidhydrochlorid und Chloramphenikol. *Z Gesamte inn Med* (1972) **27**, 63.

Hypoglycaemic agents + chlorpromazine

Summary

Chlorpromazine can raise blood sugar levels, particularly when given in doses of 100 mg or more. An increase in the dosage of the hypoglycaemic agent may be required.

Interaction

Chlorpromazine can raise blood sugar and antagonize the effects of the hypoglycaemic agents. This is a well-documented interaction, the first reports being published in the early 1950s.[1] A representative example:

> A long-term study over the period 1955–1966 on a large number of women who were treated for a year or more with chlorpromazine in daily doses of 100 mg or more showed that about 25% of them developed hyperglycaemia with glycosuria compared with only about 9% in a control group not taking phenothiazines of any kind. Of those treated with chlorpromazine, about a quarter showed complete remission of the symptoms when the chlorpromazine was withdrawn or the dosage reduced.[2]

There are numerous other reports of this response to chlorpromazine in man.[1,3-12,14,15] It has been thoroughly investigated in animals. There is one report which is out of step with all the others and claims that chlorpromazine had no effects at all on blood sugar levels.[13]

Chlorpromazine in doses of less than 100 mg appears not to cause this 'chlorpromazine-induced diabetes'

> A study on 25 normal subjects and six diabetic patients given chlorpromazine in doses of 50–75 mg daily showed that the glucose tolerance remained unaffected.[16]

Mechanism

It appears to be generally agreed that the hyperglycaemic effects of chlorpromazine are due to its inhibitory effect on the release of insulin by the pancreas, although it probably also causes the release of adrenaline from the adrenals which similarly raises blood sugar levels.

It seems possible that the precipitation of this 'chlorpromazine-diabetes' only occurs in those individuals who are normally just coping with their carbohydrate balance, and for whom the introduction of chlorpromazine is the last straw which tips the balance adversely.

Importance and management

An extremely well-documented and well-established interaction. The control of diabetes can be disturbed and prediabetics may develop overt diabetes. The study cited[2] indicates that the incidence is about 25% with daily chlorpromazine doses of 100 mg or more. Increases in the dosage requirements of the hypoglycaemic agent should be anticipated during concurrent use. Another study shows that daily doses in the 50–75 mg

range may not cause hyperglycaemia. Whether other chlorpromazine-like drugs behave similarly is uncertain; direct evidence of an interaction appears to be lacking.

References

1 Hiles B H. Hyperglycaemia and glycosuria following chlorpromazine therapy. *J Amer med Ass* (1956) **162**, 1651.
2 Thonnard-Neumann E. Phenothiazines and diabetes, hospitalized women. *Am J Psychiat* (1968) **124**, 978.
3 Dobkin A, Lamoreux L, Letienne R and Gilbert R G B. Some studies with largactil. *Canad Med Ass J* (1954) **70**, 626.
4 Lancaster N P and Jones D H. Chlorpromazine and insulin in psychiatry. *Br Med J* (1954) **2**, 565.
5 Giacobini F and Lassenius B. Chlorpromazine therapy in psychiatric practice; secondary effects and complications. *Nord Med* (1954) **52**, 1693.
6 Moyer J, Kinross-Wright V and Finney R M. Chlorpromazine as a therapeutic agent in clinical medicine. *Arch Int Med* (1955) **95**, 202.
7 Célice J, Porcher P and Plas S. Action de la chlorpromazine sur la vesicule biliaire et le colon droit. *Thérapie* (1955) **10**, 30.
8 Charatan F and Bartlett N. The effect of chlorpromazine ('Largactil') on glucose tolerance. *J Ment Sci* (1955) **101**, 351.
9 Cooperberg A A and Eidlow S. Haemolytic anaemia, jaundice and diabetes mellitus following chlorpromazine therapy. *Canad med Ass J* (1956) **75**, 746.
10 Blair D and Brady D M. Recent advances in the treatment of schizophrenia: group training and the tranquillizers. *J Ment Sci* (1958) **104**, 625.
11 Amdisen A. Diabetes mellitus as a side effect of treatment with tricyclic neuroleptics. *Acta Psychiat Scand* (1964) **40** (Suppl 180), 411.
12 Arneson G. Phenothiazine derivatives and glucose metabolism. *J. Neuropsychiat* (1964) **5**, 181.
13 Schwarz L and Munoz R. Blood sugar levels in patients treated with chlorpromazine. *Amer J Psychiat* (1968) **125**, 253.
14 Korenyi C and Lowenstein B. Chlorpromazine induced diabetes. *Dis Nerv Syst* (1968) **29**, 327.
15 Marmow A. Diabetes in chronic schizophrenia. *Dis Nerv Syst* (1971) **32**, 777.
16 Erle G, Basso M, Federspil G, Sicolo N and Scandellari C. Effect of chlorpromazine on blood glucose and plasma insulin in man. *Europ J clin Pharmacol* (1977) **11**, 15.

Hypoglycaemic agents + clofibrate

Summary

The hypoglycaemic effects of the sulphonylureas may be enhanced in some patients by clofibrate, possibly advantageously in those with poorly controlled diabetes. Dosage adjustment of the sulphonylurea may be called for.

Interaction

The hypoglycaemic effects of the sulphonylurea hypoglycaemic agents may be enhanced by the concurrent use of clofibrate in some, but not all, patients. A few examples:

> In a study on 13 maturity-onset diabetics on various

sulphonylureas (types not stated) who were given clofibrate, hypoglycaemia (serum glucose 30–40 mg %) was observed in 4 patients and the control of diabetes was improved in 6.[3]

In another study it was reported that the hypoglycaemic response to 1 g tolbutamide administered intravenously was enhanced in 6 patients with mild diabetes after 7 days' treatment with clofibrate.[4]

A report on 22 maturity-onset diabetics, treated with sulphonylureas and given 2 g clofibrate daily, stated that only in the 9 with poor diabetes control was this control improved and the incidence of glycosuria reduced.[6]

Another report states that no significant enhancement of the sulphonylurea-induced hypoglycaemia was seen when clofibrate was administered to 4 diabetic patients although 1 patient showed some improvement in fasting hyperglycaemia.[2,5]

There are a number of other reports showing that clofibrate causes a reduction in blood sugar levels and some improvement in diabetic control.[8-11]

Mechanism

The mechanism of this interaction is not known. In one study on 5 patients on chlorpropamide and clofibrate, the half-life of chlorpropamide was found to be increased from 38 to an average of 47 h by an as yet unidentified mechanism.[1] Among the suggestions put forward to account for this are that clofibrate displaces the sulphonylureas from their plasma protein binding sites and thereby increases their pharmacological availability,[5] or that some alteration in the excretion of the sulphonylurea and its metabolites takes place in the kidney.[1] A reduction in insulin resistance by clofibrate has also been mooted.[4,7] Alternatively, since it has been clearly shown that clofibrate has a hyperglycaemic action which is independent of the presence of another hypoglycaemic agent,[11] it is possible that any or all of these mechanisms might contribute towards the enhanced hypoglycaemia which has been described.

Importance and control

There appears to be no reason why clofibrate should not be given with the sulphonylurea hypoglycaemic agents, and indeed it has been suggested that it may be worthwhile to use clofibrate as a supplement to oral hypoglycaemic therapy with the sulphonylureas in poorly controlled diabetes.[6] However, since hypoglycaemia is a possibility in a few patients, it would be prudent to monitor the effects carefully if these drugs are used concurrently and to reduce the dosage of the hypoglycaemic agent where necessary.

References

1 Petitpierre B, Perrin L, Rudhardt M, Herrera A and Fabre J. Behaviour of chlorpropamide in renal insufficiency and under the effect of associated drug therapy. Int J Clin Pharmacol (1972) 6, 120.

2 Jain A K, Ryan J R and McMahon F G. Potentiation of hypoglycaemic effect of sulphonylureas by halofenate. New Eng J Med (1975) 293, 1284.

3 Daubresse J-C, Luyckx A S and Lefebvre P. Potentiation of hypoglycaemic effect of sulfonylureas by clofibrate. New Eng J Med (1976) 294, 613.

4 Ferrari C, Frezzati S, Testori G P and Bertazzoni A. Potentiation of hypoglycaemic response to intravenous tolbutamide by clofibrate. New Eng J Med (1976) 294, 1184.

5 Jain A K, Ryan J R and McMahon F G. Potentiation of hypoglycaemic effect of sulphonylureas by clofibrate. New Eng J Med (1976) 294, 613.

6 Daubresse J-C, Daigneux D, Bruwier M, Luyckx A and Lefrebvre P J. Clofibrate and diabetes control in patients treated with oral hypoglycaemic agents. Br J clin Pharmac (1979) 7, 599.

7 Ferrari C, Frezzati S, Romussi M, Bertazzoni A, Testori G P, Antonini S and Paracchi A. Effect of short-term clofibrate administration on glucose tolerance and insulin secretion in patients with chemical diabetes or hypertriglyceridaemia. Metabolism (1977) 26, 129.

8 Miller R D. Atromid in the treatment of post-climacteric diabetes. J Atheroscler Res (1963) 3, 694.

9 Csögör S I and Bornemisza P. The effect of clofibrate (Atromid) on intravenous tolbutamide, oral and intravenous glucose tolerance tests. Clin Trials J (1977) 14, 15.

10 Herriott S C, Percy-Robb I W, Strong J A and Thomson C G. The effect of Atromid on serum cholesterol and glucose tolerance in diabetes mellitus. J Atheroscler Res (1963) 3, 679.

11 Barnett D, Craig J G, Robinson D S and Rogers M P. Effect of clofibrate on glucose tolerance in maturity-onset diabetics. Br J clin Pharmac (1977) 4, 455.

Hypoglycaemic agents + colestipol

Summary

A report indicates that colestipol is active in insulin-treated diabetics, but may be ineffective in those treated with phenformin and sulphonylurea.

Interaction

A long-term double-blind controlled study in 12 patients with elevated serum cholesterol levels showed that the concurrent use of phenformin and a sulphonylurea (chlorpropamide, tolbutamide, or tolazamide) inhibited the normal hypocholesterolaemic effects of colestipol. No such antagonism was seen in 2 maturity-onset diabetics treated with insulin. The control of diabetes was not affected by the colestipol.[1]

Mechanism

Not understood.

Importance and management

The evidence is limited but it would seem that colestipol may not be a suitable agent for lowering serum cholesterol levels in diabetics treated with these oral hypoglycaemic agents. More data are required to confirm this report.

Reference

1 Bandisode M S and Boshell B R. Hypocholesterolemic activity of colestipol in diabetes. *Curr Ther Res* (1975) **18**, 276.

Hypoglycaemic agents + oral contraceptives

Summary

Some diabetic patients require a small increase in their dosage of hypoglycaemic agent while taking oral contraceptives. A few may require a decrease. It is not usual for the control of diabetes to be seriously distubed.

Interaction

Although there are a few reports[4,5,6] of individual patients who have experienced a marked disturbance of their diabetic control, the glucose-tolerance impairment induced by the oral contraceptives is usually insufficient to necessitate more than modest changes in the dosage of the hypoglycaemic agent, or none at all.

> A study on the effects of norethynodrel, 5 mg, with mestranol, 0·075 mg, on 30 postmenopausal diabetic women showed that more than half of them demonstrated abnormal glucose tolerance, but changes in their requirements of insulin or oral hypoglycaemic were described as 'few, scattered and slight in magnitude'.[1]

In another study[2] on 179 diabetic women taking a variety of oral contraceptives, 34% required an increase in insulin and 7% a decrease, whereas another report[3] on the use of *Orthonovin* (norethisterone with mestranol) stated that no insulin changes were necessary.

Mechanism

Not understood. Many mechanisms have been considered including changes in cortisol secretion, alterations in tissue glucose utilization, production of excessive amounts of growth hormone, alterations in liver function, and others.[7]

Importance and management

Well documented. Most manufacturers of oral contraceptives include a comment among their precautions about possible disturbances of the diabetic control, but there is usually no reason to avoid concurrent use. It would be prudent to watch for possible changes in the dosage requirements of the hypoglycaemic agent.

References

1 Cochran B and Pote W W H. C-19 Nor-steroid effects on plasma lipid and diabetic control of postmenopausal women. *Diabetes* (1963) **12**, 366.
2 Zeller W J, Brehm H, Schöffling K and Melzer H. Verträglichkeit von hormonalen Ovulationshemmern bei Diabetikerinnen. *Arzneim-Forsch* (1974) **24**, 351.
3 Tyler E T, Olsen H J, Gotlib M, Levin M and Behne D. Long term usage of norethindrone with mestranol preparations in the control of human fertility. *Clin Med* (1964) **71**, 997.
4 Kopera H, Dukes N G and Ijzerman G L. Critical evaluation of clinical data on Lyndiol. *Int J Fertil* (1964) **9**, 69.
5 Peterson W F, Steel M W and Coyne R Y. Analysis of the effect of ovulatory suppressants on glucose tolerance. *Amer J Obst Gyn* (1966) **95**, 484.
6 Reder J A and Tulgan H. Impairment of diabetic control by norethynodrel with mestranol. *NY State J Med* (1967) **67**, 1073.
7 Spellacy W N. A review of carbohydrate metabolism and the oral contraceptives. *Amer J Obst Gynecol* (1969) **104**, 448.

Hypoglycaemic agents + corticosteroids

Summary

The blood sugar lowering effects of the hypoglycaemic agents may be expected to be antagonized by the concurrent use of corticosteroids with glucocorticoid activity.

Interaction, mechanism, importance and management

Corticosteroids which possess glucocorticoid activity raise blood sugar levels. This can antagonize the blood sugar lowering effects of hypoglycaemic agents used in the treatment of diabetes mellitus. For example, a study on 5 diabetics showed that a single 200 mg dose of cortisone modified their glucose tolerance curves while taking an unstated amount of chlorpropamide. The blood glucose levels of 4 of them rose (3 showed an initial fall) whereas in a previous test with chlorpropamide alone the blood sugar levels of 4 of them had fallen.[1] It would seem possible that this was due to a direct antagonism between the pharmacological effects of the two drugs, because an experimental study in normal subjects showed that another corticosteroid, prednisone, had no significant effect on the metabolism or clearance of tolbutamide.[2]

There are very few studies of this interaction, possibly because the hyperglycaemic activity of the corticosteroids has been recognized for so long and the outcome of concurrent use would seem to be obvious. The effects of corticosteroid treatment on diabetic patients should be closely monitored and appropriate measures taken to maintain the diabetic control.

References

1 Danowski T S, Mateer F M and Moses C. Cortisone enhancement of peripheral utilization of glucose and the effects of chlorpropamide. *Ann NY Acad Sci* (1959) **74**, 988.
2 Breimer D D, Zilly W and Richter E. Influence of corticosteroid on hexobarbital and tolbutamide disposition. *Clin Pharmacol Ther* (1978) **24**, 208.

Hypoglycaemic agents + co-trimoxazole

Summary

Two cases of hypoglycaemia, one severe, have been reported in patients concurrently taking hypoglycaemic agents and co-trimoxazole.

Interaction, mechanism, importance and management

In a study on the effects of co-trimoxazole, 1 patient (taking an unnamed oral hypoglycaemic agent) out of 18 showed evidence of enhanced hypoglycaemia.[1] Severe hypoglycaemia has been described in another patient taking chlorpropamide and co-trimoxazole.[2] It would seem probable that the sulphonamide component of the co-trimoxazole was responsible (see p. 341). The evidence for this interaction is very limited but it would seem prudent to keep a close check on the effects of concurrent treatment.

References

1 Mihic M, Mautner L S, Feness J Z and Grant K. Effect of trimethoprim–sulfamethoxazole on blood insulin and glucose concentrations of diabetics. *Can Med Assoc J* (1975) **112**, 80s.
2 Ek I. Langvarigt klorpropamidutlöst hypoglykemitillstand Lakemedelsinteraktion? *Lakartidningen* (1974) **71**, 2597.

Hypoglycaemic agents + cyclophosphamide

Summary

Some very limited data suggest that diabetic control may be severely disturbed in some patients by the use of cyclophosphamide.

Interaction, mechanism, importance and management

Acute hypoglycaemia has been described in 2 diabetic patients under treatment with insulin and carbutamide who were concurrently treated with cyclophosphamide.[1] Three other cases of diabetes apparently induced by the use of cyclophosphamide, have also been reported.[2] These extremely limited data would suggest that a particularly close watch should be kept on the control of diabetes in patients given cyclophosphamide.

References

1 Krüger H-U. Blutzuckersenkende Wirkung von Cyclophosphamid bei Diabetikern. *Med Klin* (1966) **61**, 1462.
2 Pengelly C R. Diabetes mellitus and cyclophosphamide. *Br Med J* (1965) **1**, 1312.

Hypoglycaemic agents + diclofenac

Summary

Diclofenac has been shown not to interact with glibenclamide but as yet this has not been confirmed with the other sulphonylurea hypoglycaemic agents.

Interaction

A study on 12 glibenclamide-treated diabetic patients with rheumatic diseases showed that there were no significant changes in their blood sugar levels when they were also treated with 150 mg diclofenac a day, over a 4-day period.

Mechanism

None

Importance and management

No action appears to be necessary if diclofenac is administered to diabetics treated with glibenclamide, but as yet there appears to be no direct evidence to confirm that this is also true with the other sulphonylurea hypoglycaemic agents (chlorpropamide, tolbutamide etc).

Reference

1 Chlud K von. Untersuchungen zur Wechselwirkung von Diclofenac und Glibenclamid. *Zeit Rheumatologie* (1976) **35**, 377.

Hypoglycaemic agents + diflusinal

Summary

No interaction is reported to occur between tolbutamide and diflusinal.

Interaction, mechanism, importance and management

A preliminary report shows that when diflusinal, 375 mg twice daily, was given to diabetic patients taking tolbutamide, no alteration in their serum tolbutamide or in fasting blood glucose levels were seen.[2]

References

1 Tempero K F, Cirillo V J and Steelman S L. Diflusinal: a review of the pharmacokinetic and pharmacodynamic properties, drug interactions, and special tolerability studies in humans. *Br J Clin Pharmac* (1977) **4**, 31s.
2 McMahon F G and Ryan J R. Unpublished observations quoted in ref. 1.

Hypoglycaemic agents + disulfiram

Summary

Studies in man suggest that disulfiram does not interact with tolbutamide.

Interaction, mechanism, importance and management

Studies on 10 volunteers showed that when tolbutamide was injected intravenously following treatment with oral disulfiram (first day 400 mg three times; second day 400 mg; third and fourth days 200 mg) there was no significant alteration in the half-life or clearance rate of the tolbutamide. This indicates that an interaction during the concurrent use of these drugs is unlikely. Information about other sulphonylureas does not appear to be available.

Reference

1 Svendsen T L, Kristensen M B, Hansen J M and Skovsted L. The influence of disulfiram on the half-life and metabolic clearance rate of diphenylhydantoin and tolbutamide in man. *Europ J clin Pharmacol* (1976) **9**, 439.

Hypoglycaemic agents + ethacrynic acid

Summary

Ethacrynic acid can raise blood sugar levels in diabetic patients and oppose to some extent the effects of hypoglycaemic agents, but the importance of this appears to be limited.

Interactions

A double-blind study on 24 hypertensive patients, one third of whom were diabetic, showed that daily treatment with 200 mg ethacrynic acid over a period of 6 weeks impaired their glucose tolerance and raised the blood sugar levels of those who were diabetic.[1]

Mechanism

Not understood.

Importance and management

Although it is established that some impairment of the glucose tolerance in diabetics by ethacrynic acid can occur, there seems little evidence that it is usually an interaction of great importance, although it would clearly be prudent to be alert for changes in the requirements of the hypoglycaemic agents during concurrent use. More study is required.

Reference

1 Russell R P, Lindeman R D and Prescott L F. Metabolic and hypotensive effects of ethacrynic acid. Comparative study with hydrochlorothiazide. *J Amer Med Ass* (1968) **205**, 81.

Hypoglycaemic agents + fenclofenac

Summary

A single case report of severe hypoglycaemia suggests that fenclofenac may possibly interact with chlorpropamide.

Interaction, mechanism, importance and management

A diabetic woman, well-controlled on chlorpropamide, 500 mg, and metformin, 850 mg, daily, developed hypoglycaemia within 2 days of having her antirheumatic therapy with flurbiprofen and sustained-release indomethacin replaced by fenclofenac, 600 mg twice daily. The hypoglycaemic agents were withdrawn next day but later in the evening she went into hypoglycaemic coma. Much more study is required to confirm this possible interaction, but prescribers should be aware of this report.[1] It is suggested that in view of the known ability of fenclofenac to displace thyroxine from its binding sites, this may be a drug displacement interaction, with the fenclofenac displacing chlorpropamide from its plasma protein binding sites.

Reference

1 Allen P A and Taylor R T. Fenclofenac and thyroid function tests. *Brit Med J* (1980) **281**, 1642.

Hypoglycaemic agents + fenfluramine

Summary

Fenfluramine has inherent hypoglycaemic activity which can add to, or in some instances replace, the effects of conventional hypoglycaemic agents.

Interaction

A study on a group of obese maturity-onset diabetics who were given either fenfluramine (initially 40 mg daily increased over 4 weeks to 160 mg) or a placebo, showed that 4 of the 6 were better controlled than when previously taking a biguanide.[1]

Other reports similarly describe the hypoglycaemic effects of fenfluramine.[4]

Mechanism

Blood sugar levels are lowered by fenfluramine because it increases the uptake of glucose into skeletal muscle.[2,3]

Importance and management

A well-established and, on the whole, an advan-tageous rather than an adverse reaction, but it would be prudent to check on the extent of the response when fenfluramine is added or withdrawn from the treatment being received by diabetics.

References

1 Jackson W P U. Fenfluramine trials in a diabetic clinic. *S Afr med J* (1971) (*Suppl*), 29.
2 Turtle J R and Burgess J A. Hypoglycaemic effect of fenfluramine in diabetes mellitus. *Diabetes* (1973) 22, 858.
3 Kirby M J and Turner P. Effect of amphetamine, fenfluramine and norfenfluramine on glucose uptake into human isolated skeletal muscle. *Br J clin Pharmac* (1974) 1, 340P.
4 Dykes J R W The effect of a low-calorie diet with and without fenfluramine, and fenfluramine alone on the glucose tolerance and insulin secretion of overweight non-diabetics. *Postgrad med J* (1973) 49, 314.

Hypoglycaemic agents + frusemide

Summary

Diabetic control is not usually disturbed by the use of frusemide, although there are a few reports showing that it can sometimes elevate blood sugar levels.

Interaction, mechanism, importance and management

Although frusemide can elevate blood sugar levels[1] (but probably to a much lesser extent than the thiazide diuretics) and there are occasional reports of glycosuria and even acute diabetes in individual patients,[2] the general picture is that the control of diabetes is not usually affected by the use of frusemide.[3] It has been described as the 'diuretic of choice for the diabetic patient'.[4] Even so prescribers should be aware of its hyperglycaemic potentialities.

References

1 Hutcheon D E and Leonard G. Diuretic and antihypertensive action of frusemide. *J Clin Pharmac* (1967) 7, 26.
2 Toivonen S and Mustala O. Diabetogenic action of frusemide. *Br Med J* (1966) 1, 920.
3 Bencomo L, Fyvolent J, Kahana S and Kahana L. Clinical experience with a new diuretic, furosemide. *Curr Ther Res* (1965) 7, 339.
4 Malins J M. Diuretics in diabetes mellitus. *Practitioner* (1968) 201, 529.

Hypoglycaemic agents + guanethidine

Summary

Guanethidine has hypoglycaemic activity which can add to the effects of conventional hypoglycaemic agents.

Interaction

The insulin requirements of a diabetic woman were found to have increased from 70 units of soluble insulin per day to 94 when guanethidine was withdrawn.[1]

Other reports similarly describe the hypoglycaemic effects of guanethidine in man.[2,3]

Mechanism

Uncertain. One suggestion is that just as guanethidine lowers the blood pressure by reducing sympathetic tone, at the same time it may also impair the blood sugar homoeostatic mechanism concerned with raising blood sugar levels by the release of catecholamines. The balance of the system thus impaired tends to be tipped in favour of a reduced blood sugar level and the amounts of hypoglycaemic agent required are therefore reduced. Another idea is that the sensitivity of the tissues to insulin is increased by the guanethidine.

Importance and management
The documentation is limited, but the evidence is sufficiently strong to indicate that a check should be made on the control of the diabetes if guanethidine is added or withdrawn. The incidence is uncertain.

References
1 Gupta K K and Lillicrap C A. Guanethidine and diabetes. *Br med J* (1968) **2**, 697.
2 Gupta K K. The antidiabetic action of guanethidine. *Postgrad Med J* (1969) **45**, 455.
3 Kansal P C, Buse J and Durling F C. Effect of guanethidine and reserpine on glucose tolerance. *Curr Ther Res* (1971) **13**, 517.

Hypoglycaemic agents + halofenate

Summary
Halofenate can enhance the actions of tolbutamide, tolazamide and chlorpropamide in patients with hyperlipoproteinaemia. A reduction in the dosage of the sulphonylurea may be required to prevent excessive hypoglycaemia.

Interaction
A long-term double-blind study extending over 48 weeks on diabetic patients with type IV hyperlipoproteinaemia showed that halofenate can enhance the hypoglycaemic effects of oral sulphonylureas such as tolbutamide, tolazamide and chlorpropamide. Six out of nine diabetics taking a sulphonylurea (with or without phenformin) required a reduction in the dosage of the sulphonylurea. The daily dose of tolazamide in 4 patients was reduced from 3·25 g to 1·75 g and of chlorpropamide in 4 other patients from 1·75 g to 0·35 g daily. The daily dosages of halofenate varied with body weight (60 kg, 0·5 g; 60–110 Kg, 1·0 g; 110 Kg, 1·5 g).[1]

Mechanism
Not understood. One suggestion is that the halofenate displaces the sulphonylureas from their protein binding sites in the plasma thereby increasing their biological activity.[1] This is unlikely because although some enhancement of the hypoglycaemia was apparent after 2 weeks' concurrent use, statistically significant differences did not occur until after 4 weeks' use.

Importance and management
Information is limited, but this interaction appears to be established. Six of the 9 diabetic patients described in the report required a dosage reduction of the hypoglycaemic agent to prevent excessive hypoglycaemia, so the incidence is high. The effects of concurrent use should be monitored closely. Information about sulphonylureas other than tolbutamide, tolazamide and chlorpropamide is, as yet, lacking, but it would be prudent to be on the alert for this interaction with any sulphonylurea.

Two patients taking phenformin and halofenate, and 2 others taking insulin and halofenate who also took part in the study[1] required no adjustment in the dosage of hypoglycaemic agent, but the number of patients involved is too small to be able to make a positive statement about the significance of these results.

Reference
1 Jain A K, Ryan J R and McMahon F G. Potentiation of hypoglycaemic effect of sulphonylureas by halofenate. *New Eng J Med* (1975) **293**, 1283.

Hypoglycaemic agents + isoniazid

Summary
Some reports state that isoniazid can raise blood sugar levels in diabetics, whereas others describe a fall. The dosage of the hypoglycaemic agent may require adjustment to control the diabetes adequately.

Interactions

Both hyper- as well as hypoglycaemic effects have been reported with isoniazid.

(a) Hyperglycaemic effects

A clinical experiment on 6 diabetics being treated with insulin showed that after taking 250–400 mg isoniazid daily the fasting blood sugar levels were elevated 40% (from an average of 255 to 375 mg%), and the glucose tolerance curves rose and returned to normal levels more slowly. The effects were less marked after 6 days' treatment, the average rise in fasting blood sugar levels then being only 20%. Two other patients described in this report required an increase in their insulin dosage while taking 200 mg isoniazid daily, but a reduction when the isoniazid was withdrawn.

A case report describes a woman using insulin whose diabetes became very difficult to control while receiving isoniazid, and whose insulin requirements increased.[2]

Three out of a total of 50 non-diabetic patients on 300 mg isoniazid daily showed glycosuria, 2 of whom became frank diabetics requiring initial treatment with insulin, but later discharged on tolbutamide. The third patient showed complete remission of the diabetic symptoms when the isoniazid was withdrawn.[3]

An unsuccessful suicide attempt by a 16-year-old girl who ingested 8·75 g isoniazid caused, in addition to the usual signs of intoxication, hyperglycaemia, glycosuria and acetonuria. Frank diabetes developed.[4]

(b) Hypoglycaemic effects

Eight diabetics were tested with isoniazid and tolbutamide either alone or together. Six of them showed an average fasting blood sugar level reduction of 18% (range 5–34%) 4 h after taking 500 mg isoniazid. After 3 mg tolbutamide the average reduction was 28% (range 19–43%). And after both isoniazid and tolbutamide the average reduction was 35% (range 17–57%). The other 2 diabetics responded differently. One showed a 10% *increase* in blood sugar after the isoniazid, a 41% decrease after the tolbutamide, and a 30% decrease after taking both drugs together. The other diabetic responded to neither drug.[5]

Mechanism

Not understood. Carbohydrate metabolism is disturbed in both diabetics and non-diabetics by isoniazid.

Importance and management

An established reaction. The incidence is uncertain. Diabetics given isoniazid should be monitored closely for changes in the control of their diabetes. Appropriate dosage adjustments of the hyperglycaemic agent should be made where necessary.

References

1 Luntz G R W N and Smith S G. Effect of isoniazid on carbohydrate metabolism in controls and diabetics. *Br Med J* (1953) 1, 296.

2 Dickson I. Acute pancreatitis following administration of isonicotinic acid hydrozide. *Br J Tuberculosis* (1956) 50, 277.

3 Dickson I. Glycosuria and diabetes mellitus following INAH therapy. *Med J Aust* (1962) 49, (1) 325.

4 Tovaryš A and Siler Z. Diabetic syndrome and intoxication with INH. *Prakt Lekar* (1968) 48, 286; quoted in *Int Pharm Abs* (1968) 5, 286.

5 Segarra F O, Sherman D S and Charif B S. Experiences with tolbutamide and chlorpropamide in tuberculous diabetic patients. *Ann NY Acad Sci* (1959) 74, 656.

Hypoglycaemic agents + lithium carbonate

Summary

Limited data indicate that the control of diabetes in a few patients may be adversely affected by treatment with lithium carbonate.

Interaction

Three years after starting treatment with lithium a woman developed diabetes mellitus. Diabetic control using dietary restriction and insulin was established in the absence of lithium, but was lost soon after reintroduction of the lithium, and regained after lithium was withdrawn once again.[1]

Another report suggests some association between treatment with lithium and diabetes.[2]

Mechanism

Unknown.

Importance and management

Information about this reaction is extremely limited, but it indicates that a check should be kept on diabetic control during treatment with lithium. The incidence is uncertain.

References

1 Craig J, Abu-Saleh M, Smith B and Evans I. Diabetes mellitus in patients on lithium. *Lancet* (1977) ii, 1028.

2 Johnstone B B. Diabetes mellitus in patients on lithium. *Lancet* (1977) ii, 935.

Hypoglycaemic agents + methysergide

Summary

A preliminary study indicates that methysergide may enhance the activity of tolbutamide.

Interaction, mechanism, importance and management

A study on 8 maturity-onset diabetics showed that 2 days' pretreatment with methysergide (2 mg 6-hourly) increased the amount of insulin secreted in response to 1 g tolbutamide given intravenously by almost 40%. Whether in practice the addition or withdrawal of methysergide adversely affects the control of diabetes is uncertain, but prescribers should be aware of this interaction.

Reference

1 Baldridge J A, Quickel K E, Feldman J M and Lebovitz H E. Potentiation of tolbutamide-mediated insulin release in adult onset diabetics by methysergide maleate. *Diabetes* (1974) **23**, 21.

Hypoglycaemic agents + mianserin

Summary

The control of diabetes appears to be unaffected by the use of mianserin.

Interaction, mechanism, importance and management

Although there is some evidence[1,2,4] of a change in glucose metabolism during treatment with mianserin, the alteration failed to affect the control of diabetes in 10 patients under study and no adverse reports have yet been documented.[3]

References

1 Fell P J, Quantock D C, van der Burg W J. The human pharmacology of GB94—a new psychotropic agent. *Eur J clin Pharmac* (1973) **5**, 166.
2 Weinges A, unpublished data quoted in ref. 3.
3 Peet M and Behagel H. Mianserin: a decade of scientific development. *Br J clin Pharmac* (1978) **5**, 5s.
4 Moonie J. Unpublished data quoted by Brogden R N, Heel R C, Speight T M and Avery G S. Mianserin: a review of its pharmacological properties and therapeutic efficacy in depressive illness. *Drugs* (1978) **16**, 273.

Hypoglycaemic agents + phenylbutazone or oxyphenbutazone

Summary

The hypoglycaemic effects of tolbutamide, acetohexamide, chlorpropamide, carbutamide, glymidine and glibenclamide are enhanced by phenylbutazone which may possibly lead to severe hypoglycaemia. Other sulphonylureas probably interact similarly but this awaits confirmation. Oxyphenbutazone may be expected to behave like phenylbutazone.

Interaction

A diabetic man under treatment with tolbutamide experienced an acute hypoglycaemic attack 4 days after beginning to take 200 mg phenylbutazone three times a day, although there was no change in the diet or the dosage of tolbutamide. He was able to control the attack by eating a large bar of chocolate.[1]

There are numerous other case reports and studies of this interaction involving phenylbutazone with tolbutamide,[2-5,8,10,11,17] carbutamide,[3] acetohexamide,[6] chlorpropamide,[11] glibenclamide,[12] and glymidine,[18] some of them describing acute hypoglycaemic episodes.[2,5,6,10] There are other reports not listed here. A single report on 3 negro patients describes a paradoxical *rise* in blood sugar levels while receiving phenylbutazone and tolbutamide.[14] There is also a report suggesting that the phenylbutazone–glibornuride interaction may not be clinically important.[7] Oxyphenbutazone has been shown to interact with glycodiazine[13] and tolbutamide.[15,16]

Mechanism

Not fully resolved. There is evidence to show that phenylbutazone inhibits the renal excretion of glibenclamide,[12] tolbutamide[8] and the active metabolite of acetohexamide[6] so that the hypoglycaemic effects might be expected to be enhanced and prolonged. It has also been shown that the phenylbutazone can inhibit the metabolism of the sulphonylureas[15] as well as causing their displacement from protein binding sites,[9] but no full explanation of this interaction has yet been given.

Importance and management

Well-documented and important interactions. The incidence is uncertain. A reduction in the dosage of the sulphonylurea may be necessary if excessive hypoglycaemia is to be avoided. Not all of the sulphonylureas have been shown to interact with phenylbutazone (glibornuride probably does not[7]) but it would be prudent to assume that they all do until the contrary is proved. There is some limited evidence that the effects of tolbutamide are *reduced* in negroes[14] but whether this applies to the other sulphonylureas is not known.

It would be reasonable to expect oxyphenbutazone to interact in the same way as phenylbutazone (it is the metabolite of phenylbutazone) with most of the sulphonylureas, but confirmation of this is required.

References

1 Mahfouz M, Abdel-Maguid R and El-Dakhakhny M. Potentiation of the hypoglycaemic action of tolbutamide by different drugs. *Arzneim-Forsch* (1970) **20**, 120.

2 Dalgas M, Christiansen I and Kjerulf K. Fenylbutazoninduceret hypoglykaemitilfaelde hos klorpropamidbehandlet diabetiker. *Ugeskr Laeg* (1965) **127**, 834.

3 Kaindl F, Kretschy A, Puxkandl H and Wutte J. Zur Steigerung des Wirkungseffektes peroraler Antidiabetika durch Pyrazolonderivate. *Wien Klin Wchschr* (1961) **73**, 79.

4 Gulbrandsen R. Økt tolbutamid-effekt ved hjelp av fenylbutazon? *Tidskr Norsk Laeg* (1959) **79**, 1127.

5 Tannenbaum H, Anderson L G and Soeldner J S. Phenylbutazone-tolbutamide drug interaction. *New Eng J Med* (1974) **290**, 344.

6 Field J B, Ohata M, Boyle C and Remer A. Potentiation of acetohexamide hypoglycaemia by phenylbutazone. *New Eng J Med* (1967) **277**, 889.

7 Eckhardt W, Rudolph R, Sauer H, Schubert W R, Undeutsch D. Zur pharmakologischen Interferenz von Glibornurid mit Sulfaphenazol Phenylbutazon und Phenprocoumon beim Menschen. *Arzneim-Forsch* (1972) **22**, 2212.

8 Ober K-F. Mechanism of interaction of tolbutamide and phenylbutazone in diabetic patients. *Europ J clin Pharmacol* (1974) **7**, 291.

9 Hellman B. Potentiating effects of drugs on the binding of glibenclamide to pancreatic beta cells. *Metabolism* (1974) **23**, 839.

10 Dent L A and Jue S G. Tolbutamide + phenylbutazone; a dangerous and predictable interaction. *Drug Intell Clin Pharm* (1976) **10**, 711.

11 Schulz E. Severe hypoglycaemic reactions after tolbutamide, carbutamide and chlorpropamide. *Arch Klin Med* (1968) **214**, 135.

12 Schulz E, Koch K and Schmidt F H. Ursachen der Potenzierung der hypoglykämischen Wirkung von Sulfonylharnstoffderivaten durch Medikamente. II. Pharmakokinetik und Metabolismus von Glibanclamid (HN 419) in Gegenwart von Phenylbutazon. *Europ J Clin Pharmacol* (1971) **4**, 32.

13 Held H, Scheible G, von Olderhausen H F. Über Stoffwechsel und Interferenz von Arzneimitteln bei Gesunden und Leberkranken. *Kongress für Innere Medizin* (Wiesbaden) (1970) **76**, 1153.

14 Owusu S K and Ocran K. Paradoxical behaviour of phenylbutazone in African diabetics. *Lancet* (1972) **i**, 440.

15 Pond S M, Birkett J and Wade D N. Mechanisms of inhibition of tolbutamide metabolism: phenylbutazone, oxyphenbutazone, sulfafenazole. *Clin Pharmacol Ther* (1977) **22**, 573.

16 Kristensen M and Christensen L K. Modificazioni dell'effeto ipoglicemizzante dei farmaci ipoglicemizzanti indotte da altri farmaci. *Acta diabet lat* (Milan) (1969) **6** (Suppl 1), 116.

17 Christensen L K, Hansen J M and Kristensen M. Sulphaphenazole-induced hypoglycaemic attacks in tolbutamide-treated diabetics. *Lancet* (1963) **ii**, 1298.

18 Held H, Kaminski B and von Olderhausen H F. Die beeinflussung der Elimination von Glycodiazin durch Leber- und Nierenfunktionsstörungen und durch eine Behandlung mit Phenylbutazon, phenprocoumarol und doxycyclin. *Diabetologia* (1970) **6**, 386.

Hypoglycaemic agents + phenyramidol

Summary

The half-life of tolbutamide is prolonged by phenyramidol. The hypoglycaemic effects would be expected to be enhanced.

Interaction

When 3 normal subjects were treated with phenyramidol (400 mg three times a day) for 4 days, the half-life of a single dose of tolbutamide was found to be increased from 7 to 18 h.[1]

Mechanism

Uncertain. It is postulated that phenyramidol inhibits the metabolism of the tolbutamide, thereby prolonging its stay in the body.[1]

Importance and management

Information appears to be limited to this one study. A reduction in the dosage of tolbutamide would seem to be necessary if excessive hypoglycaemia is to be avoided. Information about other sulphonylureas is lacking.

Reference

1 Solomon H M and Schrogie J J. Effect of phenyramidol and bishydroxycoumarin on the metabolism of tolbutamide in human subjects. *Metabolism* (1967) **16**, 1029.

Hypoglycaemic agents + probenecid

Summary

The half-life of chlorpropamide is prolonged by probenecid. The hypoglycaemic effects would be expected to be enhanced.

Interaction

The half-life of chlorpropamide, but not tolbutamide, is prolonged by probenecid.

A study on 6 patients who were given single oral doses of chlorpropamide showed that the concurrent use of probenecid (1–2 g daily) increased the half-life of the hypoglycaemic agent from about 36 to 50 h.[1]

Another report claimed that the half-life of tolbutamide was also prolonged,[2] but this was not confirmed by another properly controlled study.[3]

Mechanism

It is suggested that probenecid interferes with and reduces the renal excretion of chlorpropamide, thereby prolonging its stay in the body.[1]

Importance and management

Information is very limited. A reduction in the dosage of chlorpropamide would seem to be necessary if excessive hypoglycaemia is to be avoided. Tolbutamide appears not to interact, but information about other sulphonylureas is lacking.

References

1 Petitpierre B, Perrin L, Rudhardt M, Herrera A and Fabre J. Behaviour of chlorpropamide in renal insufficiency and under the effect of associated drug therapy. *Int J clin Pharmacol* (1972) **6**, 120.
2 Stowers J M, Mahler R F and Hunter R B. Pharmacology and mode of action of the sulphonylureas in man. *Lancet* (1958) i, 278.
3 Brook R, Schrogie J J and Solomon H M. Failure of probenecid to inhibit the rate of metabolism of tolbutamide in man. *Clin Pharmacol Ther* (1968) **9**, 314.

Hypoglycaemic agents + rifampicin

Summary

Rifampicin reduces the half-life and the serum levels of tolbutamide and glycodiazine. A marked reduction in their hypoglycaemic activity would be expected.

Interaction

The half-life and serum levels of tolbutamide and glycodiazine are reduced by rifampicin.

A study on a group of 9 tuberculous patients receiving tolbutamide showed that after 4 weeks' treatment with rifampicin the half-life of tolbutamide was reduced by 43%, and the serum concentrations measured at 6 h were halved when compared with other patients not taking rifampicin.[1]

Similar results have been found in other studies with tolbutamide and rifampicin in patients with cirrhosis or cholestasis[2] and in normal subjects.[3]

The half-life of glycodiazine in man is also approximately halved by the concurrent use of rifampicin.[4]

Mechanism
The available evidence indicates that rifampicin is a potent inducer of the liver microsomal enzymes concerned with the metabolism of tolbutamide and other drugs, which hastens their clearance from the body.[1,2,3]

Importance and management
A well-established interaction. A considerable reduction in the hypoglycaemic activity of tolbutamide or glycodiazine and increased dosage requirements would be expected during concurrent use. Information about other sulphonylureas appears not to have been documented.

References
1 Syvälahti E K G, Pihlajamäki K K and Iisalo E J. Rifampicin and drug metabolism. *Lancet* (1974) **ii**, 232.
2 Zilly W, Breimer D D and Richter E. Stimulation of drug metabolism by rifampicin in patients with cirrhosis or cholestasis measured by increased hexobarbital and tolbutamide clearance. *Europ J clin Pharmacol* (1977) **11**, 287.
3 Zilly W, Breimer D D and Richter E. Induction of drug metabolism in man after rifampicin treatment measured by increased hexobarbital and tolbutamide clearance. *Europ J clin Pharmacol* (1975) **9**, 219.
4 Held H K, Schoene B, Laar H J and Fleischmann R. Die Aktivität der Bensepyrenhydroxylase im Leberpunktat des Menschen in vitro und ihre Beziehung zur Eliminationsgeschwindigkeit von Glycodiazin in vivo. *Verhandlungen der Deutschen Gesellschaft für Innere Medizin* (1974) **80**, 501.

Hypoglycaemic agents + sulindac

Summary
There appears to be no interaction between tolbutamide and sulindac in normal therapeutic doses.

Interaction
A study on 12 maturity-onset tolbutamide-treated diabetics showed that no significant changes took place in their serum tolbutamide levels, tolbutamide half-lives, time-to-peak concentration or area under the plasma tolbutamide curves when they were concurrently treated with 200 mg sulindac twice a day for a week. A slight but unimportant reduction in the fasting blood sugar levels was seen.[1]

Mechanism
None.

Importance and management
No clinically significant interaction occurs when tolbutamide and sulindac in normal doses are taken concurrently. Information about other sulphonylureas is lacking.

Reference
1 Ryan J R, Jain M D, McMahon F G and Vargas R. On the question of an interaction between sulindac and tolbutamide in the treatment of diabetes. *Clin Pharmacol Therap* (1976) **21**, 231.

Hypoglycaemic agents + sulphinpyrazone

Summary
The theoretical possibility of an interaction has yet to be realized in practice.

Interaction, mechanism, importance and management
Because of its close structural similarity sulphinpyrazone would be expected to interact in the same way as phenylbutazone with the sulphonylureas to enhance their hypoglycaemic effects, but whether in practice this actually occurs awaits confirmation.

Hypoglycaemic agents + sulphonamides

Summary

Some sulphonylurea/sulphonamide combinations interact, the result being an enhancement of the hypoglycaemic effects of the sulphonylureas. Cases of acute hypoglycaemia have been reported. Some pairs of drugs do not interact.

Interaction

The half-lives and the hypoglycaemic effects of some sulphonylureas can be enhanced by certain sulphonamides leading in some instances to the development of hypoglycaemic coma. Table 14.3 is a summary in tabular form of the information I have been able to trace.

Mechanism

By no means fully resolved. There is evidence that the sulphonamides may inhibit the metabolism of the sulphonylureas so that they accumulate in the body and their serum levels and hypoglycaemic effects are enhanced,[3,5,6] but they may also displace the sulphonylureas from their protein binding sites.[5,6,12]

Importance and management

With the possible exception of the tolbutamide/sulphaphenazole interaction, these interactions are, individually, not sufficiently well documented to form a firm basis on which to make reliable predictions about what will, and what will not, interact, but Table 14.3 can be used as a general guide.

The tolbutamide/sulphaphenazole interaction is the best documented and it would seem that these two drugs should not be given together. It would also seem prudent to avoid any of the others where an interaction is known to have occurred, but the evidence against them is much less certain. Data about other sulphonylurea/sulphonamide combinations appears to be lacking. If

Table 14.3. Interactions between sulphonylureas and sulphonamides

Drugs	Information documented	References
Tolbutamide		
+ Sulphafurazole	Three cases of severe hypoglycaemia.	1,2
(sulfisoxazole)	Two reports state no interaction	6,11
+ Sulphamethizole	Half-life of tolbutamide increased 60%.	3,4
	Metabolic clearance reduced 40%	
+ Sulphaphenazole	1 case of severe hypoglycaemia	1,5,11
	Half-life of tolbutamide increased 4–6 times	
+ Sulphadiazine	Half-life of tolbutamide increased 50%	5
+ Sulphadimethoxine	Stated to be no interaction	1,6
+ Sulphamethoxine	Stated to be no interaction	1,6
+ Sulphamethoxypyridazine	Stated to be no interaction	1,6
+ Sulphamethoxazole	Stated to be no interaction	1,6
Chlorpropamide		
+ Sulphafurazole	1 case of acute hypoglycaemia	7
(sulfisoxazole)		
+ Sulphamethazine	1 case of acute hypoglycaemia	8
+ Co-trimoxazole		
(trimethoprim +	1 case of acute hypoglycaemia.	9
sulphamethoxazole)	(see also p. 331)	
Glibornuride		
+ Sulphaphenazole	Stated to be no interaction	10

concurrent treatment is undertaken, the possibility of acute hypoglycaemia should be fully appreciated.

References

1 Soeldner J S and Steinke J. Hypoglycaemia in tolbutamide-treated diabetes. *J Amer Med Ass* (1965) **193**, 148.
2 Robinson D S. The application of basic principles of drug interaction to clinical practice. *J Urology* (1975) **113**, 100.
3 Lumholtz B, Siersbaek-Nielsen K, Skovsted L, Kampmann J and Hansen J M. Sulfamethizole-induced inhibition of diphenylhydantoin, tolbutamide, and warfarin metabolism. *Clin Pharmacol Ther* (1975) **17**, 731.
4 Siersbaek-Nielsen K, Hansen J M, Skovsted L, Lumholtz B and Kampmann J. Sulfamethizole-induced inhibition of diphenylhydantoin and tolbutamide metabolism in man. *Clin Pharmacol Ther* (1973) **14**, 148.
5 Kristensen M and Christensen L K. Drug induced changes of the blood glucose lowering effect of oral hypoglycaemic agents. *Acta diabet lat* (1969) **6**, (suppl 1) 116.
6 Christensen L K, Hansen J M and Kristensen M. Sulpha-phenazole-induced hypoglycaemic attacks in tolbutamide-treated diabetics. *Lancet* (1963) **ii**, 1298.
7 Tucker H S G and Hirsch J I. Sulfonamide-sulfonylurea interaction. *New Eng J Med* (1972) **286**, 110.
8 Dall J L C, Conway H and McAlpine S G. Hypoglycaemia due to chlorpropamide. *Scot Med J* (1967) **12**, 403.
9 Ek I. Langvarigt klorpropamidutlöst hypoglykemitillstand Läkemedelsinteraktion? *Lakartidningen* (1974) **71**, 2597.
10 Eckhardt W, Rudolph R, Sauer H, Schubert W R and Undeutsch D. Zur pharmakologischen Interferenz von Glibornurid mit Sufaphenazol, Phenylbutazon und Phenprocoumon beim Menschen. *Arsneim-Forsch* (1972) **22**, 2212.
11 Dubach U C, Bückert A and Raaflaub J. Einfluss von Sulfonamiden auf die blutzuckersenkende Wirkung oraler Antidiabetiica. *Schweiz med Wschr* (1966) **96**, 1483.
12 Hellman B. Potentiating effects of drugs on the binding of glibenclamide to pancreatic beta cells. *Metabolism* (1974) **23**, 839.

Hypoglycaemic agents + tetracyclines

Summary

A few scattered reports indicate that the hypoglycaemic effects of the sulphonylureas and insulin may be enhanced by the tetracyclines. Lactic acidosis may also be precipitated by the concurrent use of phenformin and a tetracycline.

Interaction, mechanism, importance and management

Animal studies have shown that oxytetracycline can affect blood sugar levels[1] and there are now a few reports indicating that hypoglycaemia has occurred in patients during concurrent treatment with insulin and doxycycline,[2] insulin and oxytetracycline[3] and tolbutamide with oxytetracycline.[1] The half-life of glymidine in man has also been shown to be prolonged from 4·6 to 7·6 h by doxycycline,[4] but a brief comment in another report suggests that dimethylchlortetracycline may not affect chlorpropamide.[5] All these reports suggest that a close watch should be kept for excessive hypoglycaemia during concurrent use.

Evidence is now accumulating that phenformin-induced lactic acidosis may possibly be precipitated by the use of tetracycline due, it is suggested, to some interference with the renal clearance of the phenformin. At least six cases are now on record.[6-10] Concurrent use should be avoided.

References

1 Hiatt N and Bonoriss G. Insulin response in pancreatectomised dogs treated with oxytetracyline. *Diabetes* (1970) **19**, 307.
2 New Zealand Committee on Adverse Drug Reactions. Ninth Annual Report. *NZ Dent J* (1975) **71**, 28.
3 Miller J B. Hypoglycaemic effect of tetracycline. *Br Med J* (1966) **2**, 1007.
4 Held H, Kaminski B and von Oldershausen H F. Die Beeinflussung der Elimination von Glycodiazin durch Leber- und Nierenfunktionssörungen und durch eine Behandlung mit Phenylbutazon, Phenprocoumarol und Doxycyclin. *Diabetologia* (1970) **6**, 386.
5 Petitpierre B, Perrin L, Rudhardt M, Herrera A and Fabre J. Behaviour of chlorpropamide in renal insufficiency and under the effect of associated drug therapy. *Int J clin Pharmacol* (1972) **6**, 120.
6 Aro A, Korhonen T and Halinen M. Phenformin-induced lactic acidosis precipitated by tetracycline. *Lancet* (1978) **i**, 673.
7 Tashima C K. Phenformin, tetracycline and lactic acidosis. *Br Med J* (1971) **4**, 557.
8 Blumenthal S A, Streeten D HP. Phenformin-related lactic acidosis in a 30-year-old man. *Ann intern Med* (1976) **84**, 55.
9 Korhonen T, Idänpään-Heikkilä J E and Aro A. Unpublished data quoted in ref. 6.
10 Philips P J and Pain R W. Phenformin, tetracycline and lactic acidosis. *Ann Intern Med* (1977) **86**, 111.

Hypoglycaemic agents + thiazides, chlorthalidone or related diuretics

Summary

By raising blood sugar levels the thiazide diuretics and chlorthalidone can antagonize the effects of the hypoglycaemic agents and impair the control of diabetes. Some, but by no means all, patients may require an increase in their hypoglycaemic agent dosage.

Interaction

Chlorothiazide, the first of the thiazide diuretics, was found within a year of its introduction in 1958 to have hyperglycaemic effects.[1] Since then a very large number of reports have described this same effect with other thiazides, the precipitation of diabetes in prediabetics, and the disturbance of blood sugar control in diabetics. One example from many.

A long-term study on 53 diabetics showed that treatment with either trichlormethiazole (4 or 8 mg daily) or chlorothiazide (0·5 or 1 g daily) caused a mean rise in blood sugar levels from 120 to 140 mg%. Only 7 patients required a change in their treatment: 4 required more of their oral agent, 2 an increase in insulin, and 1 was transferred from tolbutamide to insulin. The oral agents used included tolbutamide, chlorpropamide, acetohexamide and phenformin.[2]

Hyperglycaemia has also been observed with benzthiazide,[3] hydrochlorothiazide,[5] dihydroflumethiazide,[5] and chlorthalidone.[6] A full list of references is not given here for the sake of economy of space, but the documentation is very extensive.

Mechanism

Not fully understood. One study suggests that the hyperglycaemia is due to some inhibition of insulin release[9] by the pancreas. Another is that the peripheral action of insulin is affected in some way.[8]

Importance and management

An extremely well-documented interaction, of only moderate practical importance. One report of a study states that '. . . it is not of serious degree . . . and in no patient was a dramatic deterioration of diabetic control observed.'[2] The incidence in this study was about 10%, whereas another claims that it is as high as 30%.[4] There is no contraindication to concurrent use and most patients respond to an increase in the dosage of hypoglycaemia agent, or to a change from an oral drug to insulin. The adverse hyperglycaemic effects can also be reversed significantly by the use of potassium supplements.[7]

In addition to the thiazides named, the interaction may be expected to occur with the other thiazides in common use (bendrofluazide, cyclopenthiazide, cyclothiazide, methyclothiazide, polythiazide) and related diuretics such as clopamide, clorexolone, metolazone, quinethazone etc. This requires confirmation.

References

1 Wilkins R W. New drugs for the treatment of hypertension. *Ann intern Med* (1959) **50**, 1.
2 Kansal P C, Buse J and Buse M G. Thiazide diuretics and control of diabetes mellitus. *S Med J* (1969) **62**, 1374.
3 Runyan J W. Influence of thiazide diuretics on carbohydrate metabolism in patients with mild diabetes. *New Eng J Med* (1961) **267**, 541.
4 Wolff F W, Parmley W W, White K W and Okun R J. Drug-induced diabetes. Diabetogenic activity of long-term administration of benzothiadiazines. *J Amer Med Ass* (1963) **185**, 568.
5 Goldner M G, Zarowitz H and Akgun S. Hyperglycaemia and glycosuria due to thiazide derivatives administered in diabetes mellitus. *New Eng J Med* (1960) **262**, 403
6 Carliner N H, Schelling J-L, Russell R P, Okun R and Davis M. Thiazide- and phthalimidine-induced hyperglycemia in hypertensive patients. *J Amer Med Ass* (1965) **191**, 535.
7 Rapoport M I and Hurd H F. Thiazide-induced glucose intolerance treated with potassium. *Arch Int Med* (1964) **113**, 405.
8 Remenchik A P, Hoover C and Talso P J. Insulin secretion by hypersensitive patients receiving hydrochlorothiazid. *J Amer Med Ass* (1970) **212**, 869.
9 Fajans S S, Floyd J C, Knopf R F, Rull J, Guntsche E M and Conn J W. Benzothiadiazine suppression of insulin release from normal and abnormal islet tissue in man. *J Clin Invest* (1966) **45**, 481.

Hypoglycaemic agents + tolmetin

Summary

Tolmetin is reported not to interact with glibenclamide

Interaction, mechanism, importance and management

A short-term, double-blind trial extending over 5 days on 40 diabetic patients with various rheumatic disorders, and who were being treated with glibenclamide, showed that the concurrent administration of 400 mg tolmetin taken three times a day had no effect on the blood or urine glucose values.[1] There appears to be no information about the response to other sulphonylureas in the presence of tolmetin.

Reference

1 Chlud K and Kaik B. Clinical studies of the interaction between tolmetin and glibenclamide. *J Clin Pharmacol* (1977) 15, 409.

CHAPTER 15. LITHIUM CARBONATE INTERACTIONS

Lithium carbonate is used in the treatment of manic depression and depression, and is given in doses of up to 2 g daily, the dosages being adjusted to give plasma concentrations of 0·6 to 1·5 mEq/l. It should only be given under close supervision when the blood concentrations can be monitored regularly—initially weekly—to avoid the development of toxicity.

Side effects which are not serious include nausea, weakness, fine tremor, mild polydipsia and polyuria. If plasma concentrations reach about 2 mEq/l, more serious intoxication is seen: the gastrointestinal symptoms are abdominal pain, nausea, vomiting, diarrhoea, anorexia and thirst. Neurological symptoms include drowsiness, giddiness with ataxia, coarse tremor, slurred speech, blurred vision and muscular twitching. If concentrations are allowed to reach 3 mEq/l, life-threatening epileptic seizures, coma, hyperextension of the limbs, syncope and circulatory failure may occur. The lithium should be withdrawn immediately.

In addition to these side-effects, lithium can induce diabetes insipidus and hypothyroidism in some patients, and it is contraindicted in patients with renal or cardiac insufficiency.

Just how lithium exerts its beneficial effects is not known, but it may compete with sodium ions in various parts of the body and it alters the electrolyte composition of body fluids.

Other interactions involving lithium but not discussed in this chapter are to be found elsewhere in this book. The index should be consulted for a full listing.

Table 15.1. Lithium carbonate: approved and international proprietary names

Approved name	International proprietary names
Lithium carbonate	*Camcolit, Carbolith, Eskalith, Hypnorex, Lithane, Lithicarb, Lithionit, Lithium Duriles, Lithium Oligosol, Lithonate, Lithotabs, Maniprex, Neuorlithium, Phasal, Priadel, Quilonum*

Lithium carbonate + acetazolamide, chlormerodrin, spironolactone, triamterene

Summary
Some inconclusive evidence suggests that acetazolamide, spironolactone and triamterene, but not chlormerodrin, may increase the excretion of lithium

Interaction, mechanism, importance and management

There is very little information about the interaction of these diuretics with lithium. A short-term study on 6 subjects given lithium and acetazolamide demonstrated a 27–31% increase in the urinary excretion of lithium, whereas chlormerodrin had no effect.[1] This same study indicated that spironolactone had no effect on the excretion of lithium[1] whereas in another report,[2] this diuretic is said to have markedly increased the excretion of sodium and lithium. Triamterene administered to 2 patients taking lithium while on a low salt diet is also reported to have lead to a strong lithium diuresis.[2] However, none of these reports gives a clear indication of the probable outcome of using these diuretics in patients on lithium, but they emphasise the need to monitor the response to concurrent use carefully.

References
1 Thomsen K and Schou M. Renal lithium excretion in man. *Amer J Physiol* (1968) **215**, 823.
2 Baer L, Platman S and Fieve R R. Lithium and diuretics. *Symp. Rec Advan Psychological Depressive Illness*, p. 49. Williams A, Katz B and Shield D (eds). DHEW Publication (1972).

Lithium carbonate + diazepam

Summary

An isolated case has been reported of serious hypothermia during concurrent treatment with lithium and diazepam.

Interaction

A mentally retarded patient who showed occasional hypothermic episodes (below 35°C) while taking lithium and diazepam, showed no hypothermia on either drug alone. During a test of this interaction and after taking both drugs for 17 days (lithium 1 g and diazepam 30 mg daily) the patient showed a temperature fall from 35·4 to 32°C over 2 h and became comatose with reduced reflexes, dilated pupils, a systolic pressure of between 40 and 60 mmHg, a pulse rate of 40, and no piloerector response.[1]

Mechanism:
Unknown

Importance and management

Since hypothermia is potentially fatal this is clearly an important interaction if it occurs. Only one case has been reported and its general incidence is not known, but it would be prudent to watch for this interaction during concurrent treatment. There seems to be no evidence of an adverse interaction with other benzodiazepines.

Reference
1 Naylor G J and McHarg A Profound hypothermia on combined lithium carbonate and diazepam treatment. *Br Med J* (1977) **3**, 22.

Lithium carbonate + flupenthixol

Summary

Marked parkinsonian symptoms developed in a woman on lithium who was given flupenthixol, but whether this was the result of an interaction or just a toxic response to flupenthixol is not known.

Interaction, mechanism, importance and management

A psychotic woman on lithium carbonate (serum levels of 0·9 mEq/l) was additionally given 75 mg flupenthixol decanoate over a 6-week period. A few days after the last 20 mg dose, marked parkinsonian symptoms, especially akinesia, developed, but disappeared after withdrawal of both drugs. Extrapyramidal side-effects are not uncommon with flupenthixol but whether the lithium had any part to play in this reaction is unknown.

Reference
1 West A. Adverse effects of lithium treatment. *Br Med J* (1977) **2**, 642.

Lithium carbonate + frusemide or ethacrynic acid

Summary

Five cases have been described of lithium intoxication apparently induced by the concurrent use of frusemide. It seems possible that ethacrynic acid could interact similarly.

Interaction

A patient controlled on 900 mg lithium carbonate daily developed lithium intoxication when concurrently treated with frusemide.[1]

Severe lithium toxicity has also been described in 3 other patients who were concurrently treated with frusemide.[2-4] A further patient became intoxicated on lithium when concurrently given frusemide, digoxin and quinidine for congestive heart failure. Sodium intake was also restricted.[1]

Mechanism

Not fully understood. The development of lithium toxicity in the presence of frusemide would seem to be related to the rise in serum levels which can follow sodium depletion (see p. 351) associated with this diuretic. As with the thiazides (p. 352) an interaction of this kind would not be expected to be immediate, but would take a few days to develop. This might explain why a study in 6 subjects given a single dose of lithium failed to demonstrate any effect on the urinary excretion of lithium after the administration of frusemide.[5]

Importance and management

The documentation is sparse and the interaction is not fully established, but there are enough data to make it highly imprudent to administer frusemide to patients stabilized on lithium, unless the serum lithium levels can be very closely monitored and dosage adjustments made where necessary. Ethacrynic acid also causes sodium loss and may possibly interact similarly, but this requires confirmation. More study is required.

References

1 Hurtig H I and Dyson W L. Lithium toxicity enhanced by diuresis. *New Eng J Med* (1974) **290**, 748.
2 Thornton W E and Pray B J. Lithium intoxication. A report of two cases *Canad Psychiat Ass J* (1975) **20**, 281.
3. Oh, T E. Frusemide and lithium toxicity. *Anaesth Intens Care* (1977) **5**, 60.
4 Johnson G F. Lithium neurotoxicity. *Aust NZ J Psychiat* (1976) **10**, 33.
5. Thomsen K and Schou M. Renal lithium excretion in man. *Amer J Physiol* (1968) **215**, 823.

Lithium carbonate + haloperidol

Summary

Although serious adverse reactions have been described in patients treated with lithium carbonate and haloperidol, there is ample evidence that concurrent use can be uneventful and therapeutically valuable.

Interaction

Four patients with acute mania who were treated with 1500–1800 mg lithium carbonate a day and high doses of haloperidol (up to 45 mg/day), developed encephalopathic syndromes (lethargy, fever, tremulousness, confusion, extrapyramidal and cerebellar dysfunction) accompanied by leukocytosis and elevated levels of serum enzymes, blood urea nitrogen and fasting blood sugar.[1] Two of them suffered irreversible widespread brain damage and the two others were left with persistent dyskinesias.

A woman patient was observed with neuromuscular symptoms, impaired consciousness and hyperthermia after 12 days' treatment with 1500 mg lithium carbonate and 40 mg haloperidol a day. She recovered fully and uneventfully.[2]

Three patients, two of them oligophrenic, who were given 1800 mg lithium carbonate with 10–20 mg haloperidol by injection for 10 days, 27 h and 24 h respectively developed what are described as hypertonic–hypokinetic and extrapyramidal syndromes. All recovered.[3]

In contrast to these reports of adverse reactions in 8 patients, there are others describing successful and uneventful use. Cohen and Cohen who first described this interaction[1] have also written that '. . . at least 50 other patients have been similarly treated without reported adverse effects'.[1] They also say that 'a survey of the experiences of leading experts indicate that although hundreds of patients have been treated with various regimens of combined lithium carbonate/haloperidol, there have been no previous observations of substantial irreversible brain damage or persistent dyskinesia'. A retrospective search of Danish hospital records by other workers similarly showed that 425 patients had been treated with both drugs and none of them had developed this adverse reaction.[4]

Mechanism
Not understood.

Importance and management
It is clear that this drug combination is by no means contraindicated, but it would be prudent to bear in mind the possibility of this interaction if both drugs are used together, and to monitor the effects carefully. The Danish investigators offered the opinion that 'the combination of lithium and haloperidol is therapeutically useful when administered to diagnostically appropriate patients. To discourage or prohibit its use would, in our opinion, be injudicious, but treatment must be carried out under proper clinical control.'[4] This implies close monitoring.

References
1 Cohen W J and Cohen N H Lithium carbonate, haloperidol, and irreversible brain damage. *J Amer Med Ass* (1974) **230**, 1283.
2 Thornton W E and Pray B J. Lithium intoxication: a report of two cases. *Canad Psychiat Ass J* (1975) **20**, 281.
3 Marhold J, Zimanova J, Lachman M, Král J and Vojtechovsky M. To the incompatibility of haloperidol with lithium salts. *Acta Nerv Super (Praha)* (1974) **16**, 199.
4 Baastrup P C, Hollnagel P, Sørensen R and Schou M. Adverse reactions in treatment with lithium carbonate and haloperidol. *J Amer Med Ass* (1976) **236**, 2645.
5 Loudon J B and Waring H Toxic reactions to lithium and haloperidol. *Lancet* (1976) **ii**, 1088.
6 Juhl R P, Tsuang M T and Perry P J. Concomitant administration of haloperidol and lithium carbonate in acute mania. *Dis Nerv Syst* (1977) **38**, 675.

Lithium + indomethacin, diclofenac or ibuprofen

Summary
Serum lithium levels may rise during concurrent treatment with indomethacin, diclofenac or ibuprofen. Whether other antirheumatic compounds which inhibit prostaglandin synthesis interact similarly is not known.

Interaction
A single-blind study on 5 subjects taking constant daily doses of lithium carbonate (300–900 mg daily) showed that when they were concurrently treated with indomethacin (50 mg three times a day), the serum levels of lithium gradually rose until at the end of a 7-day test period they were elevated by 43%. Renal clearance fell by 31%. In an identical test on 1 subject given 400 mg ibuprofen three times a day the changes were found to be similar.[1]

Similar rises in plasma lithium levels during the use of indomethacin have been described in other reports,[2,4] and a somewhat smaller rise during the use of diclofenac.[3]

Mechanism
Not understood.

Importance and management
Information about this interaction is limited. Very few subjects were examined and the tests were of short duration; nevertheless the size of the increase in plasma lithium levels indicates that they may be of importance. Serum lithium levels should be monitored if any of these antirheumatic drugs is added to an established regimen. It is not known whether other non-steroidal antirheumatic drugs interact similarly.

Reference
1 Leftwich R B, Walker L A, Regheb M, Oates J A and Frölich J C. Inhibition of prostaglandin synthesis increases plasma lithium levels. *Clin Res* (1978) **26**, 291A.
2 Reimann I W, Leftwich R, Rhageb M and Frölich J C. Indomethacin increases plasma lithium. *Navenschmied Arch Pharmacol* (1980) **311**, R72.
3 Reimann I W. Risks of non-steroidal anti-inflammatory drug therapy in lithium treated patients. *Navenschmied Arch Pharmacol* (1980) **311**, R75.
4 Frölich J C, Leftwich R, Rhageb M, Oates J A, Riemann I and Buchanan D. Indomethacin increases plasma lithium. *Brit Med J* (1979) **2**, 1115.

Lithium carbonate + mazindol

Summary
An isolated case report describes lithium intoxication caused by the concurrent use of mazindol.

Interaction, mechanism, importance and management

A manic-depressive woman controlled for over a year on lithium carbonate (300 mg three times a day), and with serum lithium levels within the normal therapeutic range, showed signs of lithium intoxication within 3 days of starting to take 2 mg mazindol daily. Six days later she had developed twitching, limb rigidity, muscle fasciculation and was both dehydrated and stuporose. Her serum lithium levels were found to have risen to 3·2 mmol/l. The mechanism of this interaction is not understood. Although this is an isolated case report, the rapidity of the response and its potentially serious outcome indicate that these two drugs should only be given concurrently under extremely close supervision. More study is required.

Reference
1 Hendy M S, Dove A F and Arblaster P G. Mazindol-induced lithium toxicity. Br Med J (1980) 1, 684.

Lithium carbonate + methyldopa

Summary
Three cases of lithium toxicity have been reported, apparently induced by the concurrent administration of methyldopa.

Interaction

A manic-depressive woman adequately controlled for 5 years with 0·9 g lithium carbonate daily (serum levels of about 1·0 mEq/l) was hospitalized because signs of manic decompensation were beginning to occur. Later she was discharged on a daily regimen of 1·8 g lithium carbonate and 1 g methyldopa for hypertension. Despite serum levels of 0·5–0·7 mEq/l, signs of lithium toxicity were seen (blurred vision, hand tremors, diarrhoea, confusion and minimal slurring of speech). The methyldopa was therefore withdrawn and the lithium dosage reduced to 1·5 g daily. Ten days later her serum lithium was 1·4 mEq/l and accordingly the dosage was reduced to the original levels of 0·9 g daily to achieve a stable serum level of 1·0 mEq/l.[1]

A manic-depressive woman controlled for almost 3 years on lithium carbonate was additionally administered methyldopa for the treatment of hypertension. Within 2–3 weeks she complained of soreness of the mouth, swelling of the feet, tremor, slurred speech and ataxia. Both drugs were discontinued. After 2 days the serum lithium value was 1·5 mmol/l; after seven days 0·4 mmol/l; and after 11 days 0·1 mmol/l. By this time the ataxia and tremor had disappeared but the slurred speech remained. After 3 weeks all signs of toxicity had gone.[2]

A man with serious hypertension treated with 750 mg methyldopa daily began to show sluggish and apathetic behaviour within 2 days of starting to take lithium. He also showed hyperactivity of the extremities, tremors and fasciculation. The neuromuscular symptoms vanished when the lithium was withdrawn.[3]

Mechanism

Not understood. One suggestion[2] is that the methyldopa reduced the renal excretion of the lithium, thereby allowing the serum concentrations to rise to toxic levels. However, signs of intoxication remained even after the serum levels had fallen to therapeutic concentrations. Another suggestion is that the methyldopa increases the uptake of lithium into the brain.[3]

Importance and management

Although the documentation of this interaction appears to be limited to these three reports, the potentially serious outcome of this interaction indicates that any patient administered both drugs should be closely monitored for changes in serum lithium levels. There is some very limited evidence that the toxic effects may not necessarily result from elevated serum lithium levels.[4] More study is needed.

References

1 Byrd G J. Methyldopa and lithium carbonate: suspected interaction. *J Amer med Ass* (1975) **233**, 320.

2 O'Regan J B. Adverse interaction of lithium carbonate and methyldopa *Can Med Ass J* (1976) **115**, 385.

3 Osanloo E and Deglin J H. Interaction of lithium and methyldopa. *Ann Intern Med* (1980) **92**, 433.

4 Walker N, White K, Tornatore F, Boyd J L and Cohen J L. Lithium–methyldopa interactions in normal subjects. *Drug Intell Clin Pharm* (1980) **14**, 638.

Lithium + phenytoin

Summary

An isolated case report describes lithium toxicity apparently due to the concurrent use of phenytoin.

Interaction, mechanism, importance and management

A patient with a long history of depression and convulsions was treated with increasing doses of lithium carbonate and phenytoin over a period of about 12 years. Although the serum levels of both drugs remained within the therapeutic range, he eventually began to manifest thirst, polydipsia, polyuria and tremor which disappeared when the phenytoin was replaced by carbamazepine. The patient claimed that he felt normal for the first time in many years. The mechanism of this interaction, if such it is, is unknown. One suggested possibility is that the patient improved because carbamazepine has antidiuretic actions,[2] but this would not seem to be borne out by other evidence.[3] No general conclusions about the advisability of giving these two drugs together can be based on a single report but prescribers should be aware of this adverse reaction.[1]

Reference

1 MacCallum W A G. Interaction of lithium and phenytoin. *Br Med J* (1980) **280**, 10.

2 Perucca E and Richens A. Interaction between carbamazepine and lithium. *Brit Med J* (1980) **280**, 863.

3 Ghose K. Interaction between lithium and carbamazepine. *Brit Med J* (1980) **280**, 1122.

Lithium carbonate + potassium iodide

Summary

The hypothyroidic and goitrogenic effects of lithium carbonate and potassium iodide (and possibly other iodides as well) may be additive if the two drugs are used concurrently

Interaction

A patient who had been receiving lithium carbonate for over 2 years for mania and depression developed the signs and symptoms of hypothyroidism which gradually resolved once the lithium was withdrawn, but recurred when later treated with potassium iodide.[1]

A euthyroid man showed evidence of hypothyroidism after receiving 3 weeks' treatment with lithium carbonate (750–1500 mg daily). After 2 further weeks' treatment with potassium iodide as well, the hypothyroidism became even more marked, but it resolved completely within a fortnight of the withdrawal of both drugs.[1]

There are a number of other reports describing this antithyroidic effect of lithium when given on its own,[2,3,8–10] as well as with potassium iodide.[4,5] There is also a case on record involving lithium, isopropamide iodide and haloperidol.[6]

Mechanism

Lithium carbonate accumulates in the thyroid

and blocks the release of the thyroid hormones by thyroid-stimulating hormone. Precisely how this is achieved is not fully understood, but it has been suggested that it involves some inhibition of adenyl cyclase which is necessary for the synthesis of cyclic AMP which, in its turn, causes the release of the thyroid hormones.

Potassium iodide temporarily prevents the production of the thyroid hormones but, as time goes on, synthesis recommences because the amount of iodine being transported into the gland falls.

Thus, both lithium ions and iodide ions can depress the production or the release of the thyroid hormones and, as a result, generalized hypothyroidism can occur to an extent which is greater than would be seen with either drug on its own.

Importance and management
The importance and the frequency of this interaction are not easy to assess. Hypothyroidism due to lithium treatment is not infrequent: 12 out of 330 patients are said in one report[2] to have developed goitres; 20 out of 93 women and 2 out of 56 men

are described in another report[9] as having developed hypothyroidism. However there are relatively few reports of hypothyroidism due to the concurrent use of both drugs. It is clear that any patient taking both should certainly be observed for signs of hypothyroidism.

References
1 Shopsin B, Shenkman L, Blum M, and Hollander C S. Iodine and lithium-induced hypothyroidism. documentation of synergism. *Amer J Med* (1973) **55**, 695.
2 Schou, M, Amdisen A, Jensen S E and Olsen T. Occurrence of goitre during lithium treatment. *Br Med J* (1968) **3**, 710.
3 Shopsin B, Blum M and Gershon S. Lithium-induced thyroid disturbance: case report and review *Compr Psychiatry* (1969) **10**, 215.
4 Jorgensen J V, Brandrup F, Schroll M. Possible synergism between iodine and lithium carbonate. *J Amer Med Ass* (1973) **223**, 192.
5 Wiener J D. Lithium carbonate-induced myxedema. *J Amer Med Ass* (1972) **220**, 587.
6 Luby E D, Schwartz D and Rosenbaum H. Lithium carbonate-induced myxedema. *J Amer Med Ass* (1971) **218**, 1298.
7 Emerson C H, Dyson W L and Utiger R D. Serum thyrotropin and thyroxine concentrations in patients receiving lithium carbonate. *J Clin Endocrinol Metab* (1973) **36**, 338.
8 Candy J. Severe hypothyroidism—an early complication of lithium therapy. *Br Med J* (1972) **3**, 277.
9 Villeneuve A., Grantier J, Jus A and Perron D. Effect of lithium on thyroid in man. *Lancet* (1973) **ii**, 502.
10 Lloyde G.G. Rosser R. M. and Crowe M J. Effect of lithium on thyroid in man. *Lancet* (1973) **ii**, 619.

Lithium bicarbonate + sodium carbonate or chloride

Summary
Serum lithium levels are affected by the intake of sodium. The ingestion of marked amounts of sodium bicarbonate or chloride can prevent the establishment of adequate serum lithium levels. Conversely, dietary sodium restriction may result in an increase in serum lithium to toxic concentrations if not adequately controlled.

Interaction
Lithium response reduced by the presence of sodium:

A depressive man, initially given 250 mg lithium carbonate four times a day, achieved a serum lithium level of 0·5 mEq/l by the following morning. When the dosage was progressively increased to 250 mg, five, and later six times a day, the serum lithium levels failed to exceed 0·6 mEq/l because, unknown to his doctor, he was also taking sodium bicarbonate. In the words of the patient's wife: '. . . he's been taking soda bic for years for an ulcer, doctor, but since he started on that lithium he's been shovelling it in . . .'. Once the sodium bicarbonate was stopped, relatively stable serum lithium levels of 0·8 mEq/l were achieved on a dosage of 250 mg lithium carbonate four times a day.[1]

An investigation carried out to find out why a number of inpatients failed to reach, or maintain, adequate therapeutic lithium serum levels, revealed that a clinic nurse had been giving the patients doses of a proprietary effervescent saline drink (*Efferdex*) used for 'upset stomachs' containing about 50% w/w sodium bicarbonate, because the patients complained of nausea. The depression in the expected serum lithium levels was as much as 40% in some cases.[6]

Eight manic depressives and one schizophrenic were satisfactorily controlled on lithium carbonate, 2·7 g, and sodium chloride, 1·5–3·0 g, daily, with serum lithium levels ranging from 0·55–1·03 mEq/l. One of them developed signs of lithium toxicity 4 weeks after the salt supplement had been withdrawn, and another showed similar symptoms

$1\frac{1}{2}$ weeks after starting treatment with lithium, but they vanished when salt supplement was added.[4]

Lithium response increased by sodium restriction

A clinical study on 4 manic-depressive patients treated with lithium carbonate showed that serum lithium levels rose more rapidly and to a higher peak when given during salt restriction than when taking a dietary salt supplement.[2]

It is claimed in a report on 7 patients who had been given a salt substitute containing lithium chloride used for flavouring and who subsequently developed lithium intoxication, that susceptibility to the toxicity appeared to be increased by the extent of the dietary salt restriction.[7]

A manic-depressive woman, successfully controlled on 900 mg lithium carbonate daily for 6 years, developed lithium toxicity within a week of being treated for moderate congestive heart failure with digoxin, quinidine, frusemide and sodium restriction. Her serum lithium carbonate level had risen to $3 \cdot 05$ mEq/l.[5]

Mechanism

Lithium is eliminated from the body almost exclusively in the urine. The proximal tubule does not readily distinguish between sodium and lithium ions and reabsorbs 60–70% of the filtered load. A possible explanation of the interference by sodium ions with the excretion of lithium is that during sodium depletion, the extracellular volume of the body is contracted so that both ions are maximally reabsorbed, leading to an increased retention of the lithium. Conversely when the sodium levels in the body are high (due to the use of a salt supplement, for example) the extracellular volume is expanded and both sodium and lithium will be excreted rather than reabsorbed. Beyond the proximal tubule, lithium and sodium appear to be handled quite differently, but in any case lithium reabsorption is relatively small so that any interference by sodium is likely to be equally small.[3,8]

Importance and management

A well-established and important interaction. The establishment of adequate serum lithium levels can be jeopardized, as the case histories cited show, if the intake of ionic sodium is uncontrolled. Sodium bicarbonate comes in various guises and disguises (e.g. *Efferdex* (50%), *Eno's fruit salts* (56%), *Andrews Liver Salts* ($22 \cdot 6$), *Bismarex Antacid Powder* (65%), *BiSoDol Powder* (58%)). There are many similar preparations available throughout the world. Patients should seek informed advice if they feel the need to take an antacid while receiving lithium.

Since salt restriction in patients already stabilized on lithium carbonate can lead to the development of toxicity, the appearance of any of the premonitory signs (drowsiness, coarse tremor, slurred speech, loss of appetite, vomiting or diarrhoea) is an indication that serum lithium determinations should be carried out at once.

References

1 Arthur R K. Lithium levels and 'Soda Bic'. *Med J Aust* (1975) 2, 918.
2 Platman S F and Fieve R R. Lithium retention and excretion. *Arch Gen. Psychiat* (1969) 20, 285.
3 Thomsen K and Schou M. Renal lithium excretion in man. *Am J Physiol* (1968) 215, 823.
4 Bleiweiss H. Salt supplements with lithium. *Lancet* (1970) i, 416.
5 Hurtig H I and Dyson W L. Lithium toxicity enhanced by diuresis. *New Eng J Med* (1974) 290, 748.
6 McSwiggan C. Interaction of lithium and bicarbonate. *Med J Aust* (1978) 1, 38.
7 Corcoran A C, Taylor R D and Page I H. Lithium poisoning from the use of salt substitutes. *J Am Med Ass* (1949) 139, 685.
8 Singer I and Rotenberg D. Mechanisms of lithium action. *New Eng J Med* (1973) 289, 254.

Lithium carbonate + thiazides or related diuretics

Summary

Serum lithium concentrations can be increased by the concurrent use of thiazide diuretics, chlorthalidone or bumetanide. Lithium intoxication can develop.

Interaction

A patient being treated with lithium carbonate showed a rise in serum lithium concentrations from about $1 \cdot 3$ to $2 \cdot 0$ mEq/l each time he was administered 500 mg chlorothiazide a day.[4]

Two patients controlled on lithium carbonate (1200 mg daily) showed a fall in the urinary excretion of lithium accompanied by a rise in serum levels within a few days of taking 1 g chlorothiazide each day.[6]

A study carried out on 22 patients showed that long-term treatment with either hydroflumethiazide (25 mg daily) plus KCl (3·4 g daily) or benzofluazide (2·5 mg daily) led to a 24% reduction in the urinary excretion of lithium.[2]

Lithium toxicity arising from the use of thiazide diuretics given in conjuction with other diuretics has also been seen with *Moduretic* (hydrochloro-thiazide + amiloride)[1] *Aldactazide* (hydrochloro-thiazide + spironolactone)[3] and chlorothiazide with spironolactone and amiloride.[7] Chlorthali-done[9] and bumetanide[10] have also been respon-sible for the development of lithium toxicity.

Mechanism

Not fully understood. The rise in serum lithium levels would seem to result from the reduced urinary excretion already quoted.[2] The interac-tion appears to take place despite the fact that the thiazides and similar diuretics exert their major diuretic actions in the distal part of the kidney tubule, whereas lithium is reabsorbed in the proximal part.

The reason for this could be that the diuresis is accompanied by the loss of sodium. Within a few days this loss is compensated by the retention of sodium, this time in the proximal tubule. Since both sodium and lithium ions are treated virtually indistinguishably, the increased reabsorption of the sodium would include lithium as well, hence a significant and measurable reduction in its excre-tion.

This is clearly a long-term rather than an immediate effect and it is interesting to note that a short-term single-dose experiment in man with bendrofluazide and lithium failed to show any effect of the thiazide on lithium excretion[5] which is compatible with this proposed mechanism.

Importance and management

An established and potentially serious interac-tion. Thiazides and related diuretics should not be given to patients stabilized on lithium unless the serum lithium levels can be closely monitored and appropriate dosage adjustments made. However, under controlled conditions concurrent use has been advocated[8] for certain psychiatric condi-tions, and for the control of lithium-induced nephrogenic diabetes mellitus.

References

1 Macfie A C. Lithium poisoning precipitated by Diuretics. *Br Med J* (1975) **1**, 516.
2 Petersen V, Hvidt S, Thomsen K and Schou M. Effect of prolonged thiazide treatment on renal lithium excretion. *Br Med J* (1974) **2**, 143.
3 Lutz E G. Lithium toxicity precipitates by diuretics. *J Med Soc New Jersey* (1975) **72**, 439.
4 Levy S T, Forrest J N, and Heninger G R. Lithium-induced diabetes insipidus: manic symptoms, brain and electrolyte correlates, and chlorothiazide treatment. *Amer J. Psychiat* (1973) **130**, 1014.
5 Thomsen K and Schou M. Renal lithium excretion in man *Amer. J Physiol* (1968) **215**, 823.
6 Baer L, Platman S and Fieve R K. Lithium and diuretics. *Recent advances in the Psychobiology of the Depressive Illnesses*, p. 49. Williams, Katz and Shield (eds) (1972). DHEW Publications.
7 Basdevant A, Beaufils M and Corvol P. Influence des diuretiques sur l'elimination renale du lithium *Nouv Pressé med* (1976) **5**, 2085.
8 Himmelhoch J M, Forrest J, Neil J and Detre T P. Thiazide–lithium synergy in refractory mood swings. *Am J Psychiat* (1977) **134**, 149.
9 Solomon J G. Lithium toxicity precipitated by a diuretic. *Psychosomatics* (1980) **21**, 425.
10 Kerry R J, Ludlow J M and Owen G. Diuretics are dangerous with lithium. *Brit Med J* (1980) **281**, 371.

CHAPTER 16. MONOAMINE OXIDASE INHIBITOR DRUG INTERACTIONS

The observation that patients under treatment for tuberculosis with isoniazid, and more particularly with iproniazid, showed some degree of mood elevation, prompted the development and examination of other drugs which similarly showed inhibitory activity against the enzyme monoamine oxidase (MAO) and, as hoped, they proved to be effective in the treatment of psychotic and neurotic depression. Postural hypotension was noted as one of the side-effects of antidepressant therapy with iproniazid and, as a result, pheniprazine and later pargyline were introduced as antihypertensive agents. Table 16.1 is a list of the MAO inhibitors which are currently available for the treatment of depression or hypertension, as well as those which have been withdrawn.

Table 16.1. Monoamine oxidase inhibitors

Non-proprietary names	Proprietary names
Benmoxin	*Neuralex*
Etryptamine	*Monase*
Iproclozide	*Sursum*
Isocarboxazid	*Marplan*
Mebanazine	*Actomol*
Nialamide	*Niamid*
Phenelzine	*Nardil*
Phenelzine with penta-erythritol tetranitrate	*Perifenil*
Pheniprazine	*Cavodil*
Phenoxypropazine	*Drazine*
Pivhydrazine	*Tersavid*
Tranylcypromine	*Parnate*
Tranylcypromine with trifluoperazine	*Parstelin*

Furazolidone also possesses MAO inhibitory properties.
Some of the MAOI listed have been superseded.

The role of monoamine oxidase

The arrival of a nerve impulse at the end of a nerve causes the release of a small amount of chemical transmitter which, after diffusing to the receptors of the next nerve or organ, stimulates the response (Fig. 16.1). Adrenergic neurones synthesize their transmitter (noradrenaline–norepinephrine) from tyrosine by a series of biochemical steps, and this is then stored in vesicles at the nerve endings (although in the diagrams these vesicles are shown as a single 'pool' of noradrenaline). The enzyme MAO is found associated with this store of noradrenaline, its function apparently

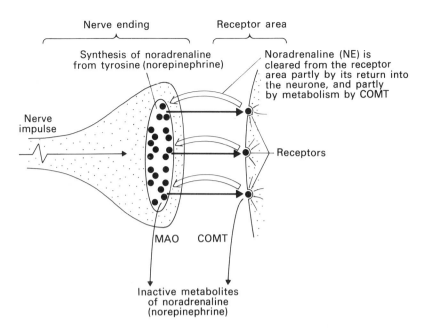

Fig. 16.1. A highly simplified diagrammatic representation of an amine-releasing (noradrenaline–norepinephrine, or 5-HT) neurone. The amine (●) which is released from the 'pool' at the nerve ending by the arrival of a nerve impulse diffuses across to the receptor and effects stimulation. The receptors are then cleared in readiness for further stimulation by the return of the amine into the neurone. A small amount is destroyed by the enzyme COMT.

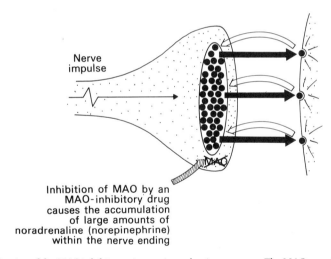

Fig. 16.2. Mode of action of the MAO inhibitors at an amine-releasing neurone. The MAO associated with the 'pool' of amine at the nerve ending is inhibited so that the amount of amine available for release by the nerve impulse is increased.

being to limit the amount of transmitter present. To use a crude analogy, the synthesis of the transmitter represents a dripping tap with the MAO acting as an enzymic leak, so that a constant level of noradrenaline is maintained. MAO is to be found in other types of neurone in the brain which use dopamine or 5-HT as transmitters where its function is essentially the same.

MAO is also found in other parts of the body, and in particularly high concentrations in the liver and gut where it acts as a protective detoxifying agent against tyramine, and possibly other potentially hazardous amines which can occur in foods which have undergone bacterial degradation. For this reason MAO was originally called tyramine oxidase.

Mode of action of the MAO-inhibitory drugs

Most of the MAO inhibitors (MAOI) inactivate MAO by forming a stable complex with the enzyme, the prime target being the MAO within the neurones of the brain. Since the normal transmitter synthesis continues unchecked but the enzymic 'leak' is blocked, the concentration of noradrenaline (and other amines in the cells) rises (see Fig. 16.2), and it is thought that the mood-elevating or antidepressant activity of the MAOI is associated with this rise. Perhaps depression represents some inadequacy in transmission between neurones in the brain? This is certainly borne out by the observation that drugs which deplete neurones of their transmitter (e.g. reserpine) can induce depression in normal individuals. Increased levels of the transmitter might therefore account for the relief of depresssion.

The effects of the MAOI are not, however, confined to the brain. The MAO in the gut and liver is also inactivated. So too is the MAO within the sympathetic nervous system, so that large amounts of noradrenaline accumulate at nerve endings and this accounts for some of the interactions with the sympathomimetic amines. Most of the MAOI also cause irreversible enzyme inhibition, resynthesis of the enzyme only taking place relatively slowly, so that the beneficial effects as well as some of the interactions can still occur up to 2–3 weeks after withdrawal of the drug. Tranylcypromine differs in being a reversible inhibitor of MAO and the onset and disappearance of its actions are much quicker than the other MAO inhibitors.

In addition to the interactions of the monoamine oxidase inhibitors described in this chapter, there are others dealt with elsewhere. A full list is to be found in the index.

Monoamine oxidase inhibitors + anticholinergics

Summary
The alleged enhancement of the effects of the anticholinergics by the MAOI in man appears to be unconfirmed.

Interaction, mechanism, importance and management
Although some books and lists of drug interactions state that the effects of the anticholinergic drugs used in the treatment of Parkinson's disease are increased by the concurrent use of the MAOI, there appears to be little or no documentary evidence describing this interaction in man, although a hyperthermic reaction has been reported in animals.[1]

Reference
1 Pedersen V and Nielsen I M. Hyperthermia in rabbits caused by interaction between MAOI's, antiparkinson drugs, and neuroleptics. *Lancet* (1975) i, 409.

Monoamine oxidase inhibitors + alcoholic drinks

Summary

Alcohol does not appear to interact with the MAOI but a serious hypertensive reaction is possible if the drink contains sufficient tyramine.

Interaction, mechanism, importance and management

No interaction seems to occur between the ethyl alcohol of alcoholic drinks and the MAOI, but a severe hypertensive reaction of the kind described in page 370 can occur if the tyramine content is high enough.

A dose of 10–25 mg tyramine is required before a serious rise in blood pressure is caused (see p. 371). The table below gives the tyramine content of various drinks analysed by two groups of workers and shows that some samples of Italian chianti, and ale and beer of Canadian origin can be relatively tyramine-rich and, in quite moderate quantities, could certainly represent a hazard to patients on MAOI. About 400 ml of one sample of chianti and roughly a litre (about 2 pints) of the samples of Canadian ale or beer analysed contained enough tyramine to reach the 10–25 mg threshold dosage.

Table 16.2 can be used as a broad general guide when advising patients on whether and what they may drink, but it should be emphasized that this table is not, and cannot be, an absolute guide because all alcoholic drinks are the end-product of a biological fermentation process and no two batches are ever absolutely identical.

References

1 Horwitz D, Lovenberg W, Engelman K and Sjoerdsma A. Monoamine oxidase inhibitors, tyramine, and cheese. *J Amer Med Ass* (1964) **188**, 1108.
2 Sen N P. Analysis and significance of tyramine in foods. *J Food Sci* (1969) **34**, 127.

Table 16.2. The tyramine content of some drinks

Drink	Tyramine (μg/ml)	Ref.
Ale (Canada)	8·8	1
Beer (USA)	1·8, 2·3, 4·4	1
Beer (Canada)	6·4, 11·1, 11·2	2
Champagne (Canada)	0·2 0·6	2
Chianti (Italy)	1·76, 12·2, 10·36, 25·4	1,2
Port	0·2	1
Reisling	0·6	1
Sauterne	0·4	1
Sherry (USA)	3·6	1
Sherry (Canada)	0·2	2
Table wine, red (Canada)	0	2
Table wine, white (Canada)	0·5	2
Wine, red (Italy)	0·4, 0·6	2

Monoamine oxidase inhibitors + barbiturates

Summary

Although the MAOI can enhance and prolong the activity of barbiturates *in animals*, only a few isolated cases have been described in man. Mebanazine appears not to interact.

Interaction

Kline has stated, without giving details, that on three or four occasions patients in his care who were taking an MAOI continued, without his knowledge, to take their usual barbiturate hypnotic and thereby '... unknowingly raised their dose of barbiturate by five to ten times, and as a consequence barely managed to stagger through the day.'[3]

A patient taking tranylcypromine was inadvertently given 250 mg sodium amylobarbitone intramuscularly for sedation. Within an hour she became ataxic, fell to the floor repeatedly hitting her head. After complaining of nausea and dizziness the patient became semicomatose and remained in that state for a further 36 h. To what extent the head trauma played a part is uncertain.[5]

Two other cases of coma attributed to concurrent use have been described.[6,7]

In contrast mebanazine is reported not to have enhanced the hypnotic activities of quinalbarbitone or butobarbitone in a number of patients, nor was there evidence of a 'hangover' effect.[8]

Mechanism

Unknown. Experiments in animals[1,2,4] suggest that the MAOI can have a general inhibitory action on the liver microsomal enzymes thereby enhancing and prolonging the activity of the barbiturates, but whether this also occurs in man occasionally, and why, is not known.

Importance and management

There appears to be little well-documented evidence that concurrent use of MAOI and barbiturates need be avoided although the existence of the cases cited indicate that some caution is appropriate. Mebanazine appears not to interact with quinalbarbitone or butobarbitone.

References

1 Wulfsohn N L and Politzer W M. 5-Hydroxytryptamine in anaesthesia. *Anaesthesia* (1962) 17, 64.
2 Lechat P. and Lemergnan A. Monoamineoxydase inhibitors and the potentiation of experimental sleep. *Biochem Phamacol* (1961) 8, 8.
3 Kline N S. Psychopharmaceuticals: effects and side effects. *Bull WHO* (1959) 21, 397.
4 Buchel L and Levy J. Mecanisme des phenomenes de synergie due sommeil experimental. II. Etude des associations iproniazide–hypnotiques, chez le rat et la souris. *Arch Sci Rech Sci Physiol* (1965) 19, 161.
5 Domino E F, Sullivan T S and Luby E D. Barbituate intoxication in a patient treated with a MAO inhibitor. *Amer J Psychiat.* (1962) 118, 941.
6 Etherington L. Personal communication (1973).
7 MacLeod I. Fatal reaction to phenelzine. *Br Med J* (1965) 1, 1554.
8 Gilmour S J G Clinical trial of mebanazine—a new monoamine oxidase inhibitor. *Br J Psychiat* (1965) 111, 899.

Monoamine oxidase inhibitors + benzodiazepines

Summary

Concurrent use of the MAOI and benzodiazepines is usually safe and effective but a very small number of adverse reactions (chorea, massive oedema) attributed to an interaction have been reported. The reports are inconclusive.

Interaction

A patient diagnosed as having endogenous depression was given phenelzine, 15 mg, and chlordiazepoxide, 10 mg, three times a day and responded well. 4–5 months later choreiform movements of moderate severity and slight dysarthria developed, both of which subsided when the drugs were withdrawn.[1]

Two patients who were being treated with chlordiazepoxide and an MAOI (one on isocarboxazid and the other on phenelzine) developed severe oedema which was attributed to the use of both drugs.[2,3]

Mechanism

Unknown.

Importance and management

The general picture portrayed by the reports in the literature is that concurrent treatment is usually effective and uneventful.[4–6] The three adverse interaction reports appear to be the exception rather than the rule and it is by no means certain that the responses described were due to a drug interaction rather than to a reaction to one or other of the drugs.

References

1 MacLeod D M. Chorea induced by transquillisers. *Lancet* (1964) i, 388.
2 Goonewardene A and Toghill P J. Gross oedema occurring during treatment for depression. *Br Med J* (1977) 2, 879.
3 Pathak S K. Gross oedema during treatment for depression. *Br Med J* (1977) 2, 1220.
4 Frommer E A. Treatment of childhood depression with antidepressant drugs. *Br Med J* (1967) 1, 729.
5 Mans J. and Senes M. L'isocarboxazide, le RO 5-0690 et

chlordizépoxide, le RO-4-0403 dérivé des thioxanthènes. Etude sur leurs effets propres et leurs possibilités d'association. *J Méd Bord* (1964) **141**, 1909.

6 Suerinck A, and Suerinck E. Etats dépressifs en milieu sana-
torial et inhibiteurs de la mono-amine oxydase. (Résultats therapeutiquespar l'association d'iproclozide et de chlordi-azépoxide). A propos de 146 observations. *J Méd Lyon* (1966) **47**, 573.

Monoamide oxidase inhibitors + beta-blockers

Summary

Despite a warning, no interaction of practical importance appears to have been documented between propranolol and a monoamine oxidase inhibitor.

Interaction, mechanism, importance and management

Although Frieden has stated[1] that 'MAO inhibitors should be discontinued at least 2 weeks prior to the institution of propranolol therapy . . .', experiments in animals[2] using mebanazine as a representative MAO inhibitor failed to show 'any undesirable property of propranolol following MAO inhibition.' There appears to be no clinical evidence with propranolol or any other beta-blocking drug of an adverse interaction with an MAO inhibitor.

References

1 Frieden J. Propranolol as an antiarrhythmic agent. *Am Heart J* (1967) **74**, 283.

2 Barrett A M and Cullum V A. Lack of interaction between propranolol and mebanazine. *J Pharm Pharmacol* (1968) **20**, 911.

Monoamine oxidase inhibitors + caffeine

Summary

A single report claims that the MAOI can enhance the CNS stimulant effects of caffeine in coffee, tea and 'cola' drinks.

Interaction, mechanism, importance and management

It is reported[1] that a patient who normally drank 10 or 12 cups of coffee a day, without adverse effects, experienced extreme jitteriness during treatment with an MAOI which subsided when the coffee consumption was reduced to 2 or 3 cups a day. The same reaction was also observed in other patients on MAOI who drank tea or some of the 'cola' drinks which also contain caffeine. Another patient claimed that a single cup of coffee taken in the morning kept him jittery all day and up the entire night as well, a reaction which occurred on three separate occasions.[1] The reason for this response is obscure.

Apart from this one report[1] and another[2] stating that the effects of caffeine *in mice* are enhanced by the presence of an MAOI, the literature appears otherwise to be silent about this interaction. Whether this reflects its mildness and unimportance, or its rarity, is not clear.

References

1 Kline N S. Psychopharmaceuticals: effects and side effects. *Bull WHO* (1959) **21**, 397.

2 Berkowitz B A, Spector S and Pool W. The interaction of caffeine, theophylline and theobromine with MAOI. *Europ J Pharmacol* (1971) **16**, 315.

Monoamine oxidase inhibitors + carbamazepine

Summary

The theoretical possibility of an MAOI–carbamazepine interaction awaits confirmation.

Interaction, mechanism, importance and management

No interaction has been described, but the manufacturers suggest that due to the close structural similarity of carbamazepine and the tricyclic antidepressants, concurrent use should be avoided.[1]

See the synopsis about the MAOI/tricyclic antidepressant interaction on page 368.

References

1 Galbraith A W, Geigy (UK) Ltd, personal communication (1968).

Monoamine oxidase inhibitors + chloral hydrate

Summary

An isolated case of fatal hyperpyrexia and another of serious hypertension have been attributed to interactions between chloral and phenelzine.

Interactions

Two adverse reaction reports:

A woman being treated with 45 mg phenelzine daily was found in bed by her family in a coma. Her doctor found her deeply comatose with marked muscular rigidity, twitching down one side, and a temperature of 41°C. She died without regaining consciousness. A postmortem did not establish the cause of death, but subsequently it came to light that she had started drinking whisky again (she had been treated for alcoholism), and she had access to chloral hydrate. She may have taken a fatal dose.[1]

A patient under treatment with 45 mg phenelzine daily and chloral hydrate for sleeping, developed an excruciating headache followed by nausea, photophobia, and a substantial rise in blood pressure.[2]

Mechanism

Unknown. There is no obvious explanation for the reaction described in the first report. The second is very similar to the 'cheese reaction' but at the time the authors of the report were unware of this type of reaction so that they failed to find out if any tyramine-rich foods had been eaten on the day of the attack.[2]

Importance and management

There is no clear evidence to show that either of these adverse reactions was due to an interaction between phenelzine and chloral and no other reports to suggest that an interaction between these drugs is normally likely.

References

1 Howarth E. Possible synergistic effects of the new thymoleptics in connection with poisoning. J Ment Sci (1961) 107, 100.
2 Dillon H and Leopold R L. Acute cerebro-vascular symptoms produced by an antidepressant. J Psychiatry (1965) 121, 1012.

Monoamine oxidase inhibitors + dextromethorphan

Summary

Two fatal cases of hyperpyrexia and coma have been reported in patients on phenelzine who ingested dextromethorphan.

Interaction

A woman who was taking 60 mg phenelzine daily drank 2 oz of a cough mixture containing dextromethorphan. Within 30 min she complained of nausea and dizziness before collapsing. She remained hyperpyrexic (42°C), hypotensive (systolic pressure of 70 mmHg) and unconscious for some time before death.[1]

A similar reaction has been described in another report,[2] although in this case the preparation used also contained phenylephrine.

Mechanism

Not understood. A similar interaction (hyperpyrexia, dilated pupils, hyperexcitability and motor restlessness) has been observed in rabbits treated with nialamide, phenelzine and pargyline.[3] The symptoms are similar to those seen in the pethidine/MAOI interaction and it has been suggested that it may similarly result from an enhanced response to 5HT.

Importance and management

Despite the limited amount of information available—two cases in man and associated animal studies—the severity of the reaction indicates that patients on MAOI should not take preparations containing dextromethorphan.

Chlorpromazine antagonizes the development of this interaction in rabbits and has been used successfully in the clinical treatment of the similar pethidine/MAOI interaction, so it may also prove to be useful for this interaction. This awaits confirmation.

References
1 Rivers N and Horner B. Possible lethal reaction between nardil and dextromethorphan. Can med Assoc J (1970) 103, 85.
2 Shamsie J C and Barriga C. The hazards of use of monoamine oxidase inhibitors in disturbed adolescents. Can med Assoc J (1971) 104, 715.
3 Sinclair J G. Dextromethorphan–monoamine oxidase inhibition interaction in rabbits. J Pharm Pharmac (1973) 25, 803.

Monoamine oxidase inhibitors + doxapram

Summary

The therapeutic effects and side-effects of doxapram are said to be enhanced by the concurrent use of MAOI.

Interaction, mechanism, importance and management

On the basis of animal studies which reportedly show that the actions of doxapram are potentiated by pretreatment with MAOI, the manufacturers[1] advise that concurrent use should be undertaken with great care. The adverse cardiovascular effects of doxapram (hypertension, tachycardia, arrhythmias) are said elsewhere[2] to be markedly increased in patients on MAOI, and it is also claimed that the pressor effects are enhanced[3] but no clinical data in support of these statements are cited.

References
1 ABPI Data Sheet Compendium 1979–80, p. 837. Pharmind Publications, London (1979).
2 Esplin D W and Zablocka-Esplin, B. Central nervous stimulants. In The Pharmacological Basis of Therapeutics, 4th edn, p. 355. Goodman L S and Gilman A (eds) Macmillan NY. (1970).
3 Martindale's Extra Pharmacopoeia, 27th edn, p. 309. 27th edn. Wade A (ed) (1977). Pharmaceutical Press, London.

Monoamine oxidase inhibitors + droperidol

Summary

An isolated and unexplained case report describes hypotension in a patient given droperidol and hyoscine 4 days after the withdrawal of phenelzine and perphenazine.

Interaction, mechanism, importance and management

Four days after withdrawal of phenelzine and per-phenazine, prior to surgery, a patient was given operative premedication with 20 mg droperidol and 0·4 mg hyoscine. About 2 h later he was observed to be pale, sweating profusely, and slightly cyanosed. His blood pressure was 75/60 mmHg and pulse rate 60. No excitement or alteration in respiration was seen. The blood pressure gradually rose to 115/80 mmHg over the next 45 min but did not return to the pre-operative figure of 160/100 mmHg for 36 h. Eleven days later (15 days after withdrawing the phenelzine) and with the same premedication, the operation was successfully undertaken without any hypotensive episodes. The response was attributed to the after-effects of the phenelzine treatment[1] but there is no obvious reason for this interaction (if indeed it *is* an interaction).

Reference

1 Penlington G N. Droperidol and monoamine oxidase inhibitors. *Br Med J* (1966) 1, 483.

Monoamine oxidase inhibitors + hypoglycaemic agents

Summary

The hypoglycaemic effects of insulin and the oral hypoglycaemic agents can be enhanced by the concurrent use of the MAOI.

Interaction

A woman diabetic, stabilized on insulin–zinc suspension, exhibited hypoglycaemic sopors and postural syncope when treated with 15–25 mg mebanazine daily, and required a 30% reduction in the dose of insulin (from 48 to 35 units daily) to achieve restabilization. The insulin requirements rose again once the mebanazine was withdrawn.[1]

A study on 35 patients with diabetes showed that the concurrent administration of mebanazine enhanced the hypoglycaemic activity of the insulin, tolbutamide or chlorpropamide with which they were being treated, and improved the control of their diabetes.[2]

There are other reports of an enhanced hypoglycaemic response in diabetics on tolbutamide treated wtih mebanazine.[3–5] A reduction in blood sugar levels has been demonstrated in man in the absence of conventional hypoglycaemic agents with mebanazine,[3] iproniazid,[6] isocarboxazid,[7] and phenelzine.[3] Experiments with animals have demonstrated similar effects.[10–12]

Mechanism

By no means fully understood. One suggestion[9,13] was that the MAOIs impair the activity of the sympathetic nervous system by replacing the normal transmitting substance, noradrenaline (norepinephrine), with a weaker substitute, octopamine. One consequence of this would be that the normal release of adrenaline from the adrenals would be impaired, and therefore the balance between the mutually opposing actions of insulin which lowers blood sugar levels, and those factors which raise them (such as adrenaline) would be upset, The result would be an exaggerated hypoglycaemic overswing. But it now seems much more likely that the MAOI have a direct action on the pancreas to release insulin.[8]

Importance and management

The evidence available shows that the MAOI can benefit the control of blood sugar levels in some diabetic patients, but a reduction in the dosage of the hypoglycaemic agent may be necessary if excessive hypoglycaemia is to be avoided. Some caution is necessary.

Only a few of the possible MAOI/hypoglycaemic agent combinations appear to have been examined, but this interaction would seem possible with any of them. This requires confirmation.

References

1 Cooper A J and Keddie K M G. Hypotensive collapse and hypoglycaemia after mebanazine—a monoamine oxidase inhibitor. *Lancet* (1964) i, 1133.
2 Wickström L and Pettersson K. Treatment of diabetics with monoamine oxidase inhibitors. *Lancet* (1964) ii, 995.
3 Adnitt P I. Hypoglycaemic action of monoamine oxidase inhibitors (MAOI's). *Diabetes* (1968) 17, 628.
4 Cooper A J. The action of mebanazine, a monoamine oxidase inhibitor antidepressant drug in diabetes—part II. *Int J Neuropsychiatry* (1966) 2, 342.
5 Adnitt P I, Oleesky S and Schneiden H. The hypoglycaemic

action of monoamine oxidase inhibitors (MAOI's) *Diabetologia* (1968) **4**, 379.

6 Weiss J, Weiss J and Weiss B. Effects of iproniazid and similar compounds on the gastrointestinal tract. *Ann NY Acad Sci* (1959) **80**, 854.

7 van Praag H M and Leijnse B. The influence of some antidepressives of the hydrazine type on the glucose metabolism in depressed patients. *Clin Chim Acta* (1963) **8**, 466.

8 Bressler R, Vargas-Cordon M and Lebovitz H E. Tranylcypromine: a potent insulin secretagogue and hypoglycaemic agent. *Diabetes* (1968) **17**, 617.

9 Cooper A J and Ashcroft G. Modification of insulin and sulfonylorea hypoglycaemia by monoamine oxidase inhibitor drugs. *Diabetes* (1967) **16**, 272.

10 Cooper A J and Ashcroft G. Potentiation of insulin hypoglycaemia by MAOI antidepressant drugs. *Lancet* (1966) **i**, 407.

11 Mahfouz M, Abdel-Maguid R and El-Dakhakhny M. Potentiation of the hypoglycaemic action of tobutamide by different drugs. *Arzneim-Forsch (Drug Res)* (1970) **20**, 120.

12 Barrett A M. Modification of the hypoglycaemic response to tolbutamide and insulin by mebanazine—an inhibitor of monoamine oxidase. *J Pharm Pharmacol* (1965) **17**, 19.

13 Kopin I J, Fischer J E. Musacchio J M, Horst W D and Weisse V K. False neurotransmitters and the mechanism of sympathetic blockade by monoamine oxidase inhibitors. *J Pharm Exp Ther* (1965) **147**, 186.

Monamine oxidase inhibitors + methadone

Summary

No adverse interaction between methadone and the MAOI has been reported and successful and uneventful concurrent use has been described.

Interaction, mechanism, importance and management

A patient on methadone maintenance therapy (30 mg daily) was successfully and uneventfully treated for depression with tranylcypromine, initially 10 mg, gradually increased to 30 mg daily.[1]

Reference

1 Mendelson G. Narcotics and monoamine oxidase inhibitors. *Med J Aust* (1979) **1**, 400.

Monamine oxidase inhibitors + methyldopa

Summary

Although animal studies suggested that an adverse interaction might occur with pargyline and methyldopa, concurrent use generally appears to be a safe although one report describes hallucinosis. The order of administration may be important. It is debatable whether a potentially depressant drug ought to be given at the same time as an antidepressant.

Interaction

Despite evidence from experiments in animals[6,7] that acute central excitation can follow the concurrent use of pargyline and methyldopa, there is only a single adverse report among a number describing no problems:

A hypertensive woman under treatment with pargyline, 25 mg four times a day, developed hallucinations about a month after starting additional treatment with methyldopa, 250 mg daily, later increased to 500 mg.[1]

This adverse reaction report contrasts with others in which no unusual reactions or toxic effects were said to have occurred.[2-5] The hypotensive response was enhanced.[5]

Mechanism

It has been clearly demonstrated[6,7] that mice treated with pargyline followed by methyldopa show extensive and prolonged central excitation. This is believed to be because methyldopa, like reserpine, causes the sudden release of accumulated catecholamines, such as noradrenaline, (norepinephrine) from nerve endings in the brain, the amounts of the catecholamines being particularly high because of the MAO inhibition. But this response appears not to have been described in man. There is no satisfactory explanation for the hallucinosis described.[1]

Importance and management

Concurrent use of pargyline and methyldopa is reported to be safe,[2-5] there being only one unexplained adverse report attributed to an interaction between them. Even so it might be prudent, wherever possible, to follow the advice of Natajaran[11] to avoid giving the methyldopa after the pargyline to prevent any possibility of the sudden release of the MAOI-accumulated stores of catecholamines.

There seems to be no documentation about the concurrent use of methyldopa and other MAOIs, but the potential depressent side-effects of methyldopa[8-10] may preclude its use in depressed patients.

References

1 Paykel E S. Hallucinosis on combined methyldopa and pargyline. *Br Med J* (1966) 1, 803.
2 Maronde R F, Haywood L J, Feinstein D and Sobel C. The monoamine oxidase inhibitor, pargyline hydrochloride, and reserpine. *J Amer Med Ass* (1963) 184, 7.
3 Herting R L. Monoamine oxidase inhibitors. *Lancet* (1965) i, 1324.
4 Kinross-Wright J and Charolampous K D. Concurrent administration of dopa decarboxylase and monoamine oxidase inhibitors in man. *Clin Res* (1963) ii, 177.
5 Gillespie L., Oates J A, Grout R and Sjoerdsma A. Clinical and chemical studies with α-methyldopa in patients with hypertension. *Circulation* (1962) 25, 281.
6 Van Rossum J M and Hurkmans J A ThM. Reversal of the effect of α-methyldopa by monoamine oxidase inhibitors. *J Pharm Pharmacol* (1963) 15, 493.
7 Van Rossum J M. Potential danger of monoamine oxidase inhibitors and α-methyldopa. *Lancet* (1963) 1, 950.
8 Pariente D. Methyldopa and depression *Br Med J* (1973) 3, 110.
9 Fleming H A. Methyldopa and depression. *Br Med J* (1973) 3, 232.
10 Bant W. Methyldopa and depression. *Br Med J* (1973) 3, 553.
11 Natajaran S. Potential dangers of monoamine oxidase inhibitors and α-methyldopa. *Lancet* (1964) i, 1330.

Monoamine oxidase inhibitors + morphine

Summary

An isolated case report describes the rapid loss of consciousness and severe hypotention in a patient on tranylcypromine who was given morphine.

Interaction

A patient with psychotic depression, well controlled on 40 mg tranylcypromine and 20 mg trifluoperazine daily, underwent a preoperative trial with morphine. 1½ h after being given 50 mg promethazine intramuscularly, she was given 1 mg morphine intravenously and several minutes later a further 2·5 mg. Five minutes later, since there were no adverse effects (the systolic pressure was 160 mmHg) and the patient was still alert and anxious, a further 2·5 mg morphine was given slowly intravenously. After approximately 3 min the patient became unconscious and unresponsive to stimuli, her pupils were pinpoint and the systolic pressure was 40 mmHg. She continued to breath, 4 mg naloxone was given intravenously and within 2 min the patient was awake and rational with a systolic pressure of 160 mmHg. (1)

Mechanism

Not understood.

Importance and management

The serious pethidine–MAOI interaction (see p. 365) also cast a shadow over morphine, and resulted in the appearance of morphine in a number of lists and charts of drugs which were said to interact with the MAOI, although there is good evidence that patients on MAOI who had reacted adversely with pethidine did not do so when given morphine.[2,3] The interaction described here is of a different character, and appears so far to represent an isolated case. Morphine cannot be regarded as totally contraindicated in patients on MAOI, but it is clear that it should be used with particular care. Naloxone proved to be a rapid and effective treatment in the case cited.

References

1 Barry B J. Adverse effects of MAO inhibitors with narcotics reversed with naloxone. *Anaesth Intens Care* (1979) 7, 194.
2 Palmer H. Potentiation of pethidine. *Br Med J* (1960) 2, 944.
3 Denton P H, Borrelli V M and Edwards N V. Dangers of monoamine oxidase inhibitors. *Br Med J* (1962) 2, 1752.

Monoamine oxidase inhibitors +
neuromuscular blockers

Summary

A single case report describes enhancement of the effects of suxamethonium (prolonged apnoea) during concurrent treatment with phenelzine.

Interaction, mechanism, importance
and management

A report[2] of a patient who showed an enhancement of the neuromuscular blocking effects of suxamethonium during treatment with phenelzine would appear to be explained by the finding[1] of a group of workers who showed that phenelzine can cause a reduction in the levels of serum pseudocholinesterase. Since the metabolism of suxamethonium depends on this enzyme, reduced levels of the enzyme would result in a reduced rate

of metabolism of the suxamethonium and in a prolongation of its effects. It is not certain whether other MAOI have a similar effect but it would be prudent to be cautious when any MAOI is being used.

References

1 Bodley P O, Halwax K, and Potts L. Low serum pseudocholinesterase levels complicating treatment with phenelzine. *Br Med J* (1969) 3, 510.
2 Bleaden F A and Czekansk G. New drugs for depression. *Br Med J* (1960) 1, 200.

Monoamine oxidase inhibitors +
pethidine (meperidine)

Summary

Concurrent use of pethidine in a few patients on MAOI can result in a serious and potentially fatal reaction: excitement, muscle rigidity, hyperpyrexia, flushing, sweating and unconsciousness can occur very rapidly; respiratory depression and hypotension are also seen. Pethidine should not be used unless a lack of sensitivity has been confirmed.

Interaction

Severe, rapid and potentially fatal toxic reactions, both excitatory and depressant, can occur in a small number of patients on MAOI treated with pethidine. Excitation, restlessness, rigidity, increased tendon reflexes, flushing, sweating, hyperpyrexia and unconsciousness can take place as well as respiratory depression, Cheyne–Stokes respiration, cyanosis and cardiovascular shock.

A woman taking iproniazid, 50 mg twice a day, was given 100 mg pethidine to treat acute precordial pain. She became restless and incoherent almost immediately and was comatose within 20 min. Within an hour she was flushed, sweating and showed Cheyne–Stokes respiration. Her pupils were dilated and unreactive. Deep reflexes could not be initiated and plantar reflexes were extensor. The

pulse rate was 82 and blood pressure 156/110 mmHg. Following the intravenous injection of 25 mg prednisolone hemi-succinate she was rousable within 10 min.[1]

A woman who, unknown to her doctor, was taking tranylcypromine, was given 100 mg pethidine. Within minutes she became unconscious, noisy and restless, having to be held down by three people. Her breathing was stertorous and the pulse impalpable. Generalized tonic spasm developed with ankle clonus, extensor plantar reflexes, shallow respiration and cyanosis. On admission to hospital she had a blood pressure of 90/60 mmHg, a pulse rate of 160, and was sweating profusely (temperature 38°C). Her condition gradually improved and 4 h after admission she was conscious but drowsy. Recovery was complete the next day.[10]

This interaction has been seen in other patients

treated with iproniazid,[1,3-5] pargyline,[2] phenelzine,[6-9] tranylcypromine[10] and mebanazine.[11] Fatalities have been reported.[6,11]

Mechanism

Not understood despite the extensive studies undertaken.[15-17] There is some evidence that the reactions may be due to an increase in levels of 5-HT within the brain, and that a critically high level must be reached before the toxicity manifests itself.

Importance and management

A well-documented, serious and potentially fatal interaction. The incidence is not know precisely but it is probably quite low. A study of this interaction on 15 patients given various MAOI failed to demonstrate it.[12] Nevertheless, patients on MAOI should not be given pethidine unless they are known not to be sensitive. Churchill-Davison has suggested[3] that this can be checked by giving patients a test dose of 5 mg pethidine after which all the vital signs (pulse, respiration, blood pressure) are checked at 5 min intervals for 20 min, and then at 10 min intervals for the rest of the hour. If no obvious change has occurred, the whole check is repeated over the next hour with 10 mg pethidine, then with 20 mg, and after 3 h with 40 mg. It is not thought necessary to carry on further because by this stage any sensitivity should have revealed itself. Churchill-Davison quotes a patient who demonstrated sensitivity after 5 mg pethidine with a systolic blood pressure fall of 30 mmHg, a pulse rate rise of 20 beats/minute, and drowsiness.

The pethidine/MAOI interaction has been successfully treated with prednisolone hemisuccinate, 25 mg[1] and chlorpromazine, 50 mg[4]. Acidification of the urine would also effectively increase the rate of clearance.[14]

References

1 Shee J C. Dangerous potentiation of pethidine by iproniazid, and its treatment. Br Med J (1960) 2, 507.
2 Vigran I M. Dangerous potentiation of meperidine hydrochloride by pargyline hydrochloride. J Amer Med Ass (1964) 187, 953.
3 Clement A J and Benazon D. Reactions to other drugs in patients taking monoamine oxidase inhibitors. Lancet (1962) ii, 197.
4 Papp C. and Benaim S. Toxic effects of iproniazid in a patient with angina. Br Med J (1958) 2, 1070.
5 Mitchell R S. Fatal toxic encephalitis occurring during iproniazid therapy in pulmonary tuberculosis. Ann Int Med (1955) 42, 417.
6 Palmer H. Potentiation of pethidine. Br Med J (1960) 2, 944.
7 Taylor D C. Alarming reaction to pethidine in patients on phenelzine. Lancet (1962) ii, 409.
8 Cocks D P. and Passemore Rowe A. Dangers of monoamine oxidase inhibitors. Br Med J (1962) 2, 1545.
9 Reid N C R W and Jones D. Pethidine and phenelzine. Br Med J (1962) 1, 408.
10 Denton P H, Borrelli V M and Edwards N V Dangers of monoamine oxidase inhibitors. Br Med J (1962) 2, 1752.
11 Anon. Death from drugs combination. Pharm J (1965) 195, 341.
12 Prosser Evans C D G. The use of pethidine and morphine in the presence of monoamine oxidase inhibitors. Br J Anesth (1968) 40, 279.
13 Churchill-Davidson H C. Anaesthesia and monoamine oxidase inhibitors. Br Med J (1965) 1, 520.
14 London D R and Milne M D. Dangers of monoamine oxidase inhibitors. Br Med J (1962) 2, 1752.
15 Leander J D, Batten J and Hargis G W. Pethidine interaction with clorgyline, pargyline or 5-hydroxytryptophan: lack of enhanced pethidine lethality or hyperpyrexia in mice. J Pharm Pharmac (1978) 30, 396.
16 Rogers K J and Thornton J A. The interaction between monoamine oxidase inhibitors and narcotic analgerus in mice. Br J Pharmal (1969) 36, 470.
17 Gessher P K and Soble A G. A study of the tranylcypromine-meperidine interaction: effects of p-chlorophenylalanine and l-5-hydroxytryptophan. J Pharmacol Exp Ther (1973) 186, 276.

Monoamine oxidase inhibitors + phenothiazines

Summary

Concurrent use of the MAOI and phenothiazines appears usually to be safe and effective, but a small number of fatal reactions attributed to an interaction have been described.

Interaction, mechanism, importance and management

Concurrent use of the MAOI and phenothiazines has been recommended[1-3] and promazine has been used safely and effectively in the treatment of overdosage with tranylcypromine.[4]

A single case report[5] describes a woman on an MAOI who experienced a severe pounding occipital headache as a result of taking 30 ml of a child's cough linctus. In the original report this interaction was attributed, by interference, to the ingestion of 9 mg promethazine, but more recently[6] it has come to light that the linctus in question was *Tixylix* containing phenylpropanolamine which is much more likely to be the cause of the response described (see p. 415).

Three unexplained fatalities, one due to the concurrent use of methotrimeprazine with pargyline,[7] another with methotrimeprazine and tranylcypromine[8] and the third with an unnamed MAOI–phenothiazine combination have been reported.[8]

References

1 Winkelman N W. Three evaluations of an MAOI and phenothiazine (a methodological and clinical study). *Dis Nerv Syst* (1965) **26**, 160.

2 Cheshrow E J and Kaplitz S E. Anxiety and depression in the geriatric and chronically ill patient. *Clin Med* (1965) **72**, 1281.

3 Janacek J, Schiele B C, Belville T and Anderson R. The effects of withdrawal of trifluoperazine on patients maintained on the combination of tranylcypromine and trifluoperazine. A double blind study. *Curr Ther Res* (1963) **5**, 608.

4 Midwinter R E. Accidental overdose with 'Parstelin'. *Br Med J* (1962) **2**, 1755.

5 Mitchell L. Psychotropic drugs. *Br Med J* (1968) **1**, 381.

6 Mitchell L (1977) Cited as a personal communication in *A Manual of Adverse Drug Interactions* 2nd edn, p. 147. Griffin J P and D'Arcy P F (1979). Wright, Bristol.

7 Barsa J A and Saunders J C. A comparative study of tranylcypromine and pargyline. *Psychopharmacologia* (1964) **6**, 295.

8 McQueen E G New Zealand committee on adverse drug reactions: fourteenth annual report, 1979. *NZ Med J* (1980) **91**, 226.

Monoamine oxidase inhibitors + rauwolfia alkaloids or tetrabenazine

Summary

The use of potentially depressive drugs such as the rauwolfia alkaloids or tetrabenazine is generally contraindicated in patients requiring treatment for depression. Central excitation and possibly hypertension can occur if the rauwolfia is added to existing MAOI therapy, but is unlikely to occur if the rauwolfia is administered first.

Interaction

Patients under treatment with MAOI who are additionally given rauwolfia alkaloids or tetrabenazine may demonstrate various manifestations of central excitation and possibly hypertension:

A chronically depressed woman treated firstly with nialamide, 100 mg three times a day, and on the third day with reserpine as well, 0·5 mg three times a day, became hypomanic on the following day and almost immediately went into frank mania.[1]

A patient who had been under treatment with nialamide, 25 mg daily, and who was subsequently given tetrabenazine 7 days after its withdrawal, collapsed 6 h later and demonstrated epileptiform convulsions, partial unconsciousness, rapid respiration and tachycardia.[2]

Other reports state that the administration of reserpine or tetrabenazine after pretreatment with iproniazid can lead to a temporary (up to 3 days) disturbance of affect and memory, associated with autonomic excitation, delerious agitation, disorientation and illusions of experience and recognition[3,4]

A delayed reserpine-reversal was seen in 3 schizophrenic patients treated firstly with phenelzine for 12 weeks, then a placebo for 16–33 weeks, and lastly reserpine. The blood pressure rose slightly and persistently and the psychomotor activity was considerably increased, lasting in two cases throughout the 12-week period of treatment.[5]

Mechanism

Rauwolfia alkaloids such as reserpine cause adrenergic nerves to become depleted of their normal stores of noradrenaline (norepinephrine). In this way they prevent the normal transmission of impulses at adrenergic nerve endings of the sympathetic nervous system and can act as antihypertensive agents. Since the brain also possesses adrenergic neurones, failure of transmission could account for the sedation and depression observed.

If these compounds are given to patients already taking MAOI, they can cause the sudden release of large amounts of accumulated noradrenaline (and in the brain of 5-HT as well) resulting in excessive stimulation of the receptors which is seen as gross central excitation and hypertension. This would account for the case reports cited and the effects seen in animals.[7–9] These stimulant effects are sometimes called 'reserpine-reversal' because instead of the expected sedation or depression, excitation or delayed depression is seen. It depends upon the order in which the drugs are given.

Importance and management

The administration of potentially depressive drugs is generally contraindicated in patients undergoing treatment for depression. If concurrent treatment for other conditions is considered desirable, it has been suggested[7] that the MAOI should be given after, and not before, the other drug so that sedation rather than excitation will occur. The documentation of this latter reaction in man is very limited.

Reference

1 Gradwell B G. Psychotic reactions and phenelzine. *Br Med J* (1960) **2**, 1018.

2 Davies T S. Monoamine oxidase inhibitors and rauwolfia compounds. *Br Med J* (1960) **2**, 739.

3 Voelkel A. Klinische Wirkung von Pharmaka mit Einfluss auf den Monoaminstoffwechsel des Gehirns. *Confinia Neurol* (1958) **18**, 144.

4 Voelkel A. Experiences with MAO inhibitors in psychiatry. *Ann NY Acad Sci* (1959) **80**, 680.

5 Esser A H. Clinical observations on reserpine reversal after prolonged MAO inhibition. *Psychiat Neurol Neurochirugica* (1967) **70**, 59.

6 Natajaran S. Potential dangers of monoamine oxidase inhibitors and α-methyldopa. *Lancet* (1964) **i**, 1330.

7 Shore P A and Brodie B B. LSD-like effects elicited by reserpine in rabbits pretreated with isonazid. *Proc Soc Exp Biol NY* (1957) **94**, 433.

8 Chessin M, Kramer R and Scott C C. Modification of the pharmacology of reserpine and serotonin by iproniazid. *J Pharmacol exp Ther* (1957) **119**, 453.

9 von Euler U S, Bygoleman S and Persson N-Å. Interaction of reserpine and monoamine oxidase inhibitors on adrenergic transmitter release. *Biochim Biol Sper* (1970) **9**, 215.

Monoamine oxidase inhibitors + tricyclic antidepressants

Summary

Because of the severe, toxic, and sometimes fatal reactions which very occasionally follow the concurrent use of MAOI and tricyclic antidepressants, this drug combination came to be regarded as contraindicated, but informed opinion now considers that with extremely careful control, combined therapy is possible and advantageous for some refractory patients.

Interaction

A highly controversial interaction because, although toxic and fatal reactions have been reported, there are many other reports describing successful and uneventful concurrent use.

Toxic reactions due to MAOI/tricyclic antidepressant combination

The toxic reactions have included (with variations) sweating, flushing, hyperpyrexia, restlessness, excitement, tremor, muscle twitching and rigidity, convulsions and coma. An illustrative example:

A depressive woman who had been taking 20 mg tranylcypromine daily for about 3 weeks, discontinued taking it 3 days before taking a single tablet of imipramine. Within a few hours she complained of an excruciating headache, and soon afterwards lost consciousness and started to convulse. The toxic reactions manifested were a temperature of 40°C, a pulse rate of 120, severe extensor rigidity, carpal spasm, opisthotonos, and cyanosis. She was treated with amobarbital and phenytoin, and her temperature was reduced with alcohol-ice soaked towels. The treatment was effective and she recovered.[11]

Similar reactions have been recorded on a number of other occasions with normal therapeutic doses of iproniazid and imipramine,[1] imipramine and tranylcypromine,[1] isocarboxazid and imipramine,[1,2] pargyline and imipramine,[3] phenelzine and imipramine[4–9] phenelzine and desipramine,[13] and clomipramine with tranylcypromine.[16]

Some other reports are confused by overdosage with one or both drugs, or the presence of other drugs and diseases. There have been fatalities.[13,16,21] There are far too many reports of these interactions to list here, but they are extensively reviewed elsewhere.[10,12,20]

Advantageous use of MAOI/tricyclic antidepressant combinations

Definite therapeutic advantages, without any particular toxic reactions, have been claimed for MAOI/tricyclic antidepressant combinations. For example, Dr G A Gander of St Thomas's Hospital, London, has stated[14] that 98 out of 149 patients on combined therapy (phenelzine, isocarboxazid or iproniazid, with imipramine or amitriptyline) over periods of 1–24 months, improved significantly and that the side-effects were 'identical in nature and similar in frequency to those seen with a single antidepressant. . . . Side effects were easily controlled by adjusting the dosage. None of the serious side effects previously reported, such as muscular twitching or loss of consciousness was seen.' Dr Gander also claimed that more than 1400 patients having combined antidepressants over a period of 4 years '. . . tend to confirm these findings described'. Dr William Sargent from the same department has also written[15] that '. . . we have used combined antidepressant drugs for nearly 10 years now on some thousands of patients. We still wait to see any of the rare dangerous complications reported.'

Other reports and reviews describing the beneficial use of MAOI/tricyclic antidepressant combinations are listed elsewhere.[12,19,20]

Mechanism

Not understood. One idea is that since both types of drug increase the levels of monoamines such as 5-HT and noradrenaline in the brain, each working in concert and reinforcing the effects of the other might raise the concentrations so high that a 'spill-over' of excessive amounts could take place into areas of the brain not concerned with mood elevation, causing the bizarre and serious reactions described. Less likely suggestions are that the MAOI inhibit enzymes concerned with the metabolism of the tricyclic antidepressants, or that active and unusual metabolites of the tricyclic antidepressants are produced.[12]

Importance and management

This interaction, when it happens, can be serious and potentially fatal but there is no precise information about its incidence. It is probably much lower than was originally thought.

No detailed clinical work has been done to find out precisely what sets the scene for a hazardous interaction to occur, but some general empirical guidelines have been suggested[10,12,18,20] so that the interaction can, as far as possible, be avoided

when concurrent treatment is thought appropriate:

1 Treatment with both types of drugs should only be undertaken by those who are well aware of the problems and can undertake adequate supervision.

2 Only patients refractory to all other types of treatment should be considered.

3 Tranylcypromine, phenelzine, clomipramine and imipramine appear to be high on the list of drugs which have interacted adversely. Amitriptyline or trimipramine and isocarboxazid are possibly safer.

4 Drugs should be given orally, not parenterally.

5 It seems safer to give the tricyclic antidepressant first, or together with the MAOI, than to give the MAOI first.

6 Small doses should be given initially, increasing the levels of each drug, one at a time, over a period of 2–3 weeks to a level generally below those used for each one individually.

One report has also suggested that patients should carry 300 mg chlorpromazine and to take it if a sudden, throbbing, radiating occipital headache occurs, and to seek medical help at once.[17]

References

1 Ayd F J. Toxic somatic and psychopathological reactions to antidepressent drugs. *J. Neuropsychiat* (1961) (*Suppl.* 1), 119.

2 Kane F J and Freeman D. Non-fatal reaction to imipramine–MAO inhibitor combination. *Amer J Psychiat* (1963) 120, 79.

3 McCurdy A and Kane A B. Transient brain syndrome as a non-fatal reaction to combined pargyline–imipramine treatment. *Amer J Psychiat* (1964) 121, 397.

4 Loeb R H. Quoted in ref. 10 below as written communication (1969).

5 Hills N F. Combining the antidepressant drugs. *Br Med J* (1965) 1, 859.

6 Davies G. Side effects of phenelzine. *Br Med J* (1960) 2, 1019.

7 Howarth E. Possible synergistic effects of the new thymoleptics in connection with poisoning. *J Ment Sci* (1961) 107, 1000.

8 Singh H. Atropine-like poisoning due to tranquillizing agents. *Amer J Psychiat* (1960) 117, 360.

9 Lockett M F and Milner G. Combining the antidepressant drugs. *Br Med J* (1965) 1, 921.

10 Schuckit M, Robins E and Feighner J. Tricyclic antidepressants and monoamine oxidase inhibitors. Combination therapy in the treatment of depression. *Arch Gen Psychiat* (1971) 24, 509.

11 Brachfeld J, Wirtschafter A and Wolfe S. Imipramine–tranylcypromine incompatibility. Near fatal toxic reaction. *J Amer Med Ass* (1963) 186, 1172.

12 Ponto L B, Perry P J, Liskow B I and Seaba H H. Drug therapy reviews: tricyclic antidepressant and monoamine oxidase inhibitor combination therapy. *Am J Hosp Pharm* (1977) 34, 954.

13 Bowen L W. Fatal hyperpyrexia with antidepressant drugs. *Br Med J* (1964) 2, 1465.

14 Gander G A. In *Antidepressant Drugs* Proc 1st Int Symp Milan (1966). Int Cong Ser, No. 122, p. 336. Excerpt Medica

15 Sargant W. Safety of combined antidepressants drugs. *Br Med J* (1971) **1**, 555.
16 Beaumont G. Drug interactions with clomipramine (Anafranil) *J Int Med Res* (1973) **1**, 480.
17 Schildkraut J J and Klein D F. The classification and treatment of depressive disorders. In *Manual of Psychiatric Therapeutics* p. 61. Shader R I (ed) (1975) Little, Brown. Boston, Mass.
18 Beaumont G. Personal communication (1978).
19 Stockley I H. Tricyclic antidepressants. Part 1. Interactions with drugs affecting adrenergic neurones. In *Drug Interactions and Their Mechanisms*, p. 14 (1974). Pharmaceutical Press, London.
20 Ananth J and Luchins D. A review of combined tricyclic and MAOI therapy. *Compr Psychiatry* (1977) **18**, 221.
21 Wright S P. Hazards with monoamine oxidase inhibitors: a persistent problem. *Lancet* (1978) **i**, 284.

Monoamine oxidase inhibitors + tyramine-rich foods

Summary

The concurrent use of monoamine oxidase inhibitors (antidepressant or antihypertensive) and tyramine-rich foods or drinks can result in a hypertensive crisis. There have been deaths from intracranial haemorrhage. Significant amounts of tyramine can occur in cheese, yeast extracts ('Marmite'), chianti wine and pickled herrings. Caviar, hydrolysed soups, chicken and beef livers have also been implicated in these interactions.

Interaction

A rapid, serious and potentially fatal rise in blood pressure can occur in patients on MAOI who ingest tyramine-rich foods and drinks. A violent occipital headache, pounding heart, neck stiffness, flushing, sweating, nausea and vomiting are usually also experienced. Two illustrative examples: the first being the first recorded observation of the interaction by Rowe, a pharmacist, in a letter after seeing the reaction in his wife who was taking *Parstelin* (tranylcypromine with trifluoperazine):

> After cheese on toast; within a few minutes face flushed, felt very ill; head and heart pounded most violently, and perspiration was running down her neck. She vomited several times, and her condition looked so severe that I dashed over the road to consult her GP. He diagnosed 'palpitations' and agreed to call if the symptoms had not subsided in an hour. In fact, the severity diminished, and after about 3 h she was normal, other than a severe headache—but 'not of the throbbing kind'. She described the early part of the attack 'as though her head must burst'.[1]

A report describes a patient who, although he had eaten Sweitzer cheese uneventfully on many occasions while being treated with pargyline, this time experienced severe substernal chest pain and palpitations within a quarter of an hour and was found on admission to hospital to have a blood pressure of 200/114 mmHg. Two other patients experienced a headache after eating aged cheese.

One of them had a severe nose bleed and was found to have a blood pressure of 240/140 mmHg.[2]

This is probably the best-documented interaction of all, there being far too many reports to list them here individually, but they are reviewed elsewhere.[1,10] Blackwell and his colleagues[6] list a total of 110 instances caused by various tyramine-rich foods which came to their attention in the period 1963–66. There have been many since. Tranylcypromine, phenelzine, mebanazine and pargyline have all been implicated in this interaction with cheese, yeast extracts, pickled herring, chicken livers, caviar, hydrolysed soups, beef livers and chianti wine. Many patients recovered uneventfully, but Blackwell and his colleagues list in their review 26 cases of intracranial haemorrhage and 9 deaths.[1] Another review lists 38 cases of haemorrhage and 21 deaths.[9]

Mechanism

Tyramine is formed in foods such as cheese by the bacterial degradation of milk and other proteins, firstly to tyrosine and other aminoacids, and the subsequent decarboxylation of the tryrosine to tyramine. (It is of interest that tyramine was first isolated from cheese in 1903 and is named after the Greek word for cheese: tyros).[21] Tyramine is an indirectly-acting sympathomimetic amine which can release noradrenaline (norepinephrine) from the adrenergic neurones associated with arterial blood vessels and causes a rise in blood pressure by stimulating their constriction (see p. 399 for an illustrated explanation of the mode of action of the sympathomimetic amines).

Normally no hypertensive reaction occurs when we ingest tyramine in cheese or other foods because both the intestinal wall and the liver, to which blood from the intestine first flows, contain the enzyme monoamine oxidase which metabolizes the tyramine before it can escape into general circulation. However, if the activity of the enzyme at these sites is inhibited, any tyramine passes freely into circulation to cause not just a rise in blood pressure, but a highly exaggerated rise due to the release from the adrenergic neurones of the large amounts of noradrenaline which accumulate there during inhibition of the MAO. This final step in the interaction is identical with the interaction which takes place with any other indirectly-acting sympathomimetic amine in the presence of an MAOI and is described on page

415. The violent headache probably occurs when the pressure reaches about 200 mmHg.

There is also evidence that other amines such as histamine and phenylethylamine may also play a part in this interaction.

Importance and management
An extremely well-documented, well-established, serious and potentially fatal interaction. The incidence is uncertain but estimates range from 1 to 20%.[7,8] Patients taking any MAOI should not eat food or take drinks which contain substantial amounts of tyramine (see Tables 16.2–16.4). As little as 6 mg can raise the blood pressure[4] and 10–25 mg would be expected to cause a serious interaction.[4] Because tyramine levels vary so much it is impossible to guess the amount present in any food or drink. An old and mature cheese may contain trivial amounts of tyramine compared with one which is innocuous looking and mild-tasting. The tyramine content can even differ significantly within a single cheese between the centre and the rind.[5] There is no guarantee that patients who have risked eating these hazar-

Table 16.3. The tyramine content of some foods

Food	Tyramine (μg/g)	Ref.
Avacado	23	17
Banana pulp	7	17
Banana (whole)	65	17
Caviar (Iranian)	680	15
Cheeses—see Table 16.4		
Figs (canned)		16
Herring (pickled)	3030	18
Liver		
chicken	94–113	19
beef	0–274	20
Orange pulp	10	17
Plum, red	6	
Sausages (fermented)		
bolognas	0–333	16
pepperoni	0–195	16
salami	0–1237	16
smoked landjaeger	396	
summer sausage	184	16
Tomato	4	17
Yeast extracts		
Barmene	157	6
Befit	419	6
Marmite	1087, 1436, 1639	6
Marmite (salt free)	187	6
Yeastrel	101	6
Yex	506	6
Yoghourt	<0·2	21

Table 16.4. The tyramine content of some cheeses. This table should not be used to predict the probable tyramine content of a cheese. It is only intended to show the extent and the variation which can occur.

Variety of cheese	Tyramine (μg/g)	Ref.
American processed	50	4
Argenti	188	13
Blue	49, 203, 266	12,13
Boursault	1116	12
Brick	194	13
Brie	180	4
Brie type (Danish)	0	12
Camembert	86, 125	4,13
Camebert type (Danish)	23	12
Cheddar		
Australian	226	6
Canadian	120, 136, 192, 251, 535, 1000, 1530	6,12
English	0·72, 182, 281, 332, 480, 953	6
Farmhouse	284	6
Kraft	214	6
New York State	1416	6
New Zealand	416, 580	4
Cream cheese	<0·2	4
Cottage	<0·2	4
Danish blue (Gorgonzola type)	31, 93, 256	12
d'Oka	158, 310	13
Edam	100,214	13
Emmental	225	4
Gouda	54, 95	13
Gouda type (Canadian)	20	12
Gourmandise	216	12
Gruyere	64 (mean of 7 samples) 514	14
Kashar	44 (mean of 7 samples)	14
Liederkrantz	1226, 1683	13
Limburger	204	13
Mozzarela	410	12
Munster	110	13
Mycelia	1340	13
Parmesan	65	12
Parmesan type (USA)	4, 5, 290	12
Provolone	38	12
Romano	197, 238	12,13
Roquefort	27, 48, 520, 267	12,13
Stilton	466, 2170	12
Swiss	50, 434	13
Tulum	208 (mean of 7 samples)	14
White (Turkish)	17·5	14

dous foodstuffs on many occasions uneventfully may not eventually experience a full-scale hypertensive crisis if all the many variables conspire together.[2]

A total prohibition should be imposed on the following: cheese and yeast extracts such as 'Marmite' and 'Bovril' (tyramine content up to 1·5 mg/g) and pickled herrings (up to 3 mg/g). Hypertensive reactions have been observed with chicken and beef livers, caviar and hydrolysed soups. Fermented bolognas and salamis, pepperoni and summer sausage, and canned figs all contain tyramine. A number of other foods are often viewed with suspicion: chocolate, yoghourt and cream. There is little reason to consider them as normally undesirable. *Whole* green bananas contain up to 65 μg/g, but the pulp contains relatively small amounts.

It is usual practice to recommend avoidance of the prohibited foods for 2–3 weeks after withdrawal of the MAOI to allow full recovery of the enzymes. If a hypertensive reaction occurs it can be reversed with an alpha-adrenoreceptor blocking agent such as phentolamine, 5 mg, given intravenously, or failing that an intramuscular injection of 50 mg chlorpromazine.

Patients prescribed MAOI should ideally be given a list of these foodstuffs, drinks and other drugs which are prohibited. See also page 357 for drinks which contain tyramine.

References

1 Blackwell B, Marley E, Price J and Taylor D. Hypertensive interactions between monoamine oxidase inhibitors and foodstuffs. *Br J Psychiat* (1967) **113**, 349.

2 Hutchison J C. Toxic effects of monoamine oxidase inhibitors. *Lancet* (1964) **ii**, 150.

3 Blackwell B. Tranylcypromine *Lancet* (1963) **i**, 167.

4 Horwitz D, Lovenberg W, Engelman K and Sjoerdsma A. Monoamine oxidase inhibitors, tyramine and cheese. *J Amer Med Ass* (1964) **188**, 1108.

5 Price K and Smith S E. Cheese reaction and tyramine. *Lancet* (1971) **i**, 130.

6 Blackwell B and Marley E. *Neuropsychopharmacology*. Proc. 5th Int Congr Coll Int Neuro-psycho-pharmacologium. Int Congr Series no. 129. Washington, March 1966. Excepta Medica Foundation

7 Anon. Hypertensive reactions to monamine oxidase inhibitors. *Br. Med J* (1964) **1**, 578.

8 Cooper A J, Magnus R V and Rose M J. A hypertensive syndrome with tranylcypromine medication. *Lancet* (1964) **i**, 527.

9 Sadusk J F. The physician and the Food and Drug Administration. *J Amer Med Ass* (1964) **190**, 907

10 Stockley I H. Drug interactions and their mechanisms, p. 55. Pharmaceutical Press, London (1974).

11 Marley E. and Blackwell B. Interactions of monoamine oxidase inhibitors, amines and foodstuffs. *Advan. Pharmacol Chemotherap.* (1970) **8**, 185.

12 Sen N P. Analysis and significance of tyramine in foods. *J Food Sci* (1969) **34**, 127.

13 Kosikowsky F V and Dahlberg A C. The tyramine content of cheese. *J Dairy Sci* (1948) **31**, 293.

14 Kayaalp S O, Renda N, Kaymarkcalan S and Ozer A. Tyramine content of some cheeses. *Toxicol app Pharmacol* (1970) **16**, 459.

15 Isaac P, Mitchell B and Grahame-Smith D G. Monoamine oxidase inhibitors and caviar. *Lancet* (1977) **ii**, 816.

16 Rice S, Eitenmiller R R and Koehler P E. Histamine and tyramine content of meat products. *J Milk Food Technol* (1975) **38**, 256.

17 Udenfriend S, Lovenberg W and Sjoerdsma A. Physiologically active amines in common fruits and vegetables. *Arch Biochem* (1959) **85**, 487.

18 Nuessle W F, Norman F C and Miller H E. Pickled herring and tranylcypromine reaction. *J Amer Med Ass* (1965) **192**, 726.

19 Hedberg D L, Gordon M W and Glueck B C. Six cases of hypertensive crisis in patients on tranylcypromine after eating chicken livers. *Amer J Psychiatry* (1966) **122**, 933.

20 Boulton A A, Cookson B and Paulton R. Hypertensive crisis in a patient on MAOI antidepressants following a meal of beef liver. *Canad Med Ass J* (1970) **102**, 1394.

21 van Slÿke L and Hart B. Conditions affecting the proportions of fat and proteins in cow's milk. *Amer Chem J* (1903) **30**, 8.

CHAPTER 17. NEUROLEPTIC AND TRANQUILLIZING DRUG INTERACTIONS

The minor tranquillizers include the benzodiazepines, loxapine, hydroxyzine and other agents which are used to treat psychoneuroses such as tension and anxiety, and are intended to induce calm without causing hypnosis. Some of the benzodiazepines are also used as anticonvulsants and hypnotics. Table 17.1 contains a list of the benzodiazepines in current use.

Table 17.1. Benzodiazepine tranquilizers

Non-proprietary names	Proprietary names
Alprazolam	
Bromazepam	
Camazepam	
Chlordiazepoxide	*Calmoden, Corix, Diapax, Librium, Libritabs, Medilium, Nack, Protensin, Solium, Viaquil*
Clobazam	*Urbanyl*
Clorazepate	*Tranxene, Tranxilen, Tranxilium*
Desmethyldiazepam	*Madar*
Diazepam	*Adozepam, Atensine, E-pam, Paxel, Sernack, Tensium, Valium*
Fosazepam	
Ketazolam	
Lorazepam	*Ativan, Tavor, Temesta*
Medazepam	*Nobrium*
Oxazepam	*Adumbran, Praxiten, Serenid, Serepax, Seresta, Sobril*
Oxazolam	*Serenal*
Ripazepam	

Other benzodiazepines such as flurazepam (*Dalmane*), temazepam (*Eurhypnos, Normison*), triazolam (*Halcion*) and nitrazepam (*Mogadon, Nitrados, Remnos, Somnased, Somnite*) are used as sedatives and hypnotics, whereas clonazepam (*Rivotril*) and diazepam have application as anticonvulsants.

The major tranquillizers are represented by chlorpromazine (and other phenothiazines), butyrophenones and thioxanthenes. Their major use is in the treatment of psychoses such as schizophrenia and mania. Some of the phenothizines are also used as antihistamines. These drugs are classified in Table 17.2.

Some of the interactions involving the neuroleptics and tranquillizers are listed in this chapter, but there are other synopses elsewhere in this book where the interacting agent is a neuroleptic or tranquillizer. A full listing is given in the Index.

Table 17.2. Phenothiazine, butyrophenone and thioxanthene neuroleptics

Non-proprietary names	Proprietary names
Phenothiazines	
Acetophenazine	*Tindal*
Butaperazine	*Randolectil, Repoise*
Carphenazine	*Proketazine*
Chlorpromazine	*Amargyl, Chloractil, Elmarine, Largactil, Thorazine*
Fluopromazine	*Psyquil, Siquil, Vesprin*
Fluphenazine	*Anatensol, Dapotum, Lyogen, Moditen, Modecate, Prolixin*
Methotrimeprazine	*Levoprome, Neurocil, Nozinan*
Pericyazine	*Decentan, Fentazin, Trilifan, Trilafon*
Pipothiazine	*Piportil L4*
Prochlorperazine	*Compazine, Stemetil*
Promazine	*Atarzine, Eliranol, Intrazine, Prazine, Sparine*
Propiomazine	*Largon*
Prothipendyl	*Dominal, Tolnate*
Thiethylperazine	*Torecan*
Thiopropazate	*Dartalan*
Thioproperazine	*Majeptil, Mayeptil*
Thioridazine	*Melleril, Novoridazine, Thioril*
Trifluoperazine	*Amylozine, Calmazine, Chemflurazine, Novoflurazine, Eskazine, Stelabid, Stelazid*

Other phenothiazines are used as antihistamines such as promethazine (*Phenergan*) isopromethazine, pyrathiazine (*Mediamer*) and isothiopendyl (*Andanol*)

Butyrophenones	
Benperidol	*Anguil, Glianimon, Frenactil*
Droperidol	*Dridol, Droleptan, Inapsin*
Haloperidol	*Haldol, Serenace*
Trifluperidol	*Psicoperidol, Triperidol*

Thioxanthenes	
Chlorprothixene	*Taractan, Tarasan, Truxal*
Flupenthixol	*Depixol, Emergil, Fluanxanol*
Thiothixene	*Navane, Orbinamon*

Benzodiazepines + antacids

Summary
The absorption of chlordiazepoxide, diazepam and clorazepate are delayed by the concurrent use of aluminium and magnesium hydroxide or trisilicate antacids, and the extent of clorazepate absorption is reduced. The clinical importance is uncertain, but probably small.

Chlordiazepoxide + aluminium magnesium hydroxide (Maalox)

A single cross-over study on 10 healthy subjects given single 25 mg doses of chlordiazepoxide with either 100 ml *Maalox* (4 g magnesium hydroxide and 4·5 g aluminum hydroxide) or 100 ml water showed that the antacid had no significant effect on the extent but reduced the rate of chlordiazepoxide absorption.[1]

Diazepam + aluminium magnesium hydroxide (Maalox) or aluminium hydroxide trisilicate (Gelusil)

A three-way cross-over study on 9 healthy subjects given diazepam with either 60 ml water, 60 ml *Maalox* or 60 ml *Gelusil* showed that the antacids caused a reduction in peak plasma concentrations and in the rate of absorption of the diazepam, but the extent of the absorption was unaffected (2)

375

Clorazepate + alumium magnesium hydroxide (Maalox)

A two-way crossover study on 10 volunteers given single 15 mg doses of clorazepate with either water or 60 ml *Maalox* showed that peak plasma concentrations of the active metabolite of clorazepate (desmethyldiazepam) were reduced about one third by the antacid, the absorption was delayed, and the amount absorbed reduced by approximately 10%. A self-assessement by the subjects taking part was that the antacid reduced the clinical effects of the clorazepate.[3]

Another study using only 30 ml *Maalox* failed to show a significant interaction with clorazepate[4]

Mechanism
The most probable mechanism for the reduction in the rate of absorption of chlordiazepoxide and diazepam is that the antacids delay the rate of gastric emptying, thereby delaying the absorption by the small intestine.

In the case of clorazepate, the interaction may depend on a different mechanism. Clorazepate is a 'prodrug' or percursor of desmethyldiazepam (the active metabolite) which is produced by hydrolysis and decarboxylation within the stomach. At the low pH values normally found in the stomach this hydrolysis is very rapid and is complete within minutes, but at higher pH values gastric emptying may occur while considerable amounts of clorazepate remain intact. Thus the poorly absorbed prodrug is moved on into the stomach instead of the much better absorbed desmethyldiazepam. Changes in pH induced by sodium bicarbonate[5] have been shown to cause a significant reduction in the absorption of desmethyldi-

azepam and the interaction described here may be due to a similar rise in the pH of the gastric contents induced by *Maalox*.

Importance and management
The delay in absorption of chlordiazepoxide and diazepam by these antacids in patients on chronic treatment is probably unimportant because these patients depend on the steady cumulative effects of these drugs which probably remain unaffected. The interaction may be less desirable in those who only take these benzodiazepines during acute episodes of anxiety and need rapid relief. Confirmation of this is needed.

The studies described here with clorazepate were made with single doses in normal subjects. The reduction in its total effects were small and probably of limited importance, but confirmation of this awaits clinical assessment in patients.

References
1 Greenblatt D J, Shader R I, Harmatz J S, Franke K, and Koch-Weser J. Influence of magnesium and aluminium hydroxide mixture on chlordiazepoxide absorption. *Clin Pharmacol Ther* (1976) 19, 234.
2 Greenblatt D J, Allen D A, MacLaughlin D S, Harmatz J S and Shader R I. Diazepam absorption: effect of antacids and food. *Clin Pharmacol Ther* (1978) 24, 600.
3 Shader R I, Georgotas A, Greenblatt D J, Harmatz J S and Allen M D. Impaired absorption of desmethyldiazepam from clorazepate by magnesium aluminium hydroxide. *Clin Pharmacol Ther* (1978) 24, 308.
4 Chun A H C, Carrigan P J, Hoffman D J, Kershner R P, Stuart J D. Effect of antacids on absorption of clorazepate. *Clin Pharmacol Ther* (1977) 22, 329.
5 Abruzzo C W, Macasieb T, Weinfeld R, Rider J A and Kaplan S A. Changes in the oral absorption characteristics in man of dipotassium clorazepate at normal and elevated gastric pH. *J Pharmacokineti Biopharm* (1977) 5, 377.

Benzodiazepines + cimetidine

Summary
The effects of diazepam may be enhanced by the concurrent use of cimetidine, possibly resulting in the development of its adverse side-effects (drowsiness, light-headedness, ataxia, incordination). Driving or handling other dangerous machinery may be made more hazardous. A similar interaction seems possible with chlordiazepoxide but not with oxazepam or lorazepam.

Interaction
Four healthy volunteers were given five 200 mg oral doses of cimetidine on one day, the last being administered half an hour before an intravenous injection of diazepam (0·1 mg/kg). Measurements of diazepam serum levels taken over the next few days showed that the elimination half-life of diazepam was prolonged by the cimetidine from 29 to 51 h, and the total plasma clearance was halved. There was also a decrease in distribution values.[1]

Similar results are described in other reports.[5] The elimination half-life of chlordiazepoxide has also been shown[6] in 8 normal subjects (taking 300 mg cimetidine, four times a day for a week) to be doubled, but oxazepam and lorazepam have been shown not to be affected.[7]

Mechanism
The reduction in the hepatic clearance of the diazepam is probably due to inhibition by the cimetidine of the liver enzymes concerned with the metabolism of the diazepam. This inhibitory effect has already been shown in rats.[2] Chlordiazepoxide similarly undergoes hydroxylation and dealkylation in the liver before glucuronidation occurs. Oxazepam and lorazepam on the other hand do not need to undergo these metabolic changes before glucuronidation can take place and therefore would not be expected to be affected by the presence of cimetidine.

Importance and management
Information is very limited, but it indicates that if diazepam is taken during treatment with cimetidine the effects of the former are likely to be enhanced and prolonged. In the report cited[1] the cimetidine was only given for a day so that on longer treatment the effects on the diazepam may be even greater than this data suggests. The side-effects of diazepam are drowsiness, light-headedness and ataxia.

Although there are no formal clinical reports of this interaction, a man who was accused of driving under the influence of drugs and who showed generalized incoordination, was absolved of blame because he was taking both drugs.[3] The defence counsel used the report cited above[1] as evidence of an interaction. Patients who drive or who handle dangerous machinery should certainly be made aware of the possible hazards. It would be reasonable to expect the effects of chlordiazepoxide to be enhanced like those of diazepam, but not those of oxazepam or lorazepam. This requires confirmation.

References
1 Klotz U, Anttila V-J and Reimann I. Cimetidine/diazepam interaction. *Lancet* (1979) ii, 699.
2 Puuvumen J and Pelkonen O. Cimetidine inhibits microsomal drug metabolism in the rat. *Eur. J Pharmacol* (1979) 55, 335.
3 Anon. Court warns on interaction of drugs. *Doctor* (1979) 9, 1.
4 Klotz U and Reimann I. Delayed clearance of diazepam due to cimetidine. *New Eng J Med* (1980) 302, 1012.
5 Dasta J, Mackichan J, Lima J and Altman M. Diazepam-cimetidine interaction. *Drug Intell Clin Pharm* (1980) 14, 633.
6 Desmond P V, Patwardhan R V, Schenker S and Speeg K V. Cimetidine impairs elimination of chlordiazepoxide (Librium) in man. *Ann Intern Med* (1980) 93, 266.
7 Patwardhan R V, Yarborough G W, Desmond P V, Johnson R F, Schenker S and Speeg K V. Cimetidine spares the glucuronidation of lorazepam. *Gastroenterology* (1980) 79, 912.

Benzodiazepines + disulfiram

Summary
The effects of chlordiazepoxide and diazepam, but not oxazepam, are increased and prolonged by the concurrent use of disulfiram. Oxazepam may therefore prove to have fewer dosage problems than either of these other two benzodiazepines.

Interaction
Towards the end of a 14–16 day period, during which they were given 0·5 g disulfiram by mouth, groups of normal subjects and alcoholic patients were also administered single doses of either 50 g chlordiazepoxide intravenously, 0·143 mg/kg diazepam orally, or 0·429 mg/kg oxazepam orally. Decreases in the plasma clearances of chlordiazepoxide (54%) and diazepam (41%), and increases in their half-lives (84% and 37%) were seen, but changes in the pharmacokinetic parameters of oxazepam were minimal[1]

Mechanism
Disulfiram inhibits a variety of liver microsomal enzymes so that the metabolism of various drugs given concurrently is reduced. The major pathway for the bio-transformation of chlordiazepoxide and diazepam involves an initial N-demethylation followed eventually by glucuronidation. If this pathway is inhibited, a slower alternative metabolic pathway is used which results in a slower clearance of the benzodiazepine from the

body and in the production of non-glucuronide (and pharmacologically active) metabolites. The eventual glucuronidation of oxazepam, on the other hand, seems to be minimally affected by disulfiram so that its clearance remains largely unaffected.[1]

Importance and management
The overall picture presented by the report cited is that the pharmacological activity of chlordiazepoxide and diazepam, but not oxazepam, are increased by disulfiram. This would be expected to

lead to enhanced sedation. Oxazepam would therefore appear to be the drug of choice in this situation and might be expected to have fewer dosage difficulties, but this requires confirmation by direct clinical studies. It should also be borne in mind that the benzodiazepines may diminish the extent of the disulfiram-alcohol interaction.

Reference
1 MacLeod S M, Sellers E M, Giles H G, Billings B J, Martin P R, Greenblatt D J and Marshman J A. Interaction of disulfiram with benzodiazepines. *Clin Pharmacol Ther* (1978) **24**, 583.

Chlorpromazine + lithium carbonate

Summary
The serum levels of chlorpromazine can be reduced to non-therapeutic levels by the concurrent administration of lithium carbonate.

Interaction
In a double-blind study on psychiatric patients it was found that 400–800 mg daily doses of chlorpromazine, which normally produced serum levels of 100–300 ng/ml, only produced levels of 0–70 ng/ml when lithium carbonate was taken at the same time.[1]

A study with 7 volunteers showed that while taking lithium carbonate (900 mg/day, giving serum lithium concentrations of 0·7 to 1·1 mEq/l) the mean peak serum levels of chlorpromazine taken at the same time were 40% lower than without lithium, and the areas under the plasma concentration time curves were 26% smaller. There was considerable individual variation.[2]

This interaction has been described in another report.[6]

Mechanism
One suggestion to account for this interaction is that because lithium delays gastric emptying time,[1] the absorption of chlorpromazine is reduced due to its being tightly bound to the gut wall where it is metabolized. This idea, however, leans very heavily on the results of animal experiments and may not necessarily apply to man.[3,4]

Importance and management
Information is limited but this interaction would

seem to be of importance. Work carried out on the relationship between plasma levels of chlorpromazine and the clinical response has shown that serum levels of less than 30 ng/ml are ineffective whereas those associated with clinical improvement are usually within the 150–300 ng/ml range or more.[5] Thus a fall in plasma levels to as little as 0–70 ng/ml (study[1] cited above) would be expected to result in a reduced therapeutic response. Increased doses may be required. Further study is required. It is not clear whether other phenothiazines behave similarly.

References
1 Kerzner B and Rivera-Calimlim L. Lithium and chlorpromazine (CPZ) interaction. *Clin Pharmacol Therap* (1976) **19**, 109.
2 Rivera-Calimlim L, Kerzner B and Karch F E. Effect of lithium on plasma chlorpromazine levels. *Clin Pharmacol Ther* (1978) **23**, 451.
3 Sundaresan P R and Rivera-Calimlim L. Distribution of chlorpromazine in the gastrointestinal tract of the rat and its effects on absorptive functions. *J Pharmacol Exp Ther* (1975) **194**, 593.
4 Curry S H, D'Mello A and Mould G P. Destruction of chlorpromazine during absorption in the rat in vivo and in vitro. *Br J Pharmacol* (1971) **42**, 403.
5 Rivera-Calimlim L, Castenada L and Lasagna L. Significance of plasma levels of chlorpromazine. *Clin Pharmacol Therap* (1973) **14**, 978.
6 Rivera-Calimlim L, Nasrallah H, Strauss J and Lasagna L. Clinical response and plasma levels: effect of dose, dosage schedules, and drug interactions on plasma chlorpromazine levels. *Clin J Psychiat* (1976) **133**, 6.

Hydroxyzine + antiparkinson drugs, atropine, lithium carbonate, phenothiazines, quinidine, procainamide, thioridazine, or tricyclic antidepressants

Summary

Hydroxyzine can cause ECG abnormalities in high doses. It has been suggested that concurrent use with other drugs which can have an adverse effect on the heart might increase the likelihood of dysrhythmias and sudden death.

Interaction, mechanism, importance and management

A study[1] on 25 elderly psychotic patients taking 300 mg hydroxyzine over a period of 9 weeks showed that ECG changes were mild except for alteration in T-waves which were definite in 9 patients and usually observed in leads 1, 2 AVL and V_{3-6}. In each case the T-waves were lower in amplitude, broadened and flattened, and somewhat notched. The QT interval was usually prolonged. A repeat of the study in a few patients, one at least given 400 mg, gave similar results, the most pronounced change being a marked attenuation of cardiac repolarization.

On the basis of these observations it has been suggested[1] that other drugs which cause ECG abnormalities (the author of the paper mentions those listed above) might aggravate and exaggerate these hydroxyzine-induced changes and increase the risk of sudden death. This potential adverse interaction awaits further study.

Reference

1 Hollister L E. Hydroxyzine hydrochloride: possible adverse cardiac interactions. *Psychopharmacol Comm* (1975) 1, 61.

Phenothiazines or butyrophenones + alcohol

Summary

A report suggests that extrapyramidal side-effects can be precipitated in patients on phenothiazines and butyrophenones by the consumption of alcohol. Enhanced CNS depression may also occur.

Interaction

A man with paranoid schizophrenic symptoms under treatment with trifluoperazine, 10 mg daily, for 7 weeks without complications, developed acute akathisia on consuming a moderate amount of beer and wine. Suppression of the symptoms was obtained by an initial intramuscular injection of benztropine mesylate 2 mg and the oral administration of 2 mg three times a day for 3 days.[1]

A patient was treated for acute undifferentiated schizophrenic reactions for a period of 8 months with chlorpromazine, 100 mg three to four times a day and trifluoperazine, 2–5 mg, three times a day. He was then treated for a further 2 months with chlorpromazine and an injection of 25 mg fluphenazine decanoate every 18 days without evidence of extrapyramidal side-effects. Within 2–3 h of consuming four cans of beer he developed an acute akathisic and dystonic reaction which subsided after treatment with biperiden hydrochloride.[1]

This same report[1] details five similar cases which the author stated were examples of numerous such alcohol-induced neuroleptic toxicity reactions, observed by him over an 18-year period, involving phenothiazines and butyrophenones.

Mechanism

Not understood. It has been suggested that alcohol may lower the threshold of resistance to the neurotoxic side-effects of these neuroleptic agents by inducing a temporary brain dysfunction.[1]

Importance and management

Information on this undesirable reaction appears

to be limited to this single report. The author claims that it has come to his attention on numerous occasions over an 18-year period, and he considers that frequent admonitions to abstain from alcohol should be routine advice during neuroleptic treatment. More study is needed.

Reference
1 Lutz E G. Neuroleptic-induced akathisia and dystonia triggered by alcohol. *J Amer Med Ass* (1977) **236**, 2422.

Phenothiazines + antacids

Summary
Concurrent administration of aluminium hydroxide and magnesium trisilicate-containing antacids such as *Aludrox* and *Gelusil* can reduce the serum levels of chlorpromazine given orally and may reduce the therapeutic response. It seems probable that the effects of this interaction can be minimized by separating their administration as much as possible, or by choosing alternative antacids.

Interaction
A psychotic patient, well controlled on chlorpromazine, relapsed within 3 days of being placed on antacid medication (type not stated). This prompted an investigation on 6 psychiatric patients which showed that when they were given 30 ml *Gelusil* (310 mg aluminium hydroxide and 620 mg magnesium trisilicate in every 5 ml) just before and just after taking a liquid suspension of chlorpromazine, their serum chlorpromazine levels measured 2 h later were reduced by about 20% (from an average of 168 to 132 ng/ml).[1,2]

A study on 10 patients taking 600–1200 mg chlorpromazine daily showed that their urinary excretion of chlorpromazine was reduced 10–45% when they were given 30 ml *Aludrox* (aluminium hydroxide gel) at the same time.[3]

Mechanism
The effects seen are most likely due to a chemical or physicochemical interaction between the chlorpromazine and the antacid within the gut which makes less chlorpromazine available for absorption. In-vitro experiments have demonstrated that chlorpromazine becomes bound to the gel structure of both aluminium hydroxide[1] and to trisilicate,[4] but that reversal of the binding takes place much more easily from the hydroxide than from trisilicate.

Importance and management
Although there seems to be only one case on record of an adverse response following this interaction, the available evidence suggests that it may be important in some cases. A simple expedient would be to space out the administration of the two drugs as much as possible to minimize their mixing in the gut. Giving the antacid at least 1 h before, or not sooner than 2 h after, the chlorpromazine has been suggested.[1] An alternative would be to give one of the ionic-type antacids such as calcium carbonate–glycine or magnesium hydroxide gel which good evidence shows do not affect the gastrointestinal absorption of chlorpromazine to any extent.[4]

Only chlorpromazine has so far been implicated in this interaction, but it would be prudent to be on the alert for it to take place with other phenothiazines.

References
1 Fann W E, Davis J M, Janowsky D S, Sekerke H J and Schmidt D M. Chlorpromazine: effects of antacids on its gastrointestinal absorption. *J Clin Pharmacol* (1973) **13**, 388.
2 Fann W E, Davis J M, Janowski D S and Schmidt D M. The effects of antacids on chlorpromazine levels. *Ann Pharmacol Ther* (1973) **14**, 135.
3 Forrest F M, Forrest I S and Serra M T. Modification of chlorpromazine metabolism by some other drugs frequently administered to psychiatric patients. *Biol Psychiat* (1970) **2**, 53.
4 Pinell O C, Fenimore D C, Davis C M and Fann W E. Drug–drug interaction of chlorpromazine and antacid. *Clin Pharmacol Ther* (1978) **23**, 125.

Phenothiazines + ascorbic acid

Summary
A single case report describes a marked reduction in serum fluphenazine levels when an ascorbic acid supplement was given.

Interaction, mechanism, importance and management
A single case report describes a man with mania who was treated with 15 mg fluphenazine daily. When 1 g ascorbic acid daily was given to correct his low ascorbic acid levels, his serum fluphenazine levels over a period of a fortnight fell by over 90%, and his manic behaviour re-emerged.[1] The reason for this reaction is not known, but it has been suggested that it may be due both to liver enzyme induction as well as to some effect on gastrointestinal absorption.

Reference
1 Dysken M W, Cumming R J, Channon R A and Davis J M. Drug interaction between ascorbic acid and fluphenazine. *J Amer med Ass* (1979) **241**, 2008.

Phenothiazines + attapulgite-pectin

Summary
An attapulgite-pectin, antidiarrhoeal preparation caused a marked reduction in the absorption of promazine in one subject.

Interaction, mechanism, importance and management
A study on a normal subject given a single 50 mg dose of promazine showed that while taking an attapulgite-pectin preparation the absorption of the promazine was delayed, and the amount reduced by about 25%, probably due to adsorption of the phenothiazine onto the attapulgite.

The data available are very limited, but suggest that attapulgite may possibly reduce the absorption of other phenothazines, and prescribers should bear this in mind.

Reference
1 Sorby D L and Liu G. Effects of adsorbents on drug absorption. II. Effect of an antidiarrhoea mixture on promazine absorption. *J Pharm Sci* (1966) **55**, 504.

Phenothiazines or butyrophenones + coffee or tea

Summary
There is some evidence that the bioavailability of the phenothiazines and the butyrophenones may be markedly reduced by tea or coffee. One report states that it is clinically unimportant.

Interaction, mechanism, importance and management
Preliminary in-vitro studies have shown that if elixirs of chlorpromazine, haloperidol, droperidol, fluphenazine, promethazine, promazine or prochlorperazine are added to tea or coffee, an insoluble precipitate forms. Analysis of these indicates that about 10% of the drug is bound, precipitated or otherwise changed by coffee, and about 90% by tea.[1,2]

A physical interaction with tea or coffee might be one explanation for the considerable variations (one hundred-fold described in one report) in plasma concentrations in patients taking equivalent doses of chlorpromazine,[3] and for the observation that schizophrenia was exacerbated in two cases by the increased consumption of tea and coffee.[4]

In contrast, a clinical report[5] claims that the serum levels of chlorpromazine, haloperidol, fluphenazine and trifluoperazine in a group of 16 mentally retarded patients were unaffected by tea or coffee. More study is needed to determine whether this possible interaction has any importance.

References
1 Kulhanek F, Linde O K and Meisenberg G. Precipitation of antipsychotic drugs in interaction with coffee or tea. *Lancet* (1979) ii, 1130.
2 Hirsch S R. Precipitation of antipsychotic drugs in interaction with coffee or tea. *Lancet* (1979) ii, 1131.
3 Lader M. Monitoring plasma concentration of neuroleptics. *Pharmakopsychiatria* (1976) 9, 170.
4 Mikkelsen E J. Caffeine and schizophrenia. *J Clin Psychiat* (1978) 39, 732.
5 Bowen S, Taylor K M and Gibb I A McL. Effect of coffee and tea on blood levels and efficacy of antipsychotic drugs. *Lancet* (1981) i, 1217.

Phenothiazines + phenobarbitone

Summary
Chlorpromazine serum levels are reduced by concurrent treatment with phenobarbitone, although the therapeutic response appears not to be significantly affected. Serum levels of thioridazine are also reduced by phenobarbitone.

Interaction
A cross-over study on 12 schizophrenic patients treated wtih 300 mg chlorpromazine/day showed that when they were additionally administered 150 mg phenobarbitione/day, there was a fall in chlorpromazine serum levels. Despite this, a general improvement in the patients condition was noted although certain physiological measurements clearly reflected a reduced response arising from the fall.[1]

In another study on 7 patients the serum levels of thioridazine were observed to be reduced by phenobarbitone.[3]

Mechanism
Biochemical studies[1] which accompanied the clinical study cited, using antipyrine as a marker of enzyme induction, indicated that chlorpromazine accelerates its own metabolism by inducing liver microsomal enzymes, and further induction occurs when phenobarbitone is added. Thus the fall in chlorpromazine serum levels can be explained. It seems likely that this also accounts for the fall in thioridazine levels.

Importance and management
The authors of the report cited[1] offer the opinion that there appear to be no practical clinical advantages in combining chlorpromazine with phenobarbitone (or other barbiturates), and possible disadvantages because the serum levels of chlorpromazine are unnecessarily diminished. There would seem to be no scientific case for prescribing these compounds together routinely.

It is not known whether phenothiazines other than chlorpromazine or thioridazine will behave similarly in the presence of barbiturates, but it would be prudent to be on the alert for a reduced therapeutic response.

Reference
1 Loga S, Curry S and Lader M. Interactions of orphenadrine and phenobarbitone with chlorpromazine: plasma concentrations and effects in man. *Br J clin Pharmac* (1975) 2, 197.
2 Ellenor G L, Musa M N and Beuthin F C. Phenobarbital-thioridazine interaction in man. *Res Comm Chem Pathol Pharmacol* (1978) 21, 185.

Phenothiazines + propranolol

Summary
The concurrent use of chlorpromazine and propranolol results in a rise in the serum levels of both drugs.

Interaction, mechanism, importance and management

A study on 7 schizophrenic patients given an average of 6·7 mg/kg chlorpromazine administered three times a day, showed that the concurrent use of propranolol (mean dosage 8·1 mg/kg) increased the serum chlorpromazine levels by 100–500%, and similarly raised the plasma levels of the active metabolites of chlorpromazine by 50–100%.[1] The mechanism is not known. This would seem to be an advantageous interaction and it possibly accounts for the value of propranolol in the treatment of schizophrenia.[2] Propranolol levels have also been shown to be raised by the use of chlorpromazine due to inhibition of its metabolism.[3]

References

1 Peet M, Middlemiss D N and Yates R A. Pharmacokinetic interaction between propranolol and chlorpromazine in schizophrenic patients. *Lancet* (1980) ii, 978.
2 Lindstrom L H and Persson E. Propranolol in chronic schizophrenia: a controlled study in neuroleptic treated patients. *Br J Psychiatr* (1980) 137, 126.
3 Vestal R E, Kornhauser D M, Hollifield J W. Inhibition of propranolol metabolism by chlorpromazine. *Clin Pharmacol Ther* (1979) 25, 19.

Phenothiazines + tricyclic antidepressants

Summary

Concurrent treatment with some combinations of tricyclic antidepressant and phenothiazine can result in a rise in serum levels of both drugs. Although proprietary fixed-dose combined preparations are available, it has been suggested that concurrent use might contribute to an increased incidence of tardive dyskinesia. Excessive weight gain has also been described.

Interaction

If a tricyclic antidepressant and a phenothiazine are administered together, the serum levels of both drugs can be increased.

Effect of phenothiazines on tricyclic antidepressant serum levels:

Imipramine + chlorpromazine or perphenazine
The urinary excretion of test doses of C14-imipramine given to 4 schizophrenic patients was reduced 30–50% during concurrent treatment with 20–48 mg perphenazine a day, and by 50% in another patient taking 300 mg chlorpromazine a day.[2]

A man who failed to respond to treatment with 300 mg chlorpromazine daily was found to recover if imipramine was added, and to relapse whenever it was withdrawn. Using C14-imipramine in other patients it was found that the plasma levels of imipramine and its active metabolite increased four-fold when chlorpromazine was given concurrently.[4]

Nortriptyline + perphenazine
A study on 3 schizophrenic patients who were administered C14-nortriptyline showed that during treatment with 36–40 mg perphenazine daily, the urinary excretion and plasma metabolite levels of nortriptyline fell, while the plasma levels of unchanged nortriptyline rose.[3]

Effect of a tricyclic antidepressant on phenothiazine serum levels:

Desipramine + butaperazine
In a controlled study on 8 schizophrenic patients taking 20 mg butaperazine daily, 6 of them on 150 mg desipramine or more daily showed a rise in butaperazine serum levels of between 50 and 300%.[1]

Mechanism

The rise in the serum levels of both groups of drugs is thought to be due to the mutual inhibition of the liver enzymes concerned with the metabolism of both drugs, resulting in the accumulation of both. The evidence which is available is consistent with this idea.[1-4]

Importance and management

Only a few of the tricyclic antidepressant/phenothiazine combinations appear to have been examined so that it is not known whether all of them interact together similarly.

These two groups of drugs are widely used together in the treatment of schizophrenic patients who show depression, and for mixed anxiety and depression. A number of fixed-dose combinations are available, for example, *Triptafen, Etrafon, Triavil* (amitriptyline and perphenazine); *Motival, Motipress* (nortriptyline and fluphenazine). However, the safety of using both drugs together has been questioned.

One of the problems associated with phenothiazine treatment is the development of tardive dyskinesia, and there is some evidence to suggest that the higher the dosage, the greater the incidence.[6] The symptoms can be transiently masked by increasing the dosage,[7] thus the presence of a tricyclic antidepressant which increases the plasma levels of the phenothiazine might not only be a factor in causing the tardive dyskinesia to develop but might also mask the condition and contribute towards the development of a chronic tardive dyskinesia syndrome, (or so it has been suggested.[1,5]) Ayd has advised[5] that until more data have been accumulated, multiple therapy of this kind should be the exception rather than the rule and these drugs should not be given together unless there are positive scientifically justified indications for doing so.

Attention has also been drawn to excessive weight gain associated with several months' use of amitriptyline with thioridazine for the treatment of chronic pain. This weight gain may be particularly undesirable for diabetic patients.[8]

References
1 El-Yousef M K and Manier D H. Tricyclic antidepressants and phenothiazines. *J Amer Med Ass* (1974) **229**, 1419.
2 Gram L F and Overø K F. Drug interaction: inhibitory effect of neuroleptics on metabolism of tricyclic antidepressants in man. *Br Med J* (1972) **1**, 463.
3 Gram L F, Overø K F and Kirk L. Influence of neuroleptics and benzodiazepines on metabolism of tricyclic antidepressants in man. *Am J Psychiatry* (1974) **131**, 8.
4 Grammer J L and Rolfe B. Interaction of imipramine and chlorpromazine in man. *Psychopharmacologia* (1972) **26**, (*Suppl*) 80.
5 Ayd F J. Pharmacokinetic interaction between tricyclic antidepressants and phenothiazine neuroleptics. *Int Drug Ther Newsletter* (1974) **9**, 31.
6 Crane G E. Persistent dyskinesia. *Brit J Psychiatry* (1973) **122**, 395.
7 Crane G E. Tardive dyskinesia in patients treated with major neuroleptics: a review of the literature. *Am J Psychiatry* (1968) **124**, (*Suppl*) 40.
8 Pfister A K. Weight gain from combined phenothiazine and tricyclic therapy. *J Amer Med Ass* (1978) **239**, 1959.

Thioridazine + lithium carbonate

Summary
Severe neurotoxicity has been described in patients treated with thioridazine and lithium carbonate.

Interaction, mechanism, importance and management
Four patients have been described, all on normal therapeutic doses of lithium and thioridazine, who developed severe neurotoxic complications characterized by seizures, encephalopathy, delerium and highly abnormal EEGs. In all cases the serum lithium levels were below 1·0 mEq/l. Three of the patients had used lithium with other phenothiazines for extended periods without problems and the fourth patient was successfully and uneventfully treated subsequently with lithium and fluphenazine. It is suggested that if this drug combination is used an EEG should be taken prior to treatment and at intervals of 1 week, 4 weeks and 8 weeks during treatment.

Reference
1 Spring G K. Neurotoxicity with combined use of lithium and thioridazine. *J Clin Psychiatry* (1979) **40**, 135.

CHAPTER 18. NEUROMUSCULAR BLOCKING DRUG INTERACTIONS

The nerve impulses which originate in the brain and are intended to cause the contraction of voluntary muscle achieve the last stage of transmission by the release from the nerve endings of acetylcholine. This neurotransmitter rapidly diffuses from the nerve endings, across the minute gap which separates it from the muscle tissues, and attaches itself to the receptors on the specialized area of the muscle called the muscle endplate. At rest this area has negative charges on the outside and positive charges inside, maintained by the energy-using activity of the cells, and is said to be polarized. The arrival of acetylcholine and its attachment to the receptors causes a local disturbance of this membrane, resulting in a reversal of the charges, or depolarization. If the localized disturbance is sufficiently large it sets in motion a much larger electrical disturbance which spreads out almost explosively across the membranes of the muscle fibre, and results in its contraction. Almost immediately—within milliseconds—the receptors are cleared of acetylcholine by the activity of a

Table 18.1 Neuromuscular blocking agents

Non-proprietary names	Proprietary names
Non-depolarizing or competitive blockers	
Alcuronium chloride	*Alloferin*
Diplacine	
Elatine	
Fazadinium bromide	*Fazadon*
Gallamine triethiodide	*Flaxedil*
Metocurine iodide	*Auxoperan, Metubine Iodide*
(dimethyl tubocurarine)	
Pancuronium bromide	*Pavulon*
Tubocurarine chloride	
(d-tubocurarine)	*Tubarine*
Depolarizing blockers	
Carbolonium bromide	*Imbretil*
(this is a dual blocker which initially has non-depolarizing activity)	
Decamethonium bromide	*Syncurine*
Decamethonium iodide (C10)	
Suxamethonium bromide (succinylcholine bromide)	*Brevidil-M*
Suxamethonium chloride (succinylcholine chloride)	*Anectine, Celocurin-Klorid, Lysthenon, Midarine Pantolax, Quelicin, Succinyl-Haf, Succinyl Asta, Succinyl Vitrum, Scoline, Sucostrin*
Suxamethonium iodide (succinylcholine iodide)	*Celocurine, Celocurin-Jodid*
Suxethonium bromide	*Brevidil-E*

localized enzyme, cholinesterase, in readiness for further stimulation, and the muscle endplate becomes repolarized.

Neuromuscular blockers are of two types, non-depolarizing and polarizing. The non-depolarizing or competitive type of blocker (e.g. tubocurarine, gallamine, etc.) competes with acetylcholine for the receptors on the muscle endplate, thereby preventing the acetycholine from acting on the receptors. Reversal of this type of blockade can be achieved by the use of one of the anticholinesterase drugs such as neostigmine which prevents the normal destruction of acetylcholine and allows its concentrations to build up. Thus the competition between the molecules of the blocker and the acetylcholine for occupancy of the receptors swings in favour of the acetylcholine and transmission is restored. Depolarizing blockers also occupy the receptors on the muscle endplate, but they differ in that they act like acetylcholine to cause depolarization. However, they are not immediately removed by cholinesterase so that the depolarization is maintained and the muscle becomes paralysed. Anticholinesterase drugs which increase the levels of acetycholine will therefore enhance and prolong the neuromuscular blockade. The type of blockade induced by some drugs can, under some circumstances, become converted to the other type. The different types of neuromuscular blocking drugs are listed in Table 18.1.

Neuromuscular blockers and anaesthetics + aminoglycoside antibiotics

Summary

The aminoglycoside antibiotics (neomycin, kanamycin, streptomycin, gentamicin, amikacin, tobramycin etc.) possess neuromuscular blocking activity so that when used with anaesthetics alone or with conventional neuromuscular blockers, serious, prolonged and potentially fatal respiratory depression can occur.

Interaction

A large number of cases have been reported in which aminoglycoside antibiotics alone or during anaesthesia have induced some degree of respiratory embarrassment or paralysis. When a surgical neuromuscular blocker has been used as well, the blockade has been deepened and recovery reversed or prolonged by the presence of the antibiotic. Often this has occurred when the antibiotic has been given during or towards the end of surgery to control possible infection, the result being that the patient who would normally have been expected to begin to recover has, quite rapidly, developed serious dyspnoea leading on to prolonged respiratory depression and, in some instances, to complete respiratory failure and death.

Pittinger and his colleagues[1] cite, in the litera-

ture over the period 1955–70, more than 50 such incidents with neomycin, 27 with streptomycin, 7 with kanamycin and 2 with dihydrostreptomycin. The cases surveyed covered virtually every route of antibiotic administration normally used in man: intraperitoneal, intrapleural, oral, intramuscular, retroperineal, oesophageal, intraluminal, cystic, beneath skin flaps, intradural and intravenous. In approximately half of the cases either d-tubocurarine, gallamine or suxamethonium had also been administered. There are far too many cases to cite each one individually here, but two typical cases will illustrate the situation, one of them involving a neuromuscular blocker and the other without a blocker:

Anaesthetic + aminoglycoside antibiotic
    A 48-year-old patient anaesthetized with cyclopro-

pane experienced severe respiratory depression following intraperitoneal irrigation with 500 ml of a 1% neomycin solution. The antibiotic-induced neuromuscular blockade was resistant to treatment with edrophonium but responded to neostigmine.[2]

Anaesthetic + aminoglycoside antibiotic + neuromuscular blocker

A 56-year-old patient, anaesthetized initially with thiopentone followed by nitrous oxide, was given a total of 160 mg gallamine as a skeletal muscle relaxant. The respiration became depressed for a period of 18 h following 2 g neomycin administered intraperitoneally.[3]

The table below (18.2) is an analysis of the interactions from the cases cited and surveyed by Pittinger:[1]

		Neomycin	Kanamycin	Streptomycin
Neuromuscular-blocking agents	d-tubocurarine	12	–	9
	gallamine	8	2	2
	suxamethonium	17	1	3

Since this extensive survey was made there have been further reports of this interaction involving other aminoglycoside antibiotics, including framycetin sulphate used to irrigate the anterior chamber of the eye,[4] gentamicin given alone[6] and with d-tubocurarine,[7] or pancuronium.[15] Amikacin,[9] tobramycin[8] and ribostamycin[5,14] with tubocurarine, but not ribostamycin with suxamethonium.[5] Dibekacin has also been shown to cause a small enhancement of the effects of tubocurarine and suxamethonium.[5,14]

Mechanism

Just why these antibiotics should act in this way is not known for certain, but two theories have been forwarded. The first is the 'chelation' hypothesis of Corrado[10] who suggested that the observed effects might result from the binding of calcium ions in the blood by the antibiotic, thereby reducing the amount of calcium available for the release of acetylcholine at the neuromuscular junction. In this way normal neuromuscular transmission would be impaired. Calcium ions are certainly antagonists of the blockade and calcium gluconate has been used effectively when edrophonium had failed to act.[11]

An alternative theory is the 'competitive hypothesis' of Brazil and Prado-Franceschi[12] which claims, on the basis of experimental evidence, that these antibiotics closely mimic the actions of magnesium ions, reducing or preventing the release of acetylcholine from nerve endings (a pre-junctional effect) and desensitizing the sites at which acetylcholine acts (a post-junctional effect).

Both of these hypotheses and the experimental evidence underlying them are too extensive to be dealt with adequately here, but they are outlined and discussed at length by Pittinger and Adams in their review.[13]

Importance and management

These are well-documented, important, and potentially serious interactions. A measure of their seriousness is that 10 out of the 111 cases cited by Pittinger[1] proved to be fatal, related directly or indirectly to the antibiotic-induced respiratory paralysis. All of the aminoglycoside antibiotics should therefore be used with extreme caution in anaesthetized patients undergoing surgery or during the postoperative recovery period, whether or not conventional neuromuscular blockers are being used as well. Patients with renal disease with hypocalcaemia who may develop higher than usual levels of the antibiotics may be particularly at risk, as well as those who already show evidence of muscular weakness.

Treatment of the respiratory paralysis has met with variable success. Neostigmine or edrophonium has been used to good effect in some cases but not in others.[1] Calcium ions are certainly antagonists of the blockade but it has been pointed out that one could not use very large amounts in clinical practice to reverse the blockade because the theoretically necessary dose (extrapolating from animal studies) would almost certainly be cardiotoxic.[1] However, as already mentioned, calcium gluconate has been used successfully on one occasion where edrophonium failed.[11] Analeptics have been found generally to be ineffective.[1]

References

1 Pittinger C B, Eryasa Y and Adamson R. Antibiotic-induced paralysis. *Anesth Analg* (1970) **49**, 487.
2 New York State Society of Anaesthesiologists Clinical Anesthesia Conference: Postoperative Neomycin Respiratory depression. *NY J Med* (1960) **60**, 1977.
3 LaPorte J, Mignault J, L'Allier R and Perron P. Un cas d'apnea à la neomycin. *Un Med Canada* (1959) **88**, 149.
4 Clark R. Prolonged curarization due to intraocular soframycin. *Anaesth Int Care* (1975) **3**, 79.
5 Arai T, Hashimoto Y, Shima T, Matsukawa S and Iwatsuki

K. Neuromuscular blocking properties of tobramycin, dibecacin and ribostamycin in man. *Jap J Antibiot* (1977) **30**, 281.

6 Holtzman J L. Gentamicin and neuromuscular blockade. *Ann Int Med* (1976) **84**, 55.

7 Warner W A and Sanders E. Neuromuscular blockade associated with gentamicin. *J Amer Med Ass.* (1971) **215**, 1157.

8 Waterman P M and Smith R B. Tobramycin–curare interaction. *Anesth Analg* (1977) **56**, 587.

9 Singh Y N, Marshall I G and Harvey A L. Some effects of the aminoglycoside antibiotic amikacin on neuromuscular and autonomic transmission. *Br J Anaesth* (1978) **50**, 109.

10 Corrado A P. Respiratory depression due to antibiotics: calcium in treatment. *Anesth Analg* (1963) **42**, 1.

11 Mullet R D and Kears A S. Apnea and respiratory insufficiency after intraperitoneal administration of kanamycin. *Surgery* (1961) **49**, 530.

12 Brazil, O V and Prado-Franceschi Y. The nature of neuromuscular block produced by neomycin and gentamicin. *Arch Int Pharmacodynam et Ther* (1969) **179**, 78.

13 Pittinger C and Adamson R. Antibiotic blockade of neuromuscular function. *Ann Rev Pharmacol* (1972) **12**, 169.

14 Hasimoto Y, Shima T, Matsukawa S and Iwatsuki K. Neuromuscular blocking properties of some antibiotics in man. *Tohoku J exp Med* (1975) **117**, 339.

15 Regan A G and Perumbetti P P V. Pancuronium and gentamicin interaction in patients with renal failure. *Anesth Analg.* (1980) **59**, 393.

Neuromuscular blockers + miscellaneous non-aminoglycoside antibiotics

Summary

Colistin, colistin sulphomethate sodium, amphotericin B, lincomycin, rolitetracycline and oxytetracycline have varying degrees of neuromuscular blocking activity which in the presence of anaesthetics and conventional surgical neuromuscular blockers may lead to respiratory paralysis.

Interaction

Pittinger and his colleagues, in their literature review[1] of references to antibiotic-induced paralysis covering the period 1955–70, found 17 cases in which colistin or colistin sulphomethate sodium, with or without anaesthetics or conventional neuromuscular blockers, were responsible for the development of respiratory paralysis. Some of the patients had renal disease. There were also 5 cases with polymyxin B and 4 with rolitetracycline or oxytetracycline in myasthenic patients.

Lincomycin has been observed to induce respiratory paralysis in a man recovering from blockade with d-tubocurarine.[4] This has been confirmed in another report[5] and demonstrated in animal experiments.[4]

Amphotericin B can induce hypokalaemia resulting in muscle weakness[3,4] which might be expected to enhance the effects of neuromuscular blockers, but there appear to be no reports of this in the literature confirming that this can actually take place.

Mechanism

Not understood.

Importance and management

Interactions with colistin and colistin sulpho-methate sodium are well established. There is limited evidence of an interaction with lincomycin. These antibiotics should be given with caution to patients undergoing surgery or during the postoperative recovery period. It seems probable that the effects of the tetracyclines may only be important in myasthenic patients.[6,7] No interaction appears to occur in these patients with either chloramphenicol or penicillin.[6,7] In some instances the presence of renal disease may be a contributory factor in the development of this adverse interaction.

References

1 Pittinger C B, Eryasa Y and Adamson R. Antibiotic-induced paralysis. *Anesth Analg* (1970) **49**, 487.

2 Holeman C W and Einstein H. The toxic effects of amphotericin B in man. *Calif Med* (1963) **99**, 90.

3 Drutz D J, Fan J H, Tai T Y, Cheng J T and Hsien W C. Hypokalemic rhabdomyolysis and myoglobinuria following amphotericin therapy. *J Amer Med Ass* (1970) **211**, 824.

4 Samuelason R J, Giesecke A H, Kallus F T and Stanley V F. Lincomycin–curare interaction. *Anesth Analg* (1975) **54**, 103.

5 Hashimoto Y, Iwatsuki N and Shima T. Neuromuscular blocking properties of lincomycin and kanamycin in man. *Jap J Anesh* (1971) **20**, 407.

6 Gibbels E. Further observations on the side-effects of intravenous administration of rolitetracycline in myasthenia gravis pseudoparalytica. *Deut Med Wschr* (1967) **92**, 1153.

7 Wullen F, Kast G and Bruck A. On the side-effects of tetracycline administration in myasthenic patients. *Deut Med Wschr* (1967) **92**, 667.

Neuromuscular blockers + azathioprine

Summary
The neuromuscular blocking effects of d-tubocurarine can be markedly reduced by pretreatment with azathioprine or lymphocytic antiglobulin.

Interaction, mechanism, importance and management
A study on 26 patients showed that the neuromuscular blocking effects of d-tubocurarine were diminished by pretreatment with either azathioprine or lymphocytic antiglobulin. The dosage requirements of the curare were increased 2–4 fold. Two of the patients who had also received guanethidine showed a particularly marked interaction. The reasons for these changes are not understood. Whether it occurs with other neuromuscular blockers is not certain. Since azathioprine is converted within the body to mercaptopurine it would seem possible that this drug may cause a similar interaction. This requires confirmation.[1]

Reference
1 Vetten K B. Immunosuppressive therapy and anaesthesia. *S Afr med J* (1973) **47**, 767.

Neuromuscular blockers + beta-blockers

Summary
There is conflicting evidence claiming that the effects of suxamethonium and tubocurarine can be slightly reduced or prolonged by the concurrent use of beta-blockers.

Interaction

Reduced neuromuscular blockade
A study undertaken with 31 patients undergoing elective surgery showed that the intravenous injection of propranolol, 1 mg/15 kg, over a 4-min period, slightly decreased the neuromuscular blocking activity of suxamethonium. The mean period of apnoea was 3·6 min compared with 4·4 minutes for the control group: not statistically significant. Propranolol also accelerated the recovery from tubocurarine-induced blockade.[1]

These results are confirmed by other studies in man with tubocurarine in which propranolol and oxprenolol shortened the recovery from blockade, but pindolol had no effect except in a few subjects.[2]

Enhanced neuromuscular blockade
A report on 2 patients with thyrotoxicosis undergoing surgery who were treated with tubocurarine and who had had 120 mg propranolol daily indicated that the activity of the neuromuscular blocker was enhanced.[3]

Mechanism
Not understood. There are animal studies describing an enhancement of the neuromuscular blocking activity by the beta-blockers.[4,5]

Importance and management
Because of the uncertainty about the outcome, care should be exercised during concurrent use, but there is no reason to regard these drugs as contraindicated. Evidence about other neuromuscular blockers and beta-blockers appears to be lacking. More study is needed.

References
1 Varma Y S, Sharma P L and Singh H W. Effect of propranolol hydrochloride on the neuromuscular blocking action of d-tubocurarine and succinylcholine in man. *Indian J med Res* (1972) **60**, 266.
2 Varma Y S, Sharma P L and Singh H W. Comparative effect of propranolol, oxprenolol and pindolol on neuromuscular blocking action of d-tubocurarine in man. *Indian J med Res* (1973) **61**, 1382.
3 Rozen M S and Whan F M. Prolonged curarization associated with propranolol. *Med J Aust* (1972) **1**, 467.
4 Usubiaga J E. Neuromuscular effects of beta-adrenergic blockers and their interaction with skeletal muscle relaxants. *Anesthesiology* (1968) **29**, 484.
5 Harrah M B, Walter L W and Katzune B C. The interaction of d-tubocurarine with anti-arrhythmic drugs *Anesthesiology* (1970) **96**, 99.

Neuromuscular blockers + aprotinin

Summary

Three cases of apnoea have been described in patients recovering from neuromuscular blockade who were given aprotinin (*Trasylol*).

Interaction

Three cases have been reported of patients who underwent surgery under general anaesthesia during which suxamethonium either alone or with tubocurarine was used. At the end of, or shortly after, the operation when spontaneous breathing had recommenced, aprotinin (*Trasylol*) in doses of 2500–5000 k.i.u. was given. In each case respiration rapidly became inadequate and apnoea lasting periods of 7, 30 and 90 min occurred.

Mechanism

Not understood. Animal studies have failed to demonstrate this interaction or throw any light on its mechanism.[2]

Importance and management

Information on this interaction appears to be limited to these three cases. Users should be on the alert for the possible development of this potentially serious interaction, but its incidence is unknown.

References

1 Chasapakis G and Dimas C. Possible interaction between muscle relaxants and the kallikrein-trypsin inactivator 'Trasylol'. *Br J Anaesth* (1966) **38**, 838.
2 Ambrus J L, Wilkens H and Ambrus C M. Effect of the protease inhibitor trasylol on cholinesterase levels and on susceptibility to succinylcholine. *Res Chem Pathol Pharmacol Commun* (1970) **1**, 141.

Neuromuscular blockers + clindamycin

Summary

Clindamycin can enhance and prolong the effects of the neuromuscular blockers

Interaction, mechanism, importance and management

Clindamycin possesses inherent neuromuscular blocking activity and has been observed in a few instances to enhance the activity of conventional neuromuscular blocking agents. This has been described in a patient given pancuronium bromide[1] and in another given suxamethonium.[2] The incidence of this response is uncertain, but it would be prudent to be on the watch for this response during concurrent use.

References

1 Fogdall R P and Miller R D. Prolongation of a pancuronium-induced neuromuscular blockade by clindamycin. *Anesthesiol* (1974) **41**, 407.
2 Avery D and Finn R. Succinylcholine. Prolonged apnea associated with clindamycin and abnormal liver function tests. *Dis Nerv Syst* (1977) **38**, 473.

Neuromuscular blockers + cyclophosphamide

Summary

Cyclophosphamide reduces serum pseudocholinesterase levels. This can result in an enhancement of the effects of suxamethonium leading to respiratory embarrassment and prolonged apnoea.

Interaction

Respiratory insufficiency and prolonged apnoea were observed in a patient on two occasions while receiving cyclophosphamide and undergoing anaesthesia, during which tubocurarine and suxamethonium were given. Plasma pseudocholinesterase levels were measured and found to be low. Anaesthesia without the suxamethonium was uneventful. Seven out of 8 patients subsequently examined also showed depressed serum pseudocholinesterase levels while taking cyclophosphamide.[1]

Respiratory depression[4] and depressed serum pseudocholinesterase levels have been described in other reports.[2,3] One indicated a 35–70% reduction.[2]

Mechanism

The removal of suxamethonium from the body depends upon the presence of pseudocholinesterase. When the levels of this enzyme are depressed, the effects of the suxamethonium are enhanced and prolonged.

Importance and management

An established interaction, and with a potentially serious outcome. The general incidence is uncertain. A cyclophosphamide-induced depression in serum pseudocholinesterase levels appears to be high, and lasts several days, possibly even weeks. Plasma pseudocholinesterase levels should be checked before using depolarizing neuromuscular blockers.[1] One group of authors has recommended that suxamethonium and cyclophosphamide should not be used concurrently,[1] whereas another has suggested an appropriate reduction in the dosage of the blocker.[2]

References

1 Walker I R, Zapf P W and Mackay I R. Cyclophosphamide, cholinesterase and anaesthesia. *Aust NZ J Med* (1972) **3**, 247.
2 Zsigmond E K and Robins G. The effect of a series of anti-cancer drugs on plasma cholinesterase activity. *Canad Anaesth Soc J* (1972) **19**, 75.
3 Mone J G and Mathie W E. Qualitative and quantitative effects of pseudocholinesterase activity. *Anaesthesia* (1967) **22**, 55.
4 Wolff H. Die Hemmung der Serumcholinesterase durch Cyclophosphamid (Endoxan) *Klin Wschr* (1965) **43**, 819.

Neuromuscular blockers + diazepam

Summary

Some reports indicate that diazepam enhances the effects of skeletal neuromuscular blockers, while others indicate that it does not. Patients given both drugs should be monitored for possible changes in the depth and duration of neuromuscular blockade.

Interaction

The evidence is inconsistent and conflicting.

Enhanced blockade

Two patients who were given diazepam as a premedication and d-tubocurarine during the anaesthesia had persistent muscle weakness and respiratory depression for 3–4 h after the operation.[1]

A subsequent study by the same authors compared 10 patients administered gallamine with 4 other patients given gallamine and diazepam (0·15–0·2 mg/kg). The duration of activity of the blocker was prolonged by a factor of three by the diazepam and the depression of the twitch response was doubled.[1,2]

There are other reports of enhanced neuromuscular blockade with diazepam and tubocurarine,[3,4] suxamethonium[5] and gallamine.[3]

Reduced blockade or no effect

A study on the force of thumb adduction in response to electrical stimulation of the ulnar nerves of 15 patients undergoing surgery showed that the intra-venous injection of 0·3–0·6 mg/kg diazepam had no effect on the neuromuscular blockade due to d-tubocurarine, gallamine or decamethonium.[6]

In one of the studies already cited the duration of paralysis due to suxamethonium was reduced by 20% by diazepam (0·15 mg/kg) and the recovery time was shortened.[2]

It has been claimed in other reports that diazepam does not enhance the actions of d-tubocurarine, suxamethonium,[7,8,11] pancuronium, fazadinium or alcuronium.[11]

Mechanism

Not understood. One suggestion which has been offered[6] is that where some alteration in response has been seen it might be a reflection of a central depressant action rather than a direct effect on the myoneural junction. In support of this idea a case is cited of a man recovering from an overdose of *Mandrax* (methaqualone and diphenhydramine) who developed apnoea with muscle relaxation after being given 10 mg diazepam.[9] In another case a man under extradural anaesthesia became apnoeic and required artificial ventilation following 10 mg diazepam.[10]

Importance and management
There is no obvious explanation for these discordant observations. Anaesthetists should be aware that in some patients diazepam may alter the response to neuromuscular blockers, but there seems to be little consistency in the response.

References
1 Feldman S A and Crawley B E. Diazepam and muscle relaxants. *Br Med J* (1970) 1, 691.
2 Feldman S A and Crawley B E. Interaction of diazepam with the muscle-relaxant drugs. *Br Med J* (1970) 2, 336.
3 Vergano F, Zaccagna C A, Zuccaro G. Muscle relaxant properties of diazepam. *Minerva Anest* (1969) 35, 91.
4 Stovner J and Endresen R. Intravenous anesthesia with diazepam. *Acta Anaesth Scand* (1965) (Suppl) 24, 223.
5 Jörgensen H. Premedicinering med diazepam. *Nord Med* (1964) 72, 1395.
6 Dretchen K, Ghoneim M M and Long J P. The interaction of diazepam with myoneural blocking agents. *Anesthesiol* (1971) 34, 463.
7 Stovner J and Endresen R. Diazepam in intravenous anaesthesia. *Lancet* (1965) ii, 1298.
8 Hunter A R. Diazepam as a muscle relaxant during general anaesthesia. *Br J Anaesth* (1967) 39, 633.
9 Doughty A. Unexpected danger of diazepam. *Br Med J* (1970) 2, 239.
10 Buskop J J, Price M and Molnar I. Untoward effect of diazepam. *New Eng J Med* (1967) 277, 316.
11 Bradshaw E G and Maddison S. Effect of diazepam at the neuromuscular junction. A clinical study. *Br J Anaesth* (1979) 51, 955.

Neuromuscular blockers + dexpanthenol

Summary
Enhanced suxamethonium-induced neuromuscular blockade attributed to dexpanthenol has been described in one patient, but further studies have failed to confirm this interaction.

Interaction
A patient developed severe respiratory embarrassment following the intramuscular injection of 500 mg dexpanthenol during the recovery period from anaesthesia with nitrous oxide and cyclopropane, and neuromuscular blockade with suxamethonium.[1]

A study on 6 patients under general anaesthesia showed that their response to suxamethonium was unaffected by the infusion of 500 mg pantothenic acid.[2]

Mechanism
Unknown.

Importance and management
Although a number of warnings about this interaction have been issued by various manufacturers of products containing pantothenic acid, they seem to be based on the single unconfirmed and unexplained report cited.[1] There seems to be little reason to avoid concurrent use, but users should be aware of this case.

References
1 Stewart P. Case reports. *J Amer Assoc Nurse Anesth* (1960) 28, 56.
2 Smith R M, Gottshall S C, and Young J A. Succinylcholine–pantothenyl alcohol: a reappraisal. *Anesth Analg* (1969) 48, 205.

Neuromuscular blockers + ecothiophate iodide

Summary
The effects of suxamethonium can be markedly enhanced and prolonged in patients under treatment with ecothiophate iodide, leading to apnoea.

Interaction

In 1965 Murray McGavi warned that the systemic absorption of ecothiophate iodide from eye drops could lower serum pseudocholinesterase levels to such an extent that '... within a few days of commencing therapy, levels are reached at which protracted apnoea could occur should these patients require general anaesthesia in which muscle relaxation is obtained with suxamethonium'.[1] Cases of apnoea were reported in the following year[2,3] and the year after.[5] In one of them a woman who had received 200 mg suxamethonium showed apnoea for $5\frac{1}{2}$ h. Other studies have confirmed that ecothiophate markedly reduces the levels of pseudocholinesterase.[4]

Mechanism

Suxamethonium depends for its metabolism on the activity of pseudocholinesterase. In the presence of ecothiophate iodide (which is an anticholinesterase), the levels of the enzyme are markedly depressed so that metabolism of the suxamethonium is reduced and its effects enhanced and prolonged.

Importance and management

An established interaction with a potentially serious outcome. Plasma pseudocholinesterase is rapidly reduced to extremely low levels (less than 5%) by ecothiophate iodide administered as eye drops, and can take about 4 weeks to return to approximately normal levels.[6] Pseudocholinesterase levels should be measured prior to surgery if it is intended to use suxamethonium. An alternative neuromuscular blocker would probably be preferable.

References

1 McGavi D D M. Depressed levels of serum-pseudocholinesterase with ecothiophate-iodide eyedrops. *Lancet* (1965) **ii**, 272.
2 Gesztes T. Prolonged apnoea after suxamethonium injection associated with eye drops containing an anticholinesterase agent. *Br J Anaesth* (1966) **38**, 408.
3 Pantuck E J. Ecothiopate iodide eye drops and prolonged response to suxamethonium. *Br J Anaesth* (1966) **38**, 406.
4 Cavallaro R J, Krumperman L W and Kugler F. Effect of ecothiophate therapy on the metabolism of succinylcholine in man. *Anesth Analg* (1974) **47**, 570.
5 Mone J G and Mathie W E. Qualitative and quantitative defects of pseudocholinesterase activity. *Anaesthesia* (1967) **22**, 55.
6 de Roetth A, Dettbarn W D, Rosenberg P, Wilensky J G and Wong A. Effect of phopholine iodide on blood cholinesterase levels of normal and glaucoma subjects. *Amer. J Ophthal* (1965) **59**, 586.

Neuromuscular blockers + frusemide

Summary

The effects of tubocurarine have been reported to be enhanced by the intravenous administration of mannitol and frusemide.

Interaction

Three patients undergoing renal transplantation showed an enhancement of neuromuscular blockade due to d-tubocurarine after being administered mannitol and frusemide intravenously.[1] In each case a pronounced decrease in the twitch tension was seen. Two of them were given 0·3 mg/kg tubocurarine and later 12·5 g mannitol and 80 mg frusemide. The third was given 0·5 mg/kg tubocurarine 12·5 g mannitol and 40 mg frusemide. The last patient also demonstrated this interaction when he was later given an additional 40 mg frusemide without the mannitol. In all 3 cases the residual blockade was easily antagonized with pyridostigmine 14 mg or neostigmine 3·0 mg with 1·2 mg atropine.

Mechanism

The mechanism of this interaction is not known but the authors of the report speculate that it might have been due to a redistribution of the tubocurarine by the diuretics, possibly in association with some direct depressant effect on the neuromuscular junction.

Importance and control

Attention has been drawn to the possibility of this interaction on a number of occasions, but the report cited seems to be the only documented clinical evidence of it. Only tubocurarine has actually been implicated but it would be prudent to be alert to the possibility of an interaction with any of the other neuromuscular blockers until further evidence is available.

Reference

1 Miller R D, Sohn Y J, and Matteo R S. Enhancement of d-tubocurarine neuromuscular blockade by diuretics in man. *Anesthesiol* (1976) **45**, 422.

Neuromuscular blockers + *Innovar*

Summary

Prolongation of the effects of suxamethonium by *Innovar* (fentanyl citrate, droperidol) has been described.

Interaction, mechanism, importance and management

A case report[1] describes the enhancement of the effects of suxamethonium in a patient treated with *Innovar* (fentanyl citrate, droperidol). The mechanism is not understood, although respiratory depression is among the recognized adverse reactions of this compound preparation. Anaesthetists should be on the alert for the development of this reaction in patients given both groups of drugs, although it should be emphasized that the incidence appears to be small.

Reference

1 Wehner R J, A case study: the prolongation of Anectine effect by *Innovar*. *AANA J* (1979) **47**, 576.

Neuromuscular blockers + lignocaine or procaine

Summary

The neuromuscular blockade due to suxamethonium can be enhanced by both lignocaine (lidocaine) and procaine. This interaction is of limited importance.

Interaction

A series of experiments in human subjects given a range of intravenous doses of lignocaine (1–36 mg/kg), or procaine (1–16 mg/kg), showed that the apnoea following the concurrent use of suxamethonium (0·7 mg/kg) was prolonged. A dose relationship was established. The duration of the apnoea was very approximately doubled by 2·2 mg/kg of both lignocaine and procaine, and tripled by 11·2 mg/kg, although the effects of procaine at higher doses were more marked.[1]

Mechanism

Uncertain. It is suggested that it may be due to displacement by the local anaesthetic of the neuromuscular blocker from its plasma protein binding sites. In the case of procaine, there may additionally be competition between the suxamethonium and the procaine for hydrolysis by cholinesterase which inactivates them both.[1]

Importance and management

The documentation is limited but the interaction involving lignocaine or procaine appears to be established. Marked enhancement does not occur with lower doses of either, although some care is clearly appropriate. The authors of the paper cited state that 'this effect only becomes significant after the administration of doses unlikely to be used in clinical anaesthesia. As a practical conclusion, it can be suggested that even after accidental overdosage of local anaesthetics, moderate doses of succinylcholine may be used to stop convulsions without an alarming prolongation of the apnea.'[1]

An enhancement of the actions of suxamethonium by procainamide has been described in animals[2] but appears not to have been reported in man.

References

1 Usubiaga J E, Wikinski J A, Morales R L and Usubiaga L E J. Interaction of intravenously administered procaine, lidocaine and succinylcholine in anesthetized subjects. *Anesth Analg* (1967) **46**, 39.
2 Cuthbert M F. The effect of quinidine and procainamide on the neuromuscular blocking action of suxamethonium. *Br J Anaesth* (1966) **38**, 775

Neuromuscular blockers + lithium carbonate

Summary

There are two case reports of patients taking lithium carbonate who showed prolonged neuromuscular blockade and respiratory difficulties after receiving standard doses of suxamethonium and pancuronium.

Interaction

Two different reactions have been seen: one is an enhancement of neuromuscular blockade, and the other may possibly not be an interaction but due to lithium toxicity.

Enhanced blockade

    A manic-depressive woman being treated with lithium carbonate and who had a serum lithium concentration of 1·2 mEq/l underwent surgery and was administered thiopentone, suxamethonium (a total of 310 mg over 2 h) and 0·5 mg pancuronium bromide. Prolonged neuromuscular blockade with apnoea occurred.[1,2]

This is similar to another case in which the presence of lithium enhanced the neuromuscular blockade due to pancuronium[3]

    The same interaction has also been demonstrated in a laboratory study in dogs where it was shown that an infusion of lithium carbonate alone reduced the electrically stimulated twitch by 5–10%, but in the presence of suxamethonium the twitch tension and recovery were prolonged 50–200%.[1,2]

Lithium toxicity?

    A depressive woman controlled on 750 mg lithium carbonate a day, undergoing electroconvulsive therapy, was anaesthetized and given 30 mg suxamethonium bromide intravenously. Spontaneous respiration returned within the time expected but the patient could not be roused for over 2 h and remained drowsy for the rest of the day. She was subsequently found to have a serum lithium concentration of 3·6 mEq/l but none of the usual signs of lithium toxicity. A week later when her serum lithium concentration was 0·5 mEq/l she was again given ECT using the same drugs and techniques and recovered uneventfully.[4]

Mechanism

Preliminary data from the study in dogs[1,2] show that prostigmine is ineffective in reversing the neuromuscular blockade. So too are calcium and potassium. But there is far too little evidence yet available to say just how lithium enhances the actions of suxamethonium or pancuronium.

Importance and management

Although there are only two reports so far of enhanced neuromuscular blockade in the presence of lithium, it would clearly be prudent to be alert to the possibility of this interaction if suxamethonium, pancuronium, or any other neuromuscular blocker is used in patients controlled on lithium carbonate.

    There is too little evidence to comment constructively on the second type of reaction described.

References

1 Hill G, Wong K C, Hodges M and Seutker C. Potentiation of succinylcholine neuromuscular blockade by lithium carbonate. *Fed Proc* (1976) **35**, 729.
2 Hill G, Wong K C, and Hodges M R. Potentiation of succinylcholine neuromuscular blockade by lithium carbonate. *Anaesthesiol* (1976) **44**, 439.
3 Borden H, Clarke M and Katz H. The use of pancuronium bromide in patients receiving lithium carbonate. *Can Anaesth Soc J* (1974) **21**, 79.
4 Jephcott G. and Kerry R J. Lithium: an anaesthetic risk. *Br J Anaesth* (1974) **46**, 389.

Neuromuscular blockers + magnesium salts

Summary

The effects of suxamethonium, tubocurarine, decamethonium and possibly other blockers can be enhanced by magnesium sulphate administered parenterally.

Interaction

A study in a number of women undergoing caesarian section showed that those who had received magnesium sulphate for toxaemia in pregnancy required less suxamethonium (4·73 compared with 7·39 mg/kg/h) than other normal patients.[1]

Prolonged neuromuscular blockade has been described in 2 woman with pre-eclampsia who were given magnesium sulphate and either tubocurarine or suxamethonium.[2] Animal experiments have demonstrated the same effect on decamethonium[2] as well as with tubocurarine and suxamethonium.[2,3]

Mechanism

Not fully resolved. Magnesium sulphate possesses neuromuscular blocking activity and can inhibit the normal release of acetylcholine from nerve endings. It would seem possible the enhanced blockade is due to the simple addition of these effects with those of the neuromuscular blockers.

Importance and management

The documentation is limited but the interaction is established. Enhancement of the activity of neuromuscular blockers should be expected in the presence of magnesium sulphate. Intravenous calcium gluconate has been used to assist recovery in one case.[2] An interaction with magnesium sulphate given orally seems very unlikely because its absorption is poor.

References

1 Morris R and Giesecke A H. Potentiation of muscle relaxants by magnesium sulphate in toxemia of pregnancy. *South Med J* (1968) **61**, 25.
2 Ghoneim M M and Long J P The interaction between magnesium and other neuromuscular blocking agents. *Anesthesiol* (1970) **32**, 23.
3 Giesecke A H, Morris R E, Dalton M D and Stephen C R. Of magnesium, muscle relaxants, toxemic parturients, and cats. *Anesth Analg* (1968) **47**, 689.

Neuromuscular blockers + meturedepa

Summary

Meturedepa reduces serum pseudocholinesterase levels which can result in an enhancement of the effects of suxamethonium, leading to prolonged apnoea.

Interaction

Two patients on meturedepa showed prolonged apnoea after treatment with suxamethonium. One failed to breathe spontaneously for 7 h after receiving 80 mg suxamethonium, and the other similarly showed apnoea for an hour after 20 mg. Subsequent studies in 4 other patients on meturedepa showed that their serum pseudocholinesterase levels were markedly depressed.[1]

Mechanism

The removal of suxamethonium from the body depends upon the presence of serum pseudocholinesterase. When the levels of this enzyme are depressed, the effects of suxamethonium are enhanced and prolonged.

Importance and management

The information is very limited, but the interaction appears to be established. Plasma pseudocholinesterase levels should be checked before using suxamethonium in patients on meturedepa.

Reference

1 Wang R I H and Ross C A. Prolonged apnea following succinylcholine in cancer patients receiving AB-132. *Anesthesiol* (1963) **24**, 363.

Neuromuscular blockers + phenothiazines

Summary

A single case report describes prolonged apnoea when promazine was given during recovery from suxamethonium-induced blockade.

Interaction

A woman who had undergone surgery, during which she had received suxamethonium, was given 25 mg promazine intravenously for sedation during the recovery period. Within 3 min she became cyanotic and apnoeic, and required assisted respiration for 4 h.[1]

Mechanism

Not understood. One suggestion is that the promazine might act as a cholinesterase depressant thereby the recovery from the neuromuscular blockade.[1]

Importance and management

There are far too few data in this single report to make any useful general statements about the use of promazine or any other phenothiazine in patients who have had suxamethonium, except to suggest that some caution might be appropriate.

Reference

1 Regan A G. Prolonged apnoea after administration of promazine hydrochloride following succinylcholine infusion. A case report. *Anesth Analg.* (1967) **46**, 315.

Neuromuscular blockers + quinidine

Summary

The effects of both depolarizing and non-depolarizing neuromuscular blockers can be enhanced by quinidine. Recurarization with apnoea has been described when quinidine was given during the recovery period from neuromuscular blockade.

Interaction

A woman underwent surgery during which she received dimethyl tubocurarine as a muscle relaxant. After the operation, when she had recovered her motor functions and was able to talk coherently, she was given 200 mg quinidine sulphate by injection. In less than 15 min she developed muscular weakness and respiratory embarrassment to such an extent that she required intubation and assisted respiration for a period of $2\frac{1}{2}$ h. Edrophonium and neostygmine were used to aid recovery.

This interaction has been described in man in other reports involving tubocurarine[2] and suxamethonium[3,4] and investigated in animals.[5–8]

Mechanism

The evidence from animal experiments indicates that quinidine has direct actions on the muscle end-plate to decrease its excitability, and it prolongs the refractory period of skeletal muscle. These neuromuscular blocking effects appear to be additive with those of the conventional blockers.[5–8]

Importance and management

Not extensively documented in man, but it appears to be an important and established interaction. The incidence is uncertain, but in one study[3] it was demonstrated to a greater or lesser degree by 5 out of the 6 patients examined. It has only been reported in man with dimethyl tubocurarine, tubocurarine and suxamethonium, but it has been described in animals with gallamine and decamethonium as well. It would seem probable that it will occur in man with any depolarizing or non-depolarizing neuromuscular blocker, but this requires confirmation. Considerable care is clearly necessary during concurrent or sequential use.

References

1 Schmidt J L, Vick N A and Sadove M S. The effect of quinidine on the action of muscle relaxants. *J Amer Med Ass* (1963) **183**, 669.
2 Way W L, Katzung B G, and Larson C P. Recurarization with quinidine. *J Amer Med Ass* (1967) **200**, 163.
3 Grogono A W. Anesthesia for atrial defibrillation. Effect of quinidine on muscular relaxation. *Lancet* (1963) **ii**, 1039.
4 Boeré L A. Fehler and Gefahren. Recurarisation nach Chinidinsulfat. *Anaesthetist* (1964) **13**, 368.
5 Miller R D, Way W L and Katzung B G. The neuromuscular effects of quinidine. *Proc Soc Exp Biol Med* (1968) **129**, 215.
6 Miller R D, Way W L and Katzung B G. The potentiation of neuromuscular blocking agents by quinidine. *Anesthesiol* (1967) **28**, 1036.
7 Cuthbert M F. The effect of quinidine and procainamide on the neuromuscular blocking action of suxamethonium. *Br J Anaesth* (1966) **38**, 775.
8 Usubiaga J E. Potentiation of muscle relaxants by quinidine. *Anaesthesiol* (1968) **29**, 1068.

Neuromuscular blockers + triethylene-melamine (TEM), methchlorethamine (nitrogen mustard) or triethylene thiophosphoramide (thiotepa)

Summary
In-vitro studies suggest that TEM, nitrogen mustard and thiotepa may possibly cause sufficient inhibition of serum pseudocholinesterase to enhance the actions of suxamethonium.

Interaction, mechanism, importance and management

In-vitro studies[1] have shown that the following cytotoxic drugs are able to inhibit human serum pseudocholinesterase, in order of decreasing effectiveness: triethylene-melamine (TEM), cyclophosphamide, methochlorethamine (nitrogen mustard) and triethylene thiophosphoramide (thiotepa). The I_{50} values (that is to say the concentrations of each drug necessary to cause a 50% inhibition of the activity of the enzyme, using benzoylcholine as the substituted substrate) were, respectively, $3 \cdot 3 \times 10^{-4}$ M, $4 \cdot 0 \times 10^{-4}$ M, 63×10^{-4} M, and $7 \cdot 9 \times 10^{-3}$ M. Of these four drugs, only cyclophosphamide appears so far to have been shown to enhance the actions of suxamethonium (see p. 390) but it would seem prudent to check the plasma pseudocholinesterase activity of patients on any of these drugs before administering suxamethonium.

Reference
1 Zsigmond E K and Robins G. The effects of a series of anti-cancer drugs on plasma cholinesterase activity. *Canad Anaesth Soc J* (1972) **19**, 75.

Neuromuscular blockers + trimetaphan

Summary
Trimetaphan (trimethaphan) may enhance the effects of neuromuscular blockers resulting in prolonged apnoea.

Interaction

A man undergoing neurosurgery who was given tubocurarine and suxamethonium showed apnoea lasting about $2\frac{1}{2}$h during the recovery period, attributed to the concurrent use of trimetaphan (4500 mg over a 90 min period). Later, when the patient underwent further surgery using essentially the same anaesthetic techniques and agents but with very much smaller doses of trimetaphan, 35 mg over a 10 min period, the recovery was normal[1]

Prolonged apnoea has been reported in previous reports on patients given suxamethonium and trimetaphan.[2,6]

Mechanism

Not fully understood. Experiments with dogs[5] and rats[3,4] indicate that trimetaphan may have direct neuromuscular blocking activity. It has also been demonstrated in vitro that trimetaphan can inhibit pseudocholinesterase[2]. If this also occurs in vivo, the metabolism of suxamethonium would be depressed, and its activity would be expected to be prolonged.

Importance and management

Information on this interaction is extremely limited. If trimetaphan and neuromuscular blockers are used concurrently, users should be on the alert for enhanced and prolonged neuromuscular blockade.

References
1 Wilson S L, Miller R N, Wright C and Hasse D. Prolonged neuromuscular blockade with trimethaphan: a case report. *Anesth Analg* (1976) **55**, 353.
2 Tewfik G I. Trimethaphan, its effect on the pseudocholinesterase level of man. *Anaesthesia* (1957) **12**, 326.
3 Pearcy W C and Wittenstein E S. The interactions of trimethaphan (Arfonad), suxamethonium and cholinesterase inhibition in the rat. *Br J Anaesth* (1960) **32**, 156.
4 Deacock A R and Davies T D W. The influence of certain ganglionic blocking agents on the neuromuscular transmission. *Br J Anaesth* (1958) **30**, 217.
5 Randall L D, Peterson W G and Lebmann G. The ganglionic blocking action of thiophan derivatives. *J Pharmacol Exp Ther* (1949) **97**, 48.
6 Poulton T J, James F M and Lockridge O. Prolonged apnea following trimethaphan and succinylcholine. *Anesthesiology* (1979) **50**, 54.

CHAPTER 19. SYMPATHOMIMETIC DRUG INTERACTIONS

The sympathomimetic amines, as their name implies, mimic the actions of the sympathetic nervous system. Since noradrenaline (norepinephrine, levarterenol) is the neurotransmitter involved in the final link between the nerve endings of the sympathetic nervous system and the receptors of the organs and tissues innervated, the effects of stimulation of the sympathetic nerves can be reproduced or mimicked by noradrenaline. The sympathomimetic amines differ from noradrenaline. and from each other, in a variety of ways and, in the context of drug interactions, it is important to recognize these differences.

Noradrenaline itself and phenylephrine have direct stimulant actions on the noradrenaline receptors. Others, such as tyramine, act indirectly by stimulating the release of noradrenaline from nerve endings which, in its turn, stimulates the receptors. Yet others possess mixed activity. This is very simply illustrated in Figure 19.1.

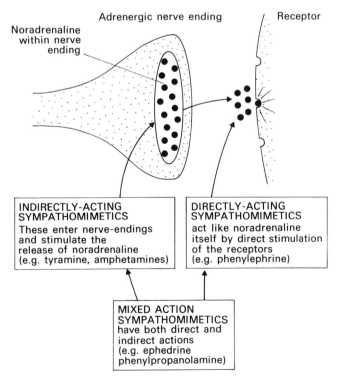

Fig. 19.1. The mode of action of directly acting, indirectly acting and mixed-action sympathomimetics at adrenergic neurones

There is also good evidence to show that the noradrenaline receptors of the sympathetic nervous system are not identical, but consist of three types, α, β_1 and β_2. It is possible to categorize the sympathomimetics into a range from those with predominantly α-stimulating activity to those with predominantly β-stimulating activity. The value of such a categorization is that the sympathomimetics can be selected for their stimulant activity on particular organs or tissues. For example, salbutamol and terbutaline selectively stimulate bronchodilator β_2-receptors and represent a significant advance on ephedrine and isoprenaline (isoproterenol) which also stimulate β_1-receptors in the heart and, in the case of ephedrine, can also stimulate α-receptors. A knowledge of the type of receptors stimulated is also important when considering the interactions of these drugs. Table 19.1 is a list indicating the activities of some of the sympathomimetics in common use.

Table 19.1. Sympathomimetic amines—a categorization with some of the therapeutic applications

Direct stimulators of alpha- and beta-receptors

Adrenaline (epinephrine)	Vasoconstrictor (α) bronchodilator (β) mydriatic ($\alpha\beta$)
Noradrenaline (norepinephrine, levarterenol)	Vasoconstrictor (α) cardiac stimulant (β)

Direct and indirect stimulantors of alpha & beta receptors

Amphetamine	Decongestant (α) CNS stimulant
Dextroamphetamine	Anorectic
Ephedrine	Decongestant (α) bronchodilator (β) vasopressor ($\alpha\beta$) mydriatic ($\alpha\beta$) CNS stimulant
Hydroxyamphetamine	Decongestant (α) vasopressor ($\alpha\beta$) mydriatic ($\alpha\beta$)
Mephentermine	Decongestant (α) vasopressor ($\alpha\beta$)
Metaraminol	Vasopressor ($\alpha\beta$)
Methamphentamine	Decongestant (α) vasopressor ($\alpha\beta$) anorectic
Phenylpropanolamine	Decongestant (α)
Pseudoephedrine	Decongestant (α) bronchodilator (β)
Tyramine	

Direct stimulantors of alpha-receptors

Methoxamine	Decongestant (α) vasopressor ($\alpha\beta$)
Phenylephrine	Decongestant (α) vasopressor ($\alpha\beta$)

Direct stimulantors of beta-receptors

Etafedrine	Bronchodilator (β)
Isoetharine	Bronchodilator (β)
Isoprenaline (isoproteronol)	Broncholdilator (β) vasodilator (β) cardiac stimulant (β)
Salbutamol	Bronchodilator (β)
Terbutaline	Bronchodilator (β)

Amphetamines and related drugs + chlorpromazine

Summary
The anorectic and other effects of amphetamines, chlorphentermine and phenmetrazine are antagonized by chlorpromazine. The antipsychotic effects of chlorpromazine can be antagonized by amphetamine

Interaction

There is mutual antagonism between the effects of chlorpromazine and amphetamines—or related anorectic agents—when taken together.

Chlorpromazine + dextroamphetamine

A study on a very large number of patients being treated with 200–600 mg chlorpromazine daily indicated that the addition of 10–40 mg amphetamine had a detrimental effect on the control of their schizophrenic symptoms.[1]

A study on schizophrenic patients being treated with phenothiazines showed that they not only failed to respond to concurrent treatment with dextroamphetamine for obesity, but the expected sleep disturbance was not seen.[3]

Antagonism of the effects of the amphetamines by chlorpromazine has been described in other reports.[2,4]

Chlorpromazine + phenmetrazine or chlorphentermine

A double-blind controlled study in patients undergoing treatment with chlorpromazine showed that the effect of phenmetrazine in reducing weight was diminished.[5]

A study in psychiatric patients given chlorphentermine or phenmetrazine for the control of obesity indicated that their effects were inhibited by concurrent treatment with chlorpromazine.[6]

Mechanism

Not understood. However, it is known that phenothiazines such as chlorpromazine are able to inhibit the 'pump' by which the amphetamines enter neurones. If this type of inhibition occurs at peripheral adrenergic neurones, and centrally at both adrenergic and dopaminergic neurones, some part of the antagonism of the amphetamines can be explained.

Importance and management

These clinical reports amply demonstrate that it is not desirable to treat patients with chlorpromazine and amphetamines, phenmetrazine or chlorphentermine concurrently. It is not clear whether this interaction takes place with phenothiazines other than chlorpromazine.

This interaction of chlorpromazine has been deliberately exploited, and with success, in the treatment of 22 children poisoned with various amphetamines (dexamphetamine, methamphetamine, phenmetrazine).[2] They were given 1 mg/kg intramuscularly initially followed by further doses as necessary.

References

1 Casey J F, Hollister L E, Klett C J, Lasky J J and Caffrey E M. Combined drug therapy of chronic schizophrenics. Controlled evaluation of placebo, dextroamphetamine, imipramine, isocarboxazid and trifluoroperazine added to maintenance doses of chlorpromazine. *Amer J Psychiatr* (1961) **117**, 997.
2 Espelin D E and Done A K. Amphetamine poisoning: effectiveness of chlorpromazine. *New Eng J Med* (1968) **278**, 1361.
3 Modell W and Hussar A E. Failure of dextroamphetamine sulphate to influence eating and sleeping patterns in obese schizophrenic patients: clinical and pharmacological significance. *J Amer Med Ass* (1965) **193**, 275.
4 Jonsson L E. Pharmacological blockade of amphetamine effects in amphetamine-dependent subjects. *Eur J Clin Pharmacol* (1972) **4**, 206.
5 Reid A A. Pharmacological antagonism between chlorpromazine and phenmetrazine in mental hospital patients. *Med J Aust* (1964) **1**, 187.
6 Sletten I W, Orgnjanov V, Menendez S, Sunderland D and El-Toumi A. Weight reduction with chlorphentermine and phenmetrazine in obese psychiatric patients during chlorpromazine therapy. *Curr Ther Res* (1967) **9**, 570.

Amphetamines + lithium carbonate

Summary

The effects of the amphetamines may be antagonized by lithium carbonate.

Interaction

Two depressed patients spontaneously abandoned abusing amphetamines because while taking lithium carbonate, they were unable to get 'high'. Another patient complained of not feeling any effects from amphetamines taken for weight reduction until the lithium carbonate was withdrawn.[1]

Another report confirms these findings.[2]

Mechanism

Not known. One suggestion is that the amphetamines and lithium seem to have mutually opposing pharmacological actions on noradrenaline uptake at adrenergic neurones.[1]

Importance and management

The data are limited but indicate that reduced

amphetamine effects are possible during concurrent treatment with lithium carbonate.

References
1 Flemenbaum A. Does lithium block the effects of amphetamine? A report of three cases. *Am J Psychiatry* (1974) **131**, 820.
2 Van Kammen D P and Murphy D. Attenuation of the euphoriant and activating effects of d- and l-amphetamine by lithium carbonate treatment. *Psychopharmacologia* (1975) **44**, 215.

Amphetamines + nasal decongestants

Summary
An isolated report describes antagonism of the effects of levoamphetamine in a hyperactive child by nasal decongestants containing phenylpropanolamine and chlorpheniramine.

Interaction
Maintenance therapy with 42 mg daily of levoamphetamine succinate in a 12-year-old hyperactive child was found to be ineffective on two occasions when he was concurrently treated with *Contac* and *Allerest* for colds. Both of these proprietary nasal decongestants contain phenylpropanolamine and chlorpheniramine.[1]

Mechanism
Not understood. One suggestion is that the phenylpropanolamine may have competitively inhibited the absorption or the action of the amphetamine.[1] There is also the possibility that chlorpheniramine may have been responsible.

Importance and management
Prescribers should be aware of this interaction, but there is too little information to make any statement about its general importance.

Reference
1 Heustis R D and Arnold L E. Possible antagonism of amphetamine by decongestant-antihistamine compounds. *J Pediatrics* (1974) **85**, 579.

Amphetamines + urinary acidifiers or alkalinizers

Summary
The loss of amphetamine in the urine is increased by urinary acidifiers, and reduced by urinary alkalinizers.

Interaction
A study in 6 normal subjects given 10–15 mg amphetamine by mouth showed that when the urine was made alkaline (approximately pH 8) by giving sodium bicarbonate, only 3% of the original dose of amphetamine was excreted in the urine over a 16 h period compared with 54% when the urine was made acid (approximately pH 5) by taking ammonium chloride.[1]

Similar results have been reported elsewhere.[3] Psychoses resulting from amphetamine retention in patients with alkaline urine have been reported.[2]

Mechanism
Amphetamine is a base which is excreted by the kidney tubules and which becomes partially ionized in solution. In alkaline solution, most of the drug exists in the un-ionized form which is readily reabsorbed by the kidney tubules so that little is lost in the urine. In acid solution, little of the drug is in the un-ionized form so that little can

be reabsorbed and much of it is lost in the urine. A more detailed and illustrated account of this interaction mechanism is given on page 9.

Importance and management
A well-established interaction. It can be usefully exploited to clear amphetamine from the body more rapidly in cases of overdose, by acidifying the urine with ammonium chloride. Conversely it can represent an undesirable interaction if therapeutic doses of amphetamine are excreted too rapidly. Care is also required to ensure that

amphetamine intoxication does not develop if the urine is made alkaline with, for example, sodium bicarbonate or acetazolamide.

References
1 Beckett A H, Rowland M and Turner P. Influence of urinary pH on excretion of amphetamine. *Lancet* (1965) i, 303.
2 Änggård E, Jönsson L-E, Hogmark A-L and Gunne L-M. Amphetamine metabolism in amphetamine psychosis. *Clin Pharmacol Ther* (1973) **14**, 870.
3 Rowland M and Beckett A H. The amphetamines: clinical and pharmacokinetic implications of recent studies of an assay procedure and urinary excretion in man. *Arzneim-Forsch* (1966) **16**, 1369.

Dopamine + ergot

Summary
An isolated case of gangrene attributed to the infusion of dopamine after ergometrine has been reported.

Interaction, mechanism, importance and management
A single case of gangrene of the extremities has been described in a patient who was given an infusion of dopamine following the administration of ergometrine.[1] This would seem to have been due to the additive peripheral vasoconstrictor effects of both drugs which reduced the

circulation to such an extent that infection became unchecked. It would seem prudent to avoid concurrent use.

Reference
1 Buchanan N, Cane R D and Miller M. Symmetrical gangrene of the extremities associated with the use of dopamine subsequent to ergometrine administration. *Intens Care Med* (1977) **3**, 55

Dopamine + phenytoin

Summary
Preliminary evidence indicates that phenytoin should not be used in patients needing dopamine to support their blood pressure because a serious hypotensive reaction may occur.

Interaction
Five patients have been described in one report who were critically ill with a variety of conditions, under treatment with a number of different drugs, and receiving dopamine hydrochloride to maintain an adequate blood pressure. When seizures developed, intravenous phenytoin sodium was given. Coincidentally their hitherto stable blood pressure fell rapidly and one patient died from cardiorespiratory arrest. A similar reaction was demonstrated in dogs made hypovolemic and hypotensive by bleeding.[1]

Mechanism
Not understood. One suggestion is that the phenytoin may have a greater myocardial depressant effect during dopamine-induced catchelamine depletion.

Importance and management
The documentation is limited to one report;[1] moreover, this suspected interaction is not fully established, but there is enough evidence to

indicate that phenytoin should only be used with great caution, or not at all, in those requiring dopamine to maintain their blood pressure.

Reference

1 Bivins B A, Rapp R P, Griffen W O, Blouin R and Bustrack J. Dopamine–phenytoin interaction. A cause of hypotension in the critically ill. *Arch Surg* (1978) **113**, 245.

Isoprenaline + tricyclic antidepressants

Summary

Although isoprenaline (isoproterenol) and amitriptyline have been used together safely and with advantage in the treatment of asthma, an isolated case has been reported of death arising from their concurrent use (or abuse?).

Interaction

A woman of 30 who was taking a mixture of theophylline, ephedrine, and phenobarbitone (*Tedral*), twice daily, died as a result of the aspiration of the gastric contents in response to cardiac arrhythmia induced by the use of amitriptyline and isoprenaline. It was esimated that she had taken more than forty 125 μg doses of isoprenaline daily for several days prior to her death. The amitriptyline was taken without the knowledge of her physician.[1]

Mechanism

It is not possible to know exactly how much of each drug this patient had taken before her death, but it seems likely that the cardiac arrhythmia was induced by the combined effects of amitriptyline (which is cardiotoxic), isoprenaline (also cardiotoxic, particularly during the hypoxia which can occur during an asthmatic attack), the fluorocarbon propellant within the inhalant (which is able to sensitize the heart muscle to adrenergic agents like isoprenaline), and ephidrine (which, like isoprenaline, has direct beta-stimulant actions on the heart). But just why cardiac arrhythmias should cause vomiting is not known.

Importance and management

There is good evidence to show that amitriptyline alone[2,3] and with isoprenaline[4] is beneficial in the treatment of asthma: moreover, in a study undertaken to find out if there was an adverse interaction between the two, no abnormalities of rhythm were seen, although one out of the four patients showed tachycardia[5]

The fatal interaction described would seem, therefore, to be due to the abuse rather than the responsible use of these agents. However, it emphasizes the risk attached to the over-use of isoprenaline inhalers if cardiotoxic drugs such as the tricyclic antidepressants are being used concurrently.

References

1 Kadar D. Amitriptyline and isoproterenol: a fatal combination. *Can Med Ass J* (1975) **112**, 556.
2 Ananth J. Antiasthmatic effect of amitriptyline. *Can Med Ass J* (1974) **110**, 1131.
3 Meares R A, Mills J E and Horvath T B. Amitriptyline and asthma. *Med J Aust* (1971) **2**, 25.
4 Matilla M J and Muittari A. Modification by imipramine of the bronchodilator response to isoprenaline in asthmatic patients. *Ann Med Int Fenn* (1968) **57**, 185.
5 Boakes A J, Laurence D R, Teoh P C, Barar F S K, Benedikter L T and Prichard B N C. Interactions between sympathomimetic amine and antidepressant agents in man. *Br Med J* (1973) **1**, 311.

Phenylephrine + monoamine oxidase inhibitors

Summary

Concurrent use of phenylephrine, taken orally, and the MAOI can result in a potentially fatal hypertensive crisis. Phenylephrine is a common constituent of many proprietary oral cough, cold and influenza preparations. The effects of parenterally administered phenylephrine may be approximately doubled.

Interaction

Concurrent use of normal oral doses of phenylephrine in patients on MAOI can result in a rapid, serious and potentially hazardous rise in blood pressure:

> A study in 4 normal subjects who were given either 45 mg phenelzine daily or 30 mg tranylcypromine daily for 7 days, showed that during this MAOI treatment the pressor response to orally administered phenylephrine was grossly enhanced. In three experiments in which 45 mg was given orally, the rise in blood pressure became potentially disasterous and had to be stopped with phentolamine. The enhancement was about 13 times in the only experiment which was not stopped, and 6–35 times in the two which were curtailed. The rise in blood pressure was accompanied by severe headache. An approximately two-fold increase was seen following parenteral administration.[2]

Another study[1] describes a two- to two-and-a-half-fold enhancement of the actions of phenylephrine given parenterally, and an exaggerated pressor response is described in a case report.[3]

Mechanism

It is normally necessary to give much larger doses of phenylephrine orally than parenterally because a large proportion of the oral dose is destroyed by the MAO/in the gut and liver, and only a small amount reaches the general circulation. But during treatment with an MAOI when the MAO is inactivated, most of the normal oral dose escapes destruction and passes freely into circulation as an overdose. Hence the gross enhancement of the pressor effects. Phenylephrine has mainly direct sympathomimetic activity, but it may also have some minor indirect actions as well as which would be expected to result in the release of some of the MAOI-accumulated noradrenaline at adrenergic nerve endings, and might account for the increased response to parenteral administration.

Importance and management

Not as extensively documented as some of the other sympathomimetic/MAOI interactions but just as serious and potentially fatal. Patients on any MAOI whether for depression or hypertension, should not take phenylephrine in normal oral doses. Phenylephrine is a common constituent of oral over-the-counter cough, cold and influenza preparations and patients should be strongly warned against them.

Whether the effects of nose drops and nasal sprays are also enhanced is not certain, but it would be prudent to avoid them until they have been shown to be safe.

The response to parenteral administration is also enhanced, $2–2\frac{1}{2}$ times so that an appropriate dosage reduction is necessary.

If a hypertensive reaction occurs, it can be controlled with an alpha-adrenoreceptor blocking agent such as phentolamine, 5 mg, given intravenously, or failing that an intramuscular injection of 50 mg chlorpromazine.

References
1 Boakes A J, Laurence D R, Teoh P C, Barar F S K, Benedikter L T and Prihard B N C. Interactions between sympathomimetic amines and antidepressant agents in man. *Br Med J* (1973) 1, 311.
2 Elis J, Laurence D R, Mattice H, and Prichard B N C. Modification by monoamine oxidase inhibitors of the effect of some sympathomimetics on blood pressure. *Br Med J* (1967) 2, 75.
3 Jenkins L C and Graves H B. Potential hazards of psychoactive drugs in association with anaesthesia. *Can Anaes Soc J* (1965) 12, 121.

Directly acting sympathomimetics + beta-adrenergic receptor blockers

Summary

In the presence of non-selective beta-blockers such as propranolol, the pressor effects of adrenaline (epinephrine) are increased and bradycardia can occur.

Interaction

Marked increases in blood pressure and bradycardia can occur following the administration of adrenaline (epinephrine) to patients under treatment with non-selective ($\beta1$ and $\beta2$) beta-blocking agents:

> Five normal subjects and 4 patients with hyperthyroidism showed a small increase in heart rate but little

change in blood pressure after the subcutaneous injection of 0·4 mg adrenaline. After pretreatment with 40 mg propranolol the same dose of adrenaline caused a 20–40 mmHg rise in blood pressure and a fall in heart rate of 23–36 beats/min.[1]

Similar marked increases in blood pressure and severe bradycardia have been described in other reports involving propranolol.[2-4] Only a small increase was seen in a comparative study with metoprolol.[4]

Mechanism
Adrenaline stimulates both the alpha- and beta-receptors of the cardiovascular system. Alpha stimulation causes vasoconstriction and beta stimulation causes both vasodilation and stimulation of the heart. The net result is usually a modest increase in heart rate and a small rise in blood pressure. If, however, the beta-receptors are blocked, the unopposed alpha vasoconstriction causes a marked rise in blood pressure, followed by bradycardia due to the unopposed increase in vagal reflex tone.[5]

Importance and management
A potentially serious interaction. Patients on non-selective beta-blockers (β_1 and β_2) such as propranolol should only be administered adrenaline (epinephrine) with caution because of the marked bradycardia and hypertension which can result. A less marked effect is likely with the selective (No, β_1) blockers such as metoprolol.[4] A list of the beta-blocking drugs is given on page 258.

References
1 Varma D R, Sharma K K and Arora R C. Response to adrenaline and propranolol in hyperthyroidism. *Lancet* (1976) **i**, 260.
2 Kram J, Bourne H R, Melmon K L and Maibach H. Propranolol. *Ann Int Med* (1974) **80**, 282.
3 Harris W S, Schoenfeld C D, Brooks R H and Weissler A M. Effect of beta adrenergic blockade on the hemodynamic responses to epinephrine in man. *Amer J Cardiol* (1966) **17**, 484.
4 van Herwaarden C L A. Effects of adrenaline during treatment with propranolol and metoprolol. *Br Med J* (1977) **2**, 1029.
5 Berchtold P and Bessman A N. Propranolol. *Ann Int Med* (1974) **80**, 119.

Directly acting sympathomimetics + guanethidine and related drugs

Summary
The pressor effects of noradrenaline (norepinephrine, levarterenol) phenylephrine, metaraminol and similar drugs can be increased two- to four-fold in the presence of guanethidine and related drugs (bethanidine, debrisoquine etc.). The mydriatic effects are similarly enhanced and prolonged.

Interactions
Pressor responses:-

Guanethidine + noradrenaline
An investigation on 6 normal subjects, given 200 mg guanethidine on the first day of the study and 100 mg a day for the next 2 days, showed that their pressor responses (one third pulse pressure + diastolic pressure) when infused with noradrenaline in a range of doses were enhanced $2\frac{1}{2}$–4 times. Moreover, cardiac arrhythmias appeared at lower doses of noradrenaline and with greater frequency than in the absence of guanethidine, and were more serious in nature.[1]

Guanethidine + metaraminol
A woman taking 20 mg guanethidine and 5 mg bendrofluazide a day had a myocardial infarct and,

although nursed flat on her back, showed a gradual decrease in her systolic blood pressure. When it had fallen to 75 mmHg she was given 10 mg metaraminol (*Aramine*) by intravenous injection. Within minutes the patient complained of a very severe headache, extreme angina, and her blood pressure was found to have risen to 220/130 mmHg.[2]

There are other reports of this enhanced pressor response involving debrisoquine with phenylephrine,[3,4] even when given orally[8] and with bretylium and noradrenaline.[5]

Mydriatic responses:-

Guanethidine + phenylephrine
The mydriasis due to phenylephrine administered in the form of a 10% eyedrop solution was observed to

be prolonged for up to 10 h in a patient who was concurrently receiving guanethidine for hypertension.[6]

This enhanced mydriatic response has been described in other studies involving guanethidine with adrenaline, phenylephrine and methoxamine,[7] and debrisoquine with phenylephrine and ephedrine.[7]

Mechanism

If sympathetic nerves are cut surgically the receptors which they normally stimulate become hypersensitive. By preventing the release of noradrenaline from adrenergic neurones, guanethidine and other adrenergic neurone blocking drugs cause a temporary 'drug-induced sympathectomy' which is also accompanied by hypersensitivity of the receptors. But just why this should be so is not certain. One suggestion is that the guanethidine prevents the removal of noradrenaline from the receptor area by blocking the normal re-uptake into the adrenergic neurone. In this way the noradrenaline accumulates and continues to stimulate the receptors so that the effects of a given dose becomes exaggerated.[8]

Importance and management

An established and potentially serious interaction. There is no clear contraindication to their concurrent use but, since the pressor effects of the sympathomimetics are exaggerated, considerable care is required. The pressor of effects of noradrenaline in the presence of guanethidine were increased two- to four-fold, and of phenylephrine two-fold. In addition the incidence and severity of heart arrhythmias was increased.[1,4] It would clearly be advisable to administer very much smaller doses of the sympathomimetics than usual. Direct evidence of this interaction seems to be limited to noradrenaline, phenylephrine and metaraminol, but dopamine, methoxamine and oxedrine all possess direct sympathomimetic acti-

vity. Bethanidine, guanoclor and guanoxan may also be expected to behave like guanethidine. If as a result of this interaction the blood pressure becomes grossly elevated, it can be controlled by the administration of an alpha-adrenergic receptor blocker such as phentolamine.[3]

Phenylephrine is contained in a number of over-the-counter cough and cold preparations, a few of which contain up to 10 mg in a dose. This is small compared with the 0·75 mg/kg (roughly 45 mg in a 10-stone individual) which was examined in one study[4,8] but it might cause some rise in blood pressure. The extent and the clinical importance of this requires further study.

An exaggeration of the pressor effects of these drugs is clearly likely to be more immediately serious than the effects of mydriasis, but enhanced and prolonged mydriasis is possible whether or not the adrenergic neurone blocker has been given systemically or topically, and the same precautions apply about using smaller amounts of the sympathomimetic drugs.

References

1 Mulheims G H, Entrup R W, Paiewonsky D and Mierzwiak D S. Increased sensitivity of the heart to catecholamine-induced arrhythmias following guanethidine. *Clin Pharmacol Ther* (1965) 6, 757.
2 Stevens F R T. A danger of sympathomimetic drugs. *Med J Aust* (1966) 2, 576.
3 Aminu J, D'Mello A and Vere D W. Interaction between debrisoquine and phenylephrine. *Lancet* (1970) ii, 935.
4 Allum W, Aminu J, Bloomfield T H, Davies C, Scales A H and Vere D W. Interaction between debrisoquine and phenylephrine in man. *Brit J Pharmacol* (1973) 47, 675P.
5 Laurence D R and Nagle R E. The interaction of bretylium with pressor agents. *Lancet* (1961) i, 593.
6 Cooper B. Neo-synephrine (10%) eye drops. *Med J Aust* (1968) 55, 420.
7 Sneddon J M and Turner P. The interactions of local guanethidine and sympathomimetic amines in the human eye. *Arch Ophthalmol* (1969) 81, 622.
8 Boura A L A and Green A F. Comparison of bretylium and guanethidine: tolerance and effects on adrenergic nerve function and responses to sympathomimetic amines. *Brit J Pharmacol* (1962) 19, 13.
9 Allum W, Aminu J, Bloomfield T H, Davies C, Scales A H and Vere D W. Interaction between debrisoquine and phenylephrine in man. *Br J clin Pharmac* (1974) 1, 51.

Directly acting sympathomimetics + methyldopa

Summary

The pressor effects of noradrenaline (norepinephrine, levarterenol) are increased and prolonged by concurrent treatment with methyldopa. It is not certain whether other directly-acting sympathomimetics interact with methyldopa similarly, but the mydriasis due to phenylephrine appears not to be affected.

Interaction

The mean blood pressure rise in 10 hypertensive patients given noradrenaline intravenously increased from 27/15 mmHg before treatment with methyldopa to 35/19 mmHg during treatment. The duration of the response was prolonged from 40 to 105 s.[1]

A patient who had received 1·25 g methyldopa daily for 6 days showed an increase in his blood pressure response to 4 μg doses of noradrenaline, administered intravenously, from about 50/25 mmHg before treatment with methyldopa, to about 80/50 mmHg during treatment. The duration of the response was prolonged from about 1 min to 3 min.[2]

Mechanism

The mechanism of this interaction is not known for certain, but there is a possible explanation. If sympathetic nerves are cut surgically the receptors which they normally stimulate become hypersensitive. Methyldopa causes a 'drug-induced sympathectomy' which also appears to be accompanied by a temporary hypersensitivity of the receptors. This may be related to some noradrenaline accumulation at the receptor area.

Importance and management

Direct information on this interaction is sparse, but it would seem prudent to begin noradrenaline administration with small doses. Dollery has suggested using one tenth of the normal dose initially.[2] Whether or not other sympathomimetic amines with direct activity (metaraminol, methoxamine etc.) interact similarly is not clear, but it would seem possible. The mydriatic activity of a 10% solution of phenylephrine was observed in one patient to be unaffected during treatment with methyldopa.[3]

References

1 Dollery C T, Harrington M and Hodge J V. Haemodynamic studies with methyldopa: effect on cardiac output and response to pressor amines. *Brit Heart J* (1963) **25**, 670.
2 Dollery C T. Physiological and pharmacological interactions of antihypertensive drugs. *Proc Roy Soc Med* (1965) **58**, 983.
3 Sneddon J M and Turner P. Ephedrine mydriasis in hypertension and the response to treatment. *Clin Pharmacol Ther* (1969) **10**, 64.

Directly and indirectly acting sympathomimetics + mianserin

Summary

No adverse interaction is likely in patients on mianserin who are treated with sympathomimetic amines

Interaction, mechanism, importance and management

Studies in depressive patients have shown that the pressor responses to tyramine and noradrenaline remain virtually unaffected after 14 days' treatment with 60 mg mianserin daily.[1–4]

The practical importance of these observations is that, unlike the situation with the tricyclic antidepressants (see p. 411), the response to noradrenaline is not increased significantly and no special precautions appear to be necessary if noradrenaline or other directly acting sympathomimetic is administered to patients on mianserin.

Similarly, none of the dietary precautions against eating foods or drinks containing tyramine, or the administration of indirectly-acting sympathomimetics such as phenylpropanolamine in cough and cold remedies which are imposed on patients taking MAOI antidepressants (see pp. 370, 404, 409) seem to be necessary with mianserin.

References

1 Ghose K, Coppen A and Turner P. Autonomic actions and interactions of mianserin hydrochloride (Org. GB 94) and amitriptyline in patients with depressive illness. *Psychopharmacol* (1976) **49**, 201.
2 Coppen A, Ghose K, Swade C and Wood K. Effect of mianserin hydrochloride on peripheral uptake mechanisms for noradrenaline and 5-hydroxytryptamine in man. *Br J clin Pharmac* (1978) **5**, 13s.
3 Ghose K. Studies on the interaction between mianserin and noradrenaline in patients suffering from depressive illness. *Br J clin Pharmal* (1977) **4**, 712.
4 Coppen A J and Ghose K. Clinical and pharmacological effects of treatment with a new antidepressant. *Arzneim-Forsch (Drug Res)* (1976) **26**, 1166.

Directly acting sympathomimetics + monoamine oxidase inhibitors

Summary

The pressor effects of adrenaline (epinephrine), noradrenaline (norepinephrine, levarterenol), isoprenaline (isoproterenol) and methoxamine may be unaltered or show some enhancement in patients taking MAOI. The enhancement may be marked in patients who show a significant hypotensive response to the MAOI.

Interaction

A slightly confused and not totally consistent picture is presented by the studies of the effects of concurrent use. Theoretically no interaction would be expected but some enhancement of the cardiovascular effects of these amines is seen, particularly if the MAOI induces hypotension:

> In an experimental study in man, 2 subjects were given phenelzine 45 mg daily, and 2 others tranylcypromine, 30 mg daily, for 7 days. No significant alterations were seen in the pressor responses to adrenaline (epinephrine) or isoprenolol (isoproteronol) but a two-fold increase in the pressor response of 1 subject on tranycypromine occurred in the mid-range of noradrenaline (norepinephrine) concentrations infused, but not in the upper or lower ranges.[1]

These results confirm those found in two other studies, one with noradrenaline and phenelzine[2] and the other with noradrenaline and methoxamine in patients taking nialamide.[3]

> A study in 3 volunteers treated with tranylcypromine showed that the effects of noradrenaline were slightly enhanced, while with adrenaline there was a two-to four-fold enhancement of heart rate and diastolic pressure, but a less marked increase in systolic pressure. Isoprenaline behaved very much like adrenaline but there was no enhancement of systolic pressure.[4]

MAOI-induced hypotension
> In a study in 7 hypertensive patients who showed postural hypotension after their blood pressure had been lowered with either pheniprazine or tranycypromine, it was demonstrated that the dose of noradrenaline required to produce a 25 mmHg rise in systolic pressure was reduced to 13–38%, and of methoxamine 30–39%.[3]

Mechanism

These sympathomimetic amines act *directly* on the receptors of the sympathetic nerve endings which innervate the arterial blood vessels so that the presence of an MAOI-induced accumulation of noradrenaline in these nerve endings would not be expected to alter the extent of this direct stimulation. The enhancement seen, particularly in those patients whose blood pressure was lowered by the MAOI, might have been due to an increased sensitivity of the receptors to stimulation which is seen if the nerves are cut, and is also seen during temporary 'pharmacological severance'.

Importance and management

The evidence from studies in man is very limited but the overall picture is that some slight to moderate enhancement of the effects of noradrenaline (levarterenol) and adrenaline (epinephrine) may occur, but the authors of two of the reports cited[1,4] are in general agreement that the extent is normally not likely to be hazardous. Some caution is, however, appropriate. Direct evidence about methoxamine is even more limited but it seems to behave similarly. None of the studies demonstrated any marked changes in the effects of isoprenaline (isoproteronol).

The situation in patients who show a reduced blood pressure due to the use of an MAOI (this would seem to apply principally to pargyline) appears to be different. A three- to seven-fold enhancement of the pressor effects of noradrenaline (levarterenol) and methoxamine was seen. Confirmation of this response is required, but what is known suggests that a considerable degree of caution should be exercised.

The interaction between the MAOI and phenylephrine is dealt with separately. See page 404.

References

1 Boakes A J, Laurence D R, Teoh P C, Barar F S K, Benedikter L T and Prichard B N C. Interactions between sympathomimetic amines and antidepressant agents in man. *Br Med J* (1973) 1, 311.
2 Elis J, Laurence D R, Mattie H and Prichard B N C. Modification by monoamine oxidase inhibitors of the effect of

some sympathomimetics on blood pressure. *Br Med J* (1967) **2**, 75.

3 Horwitz D, Goldberg L I, and Sjoerdsma A. Increased blood pressure responses to dopamine and norepinephrine pro-

duced by monoamine oxidase inhibitors in man. *J Lab and Clin Med* (1960) **56**, 747.

4 Cuthbert M F and Vere D W. Potentiation of the cardiovascular effects of some catecholamines by a monoamine oxidase inhibitor. *Brit J Pharmacol* (1971) **43**, 471P.

Directly and indirectly acting sympathomimetics + rauwolfia alkaloids

Summary

Although direct clinical evidence is sparse, the pressor and other effects of directly acting sympathomimetics (adrenaline, noradrenaline, phenylephrine) may be expected to be somewhat enhanced or remained unchanged in the presence of the rauwolfia alkaloids, while the effects of indirectly acting sympathomimetics or those with mixed activity (ephedrine, amphetamines, mephentermine, phenylpropanolamine) may be reduced or blocked.

Interaction

A patient taking reserpine who became hypotensive while undergoing surgery failed to respond to an intravenous injection of ephedrine but did so after 30 min treatment with noradrenaline during which time, presumably, the stores of noradrenaline at adrenergic neurones had become replenished.[1]

The mydriatic effects of ephedrine in man were shown to be antagonized by pretreatment with reserpine.[2]

A child who had accidentally taken reserpine in a dose thought to be about 6·5 mg failed to respond to an intramuscular injection of ephedrine (16 mg).[3]

Mechanism

The primary pharmacological action of the rauwolfia alkaloids is to cause the loss of noradrenaline (norepinephrine) from adrenergic neurones. With its transmitter gone, the adrenergic neurones cannot continue to transmit nerve impulses or to respond to sympathomimetic drug stimulation. Indirectly acting sympathomimetic amines which depend for their actions on their ability to release noradrenaline from nerve endings might be expected to have their actions blocked, whereas the effects of directly acting sympathomimetic amines should remain unchanged or possibly even enhanced because of the supersensitivity of the receptors which occurs when they are deprived of noradrenaline for any length of time. Drugs such as ephedrine which have mixed direct and indirect actions should fall somewhere between the two extremes, although the picture presented by the reports cited seem to indicate

that ephedrine has predominantly indirect activity.[1,2,3]

Experiments with dogs have demonstrated that adrenaline (epinephrine), noradrenaline (norepinephrine) and phenylephrine (all with direct actions) remain effective vasopressors after treatment with reserpine and their actions are enhanced to some extent, whereas the vasopressor actions of ephedrine, amphetamines, methamphetamine, tyramine and mephentermine (all with indirect actions) are reduced or blocked by reserpine.[5,6,7]

Importance and management

The paucity of information suggests that in practice the interactions of these sympathomimetic amines with the rauwolfia alkaloids may be of minimal importance. If a pressor drug is required, a directly acting drug such as noradrenaline (norepinephrine), or phenylephrine may be expected to be effective. Metaraminol has been used as a pressor drug with success in reserpine-treated patients.[8] The receptors may show some supersensitivity so that a dosage reduction may be required.

References

1 Ziegler C H and Lovette J B. Operative complications after therapy with reserpine and reserpine compounds. *J Amer Med Ass* (1961) **176**, 916.

2 Sneddon J M and Turner P. Ephedrine mydriasis in hypotension and the response to treatment. *Clin Pharmacol Therap* (1969) **10**, 64.

3 Phillips T. Overdose of reserpine. *Br Med J* (1955) **2**, 969.

4 Noce R H, Williams D B and Rapaport W. Reserpine (Serpasil)

in the management of the mentally ill. *J Amer Med Ass* (1955) **158**, 11.

5 Stone C A, Ross A C, Wenger H C, Ludden C T, Blessing J A, Totaro J A and Porter C C. Effect of α-methyl-3,4-dihydroxyphenylalanine (methyldopa), reserpine, and related agents on some vascular responses in the dog. *J Pharmacol Exp Ther* (1962) **136**, 80.

6 Eger EI and Hamilton W K. The effect of reserpine on the action of various vasopressors. *Anaesthesiology* (1959) **20**, 641.

7 Moore J I and Moran N C. Cardiac contractile force responses to ephedrine and other sympathomimetic amines in dogs after pretreatment with reserpine. *J Pharmacol Exp Ther* (1962) **136**, 89.

8 Smessaert A A, and Hicks R G. Problems caused by rauwolfia drugs during anaesthesia and surgery. *NY State J Med* (1961) **61**, 2399.

9 Abboud F M, and Ekstein J W. *Circulation* (1964) **29**, 219.

Directly acting sympathomimetic amines + tricyclic antidepressants

Summary

Patients being treated with tricyclic antidepressants show a grossly exaggerated response (hypertension, cardiac arrhythmias etc.) to the injection of noradrenaline (levarterenol, norepinephrine) adrenaline (epinephrine) and to a lesser extent to phenylephrine. Local anaesthetics containing these vasoconstrictors should not be used but felypressin is a safe alternative. Doxepin and maprotiline appear not to induce this interaction to the same degree as most tricyclics.

Interaction

The effects of intravenous infusions of noradrenaline were increased approximately nine-fold, and of adrenaline approximately six-fold in 6 healthy subjects who had been taking 60 mg protriptyline for 4 days.[1,2]

Several episodes have been described in another report of a marked rise in blood pressure, dilated pupils, intense malaise, violent but transitory tremor and palpitations in patients taking tricyclic antidepressants (unnamed) when they were given local anaesthetics for dental treatment containing adrenaline or noradrenaline.[3]

Five patients taking nortriptyline, desipramine or some other unnamed tricyclic antidepressant experienced adverse reactions, some of them severe (throbbing headache, chest pain), following the injection of *Xylestesin* (lignocaine with 1:25,000 noradrenaline) during dental treatment.[4]

A study carried out on 4 healthy volunteers who had been taking 75 mg imipramine a day for 5 days showed that the responses to the intravenous infusion of noradrenaline were increased four- to eightfold, to adrenaline two- to four-fold, and to phenylephrine two- to three-fold, but there were no noticeable or consistent changes in response to isoprenaline (isoproterenol).

There are other reports describing this interaction of noradrenaline, with imipramine,[6,9] desipramine,[9,10] nortriptyline,[8] protriptyline[5,10] and amitriptyline,[9,10] and of adrenaline with nortriptyline.[7]

Mechanism

One of the major actions of the tricyclic antidepressants is to block the noradrenaline (norepinephrine) 'pump' by which noradrenaline is taken up into the adrenergic neurones. (For a fuller and illustrated account of this see pages 417–419.) Thus the most important means by which noradrenaline is removed from the receptor area is inactivated and the concentration of noradrenaline outside the neurone become elevated. If, therefore, more noradrenaline or one of the other sympathomimetic amines which act directly on the receptors is infused into the body, the adrenergic receptors in the cardiovascular system which are concerned with raising blood pressure become grossly stimulated by this superabundance of amines, and the normal response is considerably magnified.

Importance and management

An established and potentially serious interaction. The parenteral administration of noradrenaline (norepinephrine, levarterenol), adrenaline (epinephrine), phenylephrine or any other sympathomimetic with predominantly direct activity should be avoided in patients under treatment with the tricyclic antidepressants. If these sympathomimetics must be used, the rate and amount injected must be very much reduced to accommodate the exaggerated responses which will occur. Local anaesthetics containing conventional vasoconstrictors should not be administered to patients taking tricyclic antidepressants, but felypressin has been shown to be a safe alternative.[11,12,16]

If an adverse interaction occurs it can be controlled by the use of one of the alpha-receptor blocking agents such as phentolamine.

Doxepin in doses of less than 200 mg daily blocks the adrenergic neurone pump much less than the other tricyclic antidepressants and so is unlikely to show this interaction to the same degree, but in larger doses it will interact like the other tricyclics.[13,15] The blocking action of maprotiline (a tetracyclic antidepressant) is also much less than most of the tricyclics and in normal therapeutic doses in one study on 3 subjects was shown not to increase the pressor response to noradrenaline.[14] The pressor response to noradrenaline is also not significantly increased in the presence of mianserin (see p. 408).

It is uncertain whether the response to oral doses of phenylephrine is enhanced.

References

1 Svedmyr N. The influence of a tricyclic antidepressive agent (protriptyline) on some circulatory effects of noradrenaline and adrenaline in man. *Life Sci* (1968) **7**, 77.

2 Svedmyr N. Potentieringsvisker vid tillförsel au katekolaminer till patienter som behandlas med tryckliska antidepressiva medel. *Svenska Läk Tidn* (1968) **65**, 72.

3 Dam W H. Personal communication cited by Kristoffersen M B. Antidepressivas potensering af Katekolaminvirkning. *Ugeskr Laeg* (1969) **131**, 1013.

4 Boakes A J, Laurence D R, Lovel K W, O'Neil R and Verrill P J.
Adverse reactions to local anaesthetic/vasoconstrictor preparations. A study of the cardiovascular responses to Xylestesin and hostacain-with-noradrenaline. *Brit dent J* (1972) **133**, 137.

5 Boakes A J, Laurence D R, Teoh P C, Barar F S K, Benedikter L T and Prichard B N C. Interactions between sympathomimetic amines and antidepressant agents in man. *Br Med J* (1973) **1**, 311.

6 Gershon S, Holmberg G, Mattsson E, Mattsson N and Marshall A. Imipramine hydrochloride. Its effects on clinical, autonomic and psychological functions. *Arch Gen Psychiat* (1962) **6**, 96.

7 Siemkowicz E. Hjertestop efter amitriptylin. *Ugeskrift Laeg* (1975) **137**, 1403.

8 Persson G and Siwers B. The rise of potentiating effect of local anaesthesia with adrenalin in patients treated with tricyclic antidepressants. *Sven Tandlak Tiskr* (1975) **68**, 9.

9 Fischbach R, Harrer G and Harrer H. Verstärkung der Noradrenalin-wirkung durch Psychopharmaka beim Menschen. *Argneim-Forsch* (1966) **16**, 263.

10 Mitchell J R, Cavanaugh J H, Arias L and Oates J A. Guanethidine and related agents. III. Antagonism by drugs which inhibit the norepinephrine pump in man. *J Clin Invest* (1970) **49**, 1596.

11 Aellig W H, Laurence D R, O'Neil R and Verrill P J. Cardiac effects of adrenaline and felypressin as vasoconstrictors in local anaesthesia for oral surgery under diazepam sedation. *Br J Anaesth* (1970) **42**, 174.

12 Goldman V, Astrom A and Evers H. The effect of a tricyclic antidepressant on the cardiovascular effects of local anaesthetic solutions containing different vasoconstrictors. *Anaesthesia* (1971) **26**, 91.

13 Fann W E, Cavanaugh J H, Kaufmann J S, Griffith J D, Davis J M, Janowsky D S and Oates J A. Doxepin: effects on transport of biogenic amines in man. *Psychopharmacologia (Berl)* (1971) **22**, 111.

14 Briant R H and George C F. The assessment of potential drug interactions with a new tricyclic antidepressant drug. *Br J clin Pharmac* (1974) **1**, 113.

15 Oates J A, Fann W E, Cavanaugh J H. Effect of doxepin on the norepinephrine pump. *Psychosomatics* (1969) **10** (suppl) 12.

16 Perovic J, Terzic M and Todorovic L. Safety of local anaesthesia induced by prilocaine with felypressin in patients on tricyclic antidepressants. *Bull Group Int Rech Sci Stomatol Odontol* (1979) **22**, 57.

Indirectly acting sympathomimetics + furazolidone

Summary

After 5–10 days' use furazolidone has MAO-inhibitory activity approximately equivalent to the antidepressant MAOI. Concurrent use with sympathomimetic amines with indirect activity (amphetamines, phenylpropanolamine, ephedrine etc.) may be expected to result in a potentially serious rise in blood pressure although direct evidence of an accidental reaction of this kind has yet to be documented.

Interaction

The pressor response to indirectly acting sympathomimetic amines such as the amphetamines is markedly increased by concurrent treatment with furazolidone:

A study in 4 patients with hypertension who were treated with furazolidone, 400 mg daily, showed

that the pressor responses to tyramine or amphetamine after 6 days' treatment had increased two- to three-fold, and after 13 days had risen about ten-fold compared with the control. These responses were approximately the same as those found in 2 other patients on pargyline.[1] The MAO inhibitiory activity of furazolidone was confirmed by measurements taken on jejunal specimens.

412

Similar findings have been reported elsewhere.[2,3]

Mechanism
Furazolidone gradually inhibits the activity of monoamine oxidase[1] in the body over a period of days so that after 5–10 days' use it will interact with amphetamine like the antidepressant MAO inhibitors. An explanation of this type of interaction is found on page 415.

Importance and management
The MAO inhibitory activity of furazolidone after 5–10 days' use is well established but reports of serious hypertensive crises with indirectly acting sympathomimetics such as the amphetamines (well documented with the antidepressant MAOI) appears to be lacking, even though the MAO-inhibitory activity of furazolidone is approximately equivalent to pargyline.[1] Notwithstanding, it would be a wise precaution for patients on furazolidone to be warned against any of the drugs prohibited to those on antidepressant and antihypertensive MAOI e.g. amphetamines, tyramine-containing foods and drinks, phenylpropanolamine, ephedrine, phenylephrine, certain cough and cold remedies, and others (see pages 370, 415).

References
1 Pettinger W A and Oates J A. Supersensitivity to tyramine during monoamine oxidase inhibition in man. Mechanism at the level of the adrenergic neurone. *Clin Pharmacol Ther* (1968) **9**, 341.
2 Pettinger W A, Soyangco F G and Oates J A. Monoamine-oxidase inhibition by furazolidone in man. *Clin Res* (1966) **14**, 258.
3 Pettinger W A, Soyangco F and Oates J A. Inhibition of monoamine oxidase in man by furazolidone. *Clin Pharmacol Ther* (1968) **9**, 442.

Indirectly acting sympathomimetics + indomethacin

Summary
An isolated case has been reported of a patient taking phenylpropanolamine who developed serious hypertension after taking a single dose of indomethacin.

Interaction
A woman who had been taking one *Trimolet* (85 mg D-phenylpropanolamine) a day for several months, as an appetite suppressant, developed a severe bifrontal headache within 15 min of taking 25 mg indomethacin. When examined 30 min later her systolic blood pressure was 210 mmHg and the diastolic was unrecordable.[1]

In a subsequent investigation it was confirmed that neither *Trimolets* nor indomethacin alone caused this response, but when taken together the blood pressure rose to a maximum of 200/150 mmHg within half an hour of taking the indomethacin, and was associated with bradycardia. The blood pressure was rapidly reduced by phentolamine.[1]

Mechanism
A possible, though unconfirmed, explanation of this interaction is as follows: phenylpropanolamine is an indirectly acting sympathomimetic amine which causes vasoconstriction. Hypertensive crises have been described with phenylpropanolamine on its own,[2–4] but in this instance it was shown that the dosage was not enough to do so in this patient. Indomethacin also raises blood pressure, one suggestion being that it does so by suppressing the synthesis of those prostaglandins normally concerned with a reduction in blood pressure, namely prostacyclin, which is a vasodilator prostaglandin within blood vessel walls, and two potent vasodilator prostaglandins, PGA and PGE, which are produced by the kidney medulla. The result would be that the phenylpropanolamine-induced vasoconstriction would be virtually unopposed, leading to a sharp rise in blood pressure, with bradycardia induced reflexly by the stimulation of the arterial baroreceptors. But just why this one individual should respond in this manner is not known.

Importance and management
This appears to be the first and only report of this interaction,[1] so that serious though it was, no conclusions can be drawn about the general inadvisability of using these two drugs together, particularly bearing in mind that several cases have been reported in which phenylpropanolamine on its own has been responsible for the development of severe hypertension.[2–4]. However

prescribers who wish to be ultracautious might prefer to use alternative (possibly better?) appetite suppressants and other anti-inflammatory agents which have not been reported to interact together.

References
1 Lee K Y, Beilin L J, and Vandongen R. Severe hypertension after ingestion of an appetite suppressant (phenylpropanolamine) with indomethacin. *Lancet* (1979) **i**, 1110.
2 Livingston P H. Transient hypertension and phenylpropanolamine. *J Am med Ass* (1966) **196**, 1159.
3 Duvernoy W F C. Positive phentolamine test in hypertension induced by a nasal decongestant. *New Eng J Med* (1969) **280**, 877.
4 Shapiro S R. Hypertension due to anorectic agent. *New Eng J Med* (1969) **280**, 1363.

Indirectly acting sympathomimetics + methyldopa

Summary

An isolated case report describes a hypertensive reaction in a patient on methyldopa and oxprenolol who took a decongestant containing phenylpropanolamine. It seems doubtful if an adverse interaction generally occurs with these sympathomimetics and methyldopa. The mydriatic effects of ephedrine are reported to be depressed by methyldopa.

Interaction

Studies in man have shown that the pressor effects of tyramine are enhanced in patients on methyldopa. In one study it was shown that after the administration of 2–3 g methyldopa daily, the pressor effects of tyramine were doubled.[1] In another study the pressor rise was found to be 50/16 mmHg compared with only 18/10 mmHg before methyldopa treatment.[2]

Phenylpropanolamine + methyldopa and oxprenolol
    A man with renal hypertension whose blood pressure was well controlled with 500 mg methyldopa and 480 mg oxprenolol daily, showed a rise in blood pressure from about 120–140/70–80 mmHg to 200/150 mmHg within 2 days of starting to take two tablets of *Triogesic* (phenylpropanolamine, 12·5 mg and paracetamol, 500 mg) three times a day. His blood pressure fell when the *Triogesic* was withdrawn.[1]

Mechanism

Uncertain. Methyldopa is believed to cause the replacement of the usual neurotransmitter at adrenergic nerve endings by methyl-noradrenaline which has a weaker pressor (alpha) activity than noradrenaline, but greater vasodilator (beta) activity. If the vasodilator activity is blocked by the presence of a beta-blocker, the alpha (pressor) activity is unopposed. So the phenylpropanolamine, by stimulating the release of the transmitter, would cause an unopposed pressor response.[1] This proposed mechanism of interaction requires confirmation.

Importance and management

Information about an adverse interaction seems to be limited to the single report cited.[3] There seems to be nothing in the literature to suggest that indirectly acting sympathomimetics normally induce an adverse reaction, although theoretically it is possible.[1,2] More data are required. One report states that the normal mydriatic effects of ephedrine are depressed by methyldopa.[3]

References
1 Pettinger W, Horwitz D, Spector S and Sjoerdsma A. Enhancement by methyldopa of tyramine sensitivity in man. *Nature* (1963) **200**, 1107.
2 Dollery C T, Harrington M and Hodge J V. Haemodynamic studies with methyldopa: effect on cardiac output and response to pressor amines. *Brit Heart J* (1963) **25**, 670.
3 Sneddon J M and Turner P. Ephedrine mydriasis in hypertension and the response to treatment. *Clin Pharmacol Ther* (1969) **10**, 64.
4 McLaren E H. Severe hypertension produced by interaction of phenylpropanolamine with methyldopa and oxprenolol. *Br Med J* (1976) **3**, 283.

Indirectly acting sympathomimetics +
monoamine oxidase inhibitors

Summary

Concurrent use of sympathomimetic amines with indirect activity (amphetamines, phenylpropanolamine, ephedrine, pseudoephedrine, metaraminol etc.) and MAOI can result in a potentially fatal hypertensive crisis. Many of these amines are found in proprietary cough, cold and influenza preparations.

Interaction

Concurrent use of sympathomimetic amines with indirect actions in patients taking MAOI, whether for depression or hypertension, can result in a sharp and serious rise in blood pressure accompanied by tachycardia, chest pains and severe occipital headache. Neck stiffness, flushing, sweating, nausea, vomiting, hypertonicity of the limbs and sometimes epileptiform convulsions are also seen. The interaction may result in fatal intracranial haemorrhage, cardiac arrhythmias and cardia arrest: Two examples from many:

A woman who, unknown to her doctors, was taking pargyline, was given phenylpropanolamine for nasal decongestion on the eve of surgery, which promptly caused a hypertensive reaction. Her blood pressure rose rapidly from 130/80 mmHg to 220/160 mmHg and she complained of occipital headache, photophobia and nausea. She also exhibited sweating, and vomited. Two intravenous injections of 5 mg phentolamine partially controlled her blood pressure.[1]

A 30-year-old depressed woman who was taking 45 mg phenelzine daily and 2 mg trifluoperazine at night, acquired some dexamphetamine tablets from a friend and took 20 mg. Within a quarter of an hour she complained of severe headache which she described as if 'her head was bursting'. An hour after taking the dexamphetamine her blood pressure was 150/100 mmHg. Later the woman became comatose and died. A post-mortem examination revealed a haemorrhage in the left cerebral hemisphere, disrupting the internal capsule and adjacent areas of the corpus striatum.[2]

This interaction has been reported and described elsewhere with amphetamine sulphate,[3] dexamphetamine,[4] methylamphetamine,[5-8] mephentermine,[20] ephedrine,[9,10], phenylpropanolamine,[12-15] pseudoephedrine[18,21] and methylphenidate,[19] in patients on tranylcypromine,[3,5,6,9,10,13] phenelzine,[2,4-9,12,15,20] isocarboxazid,[6] mebanazine[12] and pargyline.[11] There are other reports and studies of the interaction not listed here. Extrme hyperpyrexia apparently with-

out hypertension has been described with tranylcypromine and amphetamines.[16,17]

Mechanism

The symptoms of the interaction can be attributed to overstimulation of the adrenergic receptors of the cardiovascular system.

During treatment with the MAOI, large amounts of noradrenaline (norepinephrine) accumulate not only in the brain but also within the sympathetic nerve endings which innervate arterial blood vessels. Stimulation of these nerve endings by sympathomimetic amines with indirect actions causes the release of the accumulated noradrenaline and in the massive stimulation of the receptors. Consequently an exaggerated blood vessel constriction occurs and the blood pressure rise is proportionately excessive. Intracranial haemorrhage can occur if the pressure is so high that a blood vessel ruptures.

Importance and management

An extremely well-documented, serious, and potentially fatal interaction. Patients taking any MAOI, whether for depression or hypertension, should not take any sympathomimetic amine with indirect activity. These include the amphetamines (dexamphetamine, hydroxyamphetamine, methylamphetamine), mephentermine, phenylpropanolamine, ephedrine, pseudoephedrine, and metaraminol. Cyclopentamine, methylephedrine and pholedrine also have indirect sympathomimetic activity and they may be expected to interact similarly.

Some of these sympathomimetic amines occur in a considerable number of over-the-counter cough, cold and influenza preparations and patients should be strongly warned about not taking any of these without first seeking informed advice.

Direct evidence implicating benzphetamine, chlorphentermine, diethylpropion, phendimetrazine and phenmetrazine, appears not to have been documented but on the basis of their sympathomimetic activity the manufacturers warn about their concurrent administration with the MAOI.

If a hypertensive reaction occurs, it can be controlled with an alpha-adrenoreceptor blocking agent such as phentolamine, 5 mg given intravenously, or failing that an intramuscular injection of 50 mg chlorpromazine.

References

1 Jenkins L C, and Graves H B. Potential hazards of psychoactive drugs in association with anaesthesia. *Can Anaes Soc J* (1965) **12**, 121.
2 Lloyd J T and Walker D R H. Death after combined dexamphetamine and phenelzine. *Br Med J* (1965) **2**, 168.
3 Zeck P. The dangers of some antidepressant drugs. *Med J Aust* (1961) **2**, 607.
4 Tonks C M and Livingstone D. MAOI. *Lancet* (1963) **i**, 1323.
5 MacDonald R. Tranylcypromine. *Lancet* (1963) **i**, 269.
6 Mason A. Fatal reaction associated with tranylcypromine and methylamphetamine. *Lancet* (1962) **i**, 1073.
7 Dally P J. Fatal reaction associated with tranylcypromine and methylamphetamine. *Lancet* (1962) **i**, 1235.
8 Nymark M and Nielsen I M. Reactions due to the combination of MAOI's with thymoleptics, pethidine or methylamphetamine. *Lancet* (1963) **ii**, 524.
9 Elis J, Laurence D R, Mattie H and Prichard B N C. Modification by monoamine oxidase inhibitors of the effects of some sympathomimetics on blood pressure. *Br Med J* (1967) **2**, 75.
10 Low-Beer G A and Tidmarsh D. Collapse after parstelin. *Br Med J* (1963) **2**, 683.
11 Horler A R and Wynne N A. Hypertensive crisis due to pargyline and metaraminol. *Br Med J* (1965) **2**, 460.
12 Tonks C M and Lloyd A T. Hazards with monoamine oxidase inhibitors. *Br Med J* (1965) **1**, 589.
13 Cuthbert M F, Greenberg M P and Morley S W. Cough and cold remedies: potential danger to patients on monoamine oxidase inhibitors. *Br Med J* (1969) **1**, 404.
14 Mason A M S and Buckle R M. 'Cold' cures and monoamine oxidase inhibitors. *Br Med J* (1961) **1**, 845.
15 Humberstone P M. Hypertension from cold remedies. *Br Med J* (1969) **1**, 846.
16 Lewis E. Hyperpyrexia with antidepressant drugs. *Br Med J* (1965) **1**, 1672.
17 Krisko I, Lewis E, and Johnson J E. Severe hyperpyrexia due to tranylcypromine and amphetamine toxicity. *Ann Int Med* (1969) **70**, 559.
18 Wright S P. Hazards with monoamine oxidase inhibitors: a persistent problem. *Lancet* (1978) **i**, 284.
19 Sherman M, Hauser G C and Glover B H. Toxic reactions to tranylcypromine. *Ann J Psychiat* (1964) **120**, 1019.
20 Stark D C C. Effects of giving vasopressors to patients on monoamine oxidase inhibitors. *Lancet* (1962) **i**, 1405.
21 Wright S P. Hazards with monoamine oxidase inhibitors: a persistent problem. *Lancet* (1978) **i**, 284.

Indirectly acting sympathomimetics + tricyclic antidepressants

Summary

On theoretical grounds the effects of indirectly acting sympathomimetics (phenylpropanolamine, amphetamines etc.) might be expected to be reduced, but no interaction of clinical importance appears to have been reported.

Interaction, mechanism, importance and management

Compounds like tyramine exert their effects by stimulating the release of noradrenaline (norepinephrine) from adrenergic neurones rather than by a direct stimulant action on the receptors (see p. 399). In the presence of a tricyclic antidepressant their entry into the neurones is partially or totally prevented and their noradrenaline-releasing effects are therefore blocked. The reduction in the pressor response to tyramine has been used to monitor the efficacy of treatment with the tricyclic antidepressants.[1] However, tyramine itself is only used as a research tool, or as a model of the behaviour of the indirectly acting sympathomimetics. The activity of other similar sympathomimetics might be expected to be blocked by the tricyclics in the same way, but as yet there appear to be no reports of adverse interactions arising from their concurrent use, so whether there is any practical importance in this interaction is an open question.

Reference

1 Mulgirigama L D, Pare C M B, Turner P, Wadsworth J and Witts D J. Tyramine pressor responses and plasma levels during tricyclic antidepressant therapy. *Postgrad Med J* (1977) **53** (Suppl 4) 30.

CHAPTER 20. TRICYCLIC ANTIDEPRESSANT DRUG INTERACTIONS

The development of the tricyclic antidepressants arose out of work carried out on phenothiazine compounds related to chlorpromazine. They share the common features of possessing two benzene rings joined by a third ring of carbon atoms, with sometimes a nitrogen (see Fig. 20.1), and of having antidepressant activity, hence their name. Table 20.1. contains a list of the tricyclic antidepressants with some of their international proprietary names.

Although the tricyclic antidepressants have been subjected to extensive biochemical and pharmacological study, it is still not known precisely how they act within the brain to relieve depression, although several theories have been forwarded.

The antidepressant activity of the tricyclic antidepressants

The arrival of a nerve impulse at the end of a nerve causes the release of a small amount of chemical transmitter which, after diffusing to the receptors of the next nerve, or an organ, stimulates a response. In the case of neurones which use

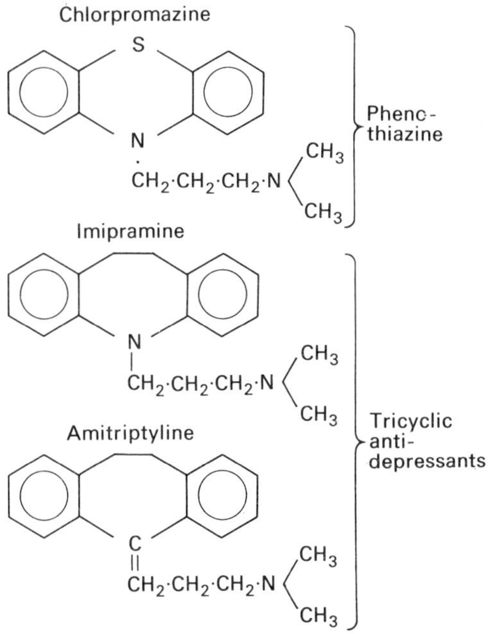

Fig. 20.1. A comparison between the chemical structures of chlorpromazine (a phenothiazine) and the chemical structures of imipramine (the first tricyclic antidepressant) and amitriptyline.

Table 20.1 Tricyclic antidepressants

Approved names	Proprietary names
Amitriptyline	*Amizol, Annolytin, Deprex, Domical, Elavil, Elatrol, Endex, Laroxyl, Larozyl, Lentizol, Levate, Mareline, Novotriptyn, Saroten, Tryptanol, Tryptizol*
Amitriptyline with chlordiazepoxide	*Limbitrol*
Amitriptyline with perphenazine	*Triptafen*
Butriptyline	*Evadyne*
Clomipramine	*Anafranil*
Desipramine	*Depramine, Norpramin, Pertofran, Pertofrin,*
Dibenzepin	*Noveril*
Dothiepin	*Prothiaden*
Doxepin	*Adapin, Aponal, Quitaxon, Sinequan, Sinquan*
Imipramine	*Anapramine, Berkomine, Censtim, Chemipramine, Dimipressin, Ethipram, Ia-Pram, Imavate, Impamin, Impranil, Imprex, Impril, Imprin, Iramil, Janimine, Melipramine, Novapramine, Norpramine, Oppanyl, Panpramine, Praminil, Presamine, Prodopress, Somipra, SK-Pramine, Thymopramine, Tofranil,*
Iprindole	*Prondol*
Melitracen	*Trausaben*
Nortriptyline	*Acetexa, Allegron, Altilev, Aventyl, Nortab, Noritren, Nortrilen, Nortrilin, Sensaval.*
Nortriptyline with fluphenazine	*Motipress, Motival*
Opipramol	*Ensidon, Insidon.*
Protriptyline	*Concordin, Maxiped, Triptil, Vivactil.*
Trimipramine	*Stangyl, Surmontil*

noradrenaline (norepinephrine) as the transmitting substance, the receptors are then 'cleared' for further stimulation by the return of the noradrenaline into the nerve endings, although a small proportion is destroyed by the enzyme catechol-O-methyl transferase (COMT). The noradrenaline which is returned to the neurone regains access by means of the noradrenaline 'pump' (see Fig. 20.2).

The tricyclic antidepressants appear to act by inhibiting the activity of this pump and in this way they raise the concentration of the transmitter in the receptor area (see Fig. 20.3). If depression represents some inadequacy in transmission between the nerves in the brain, increased amounts of transmitter may go some way towards reversing this inadequacy by improving transmission. Nerves which use 5-HT (serotonin) instead of noradrenaline appear to respond to the tricyclics in a similar way.

Other properties of the tricyclic antidepressants

The tricyclic antidepressants also possess other characteristics which are responsible for their side-effects. They have anticholinergic (atropine-like) activity and can cause dry mouth, blurred vision, constipation, urine retention and an increase in

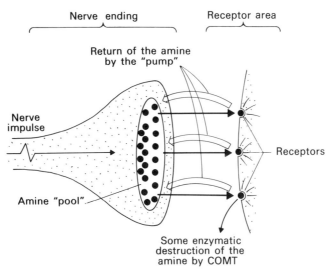

Fig. 20.2 A highly simplified diagrammatic representation of an amine-releasing (noradrenaline or serotonin) neurone. The amine (●) which is released from a 'pool' at the nerve ending by the arrival of a nerve impulse diffuses across to the receptor and effects stimulation. The receptors are then cleared in readiness for further stimulation by the return of the amine into the neurone using the 'pump'. A small amount is enzymatically destroyed by COMT.

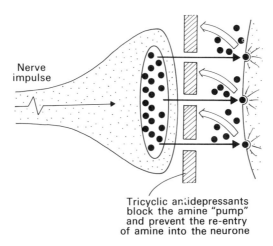

Fig. 20.3 Mode of action of the tricyclic antidepressants. The tricyclics block the 'pump' so that re-entry of the amine into the nerve ending is prevented and the amine concentration at the receptors increases.

intraocular tension. Postural hypotension occurs sometimes and there are also cardiotoxic effects. Among the central side-effects are sedation, the precipitation of seizures in certain individuals, and extrapyramidal reactions.

Other interactions involving the tricyclic antidepressants but not discussed in this chapter are to be found elsewhere in this book. The Index should be consulted.

Tricyclic antidepressants + barbiturates

Summary

The serum levels and the therapeutic response to amitriptyline, desipramine, nortriptyline, protriptyline and probably other tricyclic antidepressants may be reduced by the concurrent administration of barbiturates.

Interaction

A patient being treated with desipramine showed a 50% reduction in serum levels within a few days of beginning to take 100 mg phenobarbitone each night as a hypnotic. The side-effects of the desipramine were also markedly reduced.[1]

A comparative study on the steady-state nortriptyline levels of five pairs of twins showed that the twins taking a barbituate had considerably reduced nortriptyline serum levels, the reduction being between about 14 and 60%. The barbiturates used were not specifically named.[2]

Similar observations have been made on patients and subjects taking nortriptyline with amylobarbitone,[3] and protriptyline with sodium amylobarbitone.[4]

Mechanism

The barbiturates are potent liver enzyme-inducing agents and the most probable explanation of this interaction is that the metabolism of the tricyclics is increased resulting in a reduction in the serum levels of the antidepressant.

Importance and management

Data about this interaction are limited but it would seem to be of clinical importance. Barbiturates are well-known enzyme-inducing agents so that an interaction can be expected with any barbiturate and tricyclic antidepressant

although only a few have been documented.[1-4] Reductions in serum levels of 50% or more will almost certainly be accompanied by a reduced therapeutic response.

Toxic overdosage with tricyclics can cause convulsions and various other effects including respiratory depression which may be enhanced by phenobarbitone. It is thought[5] that diazepam maybe a better choice of anticonvulsant, although sodium amylobarbitone[6,7] and paraldehyde[8] have been used successfully.

References

1 Hammer W, Idestrom C M and Sjoqvist F. In *Antidepressant Drugs*, p. 301. Grattini S and Dukes M N G (eds) Proceedings of the 1st International Symposium, Milan (1966). International Congress Series no. 122, Excerpta Medica.
2 Alexanderson A, Evans D A P and Sjöqvist F. Steady state plasma levels of nortriptyline in twins: influence of genetic factors and drug therapy. *Br Med J* (1969) 4, 764.
3 Burrows G D and Davies B. Antidepressants and barbiturates. *Br Med J* (1971) 4, 113.
4 Moody J P, Whyte S F, MacDonald A J and Naylor G J. Pharmacokinetic aspects of protriptyline plasma levels. *Eur J Clin Pharmacol* (1977) 11, 51.
5 Crocker J and Morton B. Tricylic (antidepressant) drug toxicity. *Clinical Toxicology* (1969) 2, 397.
6 Arneson G A. A near fatal case of imipramine overdosage. *Amer J Psychiatry* (1961) 117, 934.
7 Luby E D and Domino E F. Toxicity from large doses of imipramine and MAO inhibitor in suicidal intent. *J Amer Med Ass* (1961) 117, 68.
8 Connelly J F and Venables A. A case of poisoning with 'Tofranil'. *Med J Aust* (1961) 1, 108.

Tricyclic antidepressant + benzodiazepines

Summary

Apart from 3 patients who became drowsy and forgetful and who appeared uncoordinated and drunk while taking amitriptyline and chlordiazepoxide, there is no evidence of an adverse interaction with this or any other combination of tricyclic antidepressant and benzodiazepine. One manufacturer markets a combined amitriptyline/chlordiazepoxide preparation.

Interaction

Amitriptyline + chlordiazepoxide

> A depressed patient taking 150 mg amitriptyline and 40 mg chlordiazepoxide daily became confused, forgetful and uncoordinated. He was described as giving the appearance of being drunk.[1]
>
> Two patients taking amitriptyline and 30 mg chlordiazepoxide daily showed drowsiness, memory impairment, slurring of speech and inability to concentrate. Both were unable to work and one described himself as feeling drunk.[2]

In contrast to these two adverse reports, a number of clinical trials have been carried out, involving large numbers of patients, on the efficacy of this drug combination using similar or greater dosages of each drug without any indication that the incidence of adverse reactions was greater than might have been expected with either of the drugs used singly,[3,4] and no hint of this interaction.

Other tricyclic antidepressant/benzodiazepine combinations

Studies on the effects of nitrazepam, diazepam, oxazepam and chlordiazepoxide on the steady-state plasma levels of nortriptyline and amitriptyline,[5] and of diazepam and chlordiazepoxide on nortriptyline[6] failed to show any interaction. Another study demonstrated an increase in amitriptyline serum levels during concurrent treatment with diazepam.[7]

Mechanism

Not known. The three patients described would appear to have been particularly sensitive to the combined CNS depressant effects of both drugs.

Importance and management

Apart from the three cases cited, there seem to be no other reports of adverse interactions attributed to the concurrent use of amitriptyline and chlordiazepoxide. At least one manufacturer, Roche, currently markets a combined preparation, *Limbitrol*, which contains either 5 or 10 mg chlordiazepoxide with 12·5 or 25 mg amitriptyline intended for conditions of mild anxiety with depression. The possibility of an adverse interaction cannot be entirely discounted but it is clearly highly unlikely.

There is no reason to expect any of the other tricyclic antidepressant/benzodiazepine combinations to interact adversely, except that there is the theoretical possibility that during the first few days of treatment the CNS depressants effects of the more sedative tricyclics such as amitriptyline might be slightly enhanced.

References

1 Kane F J, and Taylor T W. A toxic reaction to combined Elavil–Librium therapy. *Amer J Psychiat* (1963) **119**, 1179.
2 Abdon, F A. Elavil–Librium combination. *Amer J Psychiat* (1964) **120**, 1204.
3 Haider I. A comparative trial of RO 4-6270 and amitriptyline in depressive illness. *Brit J Psychiat* (1967) **113**, 993.
4 General Practitioner Clinical Trials. Chlordiazepoxide with amitriptyline in neurotic depression. *Practitioner* (1969) **202**, 437.
5 Silverman G and Braithwaite. Benzodiazepines and tricyclic antidepressant plasma levels. *Br Med J* (1973) **2**, 18.
6 Gram L F, Overø K F and Kirk L. Influence of neuroleptics and benzodiazepines on metabolism of tricyclic antidepressants in man. *Am J Psychiatry* (1974) **131**, 863.
7 Dugal R, Caille G, Albert J-M and Cooper S F. Apparent pharmacokinetic interaction of diazepam and amitriptyline in psychiatric patients: a pilot study. *Curr Ther Res* (1975) **18**, 679.

Tricyclic antidepressants + ethchlorvynol

Summary

Transient delirium has been attributed to the concurrent use of amitriptyline and ethchlorvynol.

Interaction, mechanism, importance and management

Hussar says that transient delirium has been reported with the combination of amitriptyline and ethchlorvynol,[1] but no further details or documentation are given, and there appear to be no other reports of this interaction.

Reference

1 Hussar D A. Tabular compilation of drug interactions. *Amer J Pharm* (1969), **141**, 109.

Tricyclic antidepressants + fenfluramine

Summary

There is contradictory evidence about whether fenfluramine should or should not be given to depressed patients receiving tricyclic antidepressants or monoamine oxidase inhibitors.

Interaction, mechanism, importance and management

Depression has been observed in some patients given fenfluramine[3] and several cases of withdrawal depression have also been observed in patients receiving amitriptyline and fenfluramine concurrently, following episodes of severe depression.[4] On the other hand one report describes a rise in the serum levels of amitriptyline when 60 mg fenfluramine was given to patients taking 150 mg amitriptyline daily for depression.[5] It has been claimed that depression is not a serious problem in most patients taking fenfluramine[6] but that it can be used safely and effectively with tricyclic antidepressants.[7,9]

Acute confusional states have been described when fenfluramine was used with phenelzine[8] but again it has been claimed that in some instances fenfluramine has been used effectively with an MAO inhibitor.[9]

The recommendation of the manufacturers and others[1,2] is that care should be exercised if fenfluramine is given to depressed patients or those on antidepressant therapy, and that fenfluramine should not be used during or within 3 weeks of stopping therapy with the MAOI. This would appear to be a practical solution to this confused situation.

References

1 ABPI Data sheet compendium, 1979–80, p. 949. Pharmind Publications, London.
2 Lockhart J D. Drugs causing weight gain. Br Med J (1974) 1, 394.
3 Gaind R. Fenfluramine (Ponderax) in the treatment of obese psychiatric out-patients. Brit J Psychiat (1969) 115, 963.
4 Harding T. Fenfluramine dependence. Br Med J (1971) 3, 305.
5 Gunne L M, Antonijevic S and Jonsson J. Effect of fenfluramine on steady state plasma levels of amitriptyline. Postgrad Med J (1975) 51 (Suppl 1) 113.
6 Pinder R M, Brogden R N, Sawyer P R, Speight T M and Avery G S. Fenfluramine: a review of its pharmacological properties and therapeutic efficacy in obesity. Drugs (1975) 10, 241.
7 Poire R, Rombach F and Crance J P. Obésité et fenfluramine (768 S). Experiences de trois ans d'utilisation prolongée et controlée du medicament en mileu psychiatrique hospitalies. Ann medicopsychologiques (1966) 1, 26.
8 Brandon S. Unusual effect of fenfluramine. Br Med J (1969) 4, 557.
9 Mason E C. Servier Laboratories Ltd. Personal Communication (1976).

Tricyclic antidepressants + furazolidone

Summary

A single case has been reported of toxic psychosis, hyperactivity, sweating, and hot and cold flashes attributed to the concurrent use of amitriptyline and furazolidone.

Interaction

A depressed woman taking daily doses of 1·25 mg conjugated oestrogenic substances and 75 mg amitriptyline, was additionally given 300 mg furazolidone and diphenoxylate with atropine sulphate. Three days later she began to experience blurred vision, profuse perspiration, followed by alternate chills and hot flashes, restlessness, motor activity, persecutory delusions, auditory hallucinations, and visual illusions. The symptoms cleared within a day of stopping the furazolidone.[1]

Mechanism

Not understood. The authors of the report point out that furazolidone has monoamine oxidase inhibitory properties and that the symptoms described were similar to those seen when the tricyclic antidepressants and MAOI interact. However, the MAO-inhibitory activity of furazolidone normally takes about 5 days or more to develop. Whether the concurrent use of atropine and amitriptyline, both of which have anticholinergic activity, may have had some part to play is not clear. The reactions seen were also similar to those of excessive anticholinergic activity.

Importance and management
No firm general conclusions can be based on such slim evidence, but prescribers should be aware of this adverse reaction if furazolidone and a tricyclic antidepressant are given concurrently.

Reference
1 Aderhold R M and Muniz C E. Acute psychosis with amitriptyline and furazolidone. *J Amer med Ass* (1970) **213**, 2080.

Tricyclic antidepressants + haloperidol

Summary
During treatment with haloperidol the serum levels of concurrently administered tricyclic antidepressants may be expected to rise. The clinical importance of this is uncertain.

Interaction
The urinary excretion of a test dose of C^{14}-imipramine given to 2 schizophrenic patients was reduced 35–40% during concurrent treatment with 12–20 mg haloperidol daily.[1,3]

A similar study on another schizophrenic patient who was administered C^{14}-nortriptyline showed that during treatment with 16 mg haloperidol daily the urinary excretion and plasma metabolite levels of nortriptyline fell, while the plasma levels of unchanged nortriptyline rose.[2]

Mechanism
On the basis of the studies described it is suggested that haloperidol inhibits the metabolism of these tricyclic antidepressants, thereby delaying their excretion from the body and resulting in an increase in their serum levels.

Importance and management
The information on this interaction is limited to these studies on imipramine and nortriptyline with haloperidol. The clinical importance of the rise in serum tricyclic antidepressant levels described has not been determined. Whether it occurs with other tricyclic antidepressants is uncertain.

References
1 Gram L F, Overø K F. Drug interaction: inhibitory effect of neuroleptics on metabolism of tricyclic antidepressants in man. *Br Med J* (1972) **1**, 463.
2 Gram L F, Overø K F and Kirk L. Influence of neuroleptics and benzodiazepines on metabolism of tricyclic antidepressants in man. *Am J Psychiatry* (1974) **131**, 8.
3 Gram L F. Laegemiddelinteraktion: haemmende virkning af neuroleptica på tricykliske antidepressivas metabolisering. *Nord Psykiatr Tidsskr* (1971) **4**, 357.

Tricyclic antidepressants + hypoglycaemic agents

Summary
There appears to be no evidence of an interaction between these two groups of drugs. A study showed that the half-life of tolbutamide was unaffected by amitriptyline.

Interaction, mechanism, importance and management
A study in 4 patients showed that after 9 days' treatment with amitriptyline, 25 mg daily, the half-life of single 500 mg oral doses of tolbutamide was unaffected. The absence of other reports in the literature would also appear to indicate that no interaction normally takes place between these two groups of drugs.

Reference
1 Pond S M, Graham G G, Birkett D J and Wade D N. Effects of tricyclic antidepressants on drug metabolism. *Clin Pharmacol Therap* (1975) **18**, 191.

Tricyclic antidepressants + methylphenidate

Summary

Methylphenidate can cause a marked increase in the blood levels of imipramine resulting in clinical improvement. Whether levels can rise to toxic concentrations appears not to be documented.

Interaction

A study in '. . . several patients . . .' demonstrated a dramatic increase in the blood levels of desipramine and imipramine during concurrent treatment with imipramine and methylphenidate. In one patient taking 150 mg imipramine daily it was observed that 20 mg methylphenidate a day increased the blood levels of the imipramine from 100 to 700 μg/l, and of desipramine from 200 to 850 μg/l over a period of 16 days.[1]

Similar effects have been described in other reports.[2,3]

Mechanism

In-vitro experiments with human liver slices indicate that methylphenidate inhibits the metabolism of imipramine resulting in its accumulation, reflected in raised blood levels.[3]

Importance and management

Information is limited. Some therapeutic improvement, as might be expected, has been seen because of the raised blood levels of the antidepressant, but whether this might also lead to tricyclic antidepressant toxicity is uncertain. This possibility should be borne in mind. Information about other tricyclic antidepressants is lacking.

References

1 Dayton P G, Perel J M, Israili Z H, Faraj B A, Rodewig K, Black N and Goldberg L I. Studies with methlphenidate: drug interactions and metabolism. In 'Clinical Phamacology of Psychoactive Drugs', p. 183. Sellers E M (ed) (1975). Alcoholism and Drug Addiction Research Foundation, Toronto.
2 Cooper T B and Simpson G M. Concomitant imipramine and methylphenidate administration: a case report. Am J Psychiat (1973) 130, 721.
3 Wharton R N, Perel J M, Dayton P G and Malitz S. A potential use for the interaction of methylphenidate with tricyclic antidepressants. Am J Psychiat (1971) 127, 1619.

Tricyclic antidepressants + oestrogens

Summary

Imipramine toxicity and a reduced antidepressant response induced by concurrent treatment with some doses of ethinyl-oestradiol have been described in 5 patients. The general importance of this interaction is not known.

Interaction

A 2-week study was carried out on 30 women with primary depression given 150 mg imipramine daily. Ten received imipramine and an oestrogen (either 50 μg or 25 μg ethinyloestradiol), 10 received imipramine and a placebo, and 10 received only a placebo. After a week of the trial the patients on imipramine and 50 μg ethinyloestradiol showed less improvement than those taking imipramine with a placebo, and 4 of the women showed signs of imipramine toxicity, which was dealt with by halving the dose of imipramine.[1,2]

This report[1] prompted a retrospective review of the clinical history of a woman who had been taking 100 mg imipramine daily with 2·5 mg conjugated oestrogen for a period of 3 years or so. She had apparently always complained of lethargy and showed signs of depersonalization and occasional tremor. More severe toxicity ensued when she doubled and then tripled the dose of oestrogen. She was later satisfactorily treated with a quarter of the original dose of oestrogen.[3]

Mechanism

Not known. It has been suggested that the ethinyloestradiol inhibits the metabolism of imipramine so that its serum levels rise, leading to the development of toxicity, but there is no direct evidence to support this idea.[4]

Importance and management

The general importance is difficult to assess. Only 5 patients have clearly demonstrated this interaction, whereas concurrent use is by no means uncommon; 50 μg of ethinyloestradiol is contained in a large number of combined oral contraceptives but there seems to be no evidence that tricyclic antidepressant toxicity is seen more often in those on the pill than those who are not. This general impression is confirmed by a retrospective study of women on various types of oral contraceptive and clomipramine.[5]

On balance it would be prudent to be on the alert for the development of toxicity during concurrent use, but the incidence is uncertain. A reduction in the dosage or withdrawal of either should control any toxic symptoms.

References
1 Prange A J, Wilson I C and Alltop L B. Estrogen may well affect response to antidepressant. *J Amer Med Ass* (1972) **219**, 143.
2 Prange A J, Wilson I C and Alltop L B. The effect of estrogen on imipramine response in depressed women. 5th World Congress of Psychiatry, Mexico City, November 1971.
3 Khurana R C. Estrogen–imipramine interaction. *J Amer Med Ass* (1972) **222**, 702.
4 Somani S M, and Khurana R C. Mechanism of estrogen–imipramine interaction. *J Amer Med Ass* (1973) **223**, 560.
5 Beamont G. Drug interactions with clomipramine (Anafranil) *J Int Med Res* (1973) **1**, 480.

Tricyclic antidepressant + neuromuscular blocker and hyoscine

Summary
Hypotension due to the concurrent use of doxepin with pancuronium and hyoscine has been reported.

Interaction, mechanism, importance and management
Hypotension attributed to the concurrent use of doxepin with pancuronium bromide and hyoscine is included among the drug interactions (1973–74) which are listed by the New Zealand Committee on Adverse Drug Reactions in their 9th Annual Report. No details are given.

Reference
1 New Zealand Committee on Adverse Drug Reactions. Ninth Annual Report. *NZ Dent J* (1975) **71**, 28.

Tricyclic antidepressants + thioxanthenes

Summary
Flupenthixol appears not to interact with imipramine.

Interaction, mechanism, importance and management
A study[1] on the possibility of an interaction between the tricyclic antidepressants and neuroleptic agents showed that unlike the situation with chlorpromazine and perphenazine (see page. 383) the concurrent administration of 3–6 mg flupenthixol had no effect on the total excretion of C14-imipramine. No other data appear to be available. On the basis of this very limited evidence it would seem that no interaction takes place.

Reference
1 Gram L F, and Overø K F. Drug interaction: inhibitory effect of neuroleptics on metabolism of tricyclic antidepressants in man. *Br Med J* (1972) **1**, 463.

Tricyclic antidepressants + thyroid preparations

Summary

The antidepressant response to imipramine, amitriptyline and possibly other tricyclic antidepressants can be accelerated by the concurrent use of thyroid preparations. An isolated case of paroxysmal atrial tachycardia and another of thyrotoxicosis induced by concurrent therapy have been described.

Interaction

Accelerated response to tricyclic antidepressant treatment

A double-blind study extending over 4 weeks on 20 patients with severe primary depression and treated with 150 mg imipramine a day showed that the addition of 25 μg tri-iodothyronine daily enhanced the speed and efficacy of the imipramine in relieving depression. The patients remained euthyroidic.[1]

Similar results have been described in other reports using imipramine[2,3,4] and amitriptyline.[5] One study failed to show this response.[6]

Adverse responses

A hospitalized patient under treatment for hypothyroidism and depression with 150 mg imipramine and 60 mg thyroid a day complained of dizziness and nausea and was found to have developed paroxysmal auricular tachycardia.[7]

A 10-year-old girl with congenital hypothyroidism was maintained for years on 150 mg desiccated thyroid daily and remained clinically euthyroid. After 5 months' treatment with 25 mg imipramine daily for enuresis she developed severe thyrotoxicosis which remitted once the imipramine was withdrawn, while continuing on the same dosage of thyroid[8]

Mechanism

Not understood. One idea, supported by animal data, is that the thyroid hormones increase the sensitivity of the adrenergic neurones in the CNS to adrenaline, perhaps by an action on adenyl cyclase. That is to say the general levels of CNS excitation are raised by (a) inhibition of the noradrenaline pump by the antidepressant, and (b) an increase in the sensitivity of the noradrenaline receptors. Certainly some increased sensitivity to imipramine has been shown in mice where the fatal dose in hyperthyroidic mice is about half that of euthyroidic mice.[7] This increased sensitivity might explain the enhanced antidepressant response cited[1-5] and possibly the paroxysmal tachycardia,[7] but just why thyrotoxicosis should be precipitated by imipramine is not clear.

Importance and management

The response to imipramine and amitriptyline can be accelerated by the concurrent use of tri-iodothyronine. A dosage of 25 μg daily has been used with good effect[1-4] with patients remaining euthyroidic. Whether other tricyclic antidepressants behave similarly is uncertain.

To what extent abnormalities of thyroid function predispose patients to an adverse response to the tricyclic antidepressants is not known, but some degree of caution would seem appropriate in non-euthyroidic patients.

References

1 Wilson I C, Prange A J, McClane T K, Rabon A M and Lipton M A. Thyroid-hormone enhancement of imipramine in non-retarded depressions. *New Eng J Med* (1970) **282**, 1063.
2 Prange A J, Wilson I C, Rabon A M and Lipton M A. Enhancement of imipramine antidepressant activity by thyroid hormone. *Amer J Psychiat* (1969) **126**, 457.
3 Copper A, Whybrow P C, Noguera R, Maggs R and Prange A J. The comparative antidepressant value of L-tryptophan and imipramine with and without attempted potentiation by tri-iodothyronine. *Arch Gen Psychiatr* (1972) **26**, 234.
4 Prange A J, Wilson I C, Rabon A M and Lipton M A. Enhancement of imipramine by tri-iodothyronine in un-selected depressed patients. *Proc. 6th Internat. Cong. CINP*, Tarragona 1968, p. 532. Excerpta Medica International Congress Series no 180 (1969).
5 Wheatly D. Potentiation of amitriptyline by thyroid hormone. *Arch Gen Psychiatr* (1972) **26**, 229.
6 Feighner J P. Hormonal potentiation of imipramine and ECT in primary depression. *Amer J Psychiat* (1972) **128**, 50.
7 Prange A J. Paroxysmal auricular tachycardia apparently resulting from combined thyroid-imipramine treatment. *Amer J Psychiat* (1963) **119**, 994.
8 Colantonio L A and Orson J M. Triiodothyronine thyrotoxicosis. Induction by desiccated thyroid and imipramine. *Am J Dis Child* (1974) **128**, 396.

Tricyclic antidepressants + urinary alkalinizers and acidifiers

Summary

Blood levels of nortriptyline and desipramine are not significantly affected by agents which alter urinary pH.

Interaction, mechanism, importance and management

The tricyclic antidepressants are bases and it might be thought that changes in urinary pH would have an effect on their excretion which would be reflected in changes in blood levels. However, a study[1] in 10 depressed patients and 4 dogs given nortriptyline or desipramine showed that the urinary excretion of unchanged drug was extremely small (less than 5%) compared with amounts excreted after metabolic inactivation. No significant changes in blood levels are likely even with agents such as acetazolamide or ammonium chloride which can have a marked effect on the pH of the urine. These results were confirmed in 12 other patients. Even in cases of poisoning '. . . vigorous procedures such as forced diuresis, peritoneal dialysis, or haemodialysis can therefore not be expected to markedly accelerate the elimination of these drugs'.[1] Only in cases of hepatic dysfunction is simple urinary clearance likely to take on a more importance role. Direct information about other tricyclic antidepressants does not appear to be available.

Reference

1 Sjöqvist F, Berglund F, Borgå O, Hammer W, Andersson S, and Thorstrand C. The pH-dependent excretion of monomethylated tricyclic antidepressants. *Clin Pharmacol Ther* (1969) 10, 826.

CHAPTER 21. MISCELLANEOUS DRUG INTERACTIONS

Anti-anaemic agents + chloramphenicol

Summary

Quite apart from the serious and potentially fatal bone marrow depression which can occur with chloramphenicol, it may also induce a milder, reversible depression which can antagonize the treatment of anaemia.

Interaction, mechanisms, importance and management

Among the toxic effects of chloramphenicol is bone marrow depression. One form of this is extremely serious and irreversible, and can result in fatal aplastic anaemia. The other form is probably unrelated, milder and reversible, and appears to be caused by antibiotic serum levels of 25 μg/ml or more. It is thought that the latter form of marrow depression may be due to inhibition of protein synthesis within the bone marrow, and is characterized by anaemia, the first sign being a fall in the reticulocyte count which reflects the suppression of red cell maturation. This response has been described in animals,[1] in normal individuals,[2] in normal individuals receiving vitamin B_{12} and folic acid,[3] and in anaemic patients being treated with iron-dextran or vitamin B_{12}.[4]

In a report on patients under treatment for anaemia who were also given chloramphenicol, 10 out of 20 on iron–dextran for iron-deficiency anaemia failed to show the expected haematological response, and all of 4 patients receiving vitamin B_{12} for pernicious anaemia were similarly refractory until the chloramphenicol was withdrawn.[4]

If chloramphenicol is to be used, the authors of one study recommend that dosages of 25–30 mg/kg are usually adequate for treating infections without running the risk of elevating serum levels to 25 μg/ml or more when bone marrow depression frequently occurs.[5] A preferable alternative would be to use a safer antibiotic.

It has been claimed that the optic neuritis which sometimes occurs with chloramphenicol can be reversed with large doses of vitamins B_6 and B_{12}.[6]

References

1 Rigdon R H, Crass G and Martin A. Anemia produced by chloramphenicol (chloromycetin) in the duck. *AMA Arch Pathol* (1954) **58**, 85.
2 McCurdy P R. Chloramphenicol bone marrow toxicity. *J Amer Med Ass* (1961) **176**, 588.
3 Jiji R M, Gangarosa E J, and de la Marcorra F. Chloramphenicol and its sulfamoly analogue. Report of reversible erythropoietic toxicity in healthy volunteers. *Arch Intern Med* (1963) **111**, 70.
4 Saidi P, Wallerstein R O and Aggeler P M. Effect of chloramphenicol on erythropoiesis. *J Lab Clin Med* (1961) **57**, 247.
5 Scott J L, Finegold S M, Belkin G A, and Lawrence I S. Chloramphenicol and bone marrow depression. *New Eng J Med* (1965) **272**, 1137.
6 Cocke J C. Chloramphenicol optic neuritis. *Amer J Dis Child* (1967) **114**, 424.

Caffeine + idrocilamide

Summary

Idrocilamide causes the caffeine contained in tea, coffee or other drinks to be retained in the body leading to insomnia, extreme nervousness, anxious agitation and other manifestations of caffeine toxicity.

Interaction

Evidence that the ingestion of caffeine in coffee might have had some part to play in the development of the neuropsychiatric disorders seen in some patients on idrocilamide, prompted a pharmacokinetic study on 4 normal subjects. It was found that while under treatment with idrocilamide, 400 mg three times a day, the half-life of caffeine from a cup of coffee containing 150–200 mg caffeine was prolonged by a factor of nine (from about 7 h to 57 h) and the overall clearance of caffeine was decreased approximately 90%.[1,2]

Mechanism

The experimental evidence indicates that idrocilamide causes a marked inhibition of the metabolism and clearance of caffeine from the body leading to its accumulation.[1]

Importance and management

The evidence is limited, but the interaction appears to be established. Patients treated with idrocilamide should be advised not to drink tea, coffee, or other caffeine-containing drinks, or to take only very small amounts, if the toxic effects of caffeine accumulation are to be avoided.

References

1 Brazier J L, Descotes J, Lery N, Ollagnier M and Evreux J-Cl. Inhibition by idrocilamide of the disposition of caffeine. *Europ J Clin Pharmacol* (1980) **17**, 37.
2 Evreux J C, Bayere J J, Descotes J, Lery N, Ollagnier M and Brazier J L. Les accidents neuropsychiques de l'idrocilamide: conséquence d'une inhibition due métabolisme de la caféine? *Lyon Médical* (1979) **241**, 89.

Carbenoxolone + diuretics

Summary

The concurrent use of thiazides or similar diuretics and carbenoxolone may result in hypokalaemia. The ulcer-healing properties of carbenoxolone are antagonized by spironolactone.

Interaction, mechanism, importance and management

Among the side-effects of carbenoxolone treatment are a rise in blood pressure, fluid retention and a reduction in serum potassium levels due, it is believed, to the mineralocorticoid-like activity of carbenoxolone. In one study in which spironolactone (an aldosterone antagonist) was used to combat these side-effects, the ulcer healing properties of carbenoxolone were also found to be inhibited as well[1]. For this reason spironolactone is not a suitable diuretic for patients on carbenoxolone.

The thiazide diuretics can be used to control the side-effects of carbenoxolone treatment without adversely affecting the ulcer healing properties, but regular checks on serum potassium levels should be carried out and, where necessary, potassium supplements should be given to control the reduction in potassium levels which can take place because both carbenoxolone and the thiazides cause potassium loss.

Similar precautions should be taken with any of the other diuretics which cause potassium loss. Severe potassium deficiency with rhabdomyolosis and tubular necrosis has been described in one patient treated with carbenoxolone and chlorthalidone without potassium supplementation.[2]

It has been suggested that triamterine might be a suitable alternative diuretic, but not amiloride which may possibly behave like spironolactone.

References

1 Doll R, Langman M J S and Shawdon H H. Treatment of gastric ulcer with carbenoxolone: antagonistic effect of spironolactone. *Gut* (1968) 9, 42.

2 Descamps C. Rhabdomyolosis and acute tubular necrosis associated with carbenoxolone and diuretic treatment. *Br Med J* (1977) 1, 272

Charcoal + other drugs

Summary

Charcoal adsorbs drugs onto its surface and can markedly reduce their availability for absorption by the gut. The administration of charcoal should be separated from other drugs by as long a time interval as possible. The effectiveness of this requires confirmation.

Interaction, mechanism, importance and management

Activated charcoal is able to adsorb gases, toxins and drugs onto its surface. Many of the reports in the literature about charcoal are concerned with the treatment of cases of poisoning where these adsorptive properties are exploited, but charcoal in doses intended to adsorb intestinal gas, or for the treatment of diarrhoea and dysentery, can also adsorb drugs given in normal therapeutic doses. In this way gastrointestinal absorption, blood levels, and the therapeutic response are all reduced. An example: in one study in man[1] it was shown that 98% of a 0·5 mg dose of digoxin, 98% of a 500 mg dose of phenytoin, and 70% of a 1 g dose of aspirin was adsorbed by 50 g activated charcoal in water. Similar levels of adsorption may be expected with many other drugs. For this reason the administration of charcoal and other drugs should be separated as much as possible to obviate their admixture in the gut, although it should be emphasised that as yet there is little or no documentation to confirm that this is effective.

Reference

1 Neuvonen P J, Elfving S M and Elonen E. Reduction of absorption of digoxin, phenytoin and aspirin by activated charcoal in man. *Europ J clin Pharmacol* (1978) 13, 213.

Cholestyramine + clofibrate

Summary

No significant interaction occurs between cholestyramine and clofibrate.

Interaction, mechanism, importance and managment

A study on 15 patients taking 1 g clofibrate twice daily showed that 16 g cholestyramine daily had no effect on the fasting plasma levels, urinary and faecal excretion, or the half-life of clofibrate.[1]

Reference

1 Sedaghat A and Ahrens E H. Lack of effect of cholestyramine on the pharmacokinetics of clofibrate in man. *Europ J clin Invest* (1975) 5, 177.

Cholinergic drugs + procainamide or quinidine

Summary
The activity of cholinergic drugs used for the treatment of myasthenia gravis can be antagonized by procainamide or quinidine.

Interaction, mechanism, importance and management
It is usual to avoid the use of procainamide in patients with myasthenia gravis because of its neuromuscular blocking activity which increases the muscular weakness.[1] For this reason antagonism of the effects of cholinergic drugs used to treat myasthenia gravis may be expected if procainamide is used concurrently. A similar interaction may occur with quinidine,[2] and with other drugs with neuromuscular blocking activity, such as the aminoglycoside antibiotics.

References
1 Drachman D A and Skom J H. Procainamide—a hazard in myasthenia gravis. *Archs Neurol* (1965) **13**, 316.
2 Aviado D M and Salem H. Drug action, reaction and interaction. I. Quinidine for cardiac arrhythmias. *J Clin Pharmac* (1975) **15**, 477.

Cimetidine + antacids

Summary
There is contradictory evidence indicating that the absorption of cimetidine is or is not reduced by the use of antacids. The clinical importance of this possible interaction has not been established.

Interaction
The evidence available is inconsistent.

Reduced absorption:
A study on 9 patients with active peptic-ulcer disease showed that if after an overnight fast they were given 200 mg cimetidine and 30 ml *Novalucol* (a suspension of 6 g aluminium hydroxide and 2·5 g magnesium hydroxide per 100 ml) the serum concentrations of cimetidine recorded over a 9-h period were reduced by an average of 22% (range 3–48%) when compared with those on cimetidine alone.[2]

Absorption unaffected:
A study on 6 healthy subjects who were given cimetidine showed that the serum concentrations and urinary output of cimetidine were unaffected by either 20 ml *Aludrox* SA (4·75 ml aluminium hydroxide gel and 100 mg magnesium hydroxide in every 5 ml) or by two *Rennies* (80 mg light magnesium carbonate and 680 mg chalk per tablet) taken at the same time.[1]

Mechanism
Not understood. Whether there is any significance in the fact that an interaction was demonstrated in patients with active peptic-ulcer disease, but not in normal subjects is uncertain.

Importance and management
Much more study is required to resolve this situation. It would, however, clearly be prudent to bear in mind the possibility of a reduced response to cimetidine if antacids are used concurrently. There is no clear case for avoiding the use of antacids. The authors of the report describing an interaction[2] confine their advice to the cautious suggestion that 'a combination of antacid and cimetidine may not always be beneficial . . .'.

References
1 Burland W L, Darkin D W, and Mills M W. Effect of antacids on absorption of cimetidine. *Lancet* (1976) **ii**, 965.
2 Bodemar G, Norlander B and Walan A. Diminished absorption of cimetidine caused by antacids. *Lancet* (1979) **i**, 444.

Cimetidine + penicillins or co-trimoxazoie

Summary

Ampicillin, benzylpenicillin and co-trimoxazole appear not to be adversely affected by the concurrent use of cimetidine.

Interaction, mechanism, importance and management

Studies in man have shown that cimetidine does not adversely affect the bioavailability of ampicillin[1] or trimethoprim and sulphamethoxazole in form of co-trimoxazole.[1] The bioavailability of benzylpenicillin may even be increased.[2]

References

1 Rogers H J, James C A, Morrison P J and Bradbrook I D. Effect of cimetidine on oral absorption of ampicillin and cotrimoxazole. *J Antimicrob chemother* (1980) **6**, 297.
2 Fairfax A J, Adam J and Pagan F S. Effect of cimetidine on absorption of oral benzylpenicillin. *Brit Med J* (1977) **2**, 820.

Clofibrate + glibenclamide

Summary

The antidiuretic effects of clofibrate in the treatment of diabetes insipidus are antagonized by glibenclamide.

Interaction

A study carried out on 11 patients with pituitary diabetes insipidus showed that clofibrate reduced the volume of urine excreted, but when given with glibenclamide the volume excreted increased once again. For example, one patient who without any treatment at all excreted 5·8 l urine daily, excreted only 2·3 l while taking 2 g clofibrate. But with glibenclamide and clofibrate he excreted 3·6 l a day.[1] The diuretic action of glibenclamide was also found to be inhibited by carbamazepine and DDAVP.[1]

Mechanism

Unknown.

Importance and management

Although some of the sulphonylureas such as chlorpropamide[2] can be used for the treatment of diabetes insipidus, glibenclamide paradoxically antagonizes the antidiuretic effects of clofibrate. Combined use of these drugs would seem to be undesirable.

References

1 Radó J P, Szende L, Marosi J, Juhos E, Sawinsky I and Takó J. Inhibition of the diuretic action of glibenclamide by clofibrate, carbamazepine and 1-deamino-8-D-arginine-vasopressin (DDAVP) in patients with pituitary diabetes insipidus. *Acta diabet lat* (1974) **11**, 179.
2 Miller M. and Moses A M. Mechanism of chlorpropamide action in diabetes insipidus. *J Clin Endocrinol Metab* (1970) **30**, 488.

Clofibrate + contraceptives

Summary

Antagonism of the effects of clofibrate by oral contraceptives has been described in 2 patients. Contraceptive-induced rises in serum triglyceride and cholesterol levels are common.

432

Interaction

A woman with hypercholesterolaemia, under treatment with clofibrate, showed a rise in serum cholesterol levels on each of two occasions when concurrently using an oral contraceptive.[1]

A similar response has been described in another report.[2] Rises in serum levels of trigylcerides and cholesterol in women taking oral contraceptives are well recognized.[3,4]

Mechanism

The reason for the rises in serum levels of triglycerides and cholesterol is not fully understood.

Importance and management

Although there appear to be only two reports of an interaction between the oral contraceptives and clofibrate, it is an expected interaction because contraceptive-induced rises in triglyceride and cholesterol levels have been extensively described. Whether oral contraceptives are therefore suitable for women requiring treatment with clofibrate is questionable.

References

1 Smith R B W and Prior I A M. Oral contraceptive opposition to hypocholesterolaemic action of clofibrate. *Lancet* (1968) i, 750.
2 Robertson-Rintoul J. Raised serum-lipids and oral contraceptives. *Lancet* (1972) ii, 1320.
3 Wynn V, Doar J W H, Mills G L and Stokes T. Fasting serum triglyceride, cholesterol and lipoprotein levels during oral contraceptive therapy. *Lancet* (1969) ii, 756.
4 Stokes T and Wynn V. Serum lipids in women on oral contraceptives. *Lancet* (1971) ii, 677.

CNS depressants + CNS depressants

Summary

The concurrent use of two or more drugs with central nervous depressant effects may be expected to result in enhanced CNS depression. This can have undesirable and even potentially serious consequences.

Interaction, mechanism, importance and management

The primary pharmacological effect of some drugs, and the unwanted side-effect of many others is central nervous depression, so that if taken together the CNS-depressant effects may be additive. It is by no means unusual for patients to be taking up to half-a-dozen drugs concurrently (possibly alcohol as well) and for the cumulative CNS-depressant effects to range from mild drowsiness through to a befuddled stupor which can make the performance of the simplest everyday task almost impossible. The importance of this will depend on the context: at home and at bedtime it may be advantageous, whereas at work, in a busy street, driving a car or handling other dangerous machinery where alertness is at a premium, it may be potentially life-threatening. Few, if any, well-controlled studies have been undertaken on the cumulative detrimental effects of CNS depressants (except with alcohol) but the potential hazards are obvious. The following is a list of some of the drugs which to a greater or lesser extent possess CNS-depressant activity, and which may be expected to interact in this way:

Alcohol, analgesics, antibiotics, anticonvulsants, antidepressents, antihistamines, antinauseants, cough and cold preparations, hypnotics, narcotics, sedatives, tranquillizers.

Some of the interactions of alcohol with these drugs are dealt with in individual synopses. The Index should be consulted.

Corticosteroids + antacids

Summary

Serum levels of prednisone or prednisolone, following oral administration, appear to be unaffected by the use of antacids containing aluminium hydroxide, magnesium hydroxide or magnesium trisilicate, but phosphate depletion can confuse the diagnostic picture. In contrast, the absorption of dexamethasone can be considerably reduced by magnesium trisilicate, but the importance of this awaits confirmation.

Interaction

Prednisone or prednisolone + 'Gastrogel', aluminium hydroxide or magnesium trisilicate

A study carried out on 5 patients with chronic neurological disorders, requiring steroid therapy, who were given a single 20 mg dose of prednisone, and on 2 healthy subjects given 10 mg, showed that the concurrent administration of 20 ml *Gastrogel* (250 mg aluminium hydroxide, 120 mg magnesium hydroxide and 120 mg magnesium trisilicate in every 5 ml) had no significant effect on the serum levels, and serum half-life or the area under the plasma concentration time curves of the corticosteroid.[1]

Another study on 8 subjects who were given an average of 20 mg prednisolone (0·3 mg/kg) and either 30 ml Magnesium Trisilicate Mixture BP or 30 ml *Aludrox* (aluminium hydroxide gel) showed that although there was a small reduction in the peak prednisolone levels and in the amounts absorbed compared with a control group of subjects, the differences were not statistically significant. In one of the test subjects taking magnesium trisilicate the levels were considerably reduced.[2]

Dexamethasone + magnesium trisilicate

A study on 6 subjects given a single 1 mg oral dose of dexamethasone showed that the concurrent administration of 5 g magnesium trisilicate in 100 ml water significantly reduced its bioavailability. Using the urinary excretion of 11-hydroxycorticosteroids as a measure, the reduction was of the order of 75%.[4]

Mechanism

The reduction in the absorption of dexamethasone has been attributed to drug adsorption onto the surface of the antacid.

Importance and management

Information is limited but it would appear that the serum levels of neither prednisone nor prednisolone are normally significantly affected by the concurrent use of the antacids cited, although it has been pointed out that there is the possibility that small doses of corticosteroid might be affected to some extent.[2] However, one of the possible problems of concurrent use is illustrated by the case of a prednisolone-dependent asthmatic man who, as a result of taking *Maalox* (magnesium-aluminium hydroxide gel) and *Mylanta* (dimethicone with aluminium hydroxide gel and magnesium hydroxide), both of which are phosphate-binding antacids, developed a phosphate-depletion syndrome which mimicked steroid-induced side-effects and confused the diagnostic picture.[3]

Magnesium trisilicate appears to cause a significant reduction in the absorption of dexamethasone, but the single-dose study described requires the confirmation of longer-term studies before the importance of this can be firmly established.

References

1 Tanner A R, Caffin J A, Halliday J W and Powell L W. Concurrent administration of antacids and prednisone: effect on serum levels of prednisolone. *Br J clin Pharmac* (1979) 7, 397.
2 Lee D A H, Taylor G M, Walker J G and James V H T. The effect of concurrent administration of antacids on prednisolone absorption. *Br J clin Pharmac* (1979) 8, 92.
3 Goodman M, Solomons C C and Miller P D. Distinction between the common symptoms of the phosphate-depletion syndrome and gluco-corticoid-induced disease. *Am J Med* (1978) 65, 868.
4 Naggar V F, Khalil S A and Gouda M W. Effect of concomitant administration of magnesium trisilicate on G I absorption of dexamethasone in humans. *J Pharm Sci* (1978) 67, 1029.

Corticosteroids + anti-infective agents

Summary

The corticosteroids can suppress the normal reactions of the body to attack by micro-organisms. Anti-infective agents used as 'cover' may not necessarily prevent the development of generalized potentially life-threatening infections.

Interaction

A patient with severe cystic acne vulgaris who had been treated with a low dose of oral tetracycline, 500 mg daily, and betamethasone, 2 mg daily, for 7 months, became toxaemic and pyrexic with severe acne and cellulitis of the face due to the emergence of the gram-negative organism not susceptible to the antibiotic.[1]

Mechanism
The corticosteroids reduce inflammation and impair antibody formation which increases the susceptibility of the body to infection. In the case cited, an organism emerged which was not controlled by the tetracycline, and in the presence of the adrenocortical insufficiency induced by the corticosteroid became disseminated throughout the body.

Importance and management
Not, strictly speaking, an interaction. The in-creased susceptibility to infection induced by corticosteroids is very well documented. The example cited amply demonstrates the importance of monitoring concurrent use very thoroughly indeed. As the author of the paper rightly points out '. . . it appears that if oral corticoids or combined therapy are ever warranted, they should be very carefully policed because of the risk of turning a benign disease into one that is potentially fatal'.

Reference
1 Paver K. Complications from combined oral tetracycline and oral corticoid therapy on acne vulgaris. *Med J Aust* (1970) i, 1059.

Corticosteroids + non-steroidal anti-inflammatory agents (aspirin, indomethacin, phenylbutazone etc.)

Summary
Concurrent use is reputed to increase the incidence of gastrointestinal ulceration, but this has yet to be conclusively demonstrated.

Interaction, mechanism, importance and management
It is usually said that since most of the non-steroidal anti-inflammatory drugs such as indomethacin, aspirin, phenylbutazone, and others can cause varying degree of gastrointestinal irritation and ulceration, the concurrent use of corticosteroids (also said to cause ulceration, but not definitely proved to do so) might be expected to increase the risk. One study[1] with patients on prednisone and indomethacin certainly suggested that this might be so, but extensive studies confirming this with indomethacin and other similar drugs appear not to have been carried out. Nevertheless in the absence of definite information, it would seem prudent to pay particular attention to this possibility if concurrent therapy is undertaken.

Reference
1 Emmanuel J H and Montgomery R D. Gastric ulcer and anti-arthritic drugs. *Postgrad Med J* (1971) **47**, 227.

Corticosteroids + barbiturates

Summary
The therapeutic effects of systemically administered corticosteroids such as dexamethasone, hydrocortisone, methylprednisolone, prednisolone and prednisone may be diminished by the concurrent use of phenobarbitone and probably other barbiturates, particularly when given in high doses.

Interaction

Although a number of pharmacokinetic studies have been done on this interaction there seem to be very few reports of genuine adverse responses to the concurrent use of these two groups of drugs:

> Three prednisone-dependent patients with bronchial asthma taking 10–40 mg prednisone daily showed a marked worsening of their symptoms within a few days of being administered 120 mg phenobarbitone daily. There was a deterioration in the results of pulmonary function tests (FEV$_1$, degree of bronchospasm) and a rise in eosinophil counts. An increase in the clearance of prednisone was observed. The deterioration was reversed when the phenobarbitone was withdrawn.[1]

> A preliminary study[6] suggested that the survival of kidney transplants in a group of 75 children who were being given azathioprine and prednisone as immunosuppressants was reduced in those receiving anticonvulsant therapy with phenobarbitone, 60–120 mg daily. Two of the 11 epileptic children were also taking phenytoin, 100 mg daily.

> Nine patients with rheumatoid arthritis being treated with prednisolone, 8–15 mg daily, showed strong evidence of clinical deterioration (as measured by changes in joint tenderness, pain, morning stiffness and fall in grip strength) when they were concurrently treated with phenobarbitone (plasma concentrations of 0–2 mg%) for an experimental period of 2 weeks. The prednisolone half-life was observed to fall 25% (from 132 to 99 minutes).[8]

Mechanism

Pharmacokinetic studies[1] on 11 patients showed that the half-life of dexamethasone was reduced by 44% by the presence of phenobarbitone and the clearance rate increased by 88%. Another clinical study[2] of 5 schizophrenic women showed that pretreatment with 350 mg phenobarbitone a day for 3 weeks markedly increased the urinary excretion of 6-hydroxycortisol following a single 300 mg dose of hydrocortisone. A study on 4 subjects showed that the half-life of methylprednisolone was reduced 56% by the presence of 120 mg phenobarbitone a day and the metabolic clearance rate rose 130%. The metabolic clearance rate of dexamethasone similarly rose 90%.[7]

All of these results are consistent with the idea that phenobarbitone, a known and potent enzyme-inducing agent, stimulates the metabolism of administered corticosteroids and thereby causes a reduction in their therapeutic effects.

It has also been shown in animal experiments[3,4] that barbiturates inhibit the release of ACTH with the results that the normal secretion of corticosteroids by the adrenal cortex is reduced, but since administered corticosteroids would themselves inhibit the release of ACTH this action of the barbiturates may not be of much significance in this context.

Importance and management

There are, as already stated, few direct reports of adverse interactions resulting from the concurrent use of these two groups of drugs, although the supporting pharmacokinetic studies indicate that this is almost certainly an important interaction. However, concurrent use is by no means contraindicated and may not be disadvantageous. A report of a group of children taking prednisone and a compound preparation containing phenobarbitone, 24 mg daily, claimed that the barbiturate appeared to have had no effect at all on the prednisone requirements.[5] On the other hand, corticosteroid-dependent individuals with suppressed adrenal function, those on high dosages of barbiturates, and those receiving steroids for immunosuppression would appear to be in a high-risk category.

The corticosteroids already mentioned (dexamethasone, hydrocortisone, methyl-prednisolone, prednisolone and prednisone) are known to be affected by the barbiturates, whereas preliminary and as yet unconfirmed work[7] suggests that methylprednisolone hemisuccinate may possibly be affected less than some of the others. It is interesting to note that a slight but significant improvement in the adrenocortical response to tetracosactrin (a synthetic corticotrophin) has been observed after phenobarbitone therapy.[8]

Phenobarbitone is the only barbiturate so far certainly implicated, but it would be prudent to suspect any barbiturate and any corticosteroid as likely candidates for this interaction. This requires direct confirmation, but the barbiturates as a group are recognized enzyme-inducing agents.

The dexamethasone adrenal suppression test may also be expected to give unreliable results in patients taking phenobarbitone,[1] but since an overnight test using 50 mg hydrocortisone instead of dexamethasone appears to give reliable results in patients taking another potent enzyme-inducing agent, phenytoin,[9] it might also be considered for those on barbiturates. (See page 438.)

References

1 Brooks S M, Werk E E, Ackerman S J, Sullivan I and Thrasher K. Adverse effects of phenobarbital on corticosteroid metabolism in patients with bronchial asthma. *New Eng J Med* (1972) **286**, 1125.
2 Burstein S and Klaiber E L. Phenobarbital-induced increase in 6β-hydroxycortisol excretion: clue to its significance in human urine. *J Clin Endocrinol Metab* (1965) **25**, 293.
3 Leonard B E. The effect of chronic administration of barbitone

sodium on pituitary-adrenal function in the rat. *Biochem Pharmacol* (1966) **15**, 263.

4 Rerup C and Hedner P. The effect of pentobarbital (Nembutal, Mebumal NFN) on corticotropin release in the rat. *Acta Endocrinol* (1962) **39**, 518.

5 Falliers C J. Corticosteroids and phenobarbital in asthma. *New Eng J Med* (1972) **287**, 201.

6 Wassner S J, Pennisi A J, Malekzadeh M H and Fine R N. The adverse effect of anticonvulsant therapy on renal allograft survival. *J Pediat* (1976) **88**, 134.

7 Stjernholm M R and Katz F H. Effects of diphenylhydantoin, phenobarbital and diazepam on the metabolism of methyl-prednisolone and its sodium succinate. *J Clin Endocrinol Metab* (1975) **41**, 887.

8 Brooks P M, Buchanan W W, Grove M and Downie W W. Effects of enzyme induction on metabolism of prednisolone. Clinical and laboratory study. *Ann Rheum Dis* (1975) **35**, 339.

9 Meikle A W, Stanchfield J B, West C D and Tyler F H. Hydrocortisone suppression test for Cushing syndrome: therapy with anticonvulsants. *Arch Int Med* (1974) **134**, 1068.

Corticosteroids + cimetidine

Summary

The concurrent use of cimetidine has been shown to have no important effect on the absorption of enteric-coated prednisolone.

Interaction, mechanism, importance and management

A randomized double-blind crossover trial on 6 healthy adults showed that treatment with cimetidine (200 mg three times a day after meals and 400 mg at bedtime) caused some minor alterations in plasma prednisolone levels following the administration of 10 mg enteric-coated prednisolone (*Deltacortril*), but no interaction of any importance was seen.[1] There would seem to be no reason to avoid their concurrent use. Information about other prednisolone formulations or corticosteroids appears to be lacking.

Reference

1 Morrison P J, Rogers H J and Bradbrook I D. Concurrent administration of cimetidine and enteric-coated prednisolone: effect on plasma levels of prednisolone. *Br J clin Pharmac* (1980) **10**, 87.

Corticosteroids + diuretics (thiazides, ethacrynic acid, frusemide)

Summary

The concurrent use of the corticosteroids and diuretics which cause the loss of potassium (ethacrynic acid, frusemide, thiazides) may cause excessive potassium depletion.

Interaction, mechanism, importance and management

The corticosteroids, particularly those which are naturally occurring, and some of the diuretics, notably ethacrynic acid, frusemide and the thiazides, cause a significant loss of potassium from the body. This is extremely well documented. Since concurrent use may be expected to increase this effect, attention should be paid to the maintenance of an adequate intake of potassium to balance this loss if members of both groups of drugs are used together.

Corticosteroids + ephedrine

Summary

Ephedrine increases the clearance of dexamethasone from the body. Theophylline appears not to interact.

Interaction

A study on 9 asthmatic patients under treatment with dexamethasone showed that concurrent treatment with 100 mg ephedrine daily for 3 weeks increased the clearance of the steroid from the body by about 40%, associated with a decrease in its half-life.[1]

Mechanism

Not understood.

Importance and management

The documentation is very limited. Although the effect of the dexamethasone would be somewhat reduced, the extent to which concurrent use reduces the overall control of asthma is uncertain. Whether ephedrine interacts with other corticosteroids is not known, but it seems possible.

Reference

1 Brooks S M, Sholiton L J, Werk E E and Altenau P. The effects of ephedrine and theophylline on dexamethasone metabolism on bronchial asthma. *J Clin Pharmacol* (1977) **17**, 308.

Corticosteroids + phenytoin

Summary

The therapeutic effects of dexamethasone and, to a lesser extent, of prednisolone, prednisone and possibly other corticosteroids may be reduced by the concurrent use of phenytoin. The results of the dexamethasone adrenal suppression test may also prove to be unreliable.

Interactions

(i) Reduction in the therapeutic response to the corticosteroids

A woman requiring corticosteroid treatment to control cerebral oedema, following surgery and radiation treatment for a brain tumour, was discharged on 6 mg dexamethasone and 300 mg phenytoin daily. She showed marked deterioration 2 months later, but responded well to increased doses of dexamethasone. She was discharged on a reduced dosage with sodium valproate replacing the phenytoin.[1]

Three other patients are described in the same report. One of them stopped taking phenytoin in error and it was found possible to reduce the dosage of the dexamethasone. The dose had to be increased when the phenytoin was restarted. In the 2 other patients, changing the anticonvulsant drug from phenytoin allowed the dosage of the dexamethasone to be reduced without relapse.[1]

The effects of phenytoin on the half-lives and clearance rates of other corticosteroids are given in Table 21.1 on p. 439.

(ii) Interference with the dexamethasone adrenal suppression test

A study carried out on 7 patients showed that in the presence of phenytoin (300–400 mg daily) their plasma cortisol levels were only reduced by dexamethasone from an average of 22 μg% to 19 μg% compared with a reduction from 18 μg% to 4 μg% in the absence of phenytoin. That is to say, the normal adrenal suppression was much less than expected. Comparable results were found with other patients when their urinary 17-hydroxycorticosteroid levels were measured.[2]

In another study[3] on 9 patients who had been taking 300–400 mg phenytoin daily for extended periods of time, it was found that their plasma cortisol and urinary 17-hydroxycorticosteroid levels were also suppressed far less than might have been expected by small doses of dexamethasone (0·5 mg every 6 h for eight doses), but with larger doses of dexamethasone (2·0 mg every 6 h for eight doses) the suppression was normal.

Mechanism

Phenytoin is a potent liver enzyme-inducing

agent and, in the case of dexamethasone, markedly increases its rate of hydroxylation to metabolites which are more water-soluble than the parent compound and so more easily cleared from the body. In this way the loss of dexamethasone is accelerated and its activity diminished. This is almost certainly the reason why the other corticosteroids are similarly affected. In the dexamethasone adrenal suppression test, this will mean that the inhibition of ACTH release from the pituitary is less than normal, and the corticosteroid response will present an unreliable picture of the functional capacity of the adrenals (see Table 21.1).

Importance and management

An established and well-documented interaction. It is clearly important if, for example, the corticosteroid is being used as an immunosuppressant during organ transplantation[7] and in other situations where treatment depends upon the circulation transporting the steroid to its site of action and which will therefore also expose the steroid to hepatic metabolism, but it has been suggested that it is unlikely to affect the response to steroid preparations administered topically, by inhalation, intra-articular injection or enema.[8] Several courses of action are open to accommodate this interaction:

(a) The dosage of corticosteroid could be increased to match the increased rate of metabolism. While it is clearly very difficult to determine the size of the increased dosage required, it has been suggested[13] that it should be considered in relation to the increase in the corticosteroid clearance rate which occurs in the presence of phenytoin (refer to Table 21.1). In the case of

prednisolone the increased dosage was found in one report[8] to average 100%, but varied in 5 individuals between 58 and 260%.

(b) Exchange the corticosteroid for another which is not affected as much. The data available suggest that the amount by which each of them is affected is related to their normal serum half-lives. Hydrocortisone appears to be affected less than either methylprednisolone or prednisolone, both of which are affected less than dexamethasone (refer to Table 21.1). There are a number of cases on record confirming the success of this method. An epileptic patient with systemic lupus erythematosus taking 300 mg phenytoin daily showed marked signs of deterioration on 16 mg dexamethasone, but was successfully controlled on 100 mg prednisone.[11] A switch from dexamethasone to equivalent doses of methylprednisolone resulted in the prompt clinical improvement of 2 patients taking phenytoin who were being treated for glioblastoma multiforme of the parietal lobes.[13]

(c) Exchange the phenytoin for another anticonvulsant. This would exclude phenobarbitone and other barbiturates which are potent enzyme-inducing agents, and probably primidone as well,[14] but sodium valproate has been shown to be a successful alternative.[1] The dexamethasone adrenal suppression test may prove to be unreliable in the presence of phenytoin, although in one of the cases already cited[3] where larger than usual doses of dexamethasone were used (2 mg every 6 h for eight doses) the suppression was normal. An overnight test using 50 mg hydrocortisone instead of dexamethasone has been examined and would appear to give reliable results even in the presence of phenytoin.[13]

Table 21.1. A comparison of the effects of phenytoin on the kinetics of different glucocorticoids (after Petereit and colleagues[8]

	Daily dosage of phenytoin (mg)	Half-life without phenytoin (min)	Decreased half-life with phenytoin (%)	Increased mean clearance rate with phenytoin (%)	Ref.
			Corticosteroid		
Hydrocortisone	300–400	60–90	−15	+25	4
Methylprednisolone	300	165	−56	+130	5
Prednisone	Prednisolone is the biologically active metabolite of prednisone so that the values for prednisone and prednisolone should be similar				6
Prednisolone	300	190–240	−45	+77	7,8
Dexamethasone	300	250	−51	+140	9,10

References

1 McLelland J and Jack W. Phenytoin/dexamethasone interaction: a clinical problem. *Lancet* (1978) **i**, 1096.

2 Werk E E, Choi Y, Sholiton L, Olinger C and Haque N. Interference in the effect of dexamethasone by diphenylhydantoin. *New Eng J Med* (1969) **281**, 32.

3 Jubiz W, Meikle A W, Levinson R A, Mizutani S, West C D and Tyler F H. Effect of diphenylhydantoin on the metabolism of dexamethasone. *New Eng J Med* (1970) **283**, 11.

4 Choi Y, Thrasher K, Werk E E, Sholiton L J and Ollinger C. Effect of diphenylhydantoin on cortisol kinetics in humans. *J Pharmacol Exp Ther* (1971) **176**, 27.

5 Stjernholm M R and Katz F H. Effects of diphenylhydantoin, phenobarbital and diazepam on the metabolism of methylprednisolone and its hemisuccinate. *J Clin Endocrinol Metab* (1975) **41**, 887.

6 Meikle A W, Weed J A, and Tyler F H. Kinetics and interconversion of prednisolone and prednisone studied with new radio-immunoassays. *J Clin Endocrinol Metab* (1975) **41**, 717.

7 Wassher S J, Pennisi A J, Malakzadeh M H and Fine R N. The adverse effects of anticonvulsant therapy on renal allograft survival. *J Paediatr* (1976) **88**, 134.

8 Petereit L B and Meikle A W. Effectiveness of prednisolone during phenytoin therapy. *Clin Pharmacol Ther* (1977) **22**, 912.

9 Brooks S M, Werk E E, Ackerman S, Sullivan I and Thrasher K. Adverse effects of phenobarbital on corticosteroid metabolism in patients with bronchial asthma. *New Eng J Med* (1972) **286**, 1125.

10 Haque N, Thrasher K, Werk E E, Knowles H C and Sholiton L J. Studies of dexamethasone metabolism in man. Effect of diphenylhydrantoin. *J Clin Endocrinol Metab* (1972) **34**, 44.

11 Boylan J J, Owen D S and Chin J B. Phenytoin interference with dexamethasone. *J Am Med Ass* (1976) **235**, 802.

12 Vincent F M. Phenytoin/dexamethasone interaction. *Lancet* (1978) **i**, 1360.

13 Meikle A W, Stanchfield J B, West C D and Tyler F H. Hydrocortisone suppression test for Cushing syndrome: therapy with anticonvulsants. *Arch Int Med* (1974) **134**, 1068.

14 Hancock K W and Levell M J. Primidone/dexamethasone interaction. *Lancet* (1978) **i**, 97.

Corticosteroids + rifampicin

Summary

The effects of the corticosteroids can be reduced by the concurrent use of rifampicin.

Interaction

A child with nephrotic syndrome taking prednisolone and who was inadvertently administered BCG vaccine was treated with rifampicin and isoniazid to prevent possible dissemination of the vaccine. Because the nephrotic condition failed to respond, the initial dosage of prednisolone was increased from 2 to 3 mg/kg/day without any evidence of corticosteroid overdosage. Later, when the rifampicin and isoniazid were withdrawn, remission of the nephrotic condition was achieved with the original dosage of prednisolone.[3]

Two patients with renal transplants receiving azathioprine and either prednisone or methylprednisolone showed a progressive deterioration in the transplant function during treatment with rifampicin. The deterioration was reversed by withdrawing the rifampicin.[4]

Two not dissimilar cases of renal transplant deterioration have also been described during rifampicin treatment, attributed by the author to possible rifampicin renal toxicity[5] but this is probably incorrect in the light of the cases cited above.[4] Another case in which the response to prednisolone appeared to have been reduced by the use of rifampicin has also been described.[3]

If the rifampicin is subsequently withdrawn, the corticosteroid requirements fall and the dosage requires reduction:

A patient found to have Addison's disease and pulmonary tuberculosis was eventually stabilized on a daily drug regimen of cortisone acetate, 100 mg, fludrocortisol 0·4 mg, streptomycin 0·75 g. isoniazid 300 mg and rifampicin 600 mg. On this regimen the patient remained clinically well for a period of 8 months, but within a month of replacing the rifampicin by ethambutol, typical signs of corticosteroid overdosage developed which only disappeared when the daily doses of cortisone acetate and fludrocortisol were reduced to 37·5 mg and 0·1 mg respectively.[1]

A similar situation has been described in another patient whose dosage of methylprednisolone could be reduced from 40 mg to 18 mg daily when rifampcin was withdrawn.[4]

Mechanism

There is good evidence to show that rifampicin, which is a potent inducer of liver microsomal enzymes, increases the metabolism and clearance—and hence reduces the effects of—both administered and endogenous corticosteroids.

In one of the studies cited[1] the half-life of cortisol in the patient described was found to be 58 min during rifampicin treatment and 82 min after withdrawal. Similarly a pharmacokinetic study on the child with nephrotic syndrome[2]

440

showed that the half-life of prednisolone was reduced from 2·17 to 1·29 h during the rifampicin treatment. Rifampicin similarly affects endogenous corticosteroids as evidenced by a more than 50% increase in cortisol production in 4 tuberculous patients during treatment with the antibiotic due, presumably, to an increase in its metabolism.[4] The urinary output of D-glutaric acid was also increased. This is another indication that enzyme induction had taken place.[4,6]

Importance and management
An important and well-established interaction. A reduction in the effects of the corticosteroids may be expected if rifampicin is administered. One suggestion put forward by Buffington and his colleagues to deal with this problem (in the context of tuberculous patients with renal transplants) is, as a first approximation, to double the daily dose of the glucocorticoid when the rifampicin therapy is started.[4] Similarly, if the rifampicin is withdrawn, it would appear to be necessary (on the basis of the limited evidence available) to reduce the corticosteroid dosages by roughly 50% to prevent overdosage.

References
1 Edwards O M, Courtnay-Evans R J, Galley J M, Hunter J and Tait A D. Changes in cortisol metabolism following rifampicin therapy. *Lancet* (1974) **ii**, 549.
2 Hendrickse W, McKiernan J, Pickup M and Lowe J. Rifampicin-induced non-responsiveness to corticosteroid treatment in nephrotic syndrome.
3 van Marle W, Woods K L and Beeley L. Concurrent steroid and rifampicin therapy. *Br Med J* (1979) **1**, 1029.
4 Buffington G A, Dominguez J H, Piering W F, Hebert L A, Kauffman H M and Lemann J. Interaction of rifampin and glucocorticoids. *J Amer Med Ass* (1976) **236**, 1958.
5 Mendez-Picon G, Murai M, Pierce J C. Tuberculosis in transplant patients: two cases of possible rifampin renal toxicity. Read before the 8th Ann. meeting of the Amer. Soc of Nephrology, Washington (1975).
6 Sotaniemi E A, Medzihradsky F, Eliasson G. Glutaric acid as an indicator of use of enzyme-inducing drugs. *Clin Pharmacol Ther* (1974) **15**, 417.

Corticosteroids + vaccines

Summary
Concurrent use is contraindicated with some live vaccines, and the immune response may be diminished in some others by the presence of a corticosteroid.

Interaction, mechanism, importance and management
The administration of the corticosteroids reduces the number of circulating lymphocytes and can block the normal immune response. For this reason immunization with some live vaccines in the presence of corticosteroids can lead to a generalized infection. However immunization can still be successfully and safely achieved if the appropriate immunoglobulin is used to give cover against a general infection while immunity develops. This has been reported in steroid-dependent patients requiring smallpox vaccination.[1]

Reference
1 Joseph M R. Vaccination of patients on steroid therapy. *Med J Aust* (1974) **2**, 181.

Disulfiram + metronidazole

Summary
Acute psychoses and confusion can result from the concurrent use of disulfiram and metronidazole.

Interaction
In a double-blind study on 58 hospitalized chronic alcoholics under treatment with disulfiram, 29 were also given metronidazole (750 mg daily for 1 month, then 250 mg daily): 6 of the 29 developed acute psychoses or confusion; 5 of them had paranoid delusions and 3 experienced visual and auditory hallucinations. The symptoms persisted and even

increased after withdrawal of the drugs but disappeared at the end of a fortnight, and did not reappear when disulfiram alone was reintroduced.[1]

This reaction has been described in another report.[2]

Mechanism

Not understood. Psychotic reactions have been described with disulfiram.

Importance and management

Although the documentation is limited it appears to be a reliably established interaction. Concurrent use should be avoided.

References

1 Rothstein E and Clancy D D. Toxicity of disulfiram combined with metronidazole. *New Eng J Med* (1969) **280,** 1006.
2 Goodhue W W. Disulfiram–metronidazole (well-identified) toxicity. *New Eng J Med* (1969) **280,** 1482.

Disulfiram + paraldehyde

Summary

Concurrent use should be avoided until more information is available.

Interaction, mechanism, importance and management

Indirect evidence[1] suggests that paraldehyde is depolymerized in the liver to acetaldehyde, and then oxidized by acetaldehyde dehydrogenase. If this is so, the concurrent use of disulfiram might be expected to result in the accumulation of acetaldehyde and in a modified 'antabuse' reaction[2], but so far there appear to be no reports of this in man. In addition alcoholics with impaired liver function are said to be sensitive to the toxic effects of paraldehyde, and may show restlessness rather than sedation when given paraldehyde. These are all good reasons for avoiding concurrent use until more is known. More study is needed.

References

1 Hitchcock P and Nelson E E. The metabolism of paraldehyde: II. *J Pharmac exp Ther* (1943) **79,** 286.
2 Keplinger M L and Wells J A. Effect of antabuse on the action of paraldehyde in mice and dogs. *Fed Proc* (1956) **15,** 445.

Disulfiram + pimozide

Summary

A toxic reaction to concurrent use has been reported

Interaction, mechanism, importance and management

An isolated case of choreoathetosis ataxia attributed to the concurrent use of disulfiram and pimozide has been reported.[1] No details were given.

Reference

1 New Zealand Committee on Adverse Drug Reactions. Ninth Annual Report. *NZ Dent J* (1975) **71,** 28.

Disulfiram or citrated calcium carbimide + tricyclic antidepressants

Summary
The effects of disulfiram and citrated calcium carbimide are increased by amitriptyline.

Interaction, mechanism, importance and management
The effects of disulfiram and citrated calcium carbimide in the treatment of alcoholism are reported[1,2] to be increased by the concurrent use of amitriptyline without any increase in the side-effects of either drug. This is due, it is suggested, to an increase in the rate of build-up of acetaldehyde and other compounds in the circula- tion. This seems to be an advantageous rather than an adverse interaction. Whether other tri- cyclic anti-depressants interact similarly appears not to have been documented.

References
1 MacCallum W A G. Drug interactions in alcoholism treat- ment. *Lancet* (1969) **i**, 313.
2 Pullar-Strecker H. Drug interactions in alcoholism treatment. *Lancet* (1969) **i**, 735.

Ergotamine tartrate + erythromycin

Summary
An isolated case report describes the development of ergotamine toxicity in a patient who took ergotamine tartrate while under treatment with erythromycin.

Interaction
A woman who had been treated for 2 days with 2 g daily of erythromycin ethylsuccinate for a dental abscess took a proprietary preparation (*Migwell*) containing 2 mg ergotamine tartrate, 91·5 mg caffeine and 50 mg cyclizine. Within an hour she began to feel drowsy and nauseated, and over the next few hours vomited several times. Later she showed pallor, cyanosis and coldness of the extremi- ties. The patient had no history of Reynaud's disease or any other similar pathological condition, and had taken the same or similar ergotamine-containing preparations on previous occasions without inci- dent.[1]

Mechanism
Not understood. The toxic symptoms observed would appear to be due to an enhancement of the effects of the ergotamine leading to toxicity.

Importance and management
Although there appears to be only one report of this interaction, a number of similar cases have been described in patients taking another macro- lide antibiotic, triacetyloleandomycin, with either ergotamine or dihydroergotamine.[1] It would therefore seem advisable to avoid the concurrent use of these drugs wherever possible, although it is clear that much more information is needed before this interaction can be firmly established.

Reference
1 Lagier G, Castot A, Riboulet G and Bosesh C. Un cas d'ergotisme mineur semblant en rapport avec une potentiali- sation de l'érgotamine par l'éthylsuccinate d'erythromycine. *Thérapie* (1979) **34**, 515.

Frusemide + chloral hydrate

Summary
The intravenous injection of frusemide following treatment with chloral may cause sweating, hot flushes, a variable blood pressure, tachycardia and uneasiness.

Interaction

Six patients who were administered a bolus of 40–120 mg frusemide intravenously and who had had chloral hydrate during the previous 24 h developed sweating, hot flushes, variable blood pressure, uneasiness and tachycardia. The reaction was immediate and lasted about 15 min or so.[1]

A retrospective study of hospital records of patients who had been given both drugs revealed that 1 patient had similarly developed this reaction and 2 others may have done so.[2]

Mechanism

Not understood. One hypothesis[1] is that the frusemide displaces from the serum protein binding sites trichloroacetic acid which is a metabolite of chloral. This in its turn either displaces thyroxine or alters the serum pH so that there is an increase in the amount of free thyroxine. There is, however, no experimental confirmation of this idea as yet.

Importance and management

The information seems to be limited to two reports. Its importance is difficult to assess but the tachycardia and variable blood pressure may be particularly undesirable in patients with acute coronary disease. One of the studies referrred to[2] found 43 patients in the records who had been exposed to both drugs in the same sequence as those who developed this reaction, but only 3 at the most experienced this interaction. The incidence is therefore apparently not high.

There is no evidence to suggest that frusemide given orally, or chloral given to patients already receiving frusemide initiates this reaction.[2] Although it is not certain, it seems likely that drugs which are variants of chloral hydrate (dichloralphenazone, petrichloral, chloral betaine etc.) will interact in the same way. Flurazepam has been shown to be a suitable noninteracting hypnotic substitute for chloral.[2]

References

1 Malach M and Berman N. Furosemide and chloral hydrate. Adverse drug interaction. *J Amer Med Ass* (1975) **232**, 638.
2 Pevonka M P, Yost R L, Marks R G, Howell W S and Stewart R B. Interaction of chloral hydrate and furosemide. A controlled retrospective study. *Drug Intell Clin Pharm* (1977) **11**, 332.

Frusemide + clofibrate

Summary

Additional treatment with clofibrate in patients with nephrotic syndrome already receiving frusemide has led to marked diuresis and muscular symptoms.

Interaction

Six patients under treatment with frusemide, 80–500 mg daily, who had hypoalbuminaemia and hyperlipoproteinaemia secondary to nephrotic syndrome, developed muscle pain, low lumbar backache, stiffness and general malaise with pronounced diuresis within 3 days of receiving additional therapy with 1–2 g clofibrate daily.[1]

Mechanism

Not understood. The marked diuresis may possibly have been due to competition and displacement of the frusemide by the clofibrate from its plasma protein binding sites. A muscular syndrome has been seen occasionally with clofibrate and this may possibly have been exacerbated by the urinary loss of Na^+ and K^+. In addition, in the patients examined, the half-life of the clofibrate was found to have been increased from 12 to 36 h which might be expected to enhance the development of toxicity by simple drug accmulation.[1]

Importance and management

The documentation is very limited and the incidence unknown. The authors suggest that serum proteins and renal function should be closely checked before using clofibrate, and if serum albumin levels are low, the total daily dose of clofibrate should not exceed 0·5 g for each 1 g per 100 ml albumin concentration.

Reference

1 Bridgman J F, Rosen S M and Thorp J M. Complications during clofibrate treatment of nephrotic-syndrome hyperlipoproteinaemia. *Lancet* (1972) **ii**, 506.

Frusemide + phenytoin

Summary

The diuretic effects of frusemide can be reduced by as much as 50% if phenytoin is being used concurrently.

Interaction

An observation made at a residential centre for epileptics that dependent oedema was higher than might have been expected, and the response to diuretic treatment appeared to be reduced, prompted a further investigation. A study on 30 patients showed that 20 and 40 mg oral doses of frusemide produced a maximal diuresis after 3–4 h instead of the more usual 2 h, and the total diuresis was reduced to 68% and 51% respectively. When 20 mg frusemide was given intravenously the total diuresis was reduced 50%. The patients were taking sodium phenytoin, 200–400 mg daily, with phenobarbitone, 60–180 mg daily, and in addition some of them were also taking carbamazepine, pheneturide, ethosuximide, diazepam or chlordiazepoxide.[1]

A further study[2] on 5 volunteers who had been pretreated with 100 mg phenytoin three times a day for 10 days, and who were then administered 20 mg frusemide orally or intravenously, showed that the maximum serum frusemide concentrations were reduced by 50%.

Mechanism

Not fully understood. The available evidence indicates that neither the renal clearance nor its metabolism is affected by the phenytoin,[2] and the interaction is probably largely due to some reduction in the absorption from the gut. One suggestion is that the phenytoin induces changes in the jejunal Na^+ pump activity.[3] This is, however, not the whole story because some diminution in the response to frusemide also occurs after intravenous administration.

Importance and management

The data are limited but the interaction appears to be well established. A reduced diuretic response may be expected in the presence of phenytoin, and larger doses of frusemide may be required.

References

1 Ahmad S. Renal insensitivity to frusemide caused by chronic anticonvulsant therapy. Br Med J (1974) 3, 657.
2 Fine A, Henderson I S, Morgan D R, and Wilstone W J. Malabsorption of frusemide caused by phenytoin. Br Med J (1977) 3, 1061.
3 Noach E L, Rees H and de Wolff P A. Effects of diphenylhydantoin (DPH) on absorptive processes in the rat jejunum. Arch Int Pharmacodynam and Therap (1973) 206, 392.

Halothane + fenfluramine

Summary

An isolated case has been reported of fatal cardiac arrest following halothane anaesthesia in a woman taking fenfluramine. Animal studies indicate that fenfluramine with halothane can cause serious heart arrhythmias and myocardial depression.

Interaction

A 23-year-old woman undergoing surgery who had been premedicated with diazepam and hyoscine, anaesthetized initially with thiopentone followed by suxamethonium and later with halothane and oxygen, became pulseless, cyanosed and showed signs of acute pulmonary oedema within 5 min of induction. She failed to respond to resuscitative measures including internal cardiac massage. It was later discovered that she had been taking fenfluramine.[1]

Studies of this possible interaction in animals showed that during the concurrent use of fenfluramine and halothane, marked ECG changes occurred and the animals showed sinus bradycardia, heart block, ventricular extrasystoles, paroxysmal ventricular tachycardia and fibrillation.[1]

Mechanism

Not known. Although fenfluramine is related chemically to both adrenaline and amphetamine

445

and might be expected to have similar pharmacological characteristics, the available evidence suggests that its effects on the heart are depressant rather than stimulant.[1,2]

Importance and management
Although there is only one case on record of this interaction, its serious nature and the results of animal studies support the recommendation[1] that patients taking fenfluramine should not undergo anaesthesia with halothane. Moreover, since the drug is not totally eliminated for several days, a week should elapse before elective anaesthesia with halothane is carried out. The use of practotolol to treat the results of this interaction appears from the animal experiments to cause further cardiac depression and the best results were obtained when no drugs at all were given, even conventional myocardial stimulants.

References
1 Bennett J A and Eltringham R J. Possible dangers of anaesthesia in patients receiving fenfluramine. *Anaesthesia* (1977) **32**, 8.
2 Gold R G, Gordon H E, Da Costa R W D, Porteus I B and Kimber K J. Fenfluramine overdosage. *Lancet* (1969) **ii**, 1306.

Halothane or fluroxene + phenytoin and phenobarbitone

Summary
A case of phenytoin intoxication followed halothane anaesthesia, and another of fatal hepatic necrosis in a woman on phenytoin, phenobarbitone and phenylbutazone who was anaesthetized with fluroxene have been reported.

Interaction
Halothane + phenytoin
    A 10-year-old epileptic girl taking 300 mg phenytoin daily and who had been taking the drug for at least 5 years was admitted to hospital for surgery. She showed slight nystagmus and her phenytoin serum levels were 25 μg/ml. Three days after anaesthesia with halothane she developed marked signs of phenytoin intoxication and was found to have a phenytoin serum level of 41 μg/ml.[1]

Fluroxene + phenytoin and phenobarbitone
    An epileptic woman taking phenylbutazone and controlled on 300 mg phenytoin and 120 mg phenobarbitone daily, required an increase in her phenytoin dosage to 2400 mg daily 1 week before surgery. She died of massive hepatic necrosis 36 h after anaesthesia with fluroxene.[2]

Mechanism
Not known. Both anaesthetics are known to be able to damage the liver. The phenytoin intoxication in the first case may have resulted from the general toxic effect of halothane on the liver which resulted in a slowing of the normal rate of phenytoin metabolism so that its serum levels rose.
    Phenytoin can stimulate drug metabolism in the liver. Pretreatment with phenobarbitone can enhance the hepatotoxicity of halogenated hydrocarbons including chloroform and carbon tetrachloride (observed in animals[3]), the toxicity of which is related to their metabolism. But whether this similarly occurs with fluroxene in man and accounts for the necrosis described in the second case is not known.

Importance and management
No firm general conclusions can be drawn from just two apparently isolated case reports like these, but they underline the potential hepatotoxicity of these anaesthetics. The authors of the second report[2] suggest that patients with similar drug histories may constitute a high-risk group for hepatic damage after halogen or vinyl–radical-containing anaesthetics, but this awaits confirmation.

References
1 Karline J M, and Kutt H. Acute diphenylhydantoin intoxication following halothane anaesthesia. *J Pediat* (1970) **76**, 941.
2 Reynolds E S, Brown B R and Vandam L D. Massive hepatic necrosis after fluroxene anesthesia—a case of drug interaction? *New Eng J Med* (1972) **286**, 530.
3 Garner R C and McLean A E M. Increased susceptibility to carbon tetrachloride poisoning in the rat after pretreatment with oral phenobarbitone. *Biochem Pharmacol* (1969) **18**, 645.

Halothane + theophylline

Summary

Cardiac arrhythmias have been described in man and animals during the concurrent use of halothane and theophylline, but the general importance of this interaction is uncertain and controversial.

Interaction, mechanism, importance and management

A report describes ventricular tachycardia in man attributed to the interaction of theophylline and halothane.[1] There are also other reports of this interaction in animals.[2,3] The authors of the first report recommend that concurrent use should be avoided,[1] but this has been disputed by another anaesthetist who has stated that '... my own experience with the liberal use of these drugs has convinced me of the efficacy and wide margin of safety associated with their use in combination'.[4]

References

1 Roizen M F and Stevens W C. Multiform ventricular tachycardia due to the interaction of aminophylline and halothane. *Anesth Analg* (1978) **57**, 738.
2 Takori M and Loehning R W. Ventricular arrhythmias induced by aminophylline during halothane anaesthesia in dogs. *Can Anaesth Soc J* (1967) **14**, 79.
3 Takori M and Loehning R W. Ventricular arrhythmias during halothane anaesthesia: effects of isoproteronol, aminophylline and ephedrine. *Can Anaesth Soc J* (1965) **12**, 275.
4 Zimmerman B L. Arrhythmogenicity of theophylline and halothane used in combination. *Anesth Analg* (1979) **58**, 259.

Iopanoic acid + cholestyramine

Summary

A single case has been reported of poor radiographic visualization of the gall bladder due apparently to an interaction between iopanoic acid and cholestyramine within the gut.

Interaction

The cholecystogram of a man with postgastrectomy syndrome, who was taking cholestyramine and who was also given oral iopanoic acid as an X-ray contrast medium, suggested that he had an abnormal and apparently collapsed gall bladder. One week after withdrawal of the cholestyramine a repeat cholecystogram gave excellent visualization of the gall bladder of normal appearance.[1]

The same effects have been observed experimentally with dogs.[2]

Mechanism

In-vitro experiments[1] with buffered solutions have shown that cholestyramine has a high affinity for iopanoic acid. It would seem probable that binding occurs within the gut before the iopanoic acid is absorbed by the gut, so that little is available for secretion in the bile, and poor visualization of the gall bladder results.

Importance and managment

Information is very limited, but the interaction would appear to be established. On the basis of other reports about drugs which similarly become bound to cholestyramine, it would seem probable that the interaction can be avoided if the administration of the iopanoic acid and cholestyramine are separated as much as possible.

Whether other orally administered acidic X-ray contrast media such as iobenzamic acid, ioglycamic acid, iophenoxic acid, iothalamic acid and others bind to cholestryramine is uncertain, but the possibility should be borne in mind.

References

1 Nelson J A. Effect of cholestryramine on teleopaque oral cholecystography. *Am J Roentgenol Radium Ther Nucl* (1974) **122**, 333.
2 Berk R N. Cited as a personal communication in ref 1.

Iron preparations + antacids

Summary

The absorption of iron and the haematological response can be reduced by the concurrent use of magnesium trisilicate. The administration of the two should be separated as much as possible.

Interaction

Arising out of a clinical observation that oral iron therapy failed to give the expected rise in haemoglobin levels until the concurrent administration of magnesium trisilicate had been discontinued, a study was undertaken on nine patients given isotopically labelled ferrous sulphate. This showed that the concurrent administration of 35 g magnesium trisilicate reduced the amount of iron absorbed from an average of 30% to 12%. The reduction was small in some patients, but one individual showed a fall in absorption from 67 to 5%.[1]

Poor absorption of iron during treatment with sodium bicarbonate has also been described.[2]

Mechanism

Uncertain. It is suggested that the magnesium trisilicate either changes the ferrous sulphate into less easily absorbed iron salts, or increases its polymerization, thereby rendering it less easily absorbed.[1] Sodium bicarbonate causes the formation of poorly absorbed iron complexes.[2]

Importance and management

The documentation is limited but the iron/magnesium trisilicate interaction is of evident clinical importance.[1] There is less information about the iron/sodium bicarbonate interaction. The administration of iron and these antacids should be separated as much as possible. Information about other antacids appears to be lacking, but it would seem prudent, and easy, to apply the same precautions.

References

1 Hall G J L, and Davis A E. Inhibition of iron absorption by magnesium trisilicate. *Med J Aust* (1969) **2**, 95.
2 Benjamin I B, Cortell S and Conrad M E. Bicarbonate-induced iron complexes and iron absorption. *Gastroenterol* (1967) **35**, 389.

Loperamide + cholestyramine

Summary

A single report indicates that cholestyramine can bind to loperamide and reduce its activity. Separating their administration as much as possible may be expected to prevent this interaction.

Interaction

A single case report describes a man who had undergone extensive surgery of the gastrointestinal tract with the creation of an ileostomy and who required treatment for excessive fluid loss. His fluid loss was observed to be 'substantially less' (not precisely quantified) when the loperamide (2 mg every 6 h) was given alone than when given in combination with cholestyramine (2 g every 4 h).[1]

Mechanism

Cholestyramine is an ion-exchange resin which can not only bind, as intended, to bile acids, but can also bind to drugs in the gut thereby making them less available for absorption, and reducing their activity. In an in-vitro study using 50 ml simulated gastric fluid, to which was added 4 g cholestyramine and 5·5 mg loperamide, it was observed that 64% of the loperamide became bound to the cholestyramine.[1] This would seem to explain why the effectiveness of the loperamide was reduced in the case described.

Importance and management

Although only one report of this interaction has been published, the fact that cholestyramine interacts in a similar way with other drugs and that it has been shown to bind to loperamide in vitro suggests that this interaction is probably of general clinical importance. It has been recommended that if the use of both drugs is thought necessary, their times of administration should be separated as much as possible. Alternatively the dosage of loperamide could be increased.[1]

Reference

1 Ti T Y, Giles H G and Sellers E M. Probable interaction of loperamide and cholestyramine. *Canad Med Ass J* (1978) 119, 607.

Methimazole + barbiturates

Summary

Animal studies indicate that an interaction may occur, but this awaits confirmation in man.

Interaction, mechanism, importance and management

Studies in rats showed that treatment with phenobarbitone increased the uptake of methimazole from the serum into the thyroid by a factor of 4, and the metabolism of methimazole was increased.[1] Whether an important interaction occurs in man is not known, but the possibility should be borne in mind during concurrent treatment.

Reference

1 Lees J F H and Alexander W D. Effect of phenobarbitone on metabolism of methimazole. *Lancet* (1973) i, 616.

Methoxyflurane + aminoglycoside antibiotics

Summary

The suggestion that methoxyflurane and aminoglycoside antibiotics might have additive nephrotoxic effects has been disputed.

Interaction, mechanism, importance and management

A very brief report[1] suggested that the nephrotoxic effect of kanamycin and gentamicin might be enhanced by the use of methoxyflurane (based on observations in patients), but a causal relationship between the concurrent use of these drugs and the toxic effects observed has been questioned.[2]

References

1 Cousins M J and Mazze R I. Tetracycline, methoxyflurane anaesthetics and renal dysfunction. *Lancet* (1972) i, 751.
2 Frascino J A. Tetracycline, methoxyflurane anesthesia and renal dysfunction. *Lancet* (1972) i, 1127.

Methoxyflurane + barbiturates

Summary

One case (possibly two) of toxic nephropathy has been described following methoxyflurane anaesthesia apparently resulting from pretreatment with a barbiturate.

Interaction

A patient who had been treated for a month with 100 mg secobarbitone daily developed a vasopressin-resistant non-oliguric renal insufficiency after receiving low-dose methoxyflurane anaesthesia, and developed high serum inorganic fluoride levels. Twelve other patients under study not treated with a barbiturate did not show this toxic reaction.[1]

A similar reaction appears to have occurred in another patient[2] and it is in line with the results of animal experiments.[1]

Mechanism
Uncertain. It is suggested that pretreatment with the secobarbital (a potent liver enzyme-inducing agent) alters the metabolism of the methoxyflurane and results in the production of metabolites which are potently nephrotoxic.[1] Marked changes in the metabolism of methoxyflurane have been clearly demonstrated in animal experiments.[1,3,4]

Importance and management
Direct evidence of this interaction in man is very limited, but it is supported by the results of animal experiments. The authors of the report cited[1] recommend that methoxyflurane should be avoided by those who are receiving, or who have recently received drugs such as the barbiturates which induce liver microsomal enzymes.

References
1 Churchill D, Yacoub J M, Siu K P, Symes A and Gault M H. Toxic nephropathy after low-dose methoxyflurane anesthesia: drug interaction with secobarbital? *Can med Assoc J* (1976) **114**, 326.
2 Cousins M J and Mazze R I. Methoxyflurane nephrotoxicity: a study of dose response in man. *J Amer Med Ass* (1973) **225**, 1611.
3 Mazze R I, Hitt B A, and Cousins M J. Effect of enzyme induction with phenobarbital on the in vivo and in vitro defluorination of isoflurane and methoxyflurane. *J Pharmacol Exp Ther* (1974) **190**, 523.
4 Son S L, Colella J J and Brown B R. The effect of phenobarbitone on the metabolism of methoxyflurane to oxalic acid in the rat. *Br J Anaesth* (1972) **44**, 1224.

Methoxyflurane + tetracyclines

Summary
Severe nephrotoxicity may occur if methoxyflurane is used in patients who are given tetracyclines.

Interaction
A report on the use of methoxyflurane on 115 patients described 7 who were given tetracycline immediately before or after surgery: 5 of them showed rises in blood urea nitrogen and creatinine, and 3 of them died. Post-mortem examination showed that they had pathological changes (oxalosis) in the kidneys. None of the other 108 patients who had not had antibiotics, or who had received penicillin, streptomycin or chloramphenicol showed renal toxicity, and none of the 9 who died from other causes showed any of the findings observed in those who had had tetracycline.[1]

There are other reports suggesting that concurrent use can cause kidney damage.[2,3,4]

Mechanism
Not understood. It seems probable that the nephrotoxic effects of both drugs may be additive.

Importance and management
The incidence of this serious reaction is not known. An association between the nephrotoxicity and the concurrent use of these drugs has not been established beyond doubt, but there is enough evidence to indicate that concurrent use should be avoided wherever possible.

References
1 Kuzucu E Y. Methoxyflurane, tetracycline and renal failure. *J Amer Med Ass* (1970) **211**, 1162.
2 Albers D D, Leverett C L and Sandin J H. Renal failure following prostatovesiculectomy related to methoxyflurane anesthesia and tetracycline–complicated by Candida infection. *J Urol* (1971) **106**, 348.
3 Proctor E A and Barton F L. Polyuric acute renal failure after methoxyflurane and tetracycline. *Br Med J* (1971) **4**, 661.
4 Stoelting R K and Gibbs P S. Effect of tetracycline therapy on renal function after methoxyflurane anaesthesia. *Anesth Analg* (1973) **52**, 431.

Metrizamide + phenothiazines

Summary

Two cases have been reported in which an adverse epileptiform reaction occurred when metrizamide was used in the presence of chlorpromazine and dixyrazine.

Interaction

A patient on long-term treatment with 75 mg chlorpromazine daily was administered metrizamide by the lumbar route (16 ml in a concentration of 170 mg of iodine/ml) as a contrast medium for myelography. Three-and-a-half hours later, and again after a further 5 h he experienced grand mal seizures.[1]

Another patient, one of a series of 34 patients, examined with metrizamide for lumbar myelography, who was also taking 10 mg dixyrazine three times a day (a phenothiazine derivative) showed epileptogenic activity on the EEG.[2]

Mechanism

Not understood. Unlike many other water-soluble contrast media, metrizamide appears normally to show no neurotoxic effects or epileptogenic activity. but experiments with dogs[3] have shown that when phenoperidine was administered concurrently in high doses (about seven times that which would be used in anaesthetic practice), the animals showed epileptogenic activity on the EEG and clinical seizures. Phenothiazines like chlorpromazine are not chemically related to phenoperidine, but both are similar in being capable of provoking epileptic activity in high doses, so that it might be that when either of them is administered with metrizamide, the combined actions provoke seizures or synergistically reduce the seizure threshold.

Clinical importance and management

Information seems to be limited to these two reports, and a direct connection between the concurrent use of these drugs and the adverse reactions described has not been firmly established. However, it would seem prudent to avoid concurrent use whenever possible.

References

1 Hindmarsh T, Grepe A and Widen L. Metrizamide–pheonothiazine interaction. Report of a case with sizures following myelography. *Acta Radiol Diag* (1975) **16**, 129.
2 Hindmarsh T. Lumbar myelography with meglumine iocarinate and metrizamide. A double-blind investigation. *Acta Radiol Diag* (1975) **16**, 24.
3 Grepe A and Widen L. Neurotoxic effect of intracranial subarachnoid application of metrizamide and meglumine iocarinate. An experimental investigation in dogs in neuroleptanalgesia. *Acta Radiol* (1973) (Suppl), **335**, 102.

Metyrapone + phenytoin

Summary

The results of the metyrapone hypothalamic-hypophyseal function test are not reliable in patients taking phenytoin. Doubling the dose of metyrapone gives results which are close to normal.

Interaction

Serum levels of metyrapone are reduced during treatment with phenytoin:

A study in 5 normal subjects and 3 patients, all on chronic treatment with 300 mg phenytoin daily, showed that compared with subjects not taking phenytoin their serum levels of metyrapone were markedly reduced. Four hours after taking the regular oral dose of metyrapone (750 mg) the serum level of the control group was 48 μg% compared with only 6·5 μg% in the phenytoin-treated subjects.

The response to metyrapone was proportionately subnormal.[1]

Other reports confirm that the urinary steroid response to the oral metyrapone test is subnormal in patients on chronic treatment with phenytoin.[3,4]

Mechanism

Evidence from studies in animals and in man suggests that the phenytoin induces the liver microsomal enzymes concerned with the metabolism of metyrapone thereby reducing its biological activity.[1,2]

Importance and management
The results of the metyrapone test for hypothalamic–hypophyseal function are not valid in patients under treatment with phenytoin. Doubling the dose of metyrapone (750 mg 2-hourly instead of 4-hourly) has been shown to give results which are similar to those found in subjects not receiving phenytoin.[1]

References
1 Meikle A W, Jubiz W, Matsukura S, West C D and Tyler F H. Effect of diphenylhydantoin on the metabolism of metyrapone and release of ACTH in man. *J Clin Endocrinol Metab* (1969) **29**, 1553.
2 Jubiz W, Levinson R A, Meikle A W, West C D, and Tyler F H. Absorption and conjugation of metyrapone during diphenylhydantoin therapy: mechanism of the abnormal response to oral metyrapone. *Endocrinology* (1970) **86**, 328.
3 Krieger D T. Effect of diphenylhydantoin on pituitary–adrenal interrelations. *J Clin Endocrinol* (1962) **22**, 490.
4 Werk E E, Thrasher K, Choi Y and Sholiton L J. Failure of metyrapone to inhibit 11-hydroxylation of 11-deoxycortisol during drug therapy. *J Clin Endocrinol* (1967) **27**, 1358.

Piperazine + chlorpromazine

Summary
An isolated case of convulsions in a child has been attributed to the use of chlorpromazine following piperazine

Interaction, mechanism, importance and management
An isolated case has been reported of a child given piperazine for pinworms who developed convulsions when treated with chlorpromazine several days later.[1] In a subsequent investigation with animals using 4·5 or 10 mg/kg chlorpromazine many of the animals died from respiratory arrest after severe clonic convulsions.[1] Another worker was unable to confirm these results.[2] It is very difficult to assess the importance of this interaction since it is by no means certain whether the convulsions in the child were due to an interaction; nevertheless there is enough evidence to warrant some caution if these drugs are used concurrently.

References
1 Boulos B M and Davis L E. Hazard of simultaneous administration of phenothiazine and piperazine. *New Eng J Med* (1969) **280**, 1245.
2 Armbrecht B H. Reaction between piperazine and chlorpromazine. *New Eng J Med* (1970) **282**, 149.

Propanidid + benzodiazepines

Summary
An isolated case report describes an enhancement of the anesthetic effects of propanidid by chlordiazepoxide.

Interaction, mechanism, importance and management
A woman who had been taking chlordiazepoxide, 20 mg daily for about 18 months and who was currently on 10 mg daily, was given atropine as an anaesthetic premedication. The injection of 100 mg propanidid (instead of the intended 500 mg) proved to be sufficient to induce adequate anaesthesia for surgery to take place.

Reference
1 Magbagbeola J A O. Interaction between chlordiazepoxide and propanidid. *Br J Anaesth* (1975) **47**, 161

Spironolactone (and other potassium-sparing diuretics) + potassium salts

Summary
Hyperkalaemia can result from the concurrent use of potassium supplements with potassium-sparing diuretics such as spironolactone or triamterene. The incidence is increased by renal impairment.

Interaction

A retrospective study of 788 patients on spironolactone showed that 1 in 5 experienced adverse effects, 41% demonstrating hyperkalaemia. The incidence of hyperkalaemia was increased four-fold by the concurrent use of potassium supplements. An increased incidence was also associated with high blood urea nitrogen levels. Thus the concurrent use of spironolactone and potassium supplements in patients with high BUN levels raised the incidence of hyperkalaemia to just over 42%.[1]

There are a number of other case reports and surveys showing a strong association between the development of hyperkalaemia and the use of potassium salts with spironolactone[2-4,7] or triamterene.[5]

Mechanism

The effects of the potassium-sparing diuretics and dietary potassium supplements are additive, resulting in a rise in serum potassium levels.

Importance and management

A well-established interaction. The survey cited indicates that the incidence is high, and that the effects are exacerbated by renal failure.[1,4]. Although concurrent administration has been used successfully to treat severe hypokalaemia[6] it should only be undertaken if the effects can be closely monitored. Amiloride may be expected to behave similarly to spironolactone and triamterene although neither diuretic is likely to interact to the same extent as spironolactone because their potassium-sparing effects are less potent.

References
1 Greenblatt D J and Koch-Weser J. Adverse reactions to spironolactone. *J Amer Med Ass* (1973) **225**, 40.
2 Kalbian V V. Iatrogenic hyperkalaemic paralysis with electrocardiographic changes. *South Med J* (1974) **67**, 342.
3 Simborg D N. Medication prescribing on a university medical service—the incidence of drug combinations with potential adverse reactions. *Johns Hopkins Med J* (1976) **139**, 23.
4 Lawson D H. Adverse reactions to potassium chloride. *Quart J Med* (1974) **43**, 433.
5 O'Reilly M V, Murnaghan D P and Williams M B. Transvenous pacemaker failure induced by hypokalaemia. *J Amer Med Ass* (1974) **288**, 336.
6 Curry P, Fitchett D, Stubbs W and Krikler D. Ventricular arrhythmias and hypokalaemia. *Lancet* (1976) **ii**, 231.
7 Spino M, Sellers E M, Kaplan H L, Stapleton C and MacLeod S M. Adverse biochemical and clinical consequences of furosemide administration. *Canad Med Ass J* (1978) **118**, 1513.

Spironolactone + salicylates

Summary
The control of hypertension by spironolactone appears to be unaffected by the concurrent use of aspirin, despite some human studies which indicate that the spironolactone-induced natriuresis is inhibited.

Interactions

The evidence is conflicting. Studies in normal subjects have shown that aspirin antagonizes the spironolactone-induced natriuresis, but in patients the antihypertensive response seems to be unaffected.

Effect on normal subjects.

A 6-week crossover study on 10 normal subjects given single doses of spironolactone (25, 50 and 100 mg), showed that 600 mg doses of aspirin reduced the urinary excretion of electrolyte (using a fixed dose of fludrocortisone as a constant mineralocorticoid stimulant against which to measure the effects).

The effectiveness of the spironolactone was reduced 70%, and the overnight sodium excretion reduced by one third in 7 out of the 10 subjects who were given 25 mg spironolactone four times a day, and a single 600 mg dose of aspirin.[1]

Reductions in sodium excretion have been described in other studies.[2,3] In one of these studies the sodium excretion was completely antagonized when aspirin was given $1\frac{1}{2}$ h after the spironolactone, but was only partially antagonized when administered in the reverse order.[3]

Effect on hypertensive patients

Five patients with low-renin essential hypertension, well controlled for 4 months or more with 100–300 mg spironolactone daily, were examined on a double-blind crossover trial. Concurrent daily doses of aspirin in the range 2·4–4·8 g daily given over 6-week periods had no effect on blood pressure, serum electrolytes, body weight, urea nitrogen or plasma renin activity.[4]

Mechanism

Uncertain. There is evidence that the active secretion by the renal tubules of canrenone (the active metabolite of spironolactone) is blocked by aspirin, but the significance of this is not entirely clear.[2]

Importance and management

The importance of this interaction is by no means clear. Despite the results of the studies in normal subjects, in practice no reduction in the antihypertensive response was seen in hypertensive patients. Concurrent use of spironolactone and aspirin or other salicylates need not be avoided but it would be prudent to monitor the response to confirm that no antagonism is taking place.

References

1 Tweedale M G, and Ogilvie R I. Antagonism of spironolactone-induced natriuresis by aspirin in man. *New Eng J Med* (1973) **289**, 198.
2 Ramsay L E, Harrison I R, Shelton J R and Vose C W. Influence of acetylsalicylic acid on the renal handling of a spironolactone metabolite in healthy subjects. *Europ J clin Pharmacol* (1976) **10**, 43.
3 Elliott H C Reduced adrenocortical steroid excretion rates in man following aspirin administration. *Metabolism* (1962) **11**, 1015.
4 Hollifield J W. Failure of aspirin to antagonize the antihypertensive effect of spironolactone in low-renin hypertension. *South Med J* (1976) **69**, 1034

Tar gel + disulfiram

Summary

A mild disulfiram reaction has been described in a patient after the application of tar gel to the skin.

Interaction

A patient with extensive psoriasis was started on treatment with tar gel (*Estar*) at night. Six days later disulfiram therapy, 125 mg orally, was commenced. On the evening of the first disulfiram dose the patient complained of queasiness and headache but denied taking any alcohol. The tar gel was replaced by crude coal tar in petrolatum and no further symptoms ensued. Four days later the patient was rechallenged with 60 g tar gel: 10 min later the patient complained of a headache and of a sensation of warmth which persisted for an hour. Blood alcohol levels were measured and found to be less than 10 mg%.[1]

Mechanism

Tar gel contains about one third of ethyl alcohol. It seems that the alcohol was either absorbed through the skin or the vapour was inhaled, thereby initiating a mild disulfiram reaction (see p. 25). It is certainly possible to initiate this reaction by the use of alcohol applied to the skin. This has been demonstrated in patients on disulfiram who used an after-shave lotion containing alcohol.[2]

Importance and management

Although this is an isolated case, it is supported by other evidence that alcohol applied to the skin can precipitate a mild disulfiram reaction in particularly sensitive individuals. This reaction is of limited importance, but prescribers should be aware that it can occur.

References

1 Ellis C N, Mitchell A J and Beardsley G R Tar gel interaction with disulfiram. *Arch Dermatol* (1979) **115**, 1367.
2 Mercurio F. Antabuse–alcohol reaction following the use of after-shave lotion. *J Amer Med Ass* (1952) **149**, 82.

Theophylline + ampicillin

Summary
Ampicillin has been shown not to interact with theophylline.

Interaction, mechanism, importance and management

A study carried out on 11 patients, all with severe asthma and aged between 3 months and 6 years, showed that the mean half life of the theophylline they were all taking was unchanged by the concurrent use of ampicillin when compared with a control group of 42 patients not taking ampicillin. So it would seem that ampicillin can be safely given to patients on theophylline.

Reference
1 Kadlec G J, Ha Le Thanh, Jarboe C H, Richard D and Karibo J M. Effect of ampicillin on theophylline half-life in infants and young children. South Med J (1978) 71, 1584.

Theophylline + barbiturates

Summary
Conflicting evidence indicates that phenobarbitone does or does not reduce serum theophylline levels.

Interaction, mechanism, importance and management

One study in man indicated that the concurrent use of phenobarbitone had no effect on the metabolism of theophylline, whereas another suggested that serum theophylline levels were reduced.[1,2] Until more data are available it would be prudent to be on the watch for a reduction in the effects of theophylline during concurrent use.

References
1 Piafsky K M, Sitar D S and Ogilvie R I. Effect of phenobarbital on the disposition of intravenous theophylline. Clin Pharmacol Ther (1977) 22, 336.
2 Landay R A, Gonzalez M A and Taylor J C. Effect of phenobarbital on theophylline disposition. J Allergy Clin Immunol (1978) 62, 27.

Theophylline + cimetidine

Summary
A case report, supported by a study in man, has shown that serum theophylline levels can be grossly elevated by the concurrent use of cimetidine. Toxicity may develop.

Interaction

The theophylline levels of an asthmatic 15-year-old girl were raised from 13·0 μg/ml to 36·7 μg/ml when she was concurrently treated for a fortnight with cimetidine (dose unstated). Theophylline levels fell to 16·9 μg/ml, on the same dosage of theophylline, when the cimetidine was withdrawn.[1]

This report is consistent with the results of a study[2] which showed that the half-life of theophylline was prolonged by 60% when cimetidine, 300 mg 6-hourly for 2 days, was given concurrently.

Mechanism

It would seem probable that cimetidine (a recognized enzyme inhibitor) depresses the metabolism of the theophylline by the liver, thereby prolonging its stay in the body and raising its serum levels.

Importance and management

The documentation is very limited, but the interaction appears to be established. Theophylline levels should be closely monitored if cimetidine is given concurrently, and suitable dosage adjustments made, to ensure that theophylline toxicity does not develop.

References

1 Weinberger M M, Smith G, Milavetz G and Hendeles L. Decreased theophylline clearance due to cimetidine. *New Eng J Med* (1981) **304**, 672.
2 Jackson J E, Powell R J, Wandell M, Bentley J and Dorr R. Cimetidine-theophylline interaction. *Pharmacologist* (1980) **22**, 231.

Theophylline + corticosteroids

Summary

Serum theophylline concentrations can be doubled by the concurrent use of hydrocortisone. Toxicity may develop.

Interaction

The development of theophylline toxicity, apparently precipitated by the intravenous administration of hydrocortisone, prompted a further study of this possible interaction on 6 patients in status asthmaticus. All the patients were given theophylline by infusion until stable serum concentrations had been attained. They were then given an intravenous bolus of hydrocortisone, followed 6 h later by three 2-hourly doses of 200 mg. In each case the theophylline concentrations rapidly climbed from about 20 μg/ml to between 30 and 50 μg/ml. At least 2 of the patients complained of nausea and headache during the use of hydrocortisone.[1]

Theophylline is reported not to affect dexamethasone.[2]

Mechanism

Unknown.

Importance and management

The data appear to be limited to these reports. The possibility of theophylline toxicity should be borne in mind during concurrent treatment with hydrocortisone and theophylline levels should be closely monitored.

Reference

1 Buchanan N, Hurwitz S and Butler P. Asthma—a possible interaction between hydrocortisone and theophylline. *S Afr Med J* (1979) **56**, 1147.
2 Brooks S M, Sholiton L J, Werk E E and Altenan P. The effects of ephedrine and theophylline on dexamethasone metabolism on bronchial asthma. *J Clin Pharmacol* (1977) **17**, 308.

Theophylline + ephedrine

Summary

The incidence of adverse side effects is increased if ephedrine and theophylline are used together, the combination being no more effective than theophylline alone.

Interaction

A double-blind randomized study on the effectiveness of ephedrine, theophylline and hydroxyzine given separately and together (conventional ephedrine/theophylline ratios of 25 : 130) to 23 children with chronic asthma showed that none of the drugs given singly caused a significant number of adverse reactions, but ephedrine/theophylline in combination was associated with the development of insomnia (14 patients), nervousness (13 patients), and gastrointestinal complaints (18 patients) including vomiting (12 patients). This combination was also no more effective than theophylline alone.[1,2]

A previous study on 12 asthmatic children produced essentially similar results[3]

Mechanism

Not known. This additive toxicity (if that is what it is) has been demonstrated in animal experiments but remains unexplained.[4]

Importance and management:

There would seem to be no advantage in the combined use of theophylline and ephedrine in the treatment of asthma, and definite disadvantages which, as the authors of the major report state, indicates that these two drugs should not be used together routinely.

References
1 Weinberger M and Bronsky E. Interaction of ephedrine and theophylline. *Clin Pharmacol Ther* (1974) **15**, 223.
2 Weinberger M, Bronsky E, Bensch G W, Brock G N and Yeckles J J. Interaction of ephedrine and theophylline. *Clin Pharmacol Ther* (1975) **17**, 585.
3 Weinberger M and Bronsky E A. Evaluation of oral bronchodilator therapy in asthmatic children *J Pediatr* (1974) **84**, 421.
4 Richards R K. Toxicity of theophylline–ephedrine–barbiturate mixtures. *J Pharmacol Exp Ther* (1942) **72**, 33.

Theophylline + erythromycin

Summary

If erythromycin is given to asthmatic patients taking high doses of theophylline, the serum levels of theophylline may be increased to toxic levels. A reduction in the dosage of theophylline may be required.

Interaction

Following the observation that 5 different patients being treated with theophylline developed nausea or vomiting within 36–48 h of starting treatment with erythromycin, a study of this interaction was carried out on 11 asthmatic patients receiving both drugs. Four showed significant increases in serum theophylline levels during treatment with erythromycin ethyl succinate, stearate or estolate. None of the patients receiving erythromycin base showed significant changes, but they were only on low doses of theophylline.[1]

A study on 5 healthy volunteers who were given single 5 mg/kg intravenous doses of theophylline (as aminophylline) showed that during treatment with erythromycin (500 mg loading dose followed by 250 mg 6-hourly) the elimination half-life of the theophylline was extended from about 7 to 11 h and its clearance was reduced.[2]

This interaction has also been described in other reports[3,5] but in a study in normal subjects given single intravenous doses of theophylline the interaction was only demonstrated in 3 out of the 9 subjects.[4]

Mechanism

Not understood.

Importance and management

An established interaction. It has been seen to take place with erythromycin stearate, estolate and succinate[1] but not so far with erythromycin base. The effects on patients taking low doses of theophylline appear to be unimportant, but the authors of the first report cited[1] recommend careful monitoring of serum theophylline levels in those taking high doses (20 mg or more/kg), and suggest that the interaction can be accommodated by reducing the dosage of theophylline during concurrent treatment with erythromycin. It seems that not all patients are likely to demonstrate this interaction[4]

References
1 Kozak P P, Cummins L H and Gillman S A. Administration of erythromycin to patients on theophylline. *J Allergy Clin Immunol* (1977) **60**, 149.
2 Pfeifer H J, Greenblatt D J and Friedman P. Effect of antibiotics on theophylline kinetics in humans. *Clin Pharmacol Ther* (1978) **23**, 124.
3 Cummins L H, Kozak P P, and Gillman S A. Erythromycin's effect on theophylline blood level. *Pediatrics* (1977) **59**, 144.
4 Pfeifer H J, Greenblatt D J and Friedman P. Effects of three antibiotics on theophylline kinetics. *Clin Pharmacol Ther* (1979) **26**, 36.
5 Cummins L H, Kozak P P and Gillman S A. Theophylline determinatons. *Ann Allergy* (1976) **37**, 450.

Theophylline + tetracycline, allopurinol or cephalexin

Summary

Preliminary evidence from tests in healthy adults suggests that tetracycline, allopurinol and cephalexin are unlikely to interact with theophylline.

Interaction, mechanism, importance and management

A trial[1] on 9 healthy adults given single intravenous doses of theophylline (5 mg/kg) showed that the concurrent administration of tetracycline or cephalexin, 250 mg every 6 h, for approximately 48 h, had no significant effects on the kinetics of theophylline. This would suggest that an interaction of importance is unlikely, although the authors of the study rightly point out that their results do not necessarily apply to children or adult patients with impairment of pulmonary, cardiac or hepatic function.

Another study [2] in 5 normal subjects showed that the apparent volume of distribution, elimination half-life and total body clearance of theophylline after a 5 mg/kg intravenous dose over 30 minutes was unaffected by 7 days' treatment with 300 mg allopurinol daily.

Reference
1 Pfeifer H J, Greenblatt D J and Friedman P. Effects of three antibiotics on theophylline kinetics. *Clin Pharmacol Ther* (1979) 26, 36.
2 Vozeh S, Powell J R, Cupit G C, Riegelman S and Sheiner L B. Influence of allopurinol on theophylline disposition in adults. *Clin Pharmacol Ther* (1980) 27, 194.

Theophylline + thiabendazole

Summary

A single case report describes grossly elevated serum theophylline levels and the development of toxicity in a patient when treated concurrently with thiabendazole for 5 days.

Interaction, mechanism, importance and management

An elderly man with chronic obstructive pulmonary disease and under multiple drug treatment (prednisone, frusemide, terbutaline, metaproteronol, theophylline) was additionally given theophylline by infusion at the rate of 40–50 mg/hr during his numerous hospitalizations. This achieved a steady-state serum theophylline concentration of 19–21 μg/ml. Although he had on a previous occasion been uneventfully (and unsuccessfully) treated for 3 days with 3 g thiabendazole daily for a *Strongloides* infestation, when given 4 g daily for 5 days he developed theophylline toxicity (severe nausea, lethargy and generalized malaise). His serum theophylline concentration was found to have more than doubled (a rise from 19·2 to 46 μg/ml).[1] The explanation put forward is that the thiabendazole inhibited the metabolism of the theophylline by the liver, thereby prolonging its stay in the body and raising the serum levels. It would seem prudent to be on the alert for this interaction in patients on theophylline if the standard 2–3 day thiabendazole treatment is extended to 5 days or more.

Reference
1 Sugar A M, Kearns P J, Haulk A A and Rushing J L. Possible thiabendazole-induced theophylline toxicity? *Amer Rev Resp Dis* (1980) 122, 501.

Theophylline + tobacco smoking

Summary

The therapeutic effects of theophylline are diminished in those who smoke.

Interaction, mechanism, importance and management

A comparative study in man showed that the mean half-life of theophylline in a group of smokers was 4·3 h compared with 7 h in a group of non-smokers, probably as a result of liver enzyme induction.[1] Almost identical results were found in another study.[2] It is estimated that those who smoke heavily (1 to 2 packs a day, 20–40 cigarettes) will need daily doses of theophylline about twice those of non-smokers.

References
1 Hunt S N, Jusko W J, and Yurchak A M. Effect of smoking on theophylline disposition. *Clin Pharmacol Ther* (1976) **19**, 546.
2 Jenne J, Nagasawa H, McHugh R, Macdonald F and Wyse E. Decreased theophylline half-life in cigarette smokers. *Life Sci* (1975) **17**, 195.

Theophylline + triacetyloleandomycin

Summary

Theophylline serum levels can rise considerably during concurrent treatment with triacetyloleandomycin (troleandomycin). In some instances this may lead to the development of theophylline toxicity.

Interaction

Eight patients with severe chronic asthma, being treated with theophylline, were concurrently given 250 mg triacetyloleandomycin four times a day. The theophylline clearance rates of 7 of them decreased by an average of 50%, and after 10 days' treatment the eighth patient suffered theophylline-induced seizure, apparently as a result of serum theophylline levels of over 40 μg/ml (normal range 10–20 μg/ml) while continuing to take a dosage of theophylline which had previously been well tolerated. The theophylline half-life of this patient was found to have increased from 4·6 to 11·3 h.[1–3]

Mechanism

Not known. It has been suggested that triacetyloleandomycin inhibits the metabolism of theophylline by the liver and hence reduces its clearance from the body.[3]

Importance and management

Increases in the serum levels of theophylline should be expected if triacetyloleandomycin is given concurrently. This may have a beneficial effect on the control of asthma in some patients, but it can also lead to the development of toxicity if the serum levels rise too high. For this reason serum theophylline levels should be monitored and suitable dosage adjustments made during combined therapy.

References
1 Weinberger M, Hudgel D, Spector S, and Chidsey C. Troleandomycin (TAO): an inhibitor of theophylline metabolism. *J Allergy Clin Immunol* (1976) **57**, 262.
2 Weinberger M, Hudgle D, Spector S, and Chidsey C. Effect of triacetyloleandomycin (TAO) on the metabolism of theophylline. *Clin Pharmacol Ther* (1976) **19**, 118.
3 Weinberger M, Hudgle D, Spector S and Chidsey C. Inhibition of theophylline clearance by troleandomycin. *J Allergy Clin Immunol* (1977) **59**, 228.

Thiazides + diflusinal

Summary

Serum levels of hydrochlorothiazide are increased by the concurrent use of diflusinal.

Interaction, mechanism, importance and management

Two preliminary reports state that the concurrent administration of 375 mg diflusinal twice a day caused a 25–30% increase in the plasma levels of hydrochlorothiazide, probably due to a decrease in the renal excretion of the diuretic.[1,2] It is doubtful if this interaction is of any practical importance. Diflusinal has uricosuric activity which counteracts the uric acid retention which occurs with hydrochlorothiazide.

References
1 Tempero K F, Cirillo V J and Steelman S L. Diflusinal: a review of the pharmacokinetic and pharmacodynamic properties, drug interactions and special tolerability studies in humans. *Br J clin Pharmac* (1977) 31s.
2 Tempero K F, Steelman S L, Besselaar G H, Smit Sibinga C Th, De Schepper P, Tjandramaga T B, Dresse A and Gribnau F W J. Special studies on diflusinal, a novel salicylate. *Clin Res* (1975) **23**, 224A.

Thiazides + propantheline

Summary

Propantheline can substantially increase the absorption of hydrochlorothiazide by the gut.

Interaction, mechanism, importance and management

A study on 6 normal volunteers showed that the absorption of hydrochlorothiazide was delayed but substantially increased (almost 40%) by the concurrent administration of 60 mg propantheline. It was suggested that this was due to a slower delivery of the drug to its areas of absorption in the small intestine. The clinical importance of this is uncertain.

Reference

1 Beerman B and Groschinsky-Grind M. Enhancement of the gastrointestinal absorption of hydrochlorothiazide by propantheline. *Europ J Clin Pharmacol* (1978) 13, 385.

Thyroxine + barbiturates

Summary

An isolated case has been reported of a reduction in the response to thyroxine due to the concurrent administration of a barbiturate hypnotic.

Interaction

An elderly woman who had been taking 0·3 mg L-thyroxine daily for many years for hypothyroidism complained of severe breathlessness within a week of reducing her regular nightly dose of *Tuinal* (quinalbarbitone sodium 199 mg and amylobarbitone sodium 100 mg) from two capsules to one. She was subsequently found to be thyrotoxic. She became symptom free once again when the dosage of L-thyroxine was halved.[1]

Mechanism

Uncertain. It seems possible that this patient had remained euthyroidic for many years because the barbiturate continually lowered the levels of circulating thyroxine. Once the dosage of barbiturate was reduced, the same dose of thyroxine became an overdose and she became thyrotoxic. It is not known why this should be, but in animals barbiturates have been show to increase the hepatocellular binding of thyroxine.[2]

Importance and management

This appears to be the only case of this interaction so far recorded. Its general importance is difficult to assess, but it serves to alert prescribers to the possibility of an interaction if a barbiturate is added to or withdrawn from the regimen of a patient requiring treatment for hypothyroidism.

References

1 Hoffbrand B I. Barbiturate/thyroid-hormone interaction. *Lancet* (1979) ii, 903.
2 Oppenheimer J H, Berstein G and Surks M I. Increased thyroxine turnover and thyroidal function after stimulation of hepatocellular binding of thyroxine by phenobarbital. *J Clin Invest* (1968) 47, 1399

Thyroid hormones + cholestyramine

Summary

The gastrointestinal absorption of thyroid hormones is reduced by the concurrent use of cholestyramine. The dosages should be separated by an interval of 4–5 h.

Interaction

The observation that a patient with hypothyroidism, controlled with thyroid extract, showed a fall in her basal metabolic rate while taking cholestyramine prompted an investigation. A study of 2 hypothyroidic patients taking 60 mg thyroid extract or 100 μg levothyroxine sodium daily, and of 5 normal subjects all given 4 g cholestyramine four times a day, showed that the absorption of radioactive thyroxine[131] was reduced and the amount remaining in the faeces was roughly doubled. One of the patients showed a worsening of her hypothyroidism. Separating the dosages by 4–5 h reduced the interference to a minium.[1]

Mechanism

The cholestyramine binds to the thyroxine within the gut thereby preventing its absorption. Since thyroxine probably also takes part in the entero-hepatic shunt (after absorption it is re-secreted in the bile), continued contact with the cholestyramine is possible.

Importance and management

An established interaction, although the documentation is very limited. The symptoms of hypothyroidism can reoccur if cholestyramine is given to patients on thyroxine. *In-vitro* tests showed that cholestyramine can also interact with tri-iodothyronine.[1] Absorption of the hormone approached normal in 3 of the 5 subjects in the study cited[1] when the dosages of the two drugs were separated by 4–5 h, and this has been recommended as a method of accommodating this interaction. Even if this precaution is taken, patients should be monitored for signs of hypothyroidism and dosage adjustments made where necessary.

References

1 Northcutt R C, Stiel J N, Hollifield J W and Stant E G. The influence of cholestyramine on thyroxine absorption. *J Amer Med Ass* (1969) **208**, 1857.

Sodium polystyrene sulphonate + antacids

Summary

The concurrent use of antacids with sodium polystyrene sulphonate may result in metabolic alkalosis

Interactions

A man with metabolic acidosis developed metabolic alkalosis when given 90 g sodium polystyrene sulphonate with 90 ml magnesium hydroxide mixture.[1]

Alkalosis has also been described in a study on a number of patients given this cation exchange resin with *Maalox* (magnesium–aluminium hydroxides) and calcium carbonate.[2]

Mechanism

It has been suggested that the sodium polystyrene sulphonate and magnesium reacted together within the gut to form magnesium polystyrene sulphonate and sodium chloride. Thus the normal neutralization of the bicarbonate ions by the gastric juice and the exchange resin within the small intestine failed to occur, resulting in absorption of the bicarbonate leading to metabolic alkalosis.

Importance and management

The documentation is very limited but the interaction appears to be established. This ion-exchange resin can be administered rectally as an enema to avoid this problem. Serum electrolyte levels should be closely monitored during its use.

References

1 Fernandez P C and Kovnat P J. Metabolic acidosis reversed by the combination of magnesium and a cation-exchange resin. *New Eng J Med* (1972) **286**, 23.
2 Schroeder E T. Alkalosis resulting from combined administration of a 'non-systemic' antacid and a cation-exchange resin. *Gastroenterology* (1969) **56**, 868.

Vitamin A + aminoglycoside antibiotics

Summary

Neomycin can markedly reduce the gastrointestinal absorption of vitamin A.

Interaction, mechanism, importance and management

A study of five healthy subjects showed that concurrent treatment with 2 g neomycin greatly reduced the absorption of test doses of vitamin A (retinyl palmitate) due, it is suggested, to a direct chemical interference between the neomycin and bile and fatty acids in the intestine which disrupts the absorption of fats and fat-soluble vitamins.[1]

The extent to which chronic treatment with neomycin (or other aminoglycosides) would impair the treatment of vitamin A deficiency has not been determined, but it would seem a possibility.

Reference

1 Barrowman J A, D'Mello A, and Herxheimer A. A single dose of neomycin impairs absorption of vitamin A (Retinol) in man. *Europ J clin Pharmacol* (1973) **5**, 199.

Warfarin + amiodarone

Summary

A single case report describes a woman who showed a marked increase in her response to warfarin, and bled, when concurrently treated with amiodarone.

Interaction

A woman showed a marked enhancement of her response to warfarin and developed gastrointestinal bleeding when concurrently treated with 200 mg amiodarone three times a day. On a later occasion the warfarin was withdrawn on the day the amiodarone was restarted. Despite this the British corrected ratio of prothrombin times (BCR) rose from 2·5 to 4·5 over the next five days, before falling in response to treatment with vitamin K.[1]

The authors of the report state that the British Committee on the Safety of Medicines has received reports suggesting that this interaction may occur. The interaction was also shown to occur in animal experiments.[1]

Mechanism
Not understood.

Importance and management
Although this is so far the only recorded case of this interaction, it would clearly be prudent to monitor closely the prothrombin times of any patient on warfarin (or any other anticoagulant) who is given amiodarone.

Reference

1 Rees A, Dalal J J, Reid P G, Henderson A H and Lewis M J. Dangers of amiodarone and anticoagulant treatment. *Brit Med J* (1981) **282**, 1756.

INDEX

In order to keep this index to a manageable size, brand names of drugs have been avoided except for compound preparations. However, tables of brand names/generic names have been included in the introductions of most chapters and these can be found by looking up the group names of the drugs in question (e.g. Anticoagulants, Benzodiazepines, Barbiturates, etc).

Most pairs of drugs known to interact (or not to interact) are indexed under their individual names as well as under their group names, with the exception of the Anticoagulants and the Monoamine Oxidase Inhibitors which are indexed under their group names only. If an individual drug is not specifically listed in the index as taking part in an interaction, some indication of its possible behaviour may be found by checking on the way the family of drugs to which it belongs is known to react.

466

Calcium carbimide (cont.)
+ tricyclic antidepressants, 443
Calcium carbonate
see also Antacids.
+ flufenamic acid, 41
+ indomethacin, 42
+ mefenamic acid, 41
+ nitrofurantoin, 95
+ oxyphenbutazone, 41
+ phenylbutazone, 41
+ phenytoin, 190
+ tetracycline, 105
Calcium carbonate glycine
see also Antacids
+ aspirin, 56
+ chlorpromazine, 380
+ quinidine, 66
Calcium chloride
+ digitalis glycosides, 299
Calcium gluconate
+ digitalis glycosides, 299
Calcium phosphate
+ tetracycline, 105
Calcium preparations
+ digitalis glycosides, 299
Carbamazepine
+ anticoagulants, 127
+ barbiturates, 187
+ benzodiazepines, 183
+ chlortetracycline, 107
+ clonazepam, 183
+ contraceptives, oral 270
+ demethyltetracycline, 107
+ dextropropoxyphene, 186
+ digitalis glycosides, 300
+ disulfiram, 199
+ doxycycline, 107
+ ethosuximide, 188
+ glibenclamide, 432
+ methacycline, 107
+ monoamine oxidase
inhibitors, 360
+ oxytetracycline, 107
+ phenobarbitone, 187
+ phenytoin, 195
+ primidone, 214
+ sodium valproate, 187
+ tetracycline, 107
+ tetraclines, 107
+ triacetyloleandomycin, 187
Carbenicillin
see also other penicillins
+ amikacin, 79
+ gentamicin, 79
+ sisomicin, 79
+ tobramycin, 79
Carbenoxolone
+ amiloride, 429
+ antihypertensives, 220
+ beta-blockers, 220
+ chlorthalidone, 429
+ clonidine, 220
+ diazoxide, 220

Carbenoxolone (cont.)
+ digitalis glycosides, 300
+ guanethidine and related
drugs, 220
+ hydrallazine, 220
+ methyldopa, 220
+ pargyline, 220
+ rauwolfia alkaloids, 220
+ spironolactone, 429
+ thiazides, 220, 429
+ triamterene, 429
Carbimazole
+ anticoagulants, 175
Carbon tetrachloride
+ anticoagulants, 127
Carbutamide
see also Hypoglycaemic
agents
+ cyclophosphamide, 331
+ phenylbutazone, 337
Cardiac glycosides, *see* Digitalis
Glycosides and individual drugs
Cardioselective Beta-blockers, *see*
Beta-blockers
Carinamide
+ heparin, 181
Carmustine
+ cimetidine, 280
+ vaccines, 284
CCNU, *see* Lomustine
Cefaclor
see also Cephalosporins
+ probenecid, 81
Cefamandole
see also Cephalosporins
+ alcohol, 15
+ probenecid, 81
Cefoperazine
see also cephalosporins
+ alcohol, 15
Cefotoxin
see also Cephalosporins
+ frusemide, 81
Cefoxitin
see also Cephalosporins
+ frusemide, 81
+ probenecid, 81
Central Nervous System
Depressants, *see* CNS
Depressants
Central Nervous System
Stimulants, *see* CNS
Stimulants
Cephacetrile
see also Cephalosporins
+ frusemide, 81
+ probenecid, 81
Cephalexin
see also Cephalosporins
+ contraceptives, 270
+ gentamicin, 74
+ probenecid, 81
+ theophylline, 457

Cephaloglycin
see also Cephalosporins
+ probenecid, 81
Cephaloridine
see also Cephalosporins
+ anticoagulants, 129
+ frusemide, 81
+ probenecid, 81
Cephalosporins
see also individual drugs
+ aminoglycosides, 74, 75
+ anticoagulants, 129
+ colistin sulphomethate
sodium (colistimethate
sodium), 80
+ frusemide, 81
+ probenecid, 81
Cephalothin
see also Cephalosporins
+ colistin sulphomethate
sodium, 80
+ frusemide, 81
+ gentamicin, 75
+ gentamicin + cis-platinum,
281
+ hydrocortisone + methotrexate,
288
+ probenecid, 81
+ tobramycin, 75
Cephazolin
+ anticoagulants, 129
Cephradine
see also Cephalosporins
+ probenecid, 81
Charcoal
+ aspirin, 430
+ digitalis glycosides, 430
+ nitrofurantoin, 95
+ phenytoin, 430
Cheese
tyramine content, 372
+ debrisoquine, 228
+ demeclocycline, 111
+ isoniazid, 91
+ monoamine oxidase
inhibitors, 370
+ procarbazine, 292
+ tetracyclines, 111
Cheese reaction, 370
Chilblain preparations (*Gon,
Amisyn, Pernivit*)
+ anticoagulants, 179
Chloral betaine
see also Chloral hydrate
+ alcohol, 21
+ anticoagulants, 130
+ frusemide, 443
Chloral hydrate
+ alcohol, 21
+ anticoagulants, 130
+ frusemide, 443
+ monoamine oxidase
inhibitors, 360

Chloramphenicol
+ ampicillin, 83
+ anti-anaemic agents, 428
+ anticoagulants, 132
+ barbiturates, 83
+ benzylpenicillin, 83
+ chlorpropamide, 326
+ contraceptives, oral, 270
+ cyclophosphamide, 282
+ folic acid, 428
+ hypoglycaemic agents, 326
+ iron, 428
+ methicillin, 83
+ methotrexate, 288
+ neuromuscular blockers, 388
+ paracetamol (acetaminophen), 82
+ penicillins, 83
+ phenobarbitone, 83
+ phenytoin, 196
+ tolbutamide, 326
+ vitamin B$_{12}$, 428
Chlordiazepoxide
see also Benzodiazepines
+ alcohol, 18
+ aluminium magnesium hydroxide, 375
+ amitriptyline, 420
+ anticoagulants, 126
+ barbiturates, 183
+ cimetidine, 376
+ disulfiram, 377
+ insulin, 324
+ levodopa, 249
+ monoamine oxidase inhibitors, 358
+ nortriptyline, 420
+ phenobarbitone, 183
+ phenytoin, 194
+ propanidid, 452
Chlorimipramine
see also Tricyclic Antidepressants
+ alcohol, 35
Chlorinated insecticides, *see* Insecticides, Lindane, Toxaphene, Gamma-benzene hexachloride
Chlormerodrin
+ lithium carbonate, 345
Chlorodyne
+ alcohol, 22
Chloroform
+ beta-blockers, 259
Chloroquine
+ azapropazone, 39
Chlorothiazide
see also Thiazides
+ anticoagulants, 175
+ lithium carbonate, 353
+ phenylbutazone, 222

Chlorphenadione, *see* Anticoagulants
Chlorpheniramine
+ alcohol, 16
+ amphetamines + phenylpropanolamine, 402
+ phenytoin, 197
Chlorphentermine
see also Sympathomimetics, indirectly-acting
+ chlorpromazine, 400
+ monoamine oxidase inhibitors, 415
Chlorpromazine
see also Phenothiazines
+ alcohol, 379, 433
+ Aludrox, 380
+ aluminium hydroxide, 380
+ amitriptyline, 244
+ amitriptyline + benztropine, 244
+ amphetamines, 400
+ antacids, 380
+ anticoagulants, 163
+ antihypertensive agents, 222
+ barbiturates, 382
+ benzhexol, 244
+ benztropine + trifluoperazine, 244
+ bethanidine, 232
+ beta-blockers, 264, 382
+ calcium carbonate-glycine, 380
+ chlorphentermine, 400
+ chlorprothixene + benztropine, 244
+ coffee, 381
+ debrisoquine, 232
+ dexamphetamine, 400
+ diazoxide, 227
+ *Gelusil*, 380
+ guanethidine and related drugs, 232
+ hypoglycaemic agents, 327
+ imipramine, 383
+ imipramine + benztropine, 244
+ levodopa, 254
+ lithium carbonate, 378
+ magnesium hydroxide, 380
+ magnesium trisilicate, 380
+ methamphetamine, 400
+ metrizamide, 451
+ nortriptyline, 244
+ orphenadrine, 244
+ phenmetrazine, 400
+ phenobarbitone, 382
+ phenytoin, 206
+ piperazine, 452
+ propranolol, 264, 382
+ sotalol, 264
+ tea, 381
+ tricyclic antidepressants, 383
+ trifluoperazine, 244

Chlorpropamide
see also Hypoglycaemic agents
+ alcohol, 317
+ allopurinol, 319
+ anticoagulants, 321
+ aspirin, 323
+ chloramphenicol, 326
+ clofibrate, 328
+ colestipol, 329
+ cortisone, 330
+ co-trimoxazole, 331, 341
+ demeclocycline, 342
+ fenclofenac, 333
+ halofenate, 335
+ monoamine oxidase inhibitors, 362
+ phenylbutazone, 337
+ probenecid, 338
+ thiazides, 343
+ salicylates, 323
+ sulphafurazole, 341
+ sulphamethazine, 341
Chlorprothixene
+ chlorpromazine + benztropine, 244
Chlortetracycline
see also Tetracyclines
+ aluminium hydroxide, 105
+ anticoagulants, 174
+ carbamazepine, 107
+ iron preparations, 109
+ penicillin, 97
+ phenobarbitone, 107
+ phenytoin, 107
Chlorthalidone
+ anticoagulants, 132
+ carbenoxolone, 429
+ digitalis glycosides, 302
+ hypoglycaemic agents, 343
+ lithium carbonate, 353
Cholestyramine
+ anticoagulants, 133
+ beta-methyl digoxin, 301
+ clofibrate, 430
+ digitalis glycosides, 301
+ digitoxin, 301
+ digoxin, 301
+ flufenamic acid, 42
+ iopanoic acid, 447
+ loperamide, 448
+ mefenamic acid, 42
+ sodium fusidate, 101
+ sulphasalazine, 102
+ thyroid hormones, 460
+ x-ray contrast media, 447
Choline salicylate
see also other salicylates
+ corticosteroids, 57
+ prednisone, 57
Cholinergic drugs
+ aminoglycoside antibiotics, 431
+ procainamide, 431

Drinks, *see* Alcohol, Coca-Cola,
    Coffee, Milk, Tea
Droperidol
    see also Butyrophenones and
        Haloperidol
    + levodopa, 254
    + monoamine oxidase inhibitors
        and hyoscine, 361
    + tea, 381
Drug biotransformation
    interactions, 5
Drug displacement interactions, 3
Drug excretion interactions, 9
Drug metabolism interactions, 5

Ecothiophate iodide
    + neuromuscular blockers, 392
    + suxamethonium, 392
Edrophonium
    + digitalis glycosides, 303
Enzyme induction interactions, 5
Enzyme inhibition interactions, 8
Ephedrine
    see also Sympathomimetics,
        indirectly-acting
    + corticosteroids, 438
    + bethanidine, 234
    + debrisoquine, 234, 406
    + dexamethasone, 438
    + furazolidone, 412
    + guanethidine and related
        drugs, 234
    + methyldopa, 414
    + monoamine oxidase
        inhibitors, 415
    + rauwolfia alkaloids, 410
    + reserpine, 410
    + theophylline, 456
Epinephrine, *see* Adrenaline and
        Sympathomimetics,
        directly-acting
Ergot and Ergot derivatives
    + beta-blockers, 262
    + dopamine, 403
    + erythromycin, 443
    + propranolol, 262
    + triacetyloleandomycin, 443
Erythromycin
    + acetazolamide, 86
    + ampicillin, 86
    + anticoagulants, 143
    + contraceptives, 270
    + ergot and its derivatives, 443
    + lincomycin, 86
    + penicillin, 86
    + sodium bicarbonate, 86
    + theophylline, 457
    + urinary acidifiers, 86
    + urinary alkalinizers, 86
Estrogen-progestogen
        contraceptives, *see*
        Contraceptives, oral

Estrogens, *see* Contraceptives, oral
    and individual agents
Ethacrynic acid
    + aminoglycosides, 77
    + anticoagulants, 144
    + corticosteroids, 437
    + digitalis glycosides, 302
    + hypoglycaemic agents, 333
    + kanamycin, 77
    + neomycin, 77
    + streptomycin, 77
Ethambutol
    + aluminium hydroxide, 87
    + antacids, 87
    + methadone, 46
Ethanol, *see* Alcohol
Ethchlorvynol
    + amitriptyline, 421
    + anticoagulants, 144
    + tricyclic antidepressants, 421
Ether
    see also Anaesthetics
    + beta-blockers, 259
    + hypoglycaemic agents, 320
Ethinamate
    + alcohol, 20
Ethinyl(o)estradiol
    see also Contraceptives, oral
    + clomipramine, 424
    + imipramine, 424
    + magnesium trisilicate, 269
Ethionamide
    + thyroid hormones, 88
Ethisterone
    + magnesium trisilicate, 269
Ethosuximide
    + barbiturates, 188
    + carbamazepine, 188
    + methylphenobarbitone, 188
    + phenobarbitone, 188
    + phenytoin, 188
    + primidone, 188
Ethylbiscoumacetate, *see*
        Anticoagulants
Ethylidene dicoumarin, *see*
        Anticoagulants
Ethyloestrenol
    + anticoagulants, 118
Ethynodiol diacetate, *see*
        Contraceptives, oral
Etryptamine, *see* Monoamine
        Oxidase Inhibitors
Excretion interactions, 9

Fazadinium
    + diazepam, 391
Felypressin
    + tricyclic antidepressants, 411
Fenbufen
    + anticoagulants, 172
Fenclofenac
    + chloropropamide, 333

Fenclofenac (cont.)
    + hypoglycaemic agents, 333
    + metformin, 333
Fenfluramine
    + amitriptyline, 422
    + anaesthetics (general), 445
    + antihypertensive agents, 221
    + beta-blockers, 221
    + bethanidine, 221
    + debrisoquine, 221
    + guanethidine and related
        drugs, 221
    + halothane, 445
    + halothane + practolol, 445
    + hypoglycaemic agents, 333
    + methyldopa, 221
    + monoamine oxidase
        inhibitors, 422
    + rauwolfia alkaloids, 221
    + reserpine, 221
    + tricyclic antidepressants, 422
Fenoprofen
    + anticoagulants, 145
Fentanyl citrate/droperidol
        (*Innovar*)
    + neuromuscular blockers, 394
Feprazone
    + anticoagulants
Ferrous compounds, *see also* Iron
        preparations
Ferrous fumarate
    + tetracycline, 109
Ferrous gluconate
    + tetracycline, 109
Ferrous sodium edetate
    + tetracyclines, 109
Ferrous succinate
    + tetracycline, 109
Ferrous sulphate
    + doxycycline, 109
    + magnesium trisilicate, 448
    + methacycline, 109
    + oxytetracycline, 109
    + tetracycline, 109
Ferrous tartrate
    + tetracycline, 109
Fish
    + isoniazid, 91
Flucloxacillin
    see also other penicillins
    + contraceptives, 272
Fludrocortisol
    see also Corticosteroids
    + rifampicin, 440
Flufenamic acid
    + aluminium hydroxide, 41
    + antacids, 41
    + bismuth oxycarbonate, 41
    + calcium carbonate, 41
    + cholestyramine, 42
    + kaolin, 41
    + magnesium oxide, 41
    + magnesium trisilicate, 41

Hypertensive crisis,
  management, 373, 416
Hypnotics
  see also individual drugs
  + alcohol, 15
  + CNS depressants (*see also*
    individual drugs), 433
  + hydroxyurea, 286
Hypoglycaemic agents
  see also individual agents
  mode of action, 314
  generic and brand names, 315
  + alcohol, 316, 317
  + allopurinol, 319
  + amiloride, 319
  + anabolic steroids, 319
  + anaesthetics, 320
  + anticoagulants, 321
  + asparaginase, 323
  + aspirin, 323
  + barbiturates, 324
  + benzodiazepines, 324
  + beta-blockers, 325
  + chloramphenicol, 326
  + chlorpromazine, 327
  + chlorthalidone, 343
  + clofibrate, 328
  + colaspase (asparaginase),
    323
  + colestipol, 329
  + contraceptives, oral, 330
  + corticosteroids, 330
  + co-trimoxazole, 331
  + cyclophosphamide, 331
  + diazoxide, 228
  + diclofenac, 332
  + diflusinal, 332
  + disulfiram, 332
  + ethacrynic acid, 332
  + ether, 320
  + fenclofenac, 333
  + fenfluramine, 333
  + frusemide, 334
  + guanethidine and related
    drugs, 334
  + halofenate, 335
  + halothane, 320
  + isoniazid, 335
  + lithium, 336
  + methoxyflurane, 320
  + methysergide, 337
  + mianserin, 337
  + monoamine oxidase
    inhibitors, 362
  + nitrous oxide, 320
  + oxyphenbutazone, 337
  + phenobarbitone, 324
  + phenothiazines, 327
  + phenylbutazone, 337
  + phenyramidol, 338
  + phenytoin, 202
  + probenecid, 339
  + rifampicin, 339

Hypoglycaemic agents (cont.)
  + salicylates, 323
  + sulindac, 340
  + sulphinpyrazone, 340
  + sulphonamides, 341
  + tetracyclines, 342
  + thiazides, 343
  + thiopentone, 320
  + tolmetin, 344
  + tricyclic antidepressants, 423
Hypoprothrombinaemia, 114
Hypotensive agents
  see also Antihypertensives and
    individual antihypertensive
    drugs, 228
  + diazoxide, 228

Ibuprofen
  + anticoagulants, 152
  + lithium carbonate, 348
  + mazindol, 43
Ice-cream
  + anticoagulants, 153
Idrocilamide
  + caffeine, 429
  + coffee, 429
  + tea, 429
Imipramine
  see also Tricyclic
    antidepressants and other
    members of the group
  + adrenaline (epinephrine), 411
  + anticholinergics, 244
  + benzhexol, 244
  + bethanidine, 235
  + chlorpromazine, 383
  + clonidine, 226
  + debrisoquine, 235
  + ethinyloestradiol, 424
  + flupenthixol, 425
  + guanethidine and related
    drugs, 235
  + haloperidol, 423
  + isoprenaline (isoproterenol),
    411
  + levodopa, 257
  + methylphenidate, 424
  + noradrenaline
    (norepinephrine), 411
  + perphenazine, 383
  + phenylephrine, 411
  + phenytoin, 212
  + rauwolfia alkaloids, 239
  + reserpine, 239
  + tri-iodothyronine, 426
Indanediones
  generic and brand names, 115
  Interactions, *see* Anticoagulants
Indomethacin
  + alcohol, 27
  + aluminium hydroxide, 42
  + antacids, 42

Indomethacin (cont.)
  + anticoagulants, 153
  + antihypertensive agents, 224
  + aspirin, 44
  + beta-blockers, 224
  + bismuth oxycarbonate, 42
  + bumetanide, 224
  + calcium carbonate, 42
  + clonidine, 224
  + corticosteroids, 435
  + diflusinal, 41
  + digitalis glycosides, 304
  + digoxin, 304
  + diuretics, 224
  + food, 43
  + frusemide, 224
  + guanethidine and related
    drugs, 224
  + kaolin, 42
  + lithium carbonate, 348
  + magnesium oxide, 42
  + magnesium trisilicate, 42
  + mazindol, 43
  + methyldopa, 224
  + neofam, 58
  + phenylbutazone, 53
  + phenylpropanolamine, 413
  + pindolol, 224
  + prednisone, 435
  + probenecid, 44
  + propranolol, 224
  + rauwolfia alkaloids, 224
  + salicylates, 44
  + sympathomimetics,
    indirectly-acting, 413
  + vaccines, 45
Innovar, see fentanyl/droperidol
Insecticides
  see also individual agents
  + anticoagulants, 154
  + phenylbutazone, 52
Insulin
  see also Hypoglycaemic
    agents
  + alcohol, 316
  + anticoagulants, 321
  + aspirin, 323
  + beta-blockers, 325
  + chlordiazepoxide, 324
  + colestipol, 329
  + contraceptives, oral, 330
  + cyclophosphamide, 331
  + doxycycline, 342
  + guanethidine and related
    drugs, 334
  + halofenate, 335
  + isoniazid, 335
  + lithium carbonate, 336
  + monoamine oxidase
    inhibitors, 362
  + nandrolone, 319
  + oxytetracycline, 342
  + phenytoin, 202

Nitrazepam (cont.)
+ amitriptyline, 420
+ anticoagulants, 126
+ levodopa, 249
+ nortriptyline, 420
+ phenytoin, 194
Nitrogen mustard
(methchloroethamine)
+ neuromuscular blockers,
398
+ suxamethonium, 398
Nitrofurantoin
+ aluminium hydroxide, 95
+ antacids, 95
+ anticholinergics, 95
+ bismuth oxycarbonate, 95
+ calcium carbonate, 95
+ charcoal, 95
+ contraceptives, 270
+ diphenoxylate, 95
+ kaolin, 95
+ magnesium oxide, 95
+ magnesium trisilicate, 95
+ naldixic acid, 94
+ propantheline, 95
+ talc, 95
Non-steroidal anti-inflammatory
agents, see individual drugs
generic and brand names, 37
Norethandrolone
see also Anabolic steroids
+ anticoagulants, 118
Nortriptyline
see also Tricyclic
antidepressants
+ alcohol, 35
+ anticoagulants, 178
+ bethanidine, 235
+ chlorpromazine, 244
+ debrisoquine, 235
+ guanethidine and related
drugs, 235
+ oxyphenbutazone, 55
+ phenothiazines, 383, 244
+ phenytoin, 212
+ perphenazine, 383
Nitrous oxide
see also Anaesthetics (general)
+ hypoglycaemic agents, 320
Noradrenaline (levarterenol,
norepinephrine)
see also Sympathomimetics,
directly-acting
+ amitriptyline, 411
+ bretylium, 406
+ desipramine, 411
+ doxepin, 411
+ guanethidine and related
drugs, 406
+ imipramine, 411
+ maprotiline, 411
+ methyldopa, 407
+ mianserin, 408

Noradrenaline (cont.)
+ monoamine oxidase
inhibitors, 409
+ nortriptyline, 411
+ protriptyline, 411
+ rauwolfia alkaloids, 410
+ reserpine, 410
+ tricyclic antidepressants, 411
Norepinephrine, see Noradrenaline
Norethindrone, see Contraceptives,
oral
Norethisterone
see also Contraceptives, oral
+ magnesium trisilicate, 269
Norethynodrel, see Contraceptives,
oral
Norgestrel, see Contraceptives, oral
Nortriptyline
see also Tricyclic
antidepressants
+ adrenaline (epinephrine), 411
+ alcohol, 35
+ amylobarbitone, 420
+ anticoagulants, 178
+ chlordiazepoxide, 420
+ clonidine, 226
+ diazepam, 420
+ haloperidol, 423
+ nitrazepam, 420
+ noradrenaline
(norepinephrine,
levarterenol), 411
+ oxazepam, 420
+ perphenazine, 383
+ phenytoin, 212
+ urinary acidifiers, 427
+ urinary alkalinizers, 427

Oestrogen-progestogen
contraceptives, see
Contraceptives, oral
Oestrogens (estrogens)
see also Contraceptives, oral and
individual agents
+ tricyclic antidepressants, 424
One-stage prothrombin time, 114
Oral anticoagulants, see
Anticoagulants, oral
Oral contraceptives, see
Contraceptives, oral
Oral hypoglycaemic agents, see
Hypoglycaemic agents and
individual drugs
Orphenadrine
+ amantadine, 244
+ chlorpromazine, 245
+ dextropropoxyphene
(propoxyphene), 39
Ouabain (strophanthin-G), see
Digitalis glycosides
Oxandrolone
see also Anabolic steroids
+ anticoagulants, 118

Oxazepam
see also Benzodiazepines
+ alcohol
+ amitriptyline, 420
+ cimetidine, 376
+ disulfiram, 377
+ levodopa, 249
+ nortriptyline, 420
Oxedrine
+ guanethidine and related
drugs, 406
Oxprenolol
see also Beta-blockers
+ anaesthetics, 259
+ halothane, 259
+ hypoglycaemic agents, 325
+ methyldopa +
phenylpropanolamine, 414
+ neuromuscular blockers, 389
+ tubocurarine, 389
Oxygen
+ bleomycin, 280
Oxymetholone
see also Anabolic steroids
+ anticoagulants, 118
Oxyphenbutazone
+ aluminium hydroxide, 41
+ anabolic steroids, 49
+ antacids, 41
+ anticoagulants, 161
+ antihypertensive agents, 222
+ bismuth oxycarbonate, 41
+ calcium carbonate, 41
+ corticosteroids, 49
+ desipramine, 55
+ dexamethasone, 49
+ glycodiazine, 337
+ guanethidine and related
drugs, 222
+ hypoglycaemic agents, 337
+ kaolin, 41
+ magnesium oxide, 41
+ magnesium trisilicate, 41
+ methandrostenolone, 49
+ methotrexate, 290
+ nortriptyline, 55
+ phenytoin, 206
+ prednisone, 49
+ tolbutamide, 337
+ tricyclic antidepressants, 55
Oxytetracycline
see also Tetracyclines
+ aluminium hydroxide, 105
+ antacids, 105
+ carbamazepine, 107
+ contraceptives, 275
+ ferrous sulphate, 109
+ insulin, 342
+ iron preparations, 109
+ milk, 111
+ phenobarbitone, 107
+ phenytoin, 107
+ tolbutamide, 342

PABA, *see* Para-aminobenzoic acid
Pamaquine
  + mepacrine, 72
Pancuronium
  see also Neuromuscular
    blockers
  + aminoglycoside antibiotics, 386
  + clindamycin, 390
  + diazepam, 391
  + doxepin + hyoscine, 425
  + gentamicin, 386
  + lithium carbonate, 395
  + morphine, 47
Pantothenic acid
  + suxamethonium, 392
Papaverine
  + levodopa, 253
Para-aminobenzoic acid (PABA)
  + sulphonamides, 104
Para-aminosalicylic acid (PAS)
  + anticoagulants, 120
  + diphenhydramine, 96
  + isoniazid, 96
  + methotrexate, 288
  + phenytoin, 205
  + probenecid, 96
  + rifampicin, 100
Paracetamol (acetaminophen)
  + alcohol, 50, 32
  + anticoagulants, 162
  + chloramphenicol, 82
  + mazindol, 43
Paraldehyde
  + alcohol, 31
  + disulfiram, 442
Pargyline
  see Monoamine oxidase
    inhibitors and
    Antihypertensive agents
Parkinson's disease and its
    treatment, 241
Paromomycin
  + anticoagulants, 119
  + 5-fluorouracil, 285
  + methotrexate, 287
PAS, *see* Para-aminosalicylic acid
PAS-Granulate
  + rifampicin, 100
Penbutolol, *see* Beta-blockers
Penicillamine
  + iron preparations
Penicillin
  see also Penicillins and
    individual drugs
  + chlortetracycline, 97
  + contraceptives, oral, 272
  + erythromycin, 86
  + neuromuscular blockers, 388
  + sulphinpyrazone, 97
Penicillin V, *see*
    Phenoxymethyl-penicillin
Penicillins
  see also individual agents

Penicillins (cont.)
  + allopurinol, 36
  + aminoglycosides, 79
  + chloramphenicol, 83
  + cimetidine, 432
  + contraceptives, 272
  + sulphinpyrazone, 97
  + tetracyclines, 97
Pentazocine
  + CNS depressants, 433
  + neofam, 58
Pentobarbitone
  see also Barbiturates
  + alprenolol, 260
  + anticoagulants, 123
  + caffeine, 183
  + lignocaine (lidocaine), 62
  + metoprolol, 260
  + promethazine + scopolamine,
    184
  + quinidine, 64, 309
Pernivit, see Chilblain preparations
Perphenazine
  + imipramine, 383
  + imipramine + benztropine,
    244
  + nortriptyline, 383
  + tricyclic antidepressants, 383
Pesticides (chlorinated)
  + phenylbutazone, 52
Pethidine (meperidine)
  + barbiturates, 51
  + CNS depressants, 433
  + furazolidone, 51
  + monoamine oxidase
    inhibitors, 365
  + phenobarbitone, 51
Petrichloral
  see also Chloral hydrate
  + anticoagulants, 130
  + frusemide, 443
Phenazone (antipyrine)
  + amylobarbitone, 52
  + anticoagulants, 162
  + barbiturates, 52
Phendimetrazine
  + monoamine oxidase
    inhibitors, 415
Phenelzine, *see* Monoamine Oxidase
    Inhibitors
Pheneturide
  + folic acid, 188
  + phenytoin, 205
Phenformin
  see also Hypoglycaemic agents
  + alcohol, 317
  + colestipol, 329
  + halofenate, 335
  + tetracyclines, 341
  + thiazides, 343
Phenindione, *see* Anticoagulants
Pheniprazine, *see* Monoamine
    Oxidase Inhibitors

Pheniramine
  + alcohol, 16
Phenmetrazine
  + chlorpromazine, 400
  + monoamine oxidase
    inhibitors, 415
Phenobarbitone (Phenobarbital)
  see also Barbiturates
  + acetazolamide, 189
  + acetyldigitoxin, 298
  + alcohol, 17
  + anticoagulants, 123
  + carbamazepine, 187
  + chloramphenicol, 83
  + chlordiazepoxide, 183
  + chlorpromazine, 382
  + chlortetracycline, 107
  + clonazepam, 183
  + contraceptives, oral, 270
  + cyclophosphamide, 282
  + demethyltetracycline, 107
  + desipramine, 420
  + dexamethasone, 435
  + digitoxin, 298
  + digoxin, 298
  + disulfiram, 199
  + doxorubicin, 284
  + doxycycline, 107
  + ethosuximide, 188
  + fluroxene + phenytoin, 446
  + folic acid, 200
  + glymidine, 324
  + griseofulvin, 88
  + hydrocortisone, 435
  + methacycline, 107
  + methimazole, 449
  + methotrexate, 287
  + methyldopa, 237
  + methylphenidate, 204
  + methylprednisolone, 435
  + prednisone, 435
  + neofam, 58
  + oxytetracycline, 107
  + pethidine, 51
  + phenothiazines, 382
  + phenylbutazone, 54
  + phenytoin, 193
  + pyridoxine, 208
  + quinidine, 64
  + quinine, 99
  + rifampicin, 184
  + sodium valproate, 185
  + sulphafurazole, 103
  + sulphasalazine, 103
  + sulphasomidine, 103
  + tetracosactrin, 435
  + tetracycline, 107
  + theophylline, 455
  + thioridazine, 382
  + triacetyloleandomycin, 186
Phenothiazines
  see also individual drugs
  generic and brand names, 375

Probenecid (cont.)
+ salicylates, 55
+ sodium salicylate, 55
+ sulphinpyrazone, 56
+ tolbutamide, 339
Procainamide
+ cholinergic drugs, 431
+ hydroxyzine, 379
+ lignocaine, 63
+ neuromuscular blockers, 394
+ suxamethonium, 394
Procaine
see also Anaesthetics, local
+ neuromuscular blockers, 394
+ sulphadiazine, 104
+ sulphonamides, 104
+ suxamethonium, 394
Procarbazine
+ alcohol, 32
+ antihypertensive agents, 292
+ cheese, 292
+ CNS depressants, 292
+ sympathomimetics, indirectly
  acting, 292
+ tyramine-rich foods, 292
+ vaccines, 284
Prochlorperazine
see also Phenothiazines
+ coffee, 381
+ guanethidine and related
  drugs, 232
+ phenytoin, 406
+ tea, 381
Progestogens, *see* Contraceptives,
  oral and individual agents
Prolintane
+ anticoagulants, 166
Promazine
see also Phenothiazines
+ attapulgite-pectin, 381
+ benztropine, 244
+ coffee, 381
+ suxamethonium, 396
+ tea, 381
Promethazine
see also Phenothiazines
+ alcohol, 16
+ coffee, 381
+ monoamine oxidase
  inhibitors, 366
+ pentobarbitone + scopolamine,
  184
+ tea, 381
Propanidid
+ chlordiazepoxide, 452
Propantheline
+ digitalis glycosides, 307
+ digoxin, 307
+ hydrochlorothiazide, 460
+ nitrofurantoin, 95
+ thiazides, 460
Propoxyphene, *see*
  Dextropropoxyphene

Propranolol
see also Beta-blockers
+ adrenaline (epinephrine), 405
+ alcohol, 20
+ aluminium hydroxide, 260
+ amiodarone, 60
+ anaesthetics, general, 259
+ antacids, 260
+ anticoagulants, 127
+ *Cafergot*, 262
+ chlorpromazine, 264, 382
+ cimetidine, 261
+ clonidine, 225
+ dextromoramide, 262
+ diazoxide, 227
+ digitalis glycosides, 299
+ doxorubicin, 285
+ ergotamine, 262
+ glucagon, 263
+ halofenate, 263
+ halothane, 259
+ indomethacin, 224
+ insulin, 325
+ isoprenaline (isoproterenol),
  265
+ levodopa, 249
+ lignocaine (lidocaine), 62
+ mianserin, 221
+ monoamine oxidase
  inhibitors, 359
+ neuromuscular blockers, 389
+ nifedipine, 263
+ phenothiazines, 382
+ quinidine, 65
+ salbutamol, 265
+ suxamethonium, 389
+ terbutaline, 265
+ tubocurarine, 389
+ verapamil, 67
Propylthiouracil
+ anticoagulants, 175
Protein binding displacement
  interactions, 3
Prothrombin time, 114
Protriptyline
see also Tricyclic
  antidepressants
+ adrenaline (epinephrine), 411
+ amylobarbitone, 420
+ bethanidine, 235
+ clonidine, 226
+ debrisoquine, 235
+ guanethidine and related
  drugs, 235
+ noradrenaline (levarterenol,
  norepinephrine), 411
Pseudoephedrine
see also Sympathomimetics,
  indirect actions
+ guanethidine and related
  drugs, 234
+ monoamine oxidase
  inhibitors, 415

Psyllium (*Metamucil*)
+ anticoagulants, 166
Pyrazolone compounds, *see*
  Kebuzone,
  Oxyphenbutazone,
  Phenylbutazone
Pyridoxine (Vitamin B_6)
+ barbiturates, 208
+ contraceptives, oral, 276
+ levodopa, 255
+ levodopa-carbidopa, 255
+ phenobarbitone, 208
+ phenytoin, 208
+ vincristine, 293
Pyrimethamine
+ co-trimoxazole, 98
+ sulphafurazole, 98
+ sulphonamides, 98

Quinacrine, *see* Mepacrine
Quinalbarbitone
see also Barbiturates
+ anticoagulants, 123
+ mebanazine, 357
+ thyroid hormones, 460
Quinethazone, *see* Thiazides
Quinidine
+ acetazolamide, 66
+ aluminium hydroxide, 66
+ *Amphogel*, 66
+ antacids, 66
+ anthraquinone laxatives, 64
+ anticoagulants, 166
+ barbiturates, 64
+ beta-blockers, 65
+ bretylium, 61
+ calcium carbonate glycine, 66
+ cholinergic drugs, 431
+ decamethonium, 397
+ digitalis glycosides, 308, 309
+ digitoxin, 308, 309
+ digoxin, 308, 309
+ digoxin + pentobarbitone, 309
+ dihydroxyaluminium
  glycinate, 66
+ dimethyl tubocurarine, 397
+ gallamine, 397
+ hydroxyzine, 379
+ lignocaine (lidocaine), 65
+ *Maalox*, 66
+ magnesium hydroxide, 66
+ metoclopramide, 64
+ *Mylanta*, 66
+ neuromuscular blockers, 397
+ pentobarbitone, 64, 309
+ phenobarbitone, 64
+ phenytoin, 64
+ primidone, 64
+ propranolol, 65
+ rifampicin (rifampin), 66
+ *Robolate*, 66
+ sodium bicarbonate, 66

489

Sodium edetate
+ digitalis glycosides, 299
Sodium fusidate
+ cholestyramine, 101
Sodium polystyrene sulphonate
+ antacids, 461
+ magnesium hydroxide, 461
Sodium salicylate
+ alprenolol, 265
+ corticosteroids, 57
+ magnesium oxide, 56
+ probenecid, 55
+ methotrexate, 291, 288
+ sulphinpyrazone, 58
Sodium valproate
+ anticoagulants, 170
+ barbiturates, 185
+ benzodiazepines, 215
+ carbamazepine, 187
+ clonazepam, 215
+ dexamethasone, 438
+ phenobarbitone, 185
+ phenytoin, 209
+ primidone, 216
Sotalol
see also Beta-blockers
+ chlorpromazine, 264
+ clonidine, 225
Spironolactone
+ anticoagulants, 170
+ aspirin, 453
+ carbenoxolone, 429
+ digitalis glycosides, 311
+ digitoxin, 311
+ digoxin, 311
+ lithium carbonate, 345
+ potassium supplements, 453
+ salicylates, 453
Stanozolol
see also Anabolic steroids
+ anticoagulants, 118
+ hypoglycaemic agents, 319
Steroids, *see* Anabolic steroids,
Contraceptives (oral) and
Corticosteroids
Streptomycin
see also Aminoglycoside
antibiotics
+ anticoagulants, 119
+ contraceptives, oral, 273
+ dimenhydrinate
(diphenhydramine), 76
+ ethacrynic acid, 77
+ gallamine, 386
+ neuromuscular blockers, 386
+ suxamethonium, 386
+ tubocurarine, 386
Stretozotocin
+ phenytoin, 293
Strophanthin-G and -K, *see* Digitalis
Glycosides
Succinylcholine, *see*
Suxamethonium

Succinylsulphathiazole
see also Sulphonamides
+ anticoagulants, 173
Sulfisoxazole, *see* Sulphafurazole
Sulfonamides, *see* Sulphonamides
and individual drugs
Sulindac
+ anticoagulants, 171
+ hypoglycaemic agents, 340
+ tolbutamide, 340
Suloctidil
+ anticoagulants, 172
Sulphadiazine
see also Sulphonamides
+ procaine, 104
+ tolbutamide, 341
Sulphadimethoxine
see also Sulphonamides
+ phenytoin, 210
+ tolbutamide, 341
Sulphafurazole (sulfisoxazole)
see also Sulphonamides
+ anticoagulants, 173
+ chlorpropamide, 341
+ phenobarbitone, 103
+ phenytoin, 210
+ pyrimethamine, 98
+ thiopentone, 103
+ tolbutamide, 341
Sulphamethazine
see also Sulphonamides
+ chlorpropamide, 341
Sulphamethizole
see also Sulphonamides
+ anticoagulants, 173
+ phenytoin, 210
+ tolbutamide, 341
Sulphamethoxazole
see also Sulphonamides
+ phenytoin, 210
+ tolbutamide, 341
Sulphamethoxine
see also Sulphonamides
+ anticoagulants, 173
+ tolbutamide, 341
Sulphamethoxydiazine
see also Sulphonamides
+ phenytoin, 210
Sulphamethoxypyridazine
see also Sulphonamides
+ contraceptives, oral, 270
+ methotrexate, 288
+ phenytoin, 210
+ tolbutamide, 341
Sulphaphenazole
see also Sulphonamides
+ anticoagulants, 173
+ cyclophosphamide, 283
+ glibornuride, 341
+ phenytoin, 210
+ tolbutamide, 341
Sulphasalazine
see also Sulphonamides

Sulphasalazine (cont.)
+ cholestyramine, 102
+ digitalis glycosides, 312
+ digitoxin, 312
+ digoxin, 312
+ folic acid, 102
+ iron salts, 103
+ phenobarbitone, 103
Sulphasomidine
see also Sulphonamides
+ phenobarbitone, 103
Sulphinpyrazone
+ anticoagulants, 172
+ hypoglycaemic agents, 340
+ penicillin, 97
+ probenecid, 56
+ salicylates, 58
+ sodium salicylate, 58
Sulphonamides
see also individual drugs
+ amethocaine, 104
+ amylocaine, 104
+ anaesthetics (local), 104
+ anticoagulants, 173
+ barbiturates, 103
+ bupivacaine, 104
+ cinchocaine, 104
+ cocaine, 104
+ contaceptives, oral, 270
+ cyclophosphamide, 283
+ hexamine compounds
(methenamine), 89
+ hypoglycaemic agents, 341
+ lignocaine (lidocaine), 104
+ mepivacaine, 104
+ methotrexate, 288
+ para-aminobenzoic acid
(PABA), 104
+ phenytoin, 210
+ prilocaine, 104
+ procaine, 104
+ pyrimethamine, 98
+ tetracaine, 104
+ tolbutamide, 341
Sulphonylureas, *see* Hypoglycaemic
agents and individual drugs
generic and brand names, 315
Suloctidil
+ anticoagulants, 172
Sulpiride
+ alcohol, 33
Sulthiame
+ phenytoin, 211
Suxamethonium (succinylcholine)
see also Neuromuscular
blockers
+ aprotinin (*Trasylol*), 390
+ clindamycin, 390
+ cyclophosphamide, 391, 398
+ dexpanthenol or pantothenic
acid, 392
+ diazepam, 391
+ dibekacin, 386

Suxamethonium (cont.)
+ digitalis glycosides, 305
+ ecothiophate iodide, 392
+ fentanyl/droperidol (*Innovar*), 394
+ kanamycin, 386
+ lignocaine, 394
+ lithium carbonate, 395
+ magnesium sulphate, 395
+ meturedepa, 396
+ monoamine oxidase inhibitors, 365
+ neomycin, 386
+ nitrogen mustard (methchlorethamine), 398
+ pantothenic acid, 392
+ phenothiazines, 396
+ procainamide, 394
+ procaine, 394
+ promazine, 396
+ propranolol, 389
+ quinidine, 397
+ ribostamycin, 386
+ streptomycin, 386
+ TEM (triethylene-melamine), 398
+ thio-tepa (triethylene thiophosphonamide), 398
+ trimetaphan, 398
Sympathomimetic amines
classification, 400
mode of action, 399
see also Sympathomimetics with direct actions, indirect actions, and individual drugs
Sympathomimetics (bronchodilators)
+ beta-blockers, 265
Sympathomimetics, direct-actions
see also individual drugs
mode of action, 399
+ beta-blockers, 405
+ doxepin, 411
+ guanethidine and related drugs, 406
+ methyldopa, 407
+ mianserin, 408
+ monoamine oxidase inhibitors, 409
+ rauwolfia alkaloids, 410
+ tricyclic antidepressants, 411
Sympathomimetics, indirect-actions
see also individual drugs
mode of action, 399
+ furazolidone, 412
+ bethanidine, 234
+ debrisoquine, 234
+ furazolidone, 412
+ guanethidine and related drugs, 234
+ indomethacin, 413

Sympathomimetics (cont.)
+ methyldopa + oxprenolol, 414
+ mianserin, 408
+ monoamine oxidase inhibitors, 415
+ procarbazine, 292
+ rauwolfia alkaloids, 410
+ tricyclic antidepressants, 416
Syringopine, *see* Rauwolfia alkaloids

Talampicillin
see also Penicillins
+ contraceptives, 272
Talc
+ nitrofurantoin, 95
Tar gel
+ disulfiram, 454
Tea
+ barbiturates, 183
+ butyrophenones, 381
+ chlorpromazine, 381
+ droperidol, 381
+ fluphenazine, 381
+ haloperidol, 381
+ idrocilamide, 429
+ monoamine oxidase inhibitors, 359
+ phenothiazines, 381
+ prochlorperazine, 381
+ promazine, 381
+ promethazine, 381
TEM (triethylene-melamine)
+ neuromuscular blockers, 398
+ suxamethonium, 398
Terbutaline
+ beta-blockers, 265
+ practolol, 265
+ propranolol, 265
Terfenadine
+ alcohol, 16
Testosterone
see also Anabolic steroids
+ anticoagulants, 118
+ hypoglycaemic agents, 319
+ insulin, 319
Tetrabenazine
+ monoamine oxidase inhibitors, 367
Tetracaine
+ sulphonamides, 104
Tetracosactrin
+ phenobarbitone, 435
Tetracycline
see also Tetracyclines
+ alcohol, 105
+ anticoagulants, 174
+ barbiturates, 107
+ carbamazepine, 107
+ cimetidine, 108
+ contraceptives, 275
+ ferrous fumarate, 109

Tetracycline (cont.)
+ ferrous gluconate, 109
+ ferrous sulphate, 109
+ ferrous tartrate, 109
+ *Maalox*, 105
+ magnesium-aluminium hydroxide, 105
+ magnesium oxide, 105
+ magnesium sulphate, 105
+ methotrexate, 288
+ methoxyflurane, 450
+ milk, 111
+ phenobarbitone, 107
+ phenytoin, 107
+ sodium bicarbonate, 105
+ theophylline, 457
+ zinc sulphate, 112
Tetracyclines
see also individual drugs
+ alcohol, 105
+ anaesthetics, 388
+ antacids, 105
+ anticoagulants, 174
+ barbiturates, 107
+ betamethasone, 434
+ bismuth carbonate, 105
+ buttermilk, 111
+ calcium carbonate, 105
+ calcium phosphate, 105
+ carbamazepine, 107
+ cheese, 111
+ cimetidine, 108
+ contraceptives, oral, 275
+ diuretics, 109
+ ferrous sodium edetate, 109
+ hypoglycaemic agents, 342
+ iron preparations, 109
+ methotrexate, 288
+ methoxyflurane, 450
+ milk, 111
+ milk products, 111
+ neuromuscular blockers, 388
+ penicillins, 97
+ phenformin, 342
+ phenytoin, 107
+ theophylline, 457
+ zinc sulphate, 112
Theophylline
+ allopurinol, 457
+ ampicillin, 455
+ anaesthetics, 447
+ barbiturates, 455
+ cephalexin, 457
+ cimetidine, 455
+ corticosteroids, 456
+ dexamethasone, 456
+ ephedrine, 456
+ erythromycin, 457
+ halothane, 447
+ hydrocortisone, 456
+ lomustine, 286
+ phenobarbitone, 455
+ phenytoin, 212